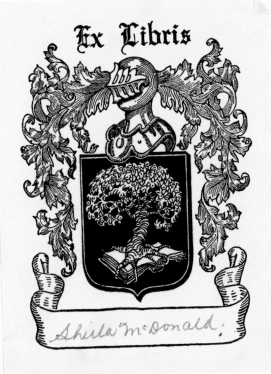

Ex Libris

Sheila McDonald.

NORMAL AND

THERAPEUTIC NUTRITION

Twelfth Edition

Fairfax T. Proudfit

Late Instructor in Nutrition and Diet Therapy, University of Tennessee College of Medicine and University of Tennessee School of Nursing, Memphis

Revised by

Corinne H. Robinson

Professor and Head, Department of Food and Nutrition, College of Home Economics, Drexel Institute of Technology, Philadelphia; Instructor, Nutrition and Diet Therapy, Jefferson Medical College Hospital School of Nursing, Philadelphia

New York

THE MACMILLAN COMPANY

First printing, May, 1961

Earlier editions: *Dietetics for Nurses* by Proudfit, copyright, 1918, 1922, 1924, 1927, by The Macmillan Company; *Nutrition and Diet Therapy* by Proudfit, copyright, 1930, 1934, 1938, 1942, by The Macmillan Company; *Nutrition and Diet Therapy* by Proudfit and Robinson, copyright, 1946, 1950, 1955, by The Macmillan Company.

Copyright renewed, 1946, 1950, 1952, 1955, 1958, by Fairfax T. Proudfit.

The illustration that appears on page 1 is reprinted with the permission of the United States Department of Agriculture; the one on page 325 is reprinted by permission from Martin, Almeda Biggs: ". . . On a Patient-centered Approach," *Am. J. Nursing,* **60:**1472–74, (Oct.) 1960; and the one on page 587 is reprinted with the permission of the United Fresh Fruit and Vegetable Association.

Library of Congress catalog card number: 61-6685

The Macmillan Company, New York
Brett-Macmillan Ltd., Galt, Ontario

Printed in the United States of America

PREFACE TO THE TWELFTH EDITION

One of the great movements toward the improvement of the health of people of all ages today, is the extension of nutrition education. The twelfth edition of this text, now under a new title, is written primarily for nursing and dietetic students, to help them better understand their role in promoting health through good nutrition, and to teach them to be competent practitioners. Professional nurses, dietitians, and physicians should find the text a useful, up-to-date reference.

The dynamic influences of research in nutrition and the related life sciences, the advances in food science and technology, the revolutionary social and economic changes, the better understanding of human behavior as a factor in food acceptance, and the growing concern for the health and well-being of the individual wherever he may live on this planet have provided the complex bases for an extensive revision of this book. Because of the volume and scope of published articles and books, it has been no easy task to select materials both suitable for the students using this book, and representative of current dietetic practice. The author earnestly hopes that this edition represents not only a synthesis of nutritional and dietetic knowledge, but also reflects a philosophy concerning nutrition and the well-being of people.

The text is presented in three sections, each of which has been subdivided into several units for convenient correlation with other studies. An occasional change of sequence of chapters and of certain materials within chapters has been made in this edition for better continuity. The dietary plans throughout the text have been rearranged to coincide with the Four Food Groups and have been compared with the 1958 Recommended Dietary Allowances. Fifty new illustrations, including many charts prepared especially for this book, have been carefully selected to supplement the text materials.

Section I, *Normal Nutrition,* includes three new chapters. "Dietary Guides and Their Uses" (Chap. 3) acquaints the student with the Recommended Dietary Allowances, the Four Food Groups, and the methods for using food composition tables before embarking upon the study of the individual nutrients. Physiologic and psychologic factors in food acceptance, and methods for effecting improved food habits are discussed in Chapter 15, "Factors Influencing Food Habits and Their Modification." The nature of local, national, and international problems in nutrition is presented in Chapter 22, "Nutrition in the Community," along with the multi-faceted approach through voluntary and official agencies, and examples of typical programs such as enrichment, emergency feeding, and international feeding programs.

The discussion about the metabolism of the nutrients has been amplified particularly to meet the needs of college nursing and dietetic students, but has been so arranged that the student in a two- or three-year program may easily omit this material without loss of continuity. The more thorough presentation of amino acids and lipids is especially pertinent to current trends in nutrition.

Chapter 16, "Cultural Food Patterns in the United States," has been completely rewritten to include an evaluation of regional dietary patterns in this country, a new description of Puerto Rican food habits, and detailed dietary patterns for Jewish, Italian, Mexican, Near Eastern, and Chinese groups. The nutrition problems of children and teenagers, the development of good food habits, the functions of the school lunch program, and nutrition education have received greater emphasis in "Nutrition for Children and Teenagers" (Chap. 19). Food additives, antibiotics, new developments in food processing, and the functions of the Food Protection Committee are among the more important revised discussions in the chapter on "Safeguarding the Food Supply" (Chap. 21).

Section II includes two new chapters: "Therapeutic Nutrition: Factors in Patient Care and Rehabilitation" (Chap. 23), with emphasis upon the effects of illness on food acceptance, the concepts of total patient care and rehabilitation, and the techniques of dietary instruction; and "Short Methods of Dietary Calculation Including Use of the Meal Exchange Lists" (Chap. 25), which should enable the student to use dietary evaluation techniques throughout the study of diet therapy. Nutritional deficiencies and their correction are discussed in Chapter 26, but the details of specific deficiency diseases have been presented in the several chapters in Section I pertaining to the nutrients. Diseases of the small intestine and colon are considered in one chapter rather than two. Likewise, the dietary management of gout has been included with the other disorders in Chapter 34, "Various Metabolic Disorders."

As in earlier editions, all therapeutic regimens have been developed as modifications of the normal diet. In each instance the student is given guidance in problems likely to be encountered in patient care, delineation of pertinent points in food selection and preparation, and a detailed description of each dietary plan. A brief discussion of clinical and pathologic findings which illustrate the use of the diet is again included so that the student may better understand the rationale for each regimen.

Detailed information has been included for the following diets not described in previous editions: High-protein, High-fat, Low-carbohydrate Diet for dumping syndrome (Chap. 29); Wheat-, Oat-, and Rye-free Diet for sprue (Chap. 31); Modified-fat Diets for prophylaxis and treatment of atherosclerosis (Chap. 36); Calcium- and Phosphorus-restricted Diet in conjunction with the treatment of urinary calculi (Chap. 37); 20-, 40-, and 60-gm Protein Diets for acute anuria and for hepatic coma (Chap. 37). The Bland Diet (Chap. 30) has been liberalized according to current concepts. The Sodium-restricted Diet (Chap. 36) has been revised to conform to the Unit lists developed for the American Heart Association. The dietary management of regional ileitis, diverticulosis, and pancreatitis is discussed in Chapter 31. Diet therapy in celiac disease, cystic fibrosis of the pancreas, phenylketonuria, and galactosemia is covered in Chapter 40, along with the management of feeding for the handicapped children such as those with cerebral palsy, cleft palate, or mental retardation.

Section III, *Practical Applications of Nutrition: Elementary Food Study,* presents a concise source of information on the characteristics and preparation of foods which will help the student give more realistic guidance to the patient. This section may be used in conjunction with courses of nutrition and diet therapy which include laboratory experiences in food preparation, or may be adapted to clinical experiences in those curricula which do not provide a nutrition laboratory. The recipes include only those dishes which require a limited time for preparation and which are suitable for many modified diets. Suggestions for the preparation of sodium-restricted diets should be particularly helpful.

The 17 tables in the Appendix are concerned with the nutritive values of foods, height-weight tables, and data for normal blood and urine constituents. Table 1 is a 1960 revision of the nutritive values of household portions of food, published by the Institute of Home Economics of the United States Department of Agriculture. The inclusion of data on saturated and unsaturated fats and on linoleic acid, in Table 1, is especially notable. A revised height-weight table for adults is also included in the Appendix.

In addition to over 200 cited references, about 700 references have been arranged according to chapter headings for the use of students during the clinical experience, for college students, and for the instructor.

The author sincerely appreciates the valuable assistance provided by many individuals and groups: instructors and students using the text who made suggestions; the author's own staff and students; publishers and authors of journal articles and books who gave permission to quote their materials; and individuals and companies who contributed illustrations. Undoubtedly, in a book of this scope, there will be some errors of commission, omission, and judgment; for these, the author is solely responsible and it is hoped that they are few and not too serious.

Most especially, recognition is given to Dr. Howard W. Robinson who has critically evaluated many sections of the text and has provided assistance in the preparation of charts and graphs. Without the patience and forbearance of both Dr. Robinson and Glenn Robinson, this edition would have been impossible. The invaluable assistance of the publishers, The Macmillan Company, is fully appreciated.

Corinne Robinson

CONTENTS

UNIT 7: Modification of the Normal Diet for Energy, Protein, and Texture

UNIT 8: Diet in Disturbances of the Gastrointestinal Tract

UNIT 9: Diet in Metabolic and Nervous Disorders

UNIT 10: Diet in Cardiovascular and Renal Disorders

UNIT 11: Diet in Miscellaneous Disorders

PRACTICAL APPLICATIONS OF NUTRITION: ELEMENTARY FOOD STUDY

UNIT 12: Foods — Their Characteristics and Preparation

APPENDIX

NORMAL NUTRITION /

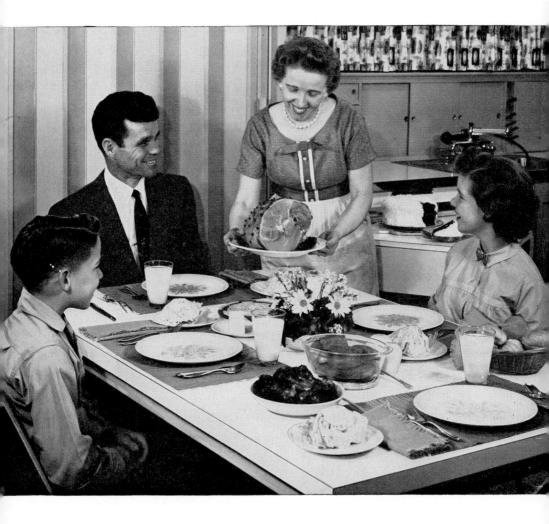

UNIT I /
Introduction to the Study
of Nutrition

CHAPTER 1

Food and Its Relation to Health

THE MEANINGS OF FOOD, NUTRITION, AND DIETETICS

What does food mean to you? When you sit down to your next meal you will have definite feelings about that meal and the specific foods which are served to you. By your eyes you will delight in the texture variations and color combinations of the food, the artistic touch of a garnish, and the beautiful table appointments; or perhaps you may be repelled because the food lacks color and is carelessly served. By your nose you will enjoy the tantalizing odors of meat or of freshly baked rolls, or the fragrance of fully ripened fruit; or possibly the odor of grease which has been too hot or of vegetables which have been cooked too long may bring about anorexia and nausea. By your sense of taste you will experience countless flavors—the salty, sweet, bitter, and sour and their variations; you will feel the textures of smooth or fibrous, crisp or soft, creamy or oily, moist or dry foods.

But your senses alone do not describe what your next meal, or any meal, means to you. Is the meal merely a way of staying alive and keeping in health; an opportunity for fellowship with your family and friends; a way to celebrate an event; an occasion for stimulating conversation; a means of satisfying your feelings when you are hurt and depressed; a display of prestige by which you show that you can afford certain foods others cannot; a token of security and love; a means of asserting your independence; a cause of concern because some foods might make you ill; an occasion of self denial; something you enjoy leisurely; taken for granted as your right; a precious gift from God for which you are thankful? What other feelings are evoked by the food you eat?

Next to the air you breathe and the water you drink, food has been basic to your existence. In fact, food has been the primary concern of man in his physical environment throughout all recorded history. By food, or its lack, the destinies of men are greatly influenced. Man must eat to live, and what he eats will affect in a high degree his ability to keep well, to work, to be happy, and to live long.

You bring to the study of nutrition and dietetics your lifetime experience with food which may serve you well in further improving your nutrition and the nutrition of your fellowmen. But it may also be that you have many incorrect ideas and such strong feelings about food that it will take much patience and perseverance on your part to change your attitudes and motivations. As you enter upon your study of nutrition and dietetics it is well for you to examine carefully your present feelings about food, as well as your knowledge of nutrition, so that you can build upon what is best in your dietary pattern and correct that which is undesirable.

Nutrition and dietetics defined. *Nutrition* is the "combination of processes by which the living organism receives and utilizes the materials necessary for the maintenance of its functions and for the growth and renewal of its components." * One of the newest of the biologic sciences, nutrition is based on and integrated with the sciences of chemistry, biochemistry, and physiology. During the last 50 years, more advances have beeen made in the understanding of nutrition than in all the preceding centuries of recorded history. (See Fig 1-1.)

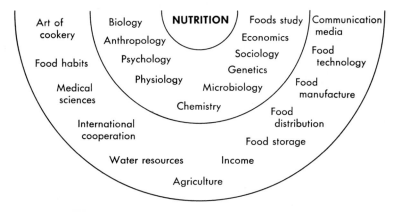

Fig. 1-1. Good nutrition for everyone is dependent upon the application of the principles of many sciences and the coordination of many disciplines.

Dietetics is "the combined science and art of feeding individuals or groups under different economic or health conditions according to the principles of nutrition and management." † It includes consideration of the planning of meals for the well and the sick, together with the selection, storage, preparation, and serving of foods with due emphasis on economic, social, and psychologic factors.

Good nutrition: what is it? The concept of health, as defined by the World Health Organization of the United Nations is the "state of complete physical,

* Turner, D. F.: *Handbook of Diet Therapy,* 3rd ed. University of Chicago Press, Chicago, 1959, p. 208.
† *Ibid.,* p. 204.

mental and social well-being and not merely the absence of disease or infirmity." * Nutrition and health are not synonymous, but without good nutrition health cannot be at its best.

Many ideas are implied in the term "good nutrition." First of all, the various *foodstuffs, nutrients,* or *food constituents,* such as protein, carbohydrates, fats, minerals, and vitamins must be supplied in optimum amounts to the body. It means further that these nutrients must be appropriately utilized in the body.

Optimum nutrition is here distinguished from merely "adequate" or "normal" nutrition in that it implies that the so-called "normal" nutritional status can be further improved upon. Thus, the optimum standards for a given nutrient may be much greater than the minimum requirements. Moreover, good nutrition, in its fullest sense, means that the numerous conditioning factors such as disease, activity, climate, etc., which may alter one's requirements for the nutrients must be carefully considered.

The achievement of good nutrition implies: (1) suitable agricultural methods which produce plant and animal foods of high nutritive value; (2) economic situations which make it possible to procure the necessary foods at a cost within the reach of all; (3) controlled industrial procedures in which foods are selected and processed with the greatest possible retention, or restoration, of their original value; and (4) conscientious and informed homemakers as well as managers of public eating places who will select, store, prepare, and serve foods every day on a safe, physiologically adequate, socially appealing, and psychologically sound basis. Only when these concepts are brought to fruition can the ultimate ideal of good nutrition and its benefits to everyone—health, happiness, efficiency, longevity—be fully realized. Obviously, individuals in any walk of life can benefit by an increased knowledge of the principles of nutrition and their application.

DIETARY TRENDS AND NUTRITIONAL PROBLEMS IN THE UNITED STATES

Dietary surveys. For approximately half a century the United States Department of Agriculture has provided data on the per capita consumption of foods. Such figures do not give information on the amount of food actually eaten, but since they represent the quantities and kinds of foods available they provide a clue to the nature of the American diet. In addition, detailed surveys of households have supplied information on practices in food buying and preparation, dietary adequacy, and points requiring emphasis in nutrition education.

In the spring of 1955, the most comprehensive survey ever undertaken was conducted by the Agricultural Research and Marketing Services of the

* *World Health Organization—What It Is, What It Does, How It Works,* Leaflet, Geneva, Switzerland, 1956.

Department of Agriculture of 6000 households of one or more persons.[1,*] The households were selected from urban, rural nonfarm, and farm families in four regions—Northeast, North Central, South, and West—in such a manner that the results of the survey would be representative of practices throughout the United States. Trained interviewers obtained information on (1) family characteristics—size, income, etc., (2) the quantities of food purchased during the preceding seven days, (3) the expenditures for food purchased, (4) practices with respect to certain foods during the preceding year, (5) the number of meals eaten away from home by each individual during the preceding week, and (6) the expenditure for food eaten away from home. Some of the results of this survey will be referred to from time to time in this and succeeding chapters.

While the data on food consumption are valuable in comparing actual practices with certain goals such as the Recommended Dietary Allowances,[2] they do not prove the absence or presence of malnutrition. The *nutritional status* of individuals can be determined only through taking a careful medical and dietary history, a thorough physical examination, and appropriate laboratory investigations, and correlating the information so obtained. Some of the specific criteria concerned with nutritional status for a given nutrient will be discussed in the succeeding chapters on the nutrients.

Changes in patterns of living. The population of the United States has shifted from rural to urban centers; but even on the farm most families now purchase much more of their food than was customary half a century ago. Americans have the benefits of many labor-saving devices in their occupations and in their homes. They work fewer hours in a week so that the way in which they spend their leisure may be decisive in determining their food needs. Leisure, to many people, means little activity—riding rather than walking, watching television rather than leading an active outdoor life, and so on.

Greater numbers of married women are working away from home than ever before, which means that there is less time for food preparation, more expensive ready-prepared foods are used, and shopping is less frequent. Husbands, as well as wives, are shopping for and preparing foods; sometimes children, especially teenagers, may be given too much freedom in their food choices thus resulting in poor nutrition. Marriages occur at an earlier age with pregnancy often presenting an additional stress on the young woman who has not fully matured and who may have been the victim of poor dietary practices.

The average American family of today has a higher income and is spending more of it for food. With this higher income, more meals are eaten in restaurants. More workers are receiving meals at their place of work rather than carrying lunches, and more children are participating in the school lunch. The family eats fewer meals together, and in far too many families some meals

* References cited in the text are listed in the Appendix on pages 791–99.

may be skipped by one or more persons. Breakfast is an often neglected meal, although some families have found that this is the one time of the day when they can plan to be together.

Variety of food choices. The scientific and technologic advances reach into every aspect of daily life, including the quantity, quality, variety, and attractiveness of the foods we eat. Frozen foods including complete meals, baked foods of all kinds, and mixes for almost every part of the meal are commonplace items in the supermarkets. The number of brands and the variety are so great that the shopper finds it difficult indeed to make wise selections.

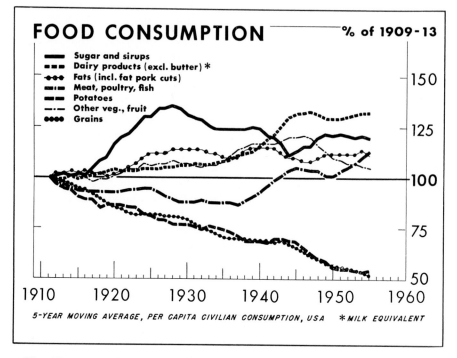

Fig. 1-2. Trends of food consumption since 1909. (*Courtesy, Agricultural Research Service, U.S. Department of Agriculture.*)

On the basis of records of per capita food consumption Americans today are eating more meat, poultry, eggs, milk and milk products, citrus fruits and tomatoes, green leafy and yellow vegetables, fats, and sugars than they did 50, or even 25, years ago. Most of these are the more costly foods. On the other hand, only half as much of two important food groups—breads and cereals, and potatoes—is eaten as 50 years ago. (See Fig. 1-2.)

Dietary adequacy. During the 1930's, a survey had indicated that a third of the diets in the United States were classed as "poor." In 1955, the diets in only 10 per cent of the households could be classed as poor. Few families had diets which provided less than two-thirds of the Recommended Dietary Allowances for one or more nutrients (see Fig. 1-3). This improvement which had occurred from the midthirties to the postwar period was the result of better economic conditions, the bread and flour enrichment program, improvements in food marketing, and nutrition education.[3] The dietary levels in 1955, however, were similar to those found in the household survey of 1948, thus indicating that little if any further improvement had occurred in spite of the fact that families spent more money for food in 1955. The challenge to nutrition education is thus obvious.

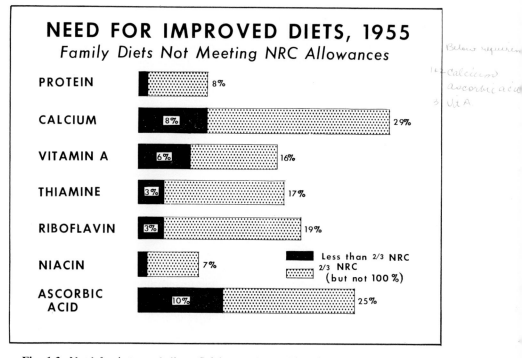

Fig. 1-3. Need for improved diets. Calcium and ascorbic acid are the nutrients most frequently supplied at levels below the Recommended Dietary Allowances according to data from the family dietary survey of 1955. (*Courtesy, Agricultural Research Service, U.S. Department of Agriculture.*)

While few families in 1955 had diets which were poor, there is still much need for improvement. The average amount of food brought into the households was ample to fully meet the Recommended Dietary Allowances for all nutrients, but the division of food was such that in many households the food supply did not fully meet the standards for one or more nutrients. Calcium and ascorbic acid were the two nutrients which were most frequently provided at less than recommended levels. From 15 to 20 per cent of households had less than recommended levels of vitamin A, thiamine, and ribo-flavin, while a tenth or less of households had less than recommended amounts of protein, iron, and niacin.

Community problems in nutrition remain. The people of the United States are probably better fed than any other people in the world. Nationwide control of deficiency disease has been realized so that overt clinical signs of nutritional deficiency are rare. Today, as never before, the American public has become aware of the importance of good nutrition. Nevertheless, there are still nutritional problems of major importance to be solved in the United States.

1. Obesity is recognized to be the chief nutritional problem in this country. It has been estimated that every fifth person over 30 years of age is overweight. Increasing numbers of children and young people are entering the overweight category. The association of obesity with degenerative diseases is well established.

2. Cardiovascular diseases, gallbladder disease, diabetes, and cirrhosis of the liver occur with frequency. The role of diet as a possible etiologic factor in cardiovascular and other degenerative diseases is receiving major attention by investigators.

3. The role of nutrition in the process of aging and in mental health is little understood.

4. Dental caries is of almost universal occurrence.

5. The extent of so-called subclinical deficiencies cannot be measured. Certainly a good deal of lowered resistance to infection, slow convalescence from illness and injury, lost time from school and work, inefficiency, and unhappiness are due to poor nutrition alone.

6. Superstitions concerning foods, fad diets, and unjustified claims for certain foods and mechanical devices by unscrupulous quacks are an increasing menace. Millions of dollars are spent annually by persons of limited income for products selling at exorbitant prices, so that there is often too little money left for the purchase of an adequate diet. Even more serious is the faith that some people place in some specific product as a cure for disease; such misplaced faith may mean that medical advice is sought too late.

GLOBAL PROBLEMS IN NUTRITION

General malnutrition. Most of the world's people today, as always, are engaged in a struggle for food. In relatively few countries, such as the United States, Canada, and western European countries, is food abundant and of great variety. Two-thirds of the world's people are caught in a relentless sequence of ignorance, poverty, malnutrition, disease, and early death. The world's population increases by approximately 100,000 persons each day, so that the expansion of food production to keep pace with, and to move ahead of, this population growth must assume staggering proportions. It is not surprising that Hundley [4] listed chronic starvation—simply not having enough to eat—as the main nutritional deficiency.

The proportion of the population of a given country which is engaged in agriculture gives a clue to the adequacy of the food supply and the standard of living. Where methods of agriculture are primitive and the food production is limited, most of the population must engage in producing food in order to survive. In the United States about 12 per cent of the workers are engaged in agriculture, which means that the remaining 88 per cent are free to diversify their occupations in science, technology, industry, and the arts so that the population enjoys the highest standard of living ever known anywhere. By contrast, 85 per cent of the workers in India, for example, are needed for food production, leaving a very small proportion available for improvement of other aspects of living.

Other deficiencies. In addition to general malnutrition, Hundley has listed protein malnutrition, anemia—especially in mothers and in young children, vitamin-A deficiency, and riboflavin deficiency as major world problems. Rickets, scurvy, pellagra, and beriberi occur in severe forms in some parts of the world but they are less prevalent than the aforementioned five. These deficiencies will be discussed in more detail in chapters related to the specific nutrients and in Chapter 26.

Responsibility for world nutrition. No thinking man or woman can afford to avoid the fact that so many of the world's people simply do not have enough to eat, nor can he, even in his own self-interest, evade the responsibility for alleviating hunger. (See Fig. 1-4.) In chronic starvation lie the frustration, tension, and envy of masses of people who will ultimately resort to violence. The political and social implications of the lack of sufficient food were expressed by President Eisenhower at the opening of the American exhibit at New Delhi, India, in December 1959, when he said:

. . . . We can eliminate the hunger that emaciates the bodies of children; that scars the souls of their parents; that stirs the passions of those who toil endlessly and earn only scraps.

Men, right now, possess the knowledge and the resources for a successful worldwide war against hunger—the sort of war that dignifies and exalts human beings. . . .*

In explanation of the American theme for the exhibit: "Food—family—friendship—freedom" he had this to say concerning food:

. . . . Food—that our bodies may be fit for every task and duty and service; our minds free from the fear of hunger; our eyes, undimmed by the tragedies of

* *The New York Times,* Saturday, December 12, 1959, p. 10.

famine, searching out new horizons; our aspirations and our plans for their achievement not frustrated by failure of crop or catastrophe of weather.*

World peace cannot be guaranteed by supplying adequate food alone, but one road to world peace is surely through a better-fed world population. Beyond this, charity and brotherhood are at the root of Christianity and indeed of all ethical systems, and to practice them should be on the conscience of mankind.

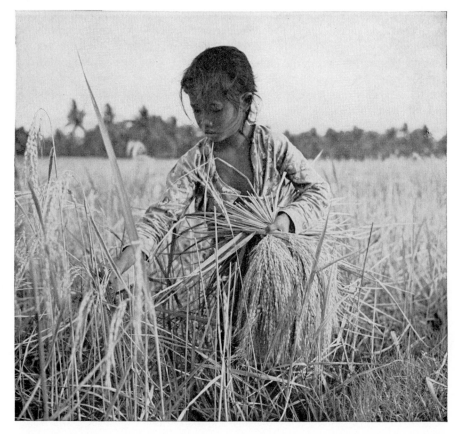

Fig. 1-4. Rice is a basic food of half of the world's population. Improvement of rice yields is an important goal of the Food and Agriculture Organization. (*Courtesy, United Nations.*)

A number of groups under the United Nations (see p. 319) are directly concerned with global problems of nutrition, namely the Food and Agriculture Organization (FAO); World Health Organization (WHO); United Nations Childrens Fund (UNICEF); United Nations Educational, Scientific and Cultural Organization (UNESCO).

* *The New York Times,* Saturday, December 12, 1959, p. 10.

SOME GOALS IN THE STUDY OF NUTRITION

Personal and family nutrition. Most of the readers of this text are contemplating professional careers in which the knowledge of nutrition, in health and in disease, and the ability to apply its principles are essential. It should be no surprise, nevertheless, to find that the first goal in the study of nutrition should be directed to oneself. If application of the principles of nutrition is important to the health of the patient, or the worker, or the child in the classroom, certainly the professional person who is responsible for such applications should be concerned about his own nutritional status. The work of a nurse, for example, is at times arduous and demanding; it is also challenging to one's best efforts. How can the nurse achieve her career goals unless she maintains her own good health of which nutrition is an integral part.

Realistically, the nurse, dietitian, and teacher are planning for life when they set good nutrition as an important goal for themselves. Most of them will marry after a few years in their chosen profession. They may continue in their professional work, or they may leave work for awhile to raise a family only to return to their work when the children are in school or are grown. The health of the entire family is more nearly assured through the application of nutritional principles by the mother. If long-range goals are considered, the nutrition of the student herself, and later of her family, together with the impact made by such an example on the community, is of fundamental importance.

Role of the nurse. A significant part of the student and graduate nurse's time is concerned with the nutrition of patients. The meals served to the patient, the acceptance of food by the patient, and the plans for rehabilitation of the patient in terms of dietary instruction suitable for the individual situation are essential components of comprehensive nursing care. Most students know people with diseases, such as diabetes or peptic ulcers, who depend upon carefully controlled diets for their well-being; all are familiar with the use of low-calorie diets for weight loss. During her years of study, the student will have ample opportunity to observe the sometimes amazing results in the recovery of patients who have been treated with diet alone. Even more important is the recognition of the principles and application of normal nutrition, for the normal diet is the need for the vast majority of patients and is the absolute basis on which the therapeutic diet should be constructed.

The nurse in nutrition education. The nurse will quickly see how her attitude toward nutrition, her feeding of the patient, and her teaching can influence the patient in the hospital to better dietary habits. She will realize that what the patient takes home with him in the way of nutrition information and in improved dietary habits can be a leaven for the patient's family as well. In the clinic she has an opportunity to follow up the patient's care in the hospital.

If she works in the schools she will, in her examination of children, note many faults which suggest the need for better nutrition, and she will realize the value of constructive lunch programs as well as of the formal classroom in improving physical status, and she may find various ways to take part in these endeavors.

The nurse in public health. The nurse may elect to work with a public health team and thus she has contacts in the home, school, industry, and other areas of community activity. The problems which home visits provoke may be challenging: perhaps she needs to show one mother how to prepare an infant formula; another person needs to know how to budget her limited income so that she can buy enough milk; another needs actual instruction in food preparation for an ill member of the family; another has been given a diet which does not fit in with the religious practices of the family; or a pregnant woman may need to know what foods she must eat and how to provide for them in her budget. It is readily seen that the nurse in public health needs a broad background in nutrition and dietetics; she also needs to know when and where to obtain advice when the problems are beyond the scope of her experience.

Objectives for the student. If the student has carefully read the preceding sections, she will no doubt be able to formulate some specific goals toward which she might aspire in the study of nutrition and diet therapy. It may help to remind her that she should strive to:

1. Acquire the proper attitude and convictions relative to the importance of nutrition in regulating her own health, that of her family, of the patient, and of the community.

2. Learn the role of food in body structure and function, and become familiar with the contributions of various foods with respect to the food constituents.

3. Obtain knowledge of the functions, digestion, absorption, and metabolism of protein, fat, carbohydrate, minerals, vitamins, and water in the body and the way in which these nutrients are interrelated.

4. Recognize the nutritive requirements of individuals and the variations which may be imposed on the food needs by activity, climate, pregnancy, lactation, growth, old age, or pathologic conditions.

5. Obtain theoretic and practical knowledge in the planning of meals together with the selection, purchase, care, preparation, and service of foods most commonly used and be able to apply the knowledge under varying circumstances.

6. Learn to appreciate the importance of economic, social, and psychologic factors in the feeding of people in health and disease.

7. Develop the ability to apply knowledge of normal nutrition to the principles of diet therapy in making modifications in the diet to meet the existing pathologic conditions.

8. Learn to teach normal and therapeutic diets to individuals and to groups, using accepted techniques of teaching and approved teaching materials.

9. Become familiar with agencies which are concerned with nutrition and health so that she may utilize their services and contribute to their functioning.

10. Know where to look for reliable sources of information, and how to evaluate publications on food and nutrition and the claims of advertising.

PROBLEMS AND REVIEW

1. What is your understanding of the following terms: nutrition; optimum nutrition; malnutrition; dietetics; foodstuff; nutrient; health; food?

2. Industrial and economic developments have been a powerful factor in the changing of our food habits. List several of these which have had an influence on our dietary habits within your lifetime.

3. Within your experience give an example of a situation in which the community has fostered better nutrition.

4. Select an article related to food from the daily newspaper or a popular magazine and discuss its merits.

5. In what ways is a knowledge of the following sciences helpful in the study of nutrition: bacteriology; chemistry; sociology; psychology?

6. What is the difference between a dietary survey and a nutritional status study?

7. *Problem.* Start a list of resources for the study of nutrition and dietetics. Add to this list as you continue in your study. Include only those books and journals which you have examined. Include the names of official and voluntary agencies in your own community, at state, federal, and international levels as you become familiar with the work they do in the area of nutrition.

8. *Problem.* Compile a list of characteristics which describe a person who is in good nutritional status. How do you measure up with this?

9. *Problem.* Review the suggested objectives for study in this chapter. Then prepare a statement in your own words which best describes the goals which you think are most important. Limit your statement to 300 words; be concise but exact.

CHAPTER 2 /

Growth of the Science of Nutrition

All recorded history shows that food has played an extraordinarily vital role in the rise and growth or the fall and decline of nations because of its effect on health and efficiency; in fact, the history of the world could probably be written in terms of food. Since earliest times food has been considered in the light of both cause and cure of disease, and few stories are more fascinating than the gradual evolution of the science of nutrition from the maze of sage philosophy, countless fads, and bizarre superstitions which have grown up through the centuries. A complete history of nutrition would occupy volumes. The material which follows merely provides some glimpses of the evolution of the science of nutrition. It is hoped that the student will find encouragement in reading detailed works on the various aspects of food and nutrition history, since such endeavors can become an absorbing hobby and inevitably strengthen the understanding of nutrition itself. The bibliography in the Appendix suggests additional readings.

Early beginnings. The ancient Egyptians chiseled drawings on stone some 5000 years ago which depicted the grinding of flour, the making of bread, and the slaughtering of cattle.[5] Grain and pottery have been found in the tombs. The most remarkable record of an ancient people is available to all who would read it, namely the record of the Hebrew people in the Old Testament of the Bible. There one can learn much of the laws and traditions for the use of food and the kinds of food available at that time.

Medical literature from the time of Hippocrates has been replete with advice for the use of food in disease and as a measure to prevent disease. There was little true understanding of what happened to food in the body until the science of physiology explained the processes of digestion, circulation, and respiration. On the other hand, the careful observations of many people gradually led to much information which proved to be fairly sound.

People are seldom reluctant to express ideas concerning diet, whether or not they are authorities on the subject. American students may be especially interested to know that one of the heroic figures in American history, namely Benjamin Franklin, expressed himself in no uncertain terms concerning the role and use of food, and that he was a close friend of the chemists who

16

founded the science of nutrition. The advice he gave with regard to food and eating typifies many comments that can be found in the literature of that period, and some of it is still good advice today. For example, we read:

Exercise should precede meals, not immediately follow them; the first promotes, the latter, unless moderate, obstructs digestion. If, after exercise, we feed sparingly, the digestion will be easy and good, the body lightsome, the temper cheerful, and all the animal functions performed agreeably. Sleep, when it follows, will be natural and undisturbed; while indolence, with full feeding, occasions horrors inexpressible; we fall from precipices, are assaulted by wild beasts, murderers and demons, and experience every variety of distress. Observe, however, that the quantities of food and exercise are relative things; those who move much may, and indeed ought to eat more; those who use little exercise should eat little. In general, mankind, since the improvements of cookery, eat about twice as much as nature requires. Suppers are not bad, if we have not dined; but restless nights naturally follow hearty suppers after full dinners. Indeed, as there is a difference in constitutions, some rest well after these meals; it costs them only a frightful dream and an apoplexy, after which they sleep till doomsday. Nothing is more common in the newspapers, than instances of people, who, after eating a hearty supper, are found dead abed in the morning.*

The science of nutrition is founded. During one of his trips to London, Franklin met Joseph Priestley (1733–1804), a Unitarian clergyman who was destined to become his lifelong friend. Through Franklin, Priestley became interested in electricity, and while attempting to write a history of this subject was led to wider experimentation. As so often happens, it was a chance experiment of his which made such a change in the course of chemistry. Seeing a lighted candle in a room he inserted it into a closed jar of "fire air" (oxygen) and found that the candle would burn more brightly for a time but would eventually be extinguished. He then inserted a mint plant into a jar and found at the end of 10 days that the air had been restored and the candle would burn as brightly as before. He not only established the necessity of oxygen for the burning candle, but he determined its importance for animals. Priestley was the victim of religious persecution and fled to America where he was widely hailed. Today, one can visit his home in Northumberland, Pa., where the chemists of America maintain a permanent memorial.

During the years when he represented this country in France, it was natural that Franklin should seek out the company of scientists. One of those whom he visited and came to know well was Antoine Laurent Lavoisier (1743–1794), who was as versatile as Franklin and who was one of the greatest men France has ever produced. Lavoisier laid the sure foundation for the

* Franklin, B.: "The Art of Procuring Pleasant Dreams, 1786," in *The Ingenious Dr. Franklin,* N. G. Goodman, ed. University of Pennsylvania Press, Philadelphia, 1931, p. 35.

knowledge of burning (oxidation), which he described as the union of the burning substance with oxygen, the name he gave to "fire air." He introduced new chemical terminology so that the confusing and often meaningless writings of earlier scientists were clarified. With his delicate balances and his thermometers he started experiments which led to our present concepts of energy metabolism, and thus he came to be known as the "Father of the Science of Nutrition." In one of these experiments together with Laplace, another French worker, he constructed a chamber for the measurement of the amount of carbon dioxide given off by a guinea pig in 10 hours. This was found to be equal to the burning of 3.33 gm of carbon in a closed vessel. He next determined the amount of ice which the guinea pig's body would melt in 10 hours. The amount of heat necessary for melting the ice was found to be almost identical with that given off in burning 3.33 gm of carbon. It was then concluded that the carbon dioxide expired by the guinea pig came from burning the equivalent of 3.33 gm of carbon. Lavoisier was in the midst of an experiment of this nature on one of his co-workers when the terrorists of the French Revolution carried him away—and thus the famous mathematician, physicist, chemist, philosopher, politician, and humanitarian became another victim of the guillotine.

Studies in metabolism. An Englishman, William Prout, in 1827 set forth the doctrine that living things need "the saccharine, the oily and the albuminous." * This teaching was challenged until a German, Justus von Liebig (1803–1873), showed beyond doubt that protein, fat, and carbohydrate are burned in the body. He developed methods for the analysis of foods, body tissues, urine, and feces and gave to the world its first idea of food composition. He knew that protein contained nitrogen and suggested that the amount of nitrogen in the urine might be a measure of the protein destruction in the body. Two other Germans, Bidder and Schmidt, showed this idea to be fact when they found that almost all of the nitrogen contained in the meat fed to dogs could be accounted for in the urine and feces. Liebig's most famous pupil was Carl von Voit, who extended the experiments on protein and who firmly established the determination of nitrogen in food and in urine and feces as a method for the measurement of protein metabolism.

In 1849 two Frenchmen, Regnault and Reiset, constructed a chamber for the measurement of oxygen intake and carbon dioxide output in small animals. At the suggestion of Voit, a Munich physicist by the name of Pettenkofer in 1862 constructed a large chamber which would accommodate a man. In the United States similar chambers were constructed, first by Atwater and Rosa and then later by Benedict.

Max Rubner, one of Voit's pupils, was the first to prove that the animal

* McCay, C. M.: "Seven Centuries of Scientific Nutrition," *J. Am. Dietet. A.,* **15**:648, 1939.

body is subject to the *law of conservation of energy*. He showed that the heat production of the animal body is proportional to the surface area. He determined the fuel values for pure protein, fat, and carbohydrate.

Thus, at the beginning of the twentieth century the science of nutrition, whose groundwork had been well laid in France, was carried forward in Germany, and destined to reach greater heights in England and America through the studies of men and women such as Chittenden, Atwater, Benedict, Carpenter, Du Bois, Lusk, Mitchell, McCollum, Hart, Osborne, Mendel, Murlin, Sherman, Rose, and many others.

Importance of minerals in the diet is recognized. That the chief compounds in bones and teeth are calcium phosphate and calcium carbonate was well known as early as 1799.[6] In fact, a book on the composition of bones appeared in 1844.

In 1840 a study by Charles J. Chossat, a physician in Genf, France, won a prize for showing that a diet of wheat and water must be supplemented with calcium carbonate if the bones of a growing pigeon are to develop.[7] For the first time the importance of calcium in the diet was thus shown. This was confirmed in 1843 by J. B. Boussingault, another Frenchman, who performed calcium-balance studies on animals.

The occurrence of goiter is as old as history itself. It apparently was always extremely common, for many paintings show individuals with the enlarged thyroid gland. In 1822, Boussingault, while on a trip to South America, observed that villagers who used salt containing iodine were free of goiter, but that those who used plain salt were afflicted. He pointed out the importance of iodine in goiter prevention and the need for keeping the intake at low levels. Because the amount subsequently used was excessive, the therapy was soon discarded, and almost 100 years elapsed before Marine and Kimball found a direct relation between the incidence of goiter and low intake of iodine.

In 1838 Berzelius, a famous Swedish chemist, concluded that the iron in hemoglobin made it possible for the blood to absorb much oxygen. Iron in its various forms had long been used as a therapeutic agent for anemia, but that it had any direct relation to diet became more apparent when Bunge in 1889 reported a case of anemia which developed in a young man on an exclusive milk diet. Bunge noted further that mice would also develop anemia on an exclusive milk diet, and that pure iron salts would not cure the anemia but that egg yolk would. He therefore concluded that some union of iron with the protein of egg was responsible for the efficiency of the cure. Thirty-five years later Hart and his associates at the University of Wisconsin again found that white rats develop anemia if fed a milk diet, that the anemia was not cured by iron salts alone, but that the ash of lettuce was an effective cure. The unknown substance present in lettuce ash was found to be copper.

Mere traces of copper added to pure iron salts were found to be adequate for cure of iron-deficiency anemia. This was another illustration of the importance of traces of certain elements in body metabolism.

Discovery of vitamins. Dr. Eijkman, a Dutch biologist, in 1897 showed that beriberi occurred when people ate rice which was polished, but that the disease could be prevented if the rice with its bran was used. He showed definitely that beriberi, or a disease showing similar symptoms of nerve disturbance, could be produced or cured at will in hens by changing the diet of unpolished rice to milled rice, or the reverse. In 1906 he wrote: "There is present in rice polishings a substance of a different nature from proteins, fats, or salts which is essential to health and the lack of which causes nutritional polyneuritis." * At the same time J. Gowland Hopkins of England and others found that laboratory animals could not live or thrive on purified mixtures of proteins, carbohydrates, fats, and inorganic salts. Fed such a diet, the animals ceased to grow, sickened, and eventually died unless the purified ration was changed. Hopkins established beyond a doubt that these "accessory factors" in foods are essential to life, and he is generally credited with the discovery of vitamins. Casimir Funk applied the name "vitamine" to these substances in 1911, the final "e" being dropped some years later when it became evident that the chemical nature of these substances was not what Funk had supposed it to be.

In the meantime Holst and Frölich, two workers in Norway, had succeeded in producing symptoms which resembled scurvy in guinea pigs by using an experimental diet which contained no fresh foods. All through history scurvy had plagued people who were forced to eat a diet devoid of fresh foods for long periods of time; the sailor, explorer, and adventurer were especially susceptible. A British physician, Dr. Lind, in 1757 had shown the efficacy of citrus fruits in both curing and preventing scurvy. The New England pioneers recognized the value of potatoes and fruits in preventing this condition. Then in the twentieth century, with the production of scurvy in the guinea pig, the way was paved for the studies on vitamin C and its later isolation and synthesis.

While the studies on the factor which would prevent beriberi were progressing, McCollum and Davis, and Osborne and Mendel had observed that animals which received diets containing lard instead of butterfat would cease to grow and would eventually develop an inflammation of the eye. When butterfat was used, the condition was corrected; cod-liver oil was found to be very effective. These discoveries led to the recognition of "fat-soluble A" and "water-soluble B" as the factors were then designated.

In the 40 years which have elapsed since the first vitamin was discovered, the growth of the vitamin family, the isolation and determination of many

* Eijkman, P., quoted in Harris, L. J.: *Vitamins in Theory and Practice.* Cambridge University Press, London, 1935.

vitamins, the partial solution of the puzzle of vitamin functions in the body, the discovery of the amazing therapeutic value of minute quantities of these vitamins in the cure of deficiency disease, the numerous determinations of food composition with respect to vitamins—all are stories which excite the imagination. It is no wonder that the subject of vitamins touched popular fancy, and that they have often been overemphasized. There is not space here to tell the story of the development of knowledge concerning vitamins, but some of these aspects will be hinted at in the chapters on vitamins (Chaps. 9, 10, and 11). Further details can be obtained by consulting references suggested in the bibliography.

Early beginnings of dietetics in America. Knowledge of food and its preparation for all in the family, whether they be well or sick, has at all times been considered a necessary training for the homemaker, to be handed down from generation to generation. The earliest cookbooks included reference to the special food needs of those who might be ill. More learned works for physicians likewise contained suggestions for diet in various disturbances. In the hospital, the feeding of patients was left to the nurses, some of whom might be especially assigned to the administration of the dietary department.

A number of cooking schools, notably in New York, Boston, and Philadelphia,[8,9] which arose during the last quarter of the nineteenth century, seem to have laid the basis for the profession of dietetics in this country. One of these, the New Century Cooking School, was founded in 1878 by a group of wealthy women in Philadelphia. Sara Tyson Rorer was graduated from the first course in this school—a course consisting of two practical lessons a week for 3 months and 24 demonstrated lectures. She succeeded Miss Devereaux, the school's first principal, after a year and worked out a "course of lectures" for the students at Woman's Medical College and the nurses at the Woman's Hospital. After 3 years she founded her own Philadelphia Cooking School. It was not long before a number of renowned physicians of Philadelphia came to her to ask if she would start a diet kitchen where food would be well prepared for special diseases so that patients who were from out-of-town and staying at hotels could be properly fed. Such a kitchen was founded and was later combined with the cooking school. Miss Rorer can, no doubt, be given the distinction of having been the first American dietitian.

One of the graduates of the first "normal class" in Miss Rorer's school, Martha G. Byerly, taught a class of senior nurses from the Pennsylvania Hospital in 1892; then, in 1893 she became superintendent of diet at the Presbyterian Hospital and continued to teach the nurses at the Pennsylvania Hospital. At the same time Mary A. Boland, who was instructor in cooking at the Johns Hopkins Hospital Training School for Nurses, wrote a *Handbook of Invalid Cookery*. These classes during the nineties seem to have been the earliest attempt to give organized instruction in dietetics to nurses.

The American Dietetic Association. At the invitation of Miss Lenna F.

Cooper of the Battle Creek Sanitarium and Miss Lulu G. Graves of Lakeside Hospital, Cleveland, a conference of 98 dietitians was held in October, 1917, in Cleveland. The purpose of this meeting was to discuss how dietitians could best serve during the war both at home and overseas, and to effect better communications among dietitians. An organization called the American Dietetic Association with the stated purpose "to benefit as many as possible" was established at this conference with 39 charter members. The membership now totals about 15,000. The four sections, Community Nutrition, Diet Therapy, Education, and Food Administration represent the varied aspects of the dietitian's work. Recently, the history of the association and its work has been written by Mary I. Barber.[10]

Growth of research. Without the faithful workers in the research laboratories and the countless numbers of experimental animals used, very little of our present nutrition knowledge would now be available. It has taken combined research in the sciences of physiology, biology, and chemistry to develop the complicated story of nutrition on a physiologic basis, but the whole program of nutrition research is even more extensive than that. For example, agriculture has undergone a remarkable change in the last few decades. Some varieties of plants are now known to be a better source of nutrients than others. Composition of the soil, fertilizers, and climate are all known to influence the amount of food produced. The control of plant pests, the adaptation of plant variety to growing conditions, the improvement of animal feeds, and the use of antibiotics to accelerate the growth of animals are but a few examples of the areas of progress.

The way in which a product is handled from the time it is gathered by the farmer until it is eaten by the consumer is known to influence nutritive value, and so there have been many studies of the effects of drying, canning, freezing, irradiation, storage, atmospheric conditions, and various methods of cookery on the retention of food values.

Dietary surveys and studies of nutritional status have been made in many parts of the United States and in other areas of the world by public health nutrition workers. Such studies serve to correlate dietary intakes with health and thus provide further evidence for the establishment of minimum requirements and adequate allowances for long-time health. These investigations are also providing a wealth of information relating to food habits and psychologic factors in feeding.

Problems in nutrition are challenging. Every question which has been answered in the science of nutrition seems to have raised a host of new ones. Of immediate interest is the question of variations in food values with changing conditions of food gathering, storage, processing, and cookery. The data now available for some nutrients such as amino acids, fatty acids, sodium, and others must be extended to give greater significance to the average values cited in food tables.

While a great deal is known about the amounts of various nutrients which are needed to prevent various deficiency diseases, complete information is lacking on the requirements of the optimum diet. Sherman has shown that improvement of an already adequate diet can prolong the length of life and the prime of life in experimental animals, but there is scarcely any research on man as yet which supports this important finding.

That nutrients cannot be put into so many convenient pigeonholes but are interrelated substances with regard to requirements and function is known. Thus, carbohydrate spares protein; tryptophan, an amino acid, can replace niacin, a vitamin; thiamine is necessary for carbohydrate metabolism, and so on. The full significance of these interrelationships is just beginning to be appreciated.

Detailed descriptions of many classic deficiency diseases have been available for a long time. On the other hand, we know little of how to diagnose deficiency at early stages either by clinical observation or by laboratory tests. Knowledge is extremely limited on the effect of nutrition on the incidence and course of degenerative diseases such as cancer, cardiovascular disease, and arthritis.

Some of the nutritional problems such as dental caries are essentially unsolved. One might also ask: What is the relation of diet to tumor development? Why do some people like certain foods and others do not? In what way might mental health be influenced by diet? What are the functions of some of the newly discovered vitamins? What are the best methods for changing the food habits of people who have been accustomed to faulty dietary patterns over long periods of time? In what ways can education be made more effective to reduce the large number of the misfed? These are but a few of the many problems waiting for solution.

CHAPTER 3 /

Dietary Guides and Their Uses

Functions of food. The nutrients which are provided to the body cells are used for energy, for building all tissues, and for the manufacture of innumerable regulatory substances. Carbohydrates, fats, and proteins supply the energy requirements. Proteins are, next to water, the chief constituents of body tissues; many other nutrients—for example, the mineral salts in bones and teeth—are equally essential structural elements although they occur in much smaller quantities than protein and water. All of the nutrients function in one way or another in the regulation of body processes. Vitamins are thought of especially in this regard, but mineral salts, amino acids, and certain carbohydrates and fats also function as such.

Metabolism. The series of processes necessary for the building of body tissues and their continuous functioning is known as *metabolism*. This broad term implies the coordination of a number of body processes:

1. Ingestion or the intake of food
2. Digestion which prepares foods for their use by the body
3. Absorption of nutrients from the gastrointestinal tract into the circulation
4. Transportation by the circulatory system of nutrients to the sites for their use, and of wastes to the points of excretion
5. Respiration, which supplies oxygen to the tissues for the oxidation of food, and which removes waste carbon dioxide. The circulatory system is again responsible for transportation of these gases
6. Use of materials: oxidation to create heat and energy; incorporation into new cells and tissues
7. Excretion of wastes: undigested food wastes and certain body wastes from the bowel; carbon dioxide by the lungs; nitrogenous, mineral salt, and other wastes from metabolism by the kidneys and by the skin

STANDARDS FOR DIETARY ALLOWANCES

Recommended Dietary Allowances. Late in 1940, the Food and Nutrition Board of the National Research Council was organized to guide the government in its nutrition program. One of the first activities of this board was the careful review of research on human requirements for the various nutrients leading to the publication of the Recommended Dietary Allowances in 1943. Since that time the board has continued to function in the evaluation of new research on nutritional needs, and has published revisions of the standards in 1945, 1948, 1953, and 1958. The title is described thus:

The title "Recommended Dietary Allowances" was selected for this standard in the effort to make it clear that the levels of nutrient intake recommended were judgments, which were not to be considered final and which should be reevaluated periodically as new information became available. Moreover, the use of this term was meant to avoid misinterpretation of the allowances as representing either minimal or optimal nutrient requirements.*

The most recent revision of the allowances is quoted in the table on page 26. The bulletin prepared by the Food and Nutrition Board [2] gives a full description of the bases for establishing these recommendations and also includes a discussion of the needs for many nutrients such as fat, carbohydrate, water, many minerals and vitamins not listed in the table. When diets are planned to meet the recommended levels set forth in the table, it is safe to assume that the body's needs for the nutrients not listed will also be met.

Uses of the table. The over-all aim of this standard has been stated thus:

The final objective of the recommended allowances must be to permit and to encourage the development of food practices by the population of the United States which will allow for greatest dividends in health and in disease prevention.†

The purposes and intended uses are further described below:

The recommended allowances for adults are given in terms of a reference man and reference woman as described in the section on calories. The body weights of the reference man and woman are 70 and 58 kilograms, respectively, and the mean environmental temperature has been taken as 20° C, a value applicable to the American population. Calorie adjustments should be made for persons who differ in body size, age, or physical activity from the reference man or woman. The ages cited are for the middle point of the decade. Allowances for boys and girls are given separately after age 12, since growth curves and customary expenditures of energy differ markedly after this age. Allowances as given in childhood are considered to apply to the middle of the age period designated. As with adults, adjustments are required for children who differ from the standard in body size or physical activity.

* Food and Nutrition Board: *Recommended Dietary Allowances—Revised 1958*. Pub. 589, National Research Council, Washington, D.C., 1958, p. 1.
† *Ibid.,* p. 28.

FOOD AND NUTRITION BOARD, NATIONAL RESEARCH COUNCIL
RECOMMENDED DAILY DIETARY ALLOWANCES,[1] REVISED 1958

DESIGNED FOR THE MAINTENANCE OF GOOD NUTRITION OF HEALTHY PERSONS IN THE U.S.A.

(Allowances are intended for persons normally active in a temperate climate)

	AGE Years	WEIGHT kg (lb.)	HEIGHT cm. (in.)	CALORIES	PROTEIN gm	CALCIUM gm	IRON mg	VITAMIN A I.U.	THIAMINE mg	RIBOFLAVIN mg	NIACIN[2] mg. equiv.	ASCORBIC ACID mg	VITAMIN D I.U.
Men	25	70 (154)	175 (69)	3200[3]	70	0.8	10	5000	1.6	1.8	21	75	
	45	70 (154)	175 (69)	3000	70	0.8	10	5000	1.5	1.8	20	75	
	65	70 (154)	175 (69)	2550	70	0.8	10	5000	1.3	1.8	18	75	
Women ..	25	58 (128)	163 (64)	2300	58	0.8	12	5000	1.2	1.5	17	70	
	45	58 (128)	163 (64)	2200	58	0.8	12	5000	1.1	1.5	17	70	
	65	58 (128)	163 (64)	1800	58	0.8	12	5000	1.0	1.5	17	70	
	Pregnant (second half)			+300	+20	1.5	15	6000	1.3	2.0	+3	100	400
	Lactating (850 ml daily)			+1000	+40	2.0	15	8000	1.7	2.5	+2	150	400
Infants[4] ..	0–1/12[4]				See Footnote 4								
	2/12–6/12	6 (13)	60 (24)	kgx120		0.6	5	1500	0.4	0.5	6	30	400
	7/12–1	9 (20)	70 (28)	kgx100		0.8	7	1500	0.5	0.8	7	30	400
Children .	1 – 3	12 (27)	87 (34)	1300	40	1.0	7	2000	0.7	1.0	8	35	400
	4 – 6	18 (40)	109 (43)	1700	50	1.0	8	2500	0.9	1.3	11	50	400
	7 – 9	27 (60)	129 (51)	2100	60	1.0	10	3500	1.1	1.5	14	60	400
	10–12	36 (79)	144 (57)	2500	70	1.2	12	4500	1.3	1.8	17	75	400
Boys	13–15	49 (108)	163 (64)	3100	85	1.4	15	5000	1.6	2.1	21	90	400
	16–19	63 (139)	175 (69)	3600	100	1.4	15	5000	1.8	2.5	25	100	400
Girls	13–15	49 (108)	160 (63)	2600	80	1.3	15	5000	1.3	2.0	17	80	400
	16–19	54 (120)	162 (64)	2400	75	1.3	15	5000	1.2	1.9	16	80	400

[1] The allowance levels are intended to cover individual variations among most normal persons as they live in the United States under usual environmental stresses. The recommended allowances can be attained with a variety of common foods, providing other nutrients for which human requirements have been less well defined. See text for more detailed discussion of allowances and of nutrients not tabulated.

[2] Niacin equivalents include dietary sources of the preformed vitamin and the precursor, tryptophan. Sixty milligrams tryptophan equals 1 milligram niacin.

[3] Calorie allowances apply to individuals usually engaged in moderate physical activity. For office workers or others in sedentary occupations they are excessive. Adjustments must be made for variations in body size, age, physical activity, and environmental temperature.

[4] See text for discussion of infant allowances. The Board recognizes that human milk is the natural food for infants and feels that breast feeding is the best and desired procedure for meeting nutrient requirements in the first months of life. No allowances are stated for the first month of life. Breast feeding is particularly indicated during the first month when infants show handicaps in homeostasis due to different rates of maturation of digestive, excretory, and endocrine functions. Recommendations as listed pertain to nutrient intake as afforded by cow's milk formulas and supplementary foods given the infant when breast feeding is terminated. Allowances are not given for protein

As with all biologic functions, nutrient requirements vary from individual to individual within a wide range. The effort has been made to afford allowances which will cover nearly the entire distribution curve of requirements, thus meeting needs of those with greatest requirements and providing a substantial margin of sufficiency for the majority of individuals. The allowances as proposed are conceived to be wholly adequate for maintaining good nutrition throughout life.

The allowances are planned for healthy, moderately active persons. The presence of acute or chronic illness may modify nutrient requirements markedly. In febrile illnesses and hyperthyroidism, needs for certain nutrients may be enhanced because of increased metabolism, while in other disorders, involving the gastrointestinal tract, absorption of nutrients provided in the diet may be impaired. These problems and the planning of diet for such persons must remain the responsibility of the physician.

Recommended dietary allowances have been provided to serve as a guide for planning adequate diets for normal healthy populations or individuals. If they are to be used for estimating the needs of population groups, the allowances must be weighted in terms of the distribution of various age, sex, and activity categories in the population. Also, if utilized for purposes of dietary surveys to determine the adequacy of food intake, it must be realized that diets affording less than recommended dietary allowances do not of necessity imply nutritional deficiency. In fact, in times of food lacks or economic stringency, it may not be possible for all segments of the population to achieve full compliance with all of the allowances. Under such circumstances, if long continued, it is possible that certain individuals with very high requirements may show signs of deterioration in health.

The values given for recommended allowances represent quantities actually consumed and do not allow for losses due to storage, cooking, or serving. Provision must be made for these losses in diet planning. The allowances, on the other hand, do provide for incomplete absorption or availability of certain nutrients such as iron and carotene. . . .

The various quantities of nutrients recommended as allowances may be readily obtained from usual portions of commonly available foods in the United States, and it should be accepted as an important precept in diet planning that variety in foods is of advantage, since it offers the potential of affording many essential nutrients in natural proportions.*

The allowances for specific nutrients will be discussed in succeeding chapters. The student should form the habit of referring to this table whenever questions arise concerning the nutritional needs for various age categories.

Dietary guides of other countries. The Committee on Nutrition of the British Medical Association has published dietary standards since 1933.[11] These standards are intended to maintain good nutrition in the *average* person, while the recommendations in the United States attempt to meet the needs of substantially all normal persons.

The Canadian Council on Nutrition has established a standard to provide

* *Ibid.*, p. 27.

"a nutritional floor beneath which maintenance of health of the people cannot be assumed." * McHenry [12] has pointed out, however, that in many respects (protein and calcium, for example) the standards are similar to, or identical with, the standards in the United States and that the Canadian standards cannot be interpreted as minimal.

Other countries have likewise set up standards and dietary guides adapted to the local needs and food resources. The Food and Agriculture Organization has made a beginning in the establishment of international standards by the publication of reports on caloric and protein requirements. [13,14]

Minimum daily requirements. For the purpose of labeling foods—especially those for which some therapeutic claims are made—the federal Food and Drug Administration has developed a table of minimum requirements (see p. 790). It is important for the student to realize that it is the FDA table, and not the Recommended Dietary Allowances, to which reference is made when food products are labeled as providing certain percentages of the minimum requirements since, in some respects, the two standards differ rather widely. The labeling of some food products includes reference to both standards, thus providing useful information to the professional person who is able to interpret the statements. However, the use of both standards can be quite confusing to the uninformed layman who conscientiously tries to interpret labeling information. Throughout this text, the Recommended Dietary Allowances, and not the FDA standards, are employed as a basis for dietary planning.

A DAILY FOOD GUIDE

Foods as sources of nutrients. Some foods are desirable because they promote all three functions of food, while others contribute primarily to energy production. Even a food like milk, which is generally considered to be the most nearly perfect food, does not contain all the food constituents in optimum amounts. Milk is an excellent source of protein for tissue building, it provides more calcium than any other food for bone and tooth formation, and it gives the most abundant supply of riboflavin. In other minerals and vitamins, too, milk is relatively rich. However, in its ascorbic acid content it is low, so that the need for citrus fruits or tomato, which are vitamin-C-rich foods, becomes readily apparent. If one goes further, one can see that additional iron is needed because milk does not supply much of it; thus, the place of egg, green leafy vegetables, fruits, and meats becomes evident. One could continue in this manner to analyze each of the foods. A variety of foods becomes one of the best guarantees that a diet will be adequate.

All foods provide for the energy needs of the body. Some foods which

* "A Dietary Standard for Canada Approved by the Canadian Council on Nutrition, Ottawa, December 7, 1948," *Bull. Canad. Council on Nutrition,* **2:**1, 1950.

have a high concentration of fats and carbohydrates are high in calories; other foods with a high proportion of water, such as fruits and vegetables, are relatively low in calories.

Four Food Groups. A standard such as the Recommended Dietary Allowances is of practical value only when it is interpreted into a selection of foods to meet the recommended levels. This may be accomplished through dietary calculations as described in the next section of this chapter. However, simple guides for the public are essential, and these have been developed by nutrition committees of government agencies and others.

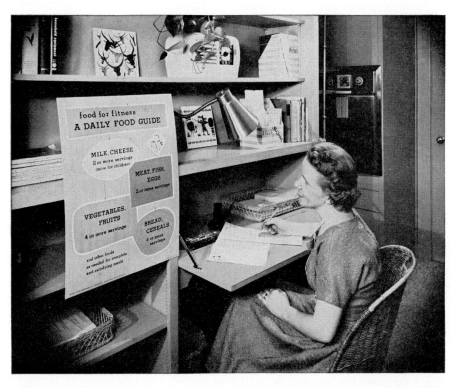

Fig. 3-1. Selecting foods from the Four Food Groups of the Daily Food Guide helps to ensure nutritious meals. (*Courtesy, Institute of Home Economics, U.S. Department of Agriculture.*)

One of these guides, "A Daily Food Guide" (Fig. 3-1), has been prepared recently by the Institute of Home Economics. The food groups are:

Milk group

    2 cups or more for adults
    3 to 4 cups for children

4 cups or more for teenagers
4 cups or more for pregnant women
6 cups or more for nursing mothers

Meat group

2 or more servings. Count as one serving:
2 to 3 ounces lean, cooked beef, veal, pork, lamb, poultry, fish—
without bone
2 eggs
1 cup cooked dry beans, dry peas, lentils
4 tablespoons peanut butter

Vegetable-fruit group

4 or more servings per day, including:
1 serving of citrus fruit, or other fruit or vegetable as a good source
of vitamin C, or 2 servings of a fair source
1 serving, at least every other day, of a dark green or deep yellow vegetable for vitamin A
2 or more servings of other vegetables and fruits, including potatoes

Bread-cereals group

4 or more servings daily (whole grain, enriched, or restored). Count as one
serving:
1 slice bread
1 ounce ready-to-eat cereal
½ to ¾ cup cooked cereal, corn meal, grits, macaroni, noodles, rice,
or spaghetti

The Four Food Groups provide a foundation for a day's meals and include
food choices which permit flexibility for seasonal, regional, and budgetary
considerations. The specific nutrient contributions made by foods in each of
the Four Food Groups will be discussed in the chapters on the nutrients (see
also table of calculations, p. 178).

The basic diet. The minimum number of servings for the adult of each of
the Four Food Groups will be used as a basis for dietary planning throughout this text. The protein, mineral, and vitamin needs are substantially met
by this plan (see p. 178), while the caloric levels are approximately sufficient
for the basal metabolism. The size of the portion will obviously need to be
modified for preschool and school children and for teenagers to provide the
correct amounts of the various nutrients.

To fully meet the energy needs, additional foods may be selected from
the fats, sweets, or from one or more of the four groups. The nutrient intake
will remain essentially at the level calculated for the basic diet if additional
energy is provided chiefly from fats and sweets, but the further selection of

foods from one or more of the four groups will substantially increase the nutritive value of the diet.

COMPOSITION OF FOODS

Factors affecting food composition. The nutritive values of foods are determined, for the most part, by chemical methods. In some instances, such as the determination of vitamin D or the evaluation of digestibility, animal feeding (bio-assay) is used. Certain of the B vitamins and some of the amino acids are best determined by observing the reproduction, or selected metabolic processes, of microorganisms (microbiologic assay).

The values for nutrients in tables of food composition are customarily expressed as averages of analyses of food samples. For some nutrients numerous analyses may have been made, while for other nutrients the number of determinations has been much more limited. Obviously, the actual nutritive value of a food may be expected to vary more or less widely from the average. Some of the more important factors which account for variation in food composition are discussed briefly below.

The nature of the soil might be expected to produce variations in the composition of foods. However, at the present time, the only correlation which has been fully established is that a low-iodine content of the soil is reflected in a low-iodine content of foods. The quantity of vitamins, or of other nutrients, has been found to be largely independent of the soil composition. Contrary to certain cultists who criticize the use of chemical fertilizers and who emphasize so-called "organic" farming, Maynard [15] presents evidence that soils which are chemically fertilized are highly productive of foods of good nutritive value.

The variety of plant and the climate are important determinants of nutritive value. The latter cannot be controlled, but nutritionists and agriculturists know that the selection of the appropriate variety of plant may be a vital consideration for dietary adequacy in those parts of the world where the food supply is otherwise poor.

The conditions of storage may modify the nutritive value of foods. Some nutrients such as ascorbic acid are rapidly lost when the temperature is high or when foods are bruised. Other nutrients may be lost to a varying degree, but not quite so readily as ascorbic acid.

Divergent procedures in food preparation are major factors which affect the nutritive value of a food as it is consumed. Losses in food preparation may be brought about through solubility of the nutrient in water, or through destruction of the nutrient. The latter is increased with high temperature, and is also dependent upon the pH of the medium in which it is cooked. The amount of peelings removed, the size of pieces subjected to cooking, the temperature used, the length of time for cooking, the amount of water used, the length of time food is held after cooking—as on a steam table—are but a few of the many variables which may result in wide differences between two foods which were identical at the start of the cooking procedure.

Processing techniques may enhance or interfere with the nutritive value of foods. Dehydration, canning, and freezing yield foods of high nutritive value, but each, in certain ways, modifies somewhat the nutrient contribution of a given food. No doubt this list could be lengthened, but it should suffice to emphasize to the student that any given value represents an approximation, and not a precise value.

Tables of food values. In view of the foregoing discussion, one might be tempted to ask what values there are in using a table of food composition. First, the tables serve as a basis for comparing one food with another; for example, milk is clearly seen to be the best source of calcium. Although we would not expect every medium-sized orange to provide *exactly* the same number of milligrams of ascorbic acid, the tables do give information which makes it safe to say that oranges, let us say, are a better source of the vitamin than applesauce. Second, the use of tables provides a means whereby the adequacy of diets may be estimated although not precisely stated. Thus, the legitimate use of tables necessitates an understanding of their values in assessing nutritive values of foods and of diets as well as an appreciation of the limitations.

The doctor, nurse, and dietitian will find consistent use of tables of food composition essential for intelligent planning of normal and therapeutic diets. Moreover, the tables provide a ready reference to answer numerous questions concerning the nutritive value of foods, and thus they are, in themselves, an effective means for counteracting food misinformation.

The several tables of food values in the Appendix have been derived from compilations made from time to time, chiefly by investigators in the Department of Agriculture. Just as the purchase of food involves certain units of measure such as ounces, pounds, pints, quarts, so the amount of nutrients in a food is expressed in certain units—grams (gm), milligrams (mg), sometimes micrograms (mcg), and international units (I.U.). In Table 1 of the Appendix (p. 720) the nutritive values are expressed for the edible part of household portions of food, thus making it simple to determine the contribution of full or fractional portions of food. Other tables give the nutritive values for 100 gm edible portion of food.

DIETARY EVALUATION

Purposes of dietary evaluation. Before beginning the evaluation of any diet, the goals to be achieved must be set, since the nature of the study is thereby determined. A dietary evaluation may be qualitative—that is, through questioning of the subject it may be established that certain kinds of foods are, or are not, being included; recommendations for dietary improvement can often be made on such a basis without the necessity of detailed calculations.

This section, however, is concerned with dietary calculations, since the student and professional worker must often resort to more quantitative approaches. Food tables may be used for the determination of the adequacy of a particular diet—either normal or therapeutic, or for the control of a specific nutrient such as sodium or fat. The student should keep a number of goals in mind as she acquires experience in the calculation of diets, since she may otherwise become discouraged at the amount of time involved in the mechanics of arithmetic! She must remember that the calculations are merely a means to an end. Among the outcomes from experience in dietary calculations are the following:

1. A greater consciousness of food habits and their relation to nutrition and health;

2. Familiarity with tables of food composition and the kinds of information which they provide;

3. Facility in using food tables whether to calculate a complete dietary, or to seek specific answers to nutritive values of a single food;

4. Knowledge concerning the important sources of each of the nutrients;

5. Ability to make recommendations for the improvement of dietaries based upon the calculation of dietary intakes;

6. Appreciation of the importance of keeping orderly and accurate records of dietary intake so that any calculations may be as reliable as possible;

7. The habits of preparing neat and concise reports which have been carefully checked for their accuracy so that co-workers may use the information provided with complete confidence.

Calculation of the nutritive value of a diet. The method which is described below may be applied to the diet for a day, for one meal, or for a recipe. It may be used for the calculation of a single nutrient such as protein, or for all nutrients listed in a given table. This method is more time consuming than shorter methods to be described in Chapter 25.

1. Study the explanation to Table 1, page 718. Become familiar with the main headings of the table: milk; eggs; meat, poultry, and fish; dry beans and peas, and nuts; vegetables; fruits; grain products; fats, sugars; and miscellaneous items. Note that the sequence of these headings is the same as that for the Four Food Groups. Note also that foods are listed in alphabetic order under each main heading. You will save much time in dietary calculation if you form the habit of listing foods in the same sequence each time.

2. Keep an accurate record, in household measures, of the foods eaten at each meal. Record the foods directly after each meal, if at all possible; do not rely on the memory. Include any foods or beverages taken between meals. Specify the exact kinds of foods eaten: for example, enriched bread, fresh orange juice, oatmeal—not bread, fruit, cereal.

3. List on your calculation sheet the total amount, in household measures, of each food eaten during the day. Enter as one item the total daily intake of any food eaten at more than one meal; for example, 1 slice enriched bread at breakfast, ¾ slice at dinner, and ½ slice at supper would be recorded as 2¼ slices bread, enriched.

4. Calculate the nutritive values for each food of the diet or recipe, multiplying the values for the stated portion in Table 1 by the amounts actually eaten. For example, 1 slice white bread, enriched (20 slices per pound) contains 60 calories, 2 gm protein, etc. Therefore, 2¼ slices would contain:

$$2\tfrac{1}{4} \times 60 = 135 \text{ calories}$$
$$2\tfrac{1}{4} \times 2 = 4\tfrac{1}{2} \text{ gm protein (recorded as 5 gm)}$$

5. When recording the results of your calculations, use only as many decimal places as appear in the original table. For example, 11.3 gm fat is recorded as 11 gm fat; but 11.5 gm fat would be recorded as 12 gm. A calculated value for thiamine of 0.074 mg would be recorded as 0.07 mg since the table lists two decimal places for thiamine.

6. Check each of your calculations to be sure it is correct before entering the result on the final calculation sheet.

7. Record all data so that numbers are legible, and digits and decimal points are aligned.

8. Total the amount of each nutrient contained in the entire diet or recipe.

9. Compare the actual totals of the diet with the Recommended Dietary Allowances of the individual for whom the evaluation was made. If there are wide deviations between the two, it is especially important to look for possible errors in calculations, misplacement of decimal points, or mistakes in additions.

10. Calculate for each of the nutrients the percentage of the Recommended Dietary Allowances which was provided by the diet.

11. Summarize the study by listing ways in which the diet can be improved.

The same calculation for a muffin recipe on page 35 illustrates some of the procedures described above.

PROBLEMS AND REVIEW

1. Distinguish between the terms *food* and *nutrient*. Give an example of each.

2. Name the three chief constituents of the body by weight.

3. What is meant by metabolism? What body processes are included in the general use of this term?

4. What is meant by the Recommended Dietary Allowances? Who has prepared this guide?

5. List the recommended allowances for yourself. If a dietary calculation indicated that you were getting less than these allowances in one or more respects, how should you interpret this?

MUFFINS

FOOD	HOUSEHOLD MEASURE	WEIGHT gm	ENERGY calories	PROTEIN gm	FAT gm	CARBOHYDRATE gm	MINERALS		VITAMINS				
							Ca mg	Fe mg	A I.U.	Thiamine mg	Riboflavin mg	Niacin mg	Ascorbic Acid mg
Milk	1 cup	244	165	9	10	12	285	0.1	390	0.08	0.42	0.2	2
Egg	1	50	80	6	6	tr	27	1.1	590	.05	.15	tr	0
Flour, enriched (all-purpose)	2 cups	220	800	24	2	168	36	6.4	0	.96	.58	7.6	0
Shortening	¼ cup	50	445	0	50	0	0	0	0	0	0	0	0
Sugar, white	¼ cup	50	195	0	0	50	0	0	0	0	0	0	0
Baking powder	3 teaspoons												
Salt	1 teaspoon												
TOTAL	12 muffins		1685	39	68	230	348	7.6	980	1.09	1.15	7.8	2
Each	1 muffin		140	3	6	19	29	0.6	80	0.09	0.10	0.7	0

6. State the characteristics of the reference woman. How do you differ?

7. Examine the labeling on a loaf of bread or a package of cereal. Calculate in milligrams the amounts of iron, thiamine, riboflavin, and niacin contained in 1 ounce of the product. What percentage of the Recommended Dietary Allowances for an adult male is provided?

8. List five reasons why two oranges may differ in ascorbic acid content.

9. Two students had hamburger for lunch, each raw hamburger weighing 4 ounces. One student received many more calories from her hamburger than did the other. Explain.

10. What is meant by: bio-assay; microbiologic assay?

Problems in the use of food tables

11. Examine the tables in the Appendix to become familiar with the information which is available.

12. Using Table 1, list the five fresh fruits which are the most outstanding sources of vitamin A. In your community, which of these, if any, are not practical for dietary planning?

13. Using Table 1, calculate the nutritive value of 35 gm nonfat dry milk; 60 gm green beans.

14. Determine from Table 1 whether whole-wheat bread is superior to enriched white bread.

15. How many eggs must you eat to provide the same amount of calcium as 1 cup of milk? What can you conclude concerning the calcium content of eggs?

16. Which is the least expensive source of ascorbic acid, canned tomato juice or frozen orange juice?

17. Keep a careful record of your food intake for a week. See page 33 for directions.

   a. Score your week's diet according to the Daily Food Guide. What food group should you emphasize each day to improve your diet?

   b. Select the day which is most nearly typical of your daily pattern and calculate the nutritive values, using Table 1. Compare your intake with your recommended allowances.

Keep your evaluation and refer to it from time to time throughout your study of nutrition.

UNIT II /

The Nutrients—Their Characteristics, Functions, Metabolism, Food Sources, Daily Allowances

CHAPTER 4 /

Proteins and Amino Acids

Importance of protein. In 1838 a Dutch chemist, Mulder, described certain organic material which is "unquestionably the most important of all known substances in the organic kingdom. Without it no life appears possible on our planet. Through its means the chief phenomena of life are produced." * Berzelius, a contemporary of Mulder suggested that this complex nitrogen-bearing substance be called *protein* from the Greek word meaning to "take the first place." [16] "Proteins" is now retained as a group name to designate the principal nitrogenous constituents of the protoplasm of all plant and animal tissues; they are necessary for tissue synthesis and in the regulation of certain body functions.

Today, as in Mulder's day, proteins still occupy first place. Protein malnutrition is probably more widespread than any other nutritional deficiency and literally millions of people in parts of Africa, South America, Central America, the West Indies, Europe, and most of Asia are dependent upon the development of more adequate protein resources before they can realize satisfactory nutrition and health. In the United States there is an abundance of protein of good quality, but even here some people do not get enough— usually because of ignorance concerning good food selection.

Chemistry and characteristics. Proteins are extremely complex organic compounds containing the elements carbon, hydrogen, oxygen, nitrogen, and, with few exceptions, sulfur. Most proteins also contain phosphorus, and some specialized proteins contain iron, iodine, copper, and other inorganic elements.

The presence of nitrogen distinguishes protein from carbohydrate and fat. Protein contains an average of 16 per cent nitrogen. The molecular weight of protein varies from 13,000 or less to several millions. These large molecules form *colloloidal* solutions which do not readily pass through membranes.

Amino acids. The units from which proteins are built are amino acids. Each of the amino acids contains a carboxyl (COOH) or acidic group and an amino (NH_2) or basic group, the latter being on the carbon next to the

---

* Mulder, G. J.: *The Chemistry of Animal and Vegetable Physiology.* Quoted in L. B. Mendel, *Nutrition: The Chemistry of Life.* Yale University Press, New Haven, 1923, p. 16.

38

carboxyl group. By varying the grouping which is attached to the carbon containing the amino group, many different amino acids are possible; for example:

$$CH_2(NH_2).COOH \quad \text{glycine}$$
$$CH_3.CH \ (NH_2).COOH \quad \text{alanine}$$
$$CH_2(NH_2).CH_2.CH_2.CH_2.CH(NH_2).COOH \quad \text{lysine}$$

Twenty different amino acids are widely distributed in proteins (p. 44), while small amounts of four or five additional amino acids have been isolated from one or more proteins.

Protein structure. Proteins are built up by linking the amino group of one amino acid to the carboxyl group of another acid. Two such amino acids linked together are known as a *dipeptide,* three as a *tripeptide,* many as *polypeptides,* whereas aggregates of polypeptides in turn are proteins. Proteins are usually grouped in three classes:

1. SIMPLE PROTEINS such as zein of corn, albumins in egg white, gliadin of wheat consist of amino acids only. An almost infinite number of proteins is possible because the number of amino acids present in the protein may vary, the 20 or so amino acids may be arranged in different sequences in different proteins, and the amount of each amino acid together with their proportions one to another may vary from protein to protein.

2. CONJUGATED PROTEINS contain protein and some nonprotein molecule. A complex iron grouping combines with protein to form hemoglobin; different groupings containing phosphoric acid result in phosphoproteins; lipids combine with protein to form lipoproteins; and vitamins such as thiamine, pantothenic acid, and many others combine with proteins to form enzymes.

3. DERIVED PROTEINS result from a partial breakdown of a native protein. Proteoses, peptones, and polypeptides which result from the action of the digestive enzymes on protein are examples of this class.

Specificity of protein. Every living organism manufactures protein which is unique and distinctive for its species. Wheat, corn, potato, beef, pork, and egg proteins, for example, are all different. Moreover, plants and animals synthesize more than one protein. Wheat, for example, contains not one but many kinds of protein. In the human body during every moment of life literally myriads of different proteins are being constructed, each intended to carry out a highly specific function.

A given protein, seemingly similar, is in fact different from one species to another. To illustrate, the hemoglobin of dog, horse, and human are all different, just as muscle proteins of each species are different. Food allergies and antibody formation are demonstrations of this specificity of proteins. Because of this fact, all proteins must be degraded to their constituent amino acids through the digestive process before they can be utilized.

Functions. Proteins constitute the chief solid matter of muscles, organs, and endocrine glands. They are major components of the matrix of bones and teeth; skin, nails, and hair; and blood cells and serum. In fact, every living cell and all body fluids, except bile and urine, contain protein. The first need for amino acids, then, is to supply the materials for the building and the continuous replacement of the cell proteins throughout life.

In addition to being the structural components of body tissues, many proteins have highly specialized functions in the regulation of body processes. Hemoglobin, an iron-bearing protein which is the chief constituent of the red blood cells, performs a vital role in carrying oxygen to the tissues. Plasma proteins are of fundamental importance in the regulation of osmotic pressure and in the maintenance of water balance. Blood proteins have a role of maintaining the normal slightly alkaline reaction of the blood. The body's resistance to disease is maintained in part by antibodies which are protein in nature.

Enzymes which are specific catalysts for metabolic processes in the body are protein in nature. Two of these, pepsin and trypsin—and others as well—are hydrolytic enzymes which participate in digestion, while numerous vitamin-protein combinations are enzymes responsible in part for the oxidation of carbohydrate, fat, and protein.

Governing the body reactions are hormones which also are protein substances—insulin, epinephrine, the thyroid hormone, and adrenocorticotropic hormone (ACTH) to name but a few. Some amino acids have specific functions: tryptophan serves as a precursor for niacin, one of the B-complex vitamins, and methionine can provide methyl groups for the synthesis of choline, another B-complex vitamin.

Proteins yield 4 calories per gram when broken down in the body. This energy is derived from the metabolism of excess food protein, or it results from the breakdown of body tissues. Because protein foods are the most expensive items of the diet, they are not an economical source of energy; moreover, the process of deamination and the excretion of the waste product urea result in additional work for the liver and kidney.

Digestion and absorption. Digestion is necessary in order to degrade the proteins to amino acids so that absorption can take place and so that the biologic specificity of the protein can be destroyed. Since saliva contains no proteolytic enzyme, the first digestive action takes place in the stomach. The hydrochloric acid in the stomach changes the inactive enzyme *pepsinogen* to the active form *pepsin,* denatures the protein so that it is more readily acted upon, and provides a suitable reaction for the optimum activity of pepsin. Pepsin acts upon specific peptide linkages to begin the digestion of protein.

Pancreatic juice contains two inactive proteolytic enzymes, *trypsinogen* and *chymotrypsinogen.* In the small intestine trypsinogen is activated to *trypsin* by *enterokinase,* an enzyme produced in the intestinal wall. Chymotrypsinogen is activated by trypsin to *chymotrypsin.* These active enzymes continue to split the proteins by attacking certain peptide linkages.

The final breakdown of proteins is effected by a group of enzymes called *peptidases* which are secreted by the intestinal mucosa. The end products of digestion, the amino acids, are absorbed from the intestinal wall into the portal circulation in a gradual and continuous manner. There is neither a large build-up of amino acids in the intestinal tract nor in the blood circulation.

About 92 per cent of the protein in the typical mixed diet eaten in the United States is normally digested. The proteins of some foods such as eggs, milk, and meat are more completely digested than are others, especially those of plant origin. A high amount of fiber such as that in the diet of vegetarians reduces the percentage of protein which is digested.

Proteins require a somewhat longer time for digestion than do carbohydrates, and thus their presence in a meal provides a feeling of satiety.

Metabolism. The absorbed amino acids are carried by the portal circulation to the liver or they may circulate directly to the tissues. (See Fig. 4-1.) At any given moment the so-called metabolic pool of amino acids includes

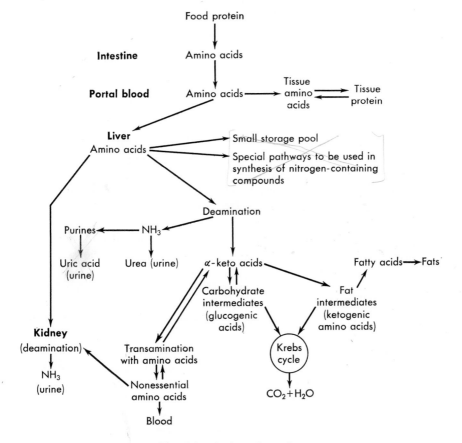

Fig. 4-1. The fate of protein.

those which have been absorbed from the small intestine and those which have been released by the breakdown of tissue proteins. From this pool amino acids can be withdrawn for the synthesis (anabolism) of any tissue proteins, including the proteins of specialized functions such as the enzymes and the hormones. The amino acids from this pool can also be broken down (catabolized), yielding the ultimate end products urea, carbon dioxide, water, and energy. Body tissues are not static, but exist in a state of *dynamic equilibrium;* that is, there is a constant and rapid breakdown of cellular material with amino acids released to the blood balanced by an equally constant and speedy synthesis of new tissues from amino acids supplied by the blood.

Nitrogen balance. One way to measure the extent of protein metabolism is to determine the nitrogen content of food, feces, and urine, since 1 gm nitrogen represents 6.25 gm protein. The difference between the nitrogen intake and the nitrogen value of the feces represents the nitrogen which has actually been absorbed, and which is therefore available for use by the body. The nitrogen content of the urine varies directly with the amount of the amino acids which are being broken down. If the nitrogen intake and the nitrogen excretion in the feces and urine are equal, the individual is said to be in *nitrogen equilibrium* or *nitrogen balance;* that is, the anabolic and catabolic activities are equal.

When the intake of nitrogen is greater than the amount excreted, the person is said to be in *positive balance;* that is, the synthesis of tissue proteins exceeds the breakdown. If, on the other hand, the excretion of nitrogen is greater than the intake, *negative balance* prevails; in other words, protein is being broken down more rapidly than it is being built up.

Catabolism of amino acids. The first step in the catabolism of amino acids is their *deamination* in the liver; that is, the amino group is removed and is subsequently synthesized into urea which is excreted as the main nitrogenous product of the urine. After the amino group has been removed, the non-nitrogenous part of the amino acid molecule has one of several fates:

1. Certain amino acids will yield glucose, which can be used immediately for energy or stored as glycogen or fat. Under severe conditions Lusk has found that 58 per cent of the amino acids could be so converted.

2. Other amino acids are converted to fat for immediate use as energy, or for storage as adipose tissue.

3. The nitrogen-free molecule may recombine with free amino groups to build new amino acids.

A negative nitrogen balance or catabolism in excess of anabolism occurs: (1) when the dietary protein level is too low to meet fully the synthetic needs; (2) when the protein fed is lacking or limited in one or more of the essential amino acids so that synthesis cannot take place; and (3) when the caloric intake is insufficient for body needs so that energy needs must be met from the body stores of fat and body reserves of protein. Protein breakdown is greatly accelerated following severe injury, burns, surgery, or illness with a high fever. The adrenocortical hormones and an excessive production of thyroxine increase the breakdown of proteins.

Synthesis of tissue proteins. Normally adults synthesize tissue proteins at a rate which is equal to their breakdown. When the protein intake is liberal, the anabolic and catabolic activities are high. All the amino acids—essential and nonessential—must be simultaneously available or no tissue building will take place. Protein cannot be manufactured if even one of the amino acids required for the cell structure is missing. If the assortment of amino acids is incomplete, the available amino acids are catabolized as described in the preceding section. The body must also have an adequate source of calories from carbohydrate and fat, because the energy requirement will take priority over tissue synthesis when there is a caloric deficit.

In certain circumstances tissues are being built beyond that required for mere replacement, namely: for growth of children; during pregnancy; for development of the muscles as in training for athletics; and during the recovery phase of an illness. This represents a state of positive nitrogen balance. Certain hormones favor tissue building: the growth hormone secreted by the pituitary, insulin, thyroxine in normal amounts, and testosterone.

Body protein reserves. The body does not store protein in the sense that it stores fat. This should not be confused with the positive nitrogen balance which prevails during growth; in this situation there is an increase in cell structure and it does not involve the addition (or storage) of nitrogen to cells already in good nutrition. However, the body does have "labile" reserves which can be mobilized in emergency. The proteins of the liver, pancreas, blood plasma, kidney, and intestinal wall have a high rate of turnover. In fact, it has been estimated that half of the protein of the liver is replaced every 10 days. The rate of turnover in muscle, skin, bone, lung, and brain is much slower. Because the muscle mass is so considerable, even a slow rate of turnover results in the mobilization of a significant amount of protein. In one sense, then, the proteins of some tissues may be loaned, as it were, to others where the need is more urgent. But just as too frequent borrowing of money without repayment leads eventually to financial ruin, so the continuous loaning of these labile proteins without their replacement ultimately leads to nutritional chaos.

Protein quality. No two food proteins are identical in their quality; that is, in the efficiency with which they can be used in the body. The quality is dependent upon the kinds and amounts of the amino acids present in the foods in relation to body needs.

Essential amino acids. The importance of the amino acid composition of proteins was shown by Osborne and Mendel in 1915, who observed that rats failed to grow or even survive if some amino acids were omitted from the diet, but that the elimination of other amino acids had no such harmful effects.

Later work by others, especially by Dr. William C. Rose,[17] established that this was also true for human beings. Thus, amino acids came to be classified as *essential* and *nonessential*. Strictly speaking, all the amino acids are essential units for the synthesis of the protein molecule. However, the body can manufacture many amino acids if it has an adequate nitrogen source, but it cannot produce certain others in adequate amounts to meet body needs. Those amino acids which cannot be synthesized in sufficient amounts by the body and which must be provided in the diet are essential. The human adult requires eight essential amino acids, while growing children require nine or perhaps ten. Arginine is classified as semiessential since growth is retarded if it is not available. The presence of cystine and tyrosine in the diet will reduce the requirement for methionine and phenylalanine respectively; hence, they are also classed as semiessential. The student should learn to recognize the names of the essential amino acids since they are being referred to more and more frequently in writings on protein nutrition.

> Essential: isoleucine, leucine, lysine, methionine, phenylalanine, threonine, tryptophan, valine
> histidine also essential for children
>
> Semiessential: arginine, cystine, tyrosine
>
> Nonessential: alanine, aspartic acid, glutamic acid, glycine, hydroxyproline, norleucine, proline, serine

Complete and incomplete proteins. Depending upon their ability to maintain life and promote growth, proteins have long been classified as *complete, partially complete,* and *totally incomplete.* A complete protein contains the essential amino acids in sufficient quantities for maintenance and a normal rate of growth. Such proteins are sometimes referred to as having a *high biologic value.* Egg, milk, and meat (including poultry and fish) proteins are all complete, but not necessarily identical in quality. Wheat germ and dried yeast have a biologic value approaching that of animal sources.

Partially incomplete proteins will maintain life, but they lack sufficient amounts of some of the amino acids necessary for growth. Gliadin, which is one of a number of proteins found in wheat, is a notable example of proteins of this class. Adults under no physiologic stress can maintain satisfactory nutrition for indefinite periods when consuming sufficient amounts of protein from certain cereals or legumes.

Totally incomplete proteins are incapable of replacing or building new tissue, and hence cannot support life, let alone promote growth. Zein, one of the proteins found in corn, and gelatin are classic examples of proteins which are incapable of even permitting life to continue.

Supplementary value of proteins. Four essential amino acids are in short supply in plant foods: lysine, methionine, threonine, and tryptophan. Just because plant foods, when fed alone, do not provide the necessary quota of essential amino acids is no reason to condemn them as protein sources. Three possibilities exist for making effective use of their protein: (1) they may be fed simultaneously with small amounts of complete protein foods; (2) the correct mixtures of several plant foods may yield all of the necessary amino acids in suitable amounts; and (3) synthetic amino acids may be added to the food to make up the deficiency.

The use of plant protein to stretch the supply of expensive animal proteins is well known. When plant proteins are fed together with a small amount of animal proteins, the quality of the mixture is likely to be as effective as if only animal protein had been fed. Therefore, a good rule in meal planning is to include some animal protein at each meal, rather than concentrating all of it in one meal. Some widely used combinations which effectively supplement one another are: cereal and milk; macaroni and cheese; eggs and toast; egg, cheese, or meat sandwiches. Bread, so important in low-cost diets, is considerably improved in its biologic value when it is made with nonfat dry milk.

To supplement plant proteins with complete proteins is not practical for most of the world's population since milk, eggs, and flesh foods are indeed scarce. The fact that some vegetarians get along quite well suggests that all the amino acids can be made available to man from plants alone if the right combinations can be found.[18] To use a variety of plant foods is a safer procedure than to depend on one plant source, since one food tends to make up for the deficiencies of another. To illustrate, corn and dry beans are not very satisfactory for protein quality when eaten separately, but in combination the biologic value is considerably improved. One of the tremendously important areas of nutrition research today is directed toward the development of mixtures of plant proteins whereby the limiting amino acid of one food is provided by another. Preliminary trials have shown that some of these mixtures when used for infant and child feeding approach the biologic value of milk.[18]

Some investigators have suggested that synthetic amino acids can be added to cereals and legumes to supply the limiting amino acids. (See Fig. 4-2.) If they can be supplied cheaply enough, and if the correct proportions can be determined, this may ultimately be one way to improve the quality of plant foods. However, certain experiments on animals have shown that the addition of a limiting amino acid to a low-protein diet increases the requirement for the second most limiting amino acid, resulting in a further decrease of growth and in liver damage.[19] Consequently, much more information must be gained on the problems of amino acid imbalance before widespread supplementation of foods with amino acids is attempted.

One may question the advisability or the need for amino acid supplementation of foods in the United States since the "average" diet exceeds by a wide margin the minimum requirements for amino acids (see table, p. 48). Lysine, the amino acid being currently added to specialty breads and some cereals, is abundantly supplied. Because of their higher cost these fortified foods fail to help persons on a restricted budget who might be in most need of them.

Daily protein needs. Many factors enter into the level of protein which is desirable for the individual, including: (1) body size; (2) the quality of

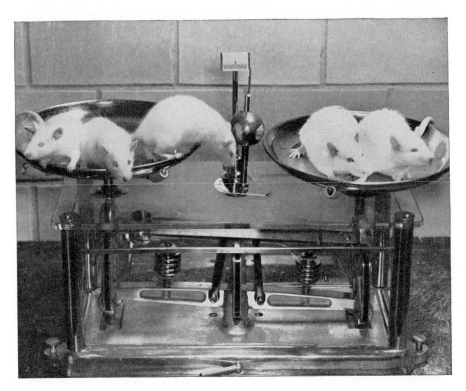

Fig. 4-2. Effect of protein quality. These rats of the same age were fed a bread diet. The two rats on the right received bread to which lysine, the limiting amino acid in grains, had been added. This improvement of the protein quality led to the greater gain. (*Courtesy, E. I. DuPont de Nemours and Company, Inc.*)

protein fed; (3) the adequacy of the caloric intake; (4) the previous state of nutrition; (5) the efficiency of digestion; and (6) the special physiologic needs as during growth (see Fig. 4-3), pregnancy, or recovery from illness.

The nitrogen-balance technique has been most widely used to determine amino acid and protein requirements. By this method the minimum protein requirement is that level of protein intake at which nitrogen equilibrium is just barely maintained on a diet adequate in essential nutrients and in calories.

Essential amino acid requirements. Dr. Rose [20,21] has determined the quantitative requirements of the essential amino acids for healthy young men by feeding a controlled diet which included a mixture of pure amino acids flavored with lemon juice and sugar, and wafers made of cornstarch, sucrose, centrifuged butterfat, corn oil, and vitamins. Similar studies have been reported for young women and for infants.[22,23] The minimum requirements on the basis of these studies are summarized in the table on page 48; they suffice only when the diet provides enough nitrogen for the synthesis of the nonessential amino acids so that the essential amino acids will not be used for this purpose. On a weight basis, it will be noted that the infant requirements are several times as high—a fact one would expect in view of the high rate of tissue synthesis during infancy.

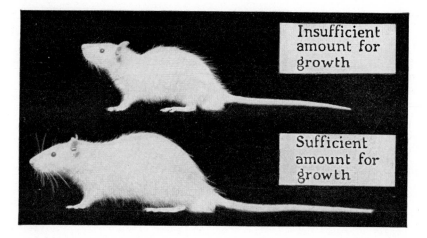

Insufficient amount for growth

Sufficient amount for growth

Fig. 4-3. Effect of different amounts of an efficient protein. Litter mates of the same sex, 18 weeks old. Weight of smaller, 135 gm; of larger, 283 gm. (*Courtesy, Bureau of Home Economics, U.S. Department of Agriculture.*)

Recommended Dietary Allowances. Because foods vary in their protein quality and because individuals may vary somewhat in their actual needs, it is wise to allow a margin of safety in the diet. An allowance of 1 gm per kg (about ½ gm per pound) of desirable body weight, or 70 and 58 gm for the reference man and woman respectively, has long been accepted.[2] It is good nutritional practice to select at least one-third of the adult protein intake from complete protein foods.

Contrary to popular beliefs, exercise does not increase the protein requirement. However, since the caloric requirement increases with activity, most people are likely to select foods for calories which also contain some protein, so that the protein intake is increased.

During pregnancy and lactation the protein allowance for the woman should be increased by 20 gm and 40 gm over the basic level, respectively. The greatest amount of protein per unit of body weight is needed during childhood. Between the ages of 1 and 12 years the allowances gradually decrease from about 3.5 gm to 2 gm per kg body weight. An allowance of 75 to 80 gm protein is recommended for adolescent girls, and 85 to 100 gm for boys. One-half to two-thirds of the protein during childhood should be selected from complete protein sources.

On a caloric basis, the protein allowances range from 10 to 15 per cent of the caloric requirement, the higher percentage being more satisfactory for children.

MINIMUM ESSENTIAL AMINO ACID REQUIREMENTS COMPARED WITH AMINO ACIDS IN THE UNITED STATES PER CAPITA FOOD SUPPLY *

	MINIMAL REQUIREMENTS			U.S. PER CAPITA
ESSENTIAL AMINO ACID	Infants mg per kg	Men gm per day	Women gm per day	FOOD SUPPLY 1953 † gm
Histidine	32			
Isoleucine	90	0.70	0.45	5.2
Leucine	120	1.10	.62	8.0
Lysine	90	.80	.50	6.1
Methionine				
In absence of cystine		1.10		
In presence of 15 mg cystine per kg	85			
In presence of 50 mg cystine per kg	65			
In presence of 200 mg cystine			.35	
In presence of 810 mg cystine		.20		
Phenylalanine				4.6
In absence of tyrosine		1.10		
In presence of 175 mg tyrosine per kg	90			
In presence of 1100 mg tyrosine		.30		
In presence of 900 mg tyrosine			.22	
Threonine	60	.50	.30	3.9
Tryptophan	30	.25	.16	1.2
Valine	93	.80	.65	5.5

* Table arranged from data summarized by: Williams, H. H.: "Amino Acid Requirements," *J. Am. Dietet. A.*, **35**:929, 1959.
† Phipard, E. F.: "Protein and Amino Acids in Diets," *Nutrition Committee News*, U.S. Department of Agriculture, Washington, D.C., May, 1959.

Minimum protein requirement. Because protein supplies throughout the world are not fully adequate, it is of the greatest importance to know what minimum levels are safe. Moreover, in certain disease conditions a temporary restriction of protein at minimum levels is desirable.

A number of studies under carefully controlled conditions have shown that the minimum protein for nitrogen equilibrium ranges from approximately

25 to 40 gm depending upon the quality of protein fed. One study [24] reports that adults can be kept in nitrogen equilibrium and in apparent good health on diets providing 0.5 gm per kg body weight when only one-tenth of the total protein is of animal origin. "Safe practical allowances" have been suggested to allow for individual variation, the quality of the protein, and to provide for adequate protein reserves in the body.[2] In a country where the quality of the protein is good, such as in the United States, such a practical adult allowance is estimated at 0.66 gm per kg, and for a country with a poor quality of protein, the practical allowance is increased to 0.84 gm per kg.

Food sources. It is now possible to compute the amino acid composition of a diet by using tables compiled by Orr and Watt [25] and to compare the values with the amino acid requirements. Such evaluations are of immense worth to the investigator who is studying effective food combinations. For practical purposes the student will continue to rely on the broad classifications of complete and incomplete proteins.

On the basis of the household survey conducted in 1955, the protein content of household supplies averaged 103 gm per person, with two-thirds of this coming from animal sources. Three of the Four Food Groups are significant for their contribution of protein. The average protein values of common foods together with a rating of their quality are presented in the table on page 51. Nonfat dry milk and meat are especially high in protein concentration, but the amounts of liquid milk and of breads and cereals consumed result in important additions to the daily total. The protein contributions of the basic diet plan may be seen in Figure 4-4.

Food preparation related to protein characteristics. Certain properties of proteins must be borne in mind in food processing and preparation. Coagulation of native proteins occurs at relatively low temperatures. As the temperature is increased and the length of heating time is prolonged, the coagulated protein becomes increasingly dry and tough. Thus, meats and eggs which are boiled are tougher than those which are cooked at a temperature below the boiling point. A roasted meat is much drier and tougher if roasted at a high temperature until well done. Since so much water has been removed during roasting, such meats have a higher protein content per unit of weight.

Minute protein films are utilized in some cookery processes. For example, whipped egg whites provide protein films about air so that leavening or lightness of the product results. In the preparation of mayonnaise, a thin film of egg protein encases the tiny oil droplets so that the emulsion remains stable. The light texture of bread is possible because of the elasticity of gluten.

When acid is added to a protein solution, a point is reached where the protein is least soluble and precipitation takes place. The addition of lactic acid to milk precipitates out the casein—an essential step in the manufacture of cheese.

The use of dry heat, when prolonged, results in a linkage of some amino acids which is not easily broken down by the digestive enzymes. Lysine, for example, combines with carbohydrates so that in the process of digestion it may not be released for absorption at the time the other amino acids are being absorbed; thus, it becomes limiting to the effectiveness of the protein eaten. In bread the brown crust contains less available lysine than does the white crumb; dry bread contains less than fresh; and toasting results in some loss. Breakfast cereals processed at high temperatures are likewise subject to such lysine losses. While these losses are not serious in the American diet which provides such abundant supplies of lysine, they could be serious when cereal foods constitute the mainstay of the diet.

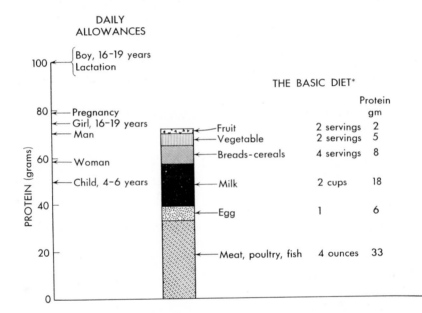

* See page 178 for complete calculations.

Fig. 4-4. The Four Food Groups of the Basic Diet meet the recommended allowances for protein for the man and woman. The addition of 1 pint milk and 1 ounce meat, or their equivalent, will fulfill increased needs. Note that the milk and meat groups provide a high proportion of complete protein.

Heating improves the nutritive value of some proteins. Egg white, soybeans, and navy beans are more efficiently used when cooked because mild heating inactivates an enzyme in these foods which inhibits the action of trypsin. Marked heating of soybean protein decreases the availability of the protein.

Protein deficiency. Because the protein intake in the United States is high, and because the quality is exceptionally good, one would not expect to see many individuals exhibiting the clinical symptoms of severe deficiency. A reduced protein intake over an extended period of time leads eventually to depletion of the labile tissue reserves and then to the lowering of blood protein levels. The speed with which the deficiency develops depends upon the quality and quantity of the protein intake, the caloric intake, the age of

AVERAGE PROTEIN CONTENT OF FOODS IN FOUR FOOD GROUPS *

FOOD	AVERAGE SERVING	PROTEIN gm	PROTEIN QUALITY LIMITING AMINO ACIDS
Milk group			
Milk, whole or skim	1 cup	9	Complete
Nonfat dry milk	⅞ ounce (3– 5 tablespoons)	9	Complete
Cottage cheese	2 ounces	10	Complete
American cheese	1 ounce	7	Complete
Ice cream	⅛ quart	3	Complete
Meat group			
Meat, fish, poultry	3 ounces, cooked	15–25	Complete; higher protein for lean cuts
Egg	1 whole	6	Complete
Dried beans or peas	½ cup cooked	7–8	Incomplete; methionine
Peanut butter	1 tablespoon	4	Incomplete; several amino acids borderline
Vegetable-fruit group			
Vegetables	½ cup	1–3	Incomplete
Fruits	½ cup	1–2	Incomplete
Bread-cereals group			
Breakfast cereals, wheat	½ cup cooked ¾ cup dry	2–3	Incomplete; lysine
Bread, wheat	1 slice	2–3	Incomplete; lysine
Macaroni, noodles, spaghetti	½ cup cooked	2	Incomplete; lysine
Rice	½ cup cooked	2	Incomplete; lysine and threonine
Corn meal and cereals	½ cup cooked	2	Incomplete; lysine and tryptophan

* These values represent approximate group averages. For specific food items, consult Table 1, in the Appendix, page 720.

the individual, and other factors. According to Youmans [26] edema (known as "nutritional edema" as distinct from edema of circulatory origin) is the first clinical sign; this is dependent upon posture and becomes more marked in the legs at the end of the day. As the condition becomes more severe, edema becomes generalized.

Protein deficiency is more likely to be seen among pregnant women from low-economic groups ignorant of the essentials of a good diet; the elderly who have too little income to secure food, insufficient understanding of the importance of diet, lack of incentive to eat, or poor health; and the chronically ill who have poor appetites but increased protein requirements. While symptoms of protein deficiency may not be detectable, the stress of an infection or surgery on such an individual may result in delayed convalescence or poor wound healing.

Kwashiorkor, a global problem in malnutrition. A major public health problem in some sixty underdeveloped countries or territories of the world is kwashiorkor (see Fig. 4-5).[18] Whether the disease is observed in Africa, Ceylon, Indonesia, Jamaica, Central America, Brazil, Spain, Greece, or elsewhere one striking fact stands out, namely, that the protein intake is severely restricted with animal protein being scarcely ever eaten.

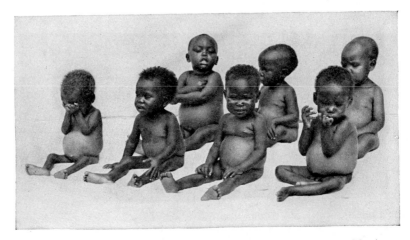

Fig. 4-5. Children suffering from kwashiorkor—Africa. (*Courtesy, M. Autret and the Food and Agriculture Organization.*)

Kwashiorkor occurs most commonly in the infant after weaning when the diet which replaces the mother's milk is markedly deficient in protein but high in carbohydrate. The calories may often be adequate as in the "sugar-baby" type of kwashiorkor seen in Jamaica. In other instances the calories may be inadequate, but not as severely deficient as the protein, thus resulting in some degree of tissue wasting.

Scrimshaw has estimated that perhaps at least 100 cases of protein malnutrition, sometimes called prekwashiorkor, exist for every child with kwashiorkor. This manifests itself by retarded growth and development and poor resistance to infection. When an infection occurs, such children succumb rapidly to the acute symptoms of kwashiorkor. Death rates for children in these areas are 10 to 40 times higher than in the United States.

Kwashiorkor has its highest incidence between the ages of 1 and 4 years when the needs for essential amino acids for tissue synthesis are great. The classic symptoms include: growth failure; retarded development; loss of

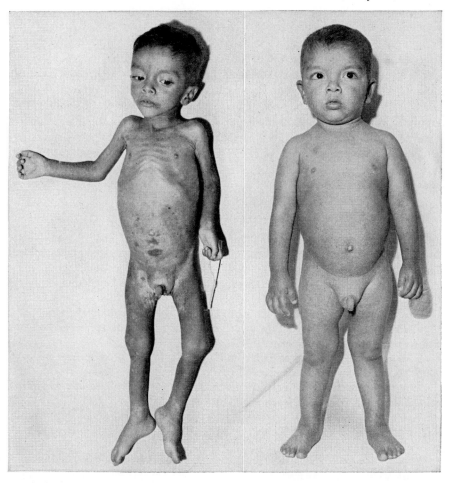

Fig. 4-6. Two-year-old child 2 weeks after admission and 10 weeks after treatment with INCAPARINA. (*Courtesy, Institute of Nutrition of Central America and Panama, and the* Journal of the American Dietetic Association.)

appetite; mental apathy; edema; diarrhea; pellagrous skin lesions; and color and texture changes of the hair. There may also be manifestations of various vitamin deficiencies.

Laboratory studies show low blood protein levels, and low vitamin-A and carotene levels. The production of digestive enzymes such as amylase, trypsin, and lipase is decreased so that digestion and absorption of food are poor. Anemia is not infrequent, and may be aggravated by malaria or hookworm infestation. Pathologic studies have shown fatty infiltration of the liver, and atrophy of the pancreas.

The treatment of kwashiorkor in most cases has consisted of reconstituted nonfat dry milk. Within a few days striking improvement may be seen and in a matter of weeks the child appears well nourished. More recently, vegetable protein mixtures have been used satisfactorily in place of milk in Central America, India, South Africa, and the Congo (see Fig. 4-6).[18]

The prevention of kwashiorkor must be directed toward the education of mothers with respect to infant feeding and the provision of protein of high biologic value within economic reach of the population group. Since the supply of nonfat dry milk is inadequate to meet the needs of all preschool children in underdeveloped areas, it is necessary to look to the further development and manufacture of inexpensive plant protein mixtures which supply the kinds and amounts of essential amino acids required by this age group.

PROBLEMS AND REVIEW

1. Proteins are essential for building and replacement of body tissues. Name three circumstances in which the protein allowance in the diet should be increased above the normal adult need.

2. Name four ways in which proteins are used in the regulation of body functions.

3. Explain why proteins are considered to be a wasteful source of energy.

4. *Problem.* Prepare an outline or diagram which shows the steps in the digestion of protein.

5. What is meant by an essential amino acid; complete protein; high biologic value; supplementary value of protein?

6. What is meant by positive nitrogen balance; negative nitrogen balance; nitrogen equilibrium? When does each condition occur?

7. How can you explain the fact that a person on a low-protein high-calorie diet is less likely to go into negative nitrogen balance than one who is on a low-calorie diet of the same protein level?

8. How can you explain the fact that some vegetarians maintain good protein nutrition while others do not?

9. *Problem.* Plan a diet for a woman which provides 60 gm of protein, of which not more than one-third is in the form of animal protein. What foods are especially important in such a diet plan?

10. What happens to protein which is eaten in excess of body requirements? Why is it important to provide a margin of safety in planning for the daily protein allowance?

11. What foods would you include in your own diet to ensure an adequate protein intake? How would you modify this plan for a growing child?

12. *Problem.* A diet contains 3000 calories and 150 gm of protein. What percentage of the calories are supplied by protein?

13. *Problem.* One pint of milk supplies 17 gm of protein. What amounts of these foods would be required to replace the protein of the milk: buttermilk; nonfat dry milk; evaporated milk; ice cream; Cheddar cheese; eggs; halibut; beef liver;

sirloin steak; peanut butter; oatmeal? How does the quality of protein in the various foods listed above compare?

14. *Problem.* On the basis of current market prices, calculate the cost for the amounts of foods which were needed to replace the protein of 1 pint milk (Problem 13). What conclusions can you draw from this calculation?

15. A friend asks you whether she should buy lysine-enriched bread in preference to the usual enriched loaf of bread. How would you reply?

16. What are the effects of insufficient protein in the diet?

17. Describe kwashiorkor with respect to its incidence, symptoms, treatment, and prevention.

CHAPTER 5 /

Carbohydrates

All living organisms ultimately derive their energy from the sun. In a highly complex manner, chlorophyll, the coloring matter in leaves, utilizes the energy of the sun to synthesize carbohydrate from the carbon dioxide of the air and the water of the soil. This process of photosynthesis is probably the most important reaction for the continuance of life, for the energy thus stored in the plant is used in turn by other species. Animal foods which are used so abundantly by people in the United States represent the conversion of carbohydrate and other nutrients of the plant world by the animal into protein and fat.

Man can utilize certain but not all of the carbohydrates produced by plants. Carbohydrates, notably from cereal grains, represent the primary source of energy for the world's population. In the United States man obtains about half of his energy needs from the carbohydrates, but in other parts of the world far greater proportions of the caloric requirement are met by carbohydrate. As the income decreases and as the available land for producing food becomes more limited in terms of the population, the cereal foods become increasingly important for providing the caloric requirement. When properly chosen, these foods also constitute significant sources of protein and of some of the B-complex vitamins.

Composition. Carbohydrates are simple sugars or substances which can be reduced to simple sugars by hydrolysis. Such breakdown of complex carbohydrates is accomplished by digestive enzymes or by heating with dilute acids.

Carbohydrates are composed of carbon, hydrogen, and oxygen, the last two being in the proportion to form water—hence the term "carbohydrate." The general formula is $C_nH_{2n}O_n$.

Classification. The carbohydrates of significance in nutrition may be classed in the following three groups:

I. *Monosaccharides, simple sugars, or hexoses,* $C_6H_{12}O_6$, are more or less sweet, water soluble, diffusible, crystallizable, and not affected by digestive enzymes.

   A. GLUCOSE, sometimes called dextrose, grape sugar, or corn

56

sugar, is found in sweet fruits such as grapes, in vegetables such as sweet corn, and in certain roots. It is prepared commercially in its crystalline form, or in corn sirup, by the hydrolysis of starch with acids.

Glucose is physiologically the most important sugar of this class. It is the chief end product of hydrolysis of di- and poly-saccharides during digestion. It is the form of carbohydrate circulating in the blood, and is utilized by the tissues for energy.

B. FRUCTOSE, also known as levulose or fruit sugar, is the sweetest of all sugars and does not easily crystallize. It occurs especially in honey, ripe fruits, and many vegetables, and also results from the hydrolysis of sucrose.

C. GALACTOSE results from the hydrolysis of lactose or milk sugar. It does not occur in the free state in nature.

II. *Disaccharides* or double sugars, $C_{12}H_{22}O_{11}$, are water soluble, diffusible, crystallizable, and of varying sweetness. They are split to simple sugars by acid hydrolysis or by the digestive enzymes.

A. SUCROSE, the table sugar with which we are familiar, is found in sugar cane, sugar beets, in the sap of sugar maples, sorghum cane, and in many fruits and vegetables.

B. MALTOSE, or malt sugar, is found in malted products such as cereals and beer as the result of the action of the enzyme, diastase, on the starch of the cereal grain. It is also an intermediate product in the digestion of starch to glucose.

C. LACTOSE, or milk sugar, is produced only by mammals. The concentration of lactose in milk varies from about 2 to 8 per cent, depending upon the species. It is not very soluble, and is much less sweet than the other single or double sugars.

III. *Polysaccharides,* $(C_6H_{10}O_5)_n$, are complex compounds with relatively high molecular weights. They are amorphous rather than crystalline, not sweet, generally insoluble, and are digested in the body with varying degrees of completeness.

A. STARCH is the form in which plants store carbohydrate, and thus is the primary source of energy in the diet. Cereal grains, seeds, roots, potatoes, green bananas, and other plants contain considerable starch. It is insoluble in cold water, but in boiling water the cell walls of the starch granule are ruptured, the starch absorbs water, and thickening results. The action of heat, enzymes, or acid on starch leads to the production of *dextrins* which are intermediate products in the breakdown of starch. The eventual product of starch hydrolysis is glucose.

B. GLYCOGEN, the so-called animal starch, is the form in which the animal body stores carbohydrate. Oysters when freshly opened, and liver immediately after removal from the slaughtered animal are sources of glycogen; however, this glycogen is rapidly broken down so that the diet ordinarily contains none.

C. CELLULOSE is the most abundant organic compound in the world, comprising at least 50 per cent of the carbon in vegetation. Wood and cotton are chiefly cellulose, but the skins of fruits, the coverings of seeds, and the structural parts of edible plants are the only forms of cellulose and hemicellulose with which we are concerned in the study of nutrition. Ruminants are able to utilize cellulose for energy because of enzymes in the rumen, but for man cellulose is a nondigestible dietary constituent. It is insoluble in hot or cold water. *Pectins* are indigestible carbohydrates occurring in ripe fruits; they have the ability to absorb water, and to form gels, a property utilized in making fruit jellies.

Functions. Unlike fats and proteins, carbohydrates are present in the body in very limited amounts. Glucose is directly, or indirectly, used for certain tissue components such as nucleic acids, the galactosides of nervous tissue, the matrix of connective tissue, and the production of lactose during lactation.

The majority of the carbohydrate in the body exists in the form of glycogen. The liver contains the greatest concentration, and at any given time the amount may range from practically none to 100 gm or more; muscle tissue, while containing a much lower concentration of glycogen than the liver, accounts for 200 gm, more or less. Thus, it may be seen that the 300 gm or so of glycogen in the healthy adult at any given time would be sufficient for the caloric needs of the individual for no more than half a day.

The chief function of carbohydrate is to furnish the primary source of energy for the work of the body. Each gram of carbohydrate burned will yield 4 calories. Carbohydrate may be used directly as energy, it may be stored as glycogen as described above, or it may be converted to adipose tissue and thus stored for later conversion to energy. Glucose is the sole form of energy for the brain and nervous tissue, and must be available, minute by minute, for the functioning of these tissues.

Dietary carbohydrate has a protein-sparing action. When the caloric level through a liberal intake of carbohydrate is adequate for the body's needs, dietary protein will not be used as a source of energy. The glucose in the body may also serve as the starting point for the synthesis of certain nonessential amino acids when a source of nitrogen is also available.

Lactose, being less soluble than other sugars, remains in the intestine long enough to encourage the growth of desirable bacteria and has been observed to enhance the absorption and utilization of calcium. It is undoubtedly no accident of nature that milk which is the outstanding source of calcium is the only dietary source of lactose.

fat-sparing effect - decrease ox of fats.

(3) A certain amount of carbohydrate is necessary in the diet so that excessive oxidation of fat will not be necessary. When carbohydrate is severely restricted, fats will be metabolized faster than the body is able to take care of the intermediate products. The piling up of these incompletely oxidized products leads to acidosis or ketosis. Carbohydrate must be almost entirely lacking from the diet for such acidosis to occur under normal conditions, but in uncontrolled diabetes mellitus (Chap. 33) ketosis is common.

For all practical purposes, cellulose, hemicellulose, and pectins yield no nutrients to the body. These indigestible substances do serve a useful purpose in facilitating the elimination of intestinal wastes. They stimulate the peristaltic movements of the gastrointestinal tract and they also have the property of absorbing water thus giving bulk to the intestinal contents.

Digestion and absorption. Simple sugars require no preparation in digestion and are ready to pass through the absorbing walls of the digestive tract as soon as they reach the small intestine. The double sugars are carried through one step in digestion to become simple sugars; and the complex sugars, the chief of which is starch, require two steps in digestion before they can be absorbed.

The cooking of foods containing starches is a valuable aid to the digestive process, for the walls of the starch cell are thereby ruptured and the material can be more quickly acted upon by the enzymes. Salivary amylase has no action on raw starch, but pancreatic amylase hydrolyzes both raw and cooked starch.

The accompanying table gives a brief outline of the digestive processes which prepare all carbohydrates for their work in the body.

HYDROLYSIS OF CARBOHYDRATES TO SIMPLE SUGARS BY ENZYMES

ENZYME	WHERE FOUND	DIGESTIVE CHANGES
Starch-splitting salivary amylase (ptyalin)	In saliva	Cooked starch split to dextrins and maltose
pancreatic amylase (amylopsin)	In pancreatic juice	Cooked and raw starch split to dextrins and maltose
Sugar-splitting sucrase (invertase)	In intestinal juice	Sucrose split to glucose and fructose
maltase	In intestinal juice	Maltose split to 2 molecules of glucose
lactase	In intestinal juice	Lactose split to glucose and galactose

There is no chemical change in fiber in the human digestive tract. Some of the tender fibers of young plants may disappear during their passage down the tract, but this is probably due to the action of bacteria rather than to the action of enzymes. During the process of digestion of foods, tough fibers such as skins of fruits and vegetables or the outer coating of the cereal grains are softened by coming into contact with acids in the stomach. They are not dissolved but are broken into smaller pieces as the result of muscular contractions of the walls of the stomach and intestines, and they pass unchanged down the tract. The fiber in cooked foods is softer and partially disintegrated, and it absorbs less water than that in uncooked foods.

Digestibility. The values for total carbohydrate listed in most food tables include that which can be digested and absorbed, and that which is non-utilizable. Separate values for fiber are often listed, although these are not necessarily comparable to the nonutilized material in the digestive tract. About 97 to 98 per cent of the carbohydrate in the diversified American diet is completely digested and absorbed. The fuel factor, 4 calories per gm, is based on this degree of digestibility. In countries where plant foods comprise most of the diet so that the fiber intake is correspondingly higher, the percentage of carbohydrate which is digested and absorbed is somewhat lower. Thus, the energy value per gram of carbohydrate ingested is somewhat less than 4 calories.

Absorption. The simple sugars resulting from the digestion of carbohydrate may diffuse directly into the capillaries in the walls of the small intestine, or they may first combine with phosphate through the action of an enzyme in the intestinal wall for more rapid absorption. The simple sugars are then carried in the blood stream to the liver and to the tissues.

Metabolism. Blood contains glucose, as it does other nutrients, in order to maintain the environment for the nourishment of every cell and tissue in the body (see Fig. 5-1). As rapidly as glucose is removed from the circulation by the various tissues, it is fed into the circulation chiefly by the liver. This is a continuous process of input and outgo, in which the necessary chemical transformations which take place are made possible by a series of enzymes and are controlled by hormonal action.

The blood glucose level in the fasting state is 70 to 90 mg per 100 ml of blood. Following a meal, the glucose level rises more or less rapidly. If one eats a sweet or drinks some fruit juice, the sugars require little digestion, absorption proceeds rapidly, and there is an early increase in the blood sugar level; the person who has been hungry just before eating such a sweet thereby experiences a prompt sense of well-being. If the food eaten had contained protein and fat, more time would be required for digestion, the rate of absorption would be more gradual, and the rise in blood sugar level would also be more gradual.

When the portal circulation brings the simple sugars from the gastrointestinal tract to the liver, galactose must first be converted to glucose since the tissues do not oxidize it as such. Fructose and glucose are combined with phosphate in the liver and then proceed to the formation of glycogen. Insulin, a hormone secreted by the islands of Langerhans in the pancreas, is essential for this conversion. When the blood sugar level drops, the glycogen in the

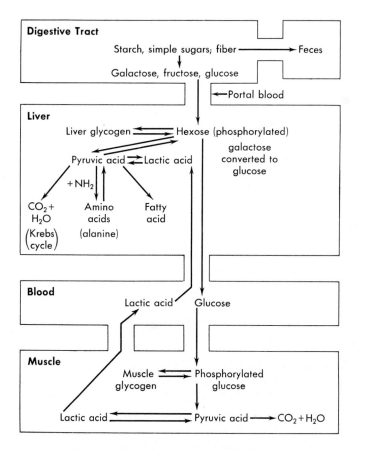

Fig. 5-1. The utilization of carbohydrates.

liver will be broken down to glucose in order to maintain the relatively constant concentration in the circulation. Three hormones have been shown to possess the ability to facilitate the breakdown of glycogen to glucose, namely, (1) epinephrine, secreted by the adrenal gland, (2) thyroxine, secreted by the thyroid gland, and (3) glucagon, a recently isolated hormone produced by the alpha cells in the pancreas.

The rate of synthesis of glycogen and its breakdown is obviously dependent upon the speed with which the tissues remove glucose from the circulation, and this, in turn, is governed by the rate of energy metabolism of the body. The uptake of glucose by the tissues is facilitated by insulin. Glucose which is withdrawn from the circulation is also converted to glycogen in the tissues. Subsequently, the glycogen is broken down to lactic and pyruvic acids, either of which may be further oxidized to provide energy for muscle contraction, with the waste products, carbon dioxide and water, being excreted by the lungs and kidney. Instead of being oxidized for energy, lactic acid might also re-enter the blood circulation, be carried to the liver, and there again be converted into glycogen.

Pyruvic acid, instead of being oxidized directly to provide energy, may be degraded to acetic acid by means of an enzyme of which thiamine, a B-complex vitamin, is a component. The acetic acid, in turn, is oxidized to provide energy, carbon dioxide, and water; or the acetate unit may be used for the synthesis of fats and cholesterol (see p. 72). Pyruvic acid could also serve as a nucleus for building the nonessential amino acid, alanine, through the addition of an amino group from another source.

So far it has been assumed that the source of glucose for metabolism was derived solely from the simple sugars absorbed from the intestinal tract. The body also realizes glucose from two additional sources, namely fats and certain amino acids. The glycerol resulting from the hydrolysis of fats is metabolized as carbohydrate; about 10 per cent of the dietary fat is so used. Certain amino acids, following their deamination, are also utilized as glucose; roughly half of the protein in the diet is a potential source of glucose in the body. Thus, a diet consisting solely of meat would yield appreciable amounts of glucose for glycogen formation in the body.

During starvation, body fat and protein may be broken down to meet the energy needs—the glucose again being realized from the same proportions of fat and amino acids as if they were of dietary origin. This concept of glucose formation from proteins and fats is essential to the understanding of the role of these three major nutrients in various therapeutic regimens, such as weight loss, weight gain, diabetes mellitus.

Normally, only trace amounts of sugar are present in the urine. However, when the glucose level of the blood exceeds approximately 160–180 mg per 100 ml, the so-called renal threshold for glucose, glucose is excreted in the urine. Urinary sugar may be found in a number of situations, including diabetes mellitus (Chap. 33).

Daily allowances. No specified dietary levels for carbohydrate are included in the Recommended Dietary Allowances. The low-carbohydrate diet of the Eskimos and the high-carbohydrate diets of many Oriental peoples indicate that man can be healthy with wide variations in carbohydrate intake. That this wide variation is compatible with good health is apparent when one realizes how readily protein, fat, and carbohydrate are interchangeable in providing the energy needs of the body.

In the United States about 45 to 50 per cent of the available calories are derived from carbohydrate. The amount of carbohydrate in the American diet has been gradually decreasing during the last 50 years because of the decreased consumption of cereal foods and potatoes.

A liberal use of carbohydrate foods is advantageous because (1) they are easily digested and almost completely absorbed for efficient use in producing energy, (2) they are protein-sparing in action, (3) when selected from enriched and whole-grain sources, or potatoes, the B-complex vitamin and iron intakes are appreciably increased, (4) they are widely distributed and economical, and (5) they enhance the palatability of the diet. For maximum protein-sparing action, some carbohydrate foods should accompany protein at each meal.

Enrichment. Refined cereals and breads are deficient in certain B-complex vitamins, especially thiamine, and in iron. Enrichment is now employed for more than 80 per cent of all refined cereals and breads which are produced in this country (see p. 315). The inclusion of four or more servings of enriched or whole-grain breads and cereals, as suggested in the Daily Food Guide, provides substantial amounts of the B vitamins and iron.

Fiber. Although it is generally conceded that some fiber is essential in the diet for normal laxation, the exact amounts required cannot be stated. Cowgill [27] considers 100 mg of fiber per kilogram, or about 5 to 6 gm per day for the adult, to be a sufficient allowance. For most persons, the average mixed diet including each day a raw vegetable and some fresh fruit with skins in addition to cooked fruits and vegetables will provide sufficient fiber. Others need to increase their intake of fiber by including some whole-grain cereals or bread. A recent study [28] including pure vegetarians, lacto-ovo-vegetarians, and nonvegetarians showed that the fiber intake could vary widely over a period of years without adverse effects on the digestive tract; the vegetarians had fiber intakes four times as high as the nonvegetarians, while the latter equaled or exceeded Cowgill's recommended allowance.

Concentrated sweets in the diet. Pure sugars are the most concentrated form of carbohydrate, providing 1 gm carbohydrate per gm of sugar. Jellies, jams, sirups, and candies, likewise, are made up largely of carbohydrate. In terms of the total energy value of the American diet, sugars and sweets account for about 10 per cent of the calories, but contribute only trace amounts of any nutrients.[29] Hence, they are sometimes referred to as "empty" calories. The dietitian and nurse must consider carefully the appropriate uses of sugar in the diet, as well as the problems inherent in excessive use.

Sugar is an important ingredient of practically all baked goods and desserts, many of which contribute essential nutrients in the milk, eggs, and enriched flour which are used in their preparation. Frozen and canned fruits are more acceptable when preserved with some sugar. Few people completely shun an occasional piece of candy. Costwise, sugar is a very inexpensive source of calories. When a high-calorie diet is required for a patient, one of the ways used to increase the caloric intake is to add one or another sugar to the food and beverages, thus keeping the bulk of the diet to a minimum. When fat intake in any diet is severely restricted, the use of sugars and starches must be increased to maintain caloric equilibrium.

On the other hand, an excessive intake of concentrated sweets by some may lead to irritation of the gastrointestinal mucosa, and may, in certain disorders, favor excessive fermentation and gas production. The person of any age who indulges in sweets to the point of reducing the intake of necessary protein, mineral, and vitamin-rich foods below recommended levels cannot expect to maintain optimal nutritional status; in fact, marked diversion from the recommended dietary levels could contribute to nutrient deficiencies and also to overweight.

The role of sugars in the incidence of dental caries is by no means sharply defined. Certainly, the occurrence of tooth decay cannot be explained solely on the basis of excessive intake of sugars. However, if the consumption of sweets by the child leads to reduced intake of other foods, dental decay may result from failure to provide the essential nutrients for tooth development. Experimental work has also established that the contact of carbohydrate with the teeth provides a favorable medium for rapid growth of bacteria; candies which are sticky and which adhere to the teeth are more likely to be harmful. Obviously, brushing the teeth following the eating of candy or other sweets, or rinsing the mouth with water, at the very least, is a helpful measure.

Certain misguided persons and unscrupulous promoters recommend the use of raw sugar, crude sugar, black strap molasses, and similar products in the place of cane or beet sugar. While the impurities in these products may contribute some mineral elements to the diet, the amount is insignificant and cannot be justified in terms of the considerable added cost usually involved.

When good food habits are developed in childhood, sugars and sweets may have a legitimate place in the diet. The sweet will not become a "good food" (in taste) which is "bad" for one; nor will it be used as a reward or a bribe. Many Americans, undoubtedly, would benefit by shifting some of their carbohydrate intake from sugars and sweets to enriched and whole-grain cereals and breads.

Food sources. In the 1955 dietary survey of American households the consumption of carbohydrate-rich foods per person per week in pounds was as follows: bakery products, 2.0; flour and other cereal products, 1.8; potatoes, sweet potatoes, 1.9; sugars and sweets, 1.2. A comparison of some carbohydrate-rich foods is presented in the table on page 65.

Carbohydrates in food preparation. Sugars in general are useful for increasing the caloric level of beverages. Gram for gram all sugars provide the same number of calories, but more of some sugars can be used because they are less sweet. If the sweetness of sucrose, the most widely used sugar, is assigned an arbitrary value of 100, the sweetening power of other sugars is as follows: fructose, 173; glucose, 74; maltose and galactose, 33; and lactose, 16. It would appear that lactose, being only one-sixth as sweet as cane sugar, would be the sugar of choice for increasing the caloric value of beverages. However, lactose is rather expensive, it dissolves less readily than other sugars, and it may provoke diarrhea if taken in excess. When its use is prescribed, the lactose should first be dissolved in a little hot water before it is mixed with cold beverages; it may tend to settle out, in which case the beverage should be well stirred before it is served.

CARBOHYDRATE CONTENT OF SOME TYPICAL FOODS

| FOOD | Measure | PER SERVING PORTION | | PER 100 GRAMS OF FOOD gm |
		Weight gm	Carbohydrate gm	
Bread, all kinds	1 slice	23	12	46–58
Cereals, breakfast, dry	1 ounce	30	22	66–88
Crackers, all kinds	2 graham	14	10	71–75
Flour, all kinds				71–80
Macaroni, noodles, rice, spaghetti	½ cup cooked	70	16	73–78 (dry basis)
Cake, plain and iced	⅟₁₆ layer	120	70	49–62
Sugar, all kinds	1 teaspoon	4	4	100
Sirups, molasses, honey	1 tablespoon	20	15	60–80
Jams, jellies	1 tablespoon	20	13	65–71
Candy	1 ounce (caramel)	30	22	50–99
Beverages, carbonated	8 ounces	240	21–28	9–12
Fruits, fresh, unsweet	1 exchange *		10	4–23
Fruits, dried	4 prunes	32	19	67–75
Potatoes, white	1 medium boiled	122	21	19 (raw)
Sweet potatoes	1 medium baked	110	36	28 (raw)
Vegetables	½ cup (peas)	80	10	4–20
Legumes	½ cup cooked	130	30	60–62 (dry)
Nuts	1 ounce (peanuts)	30	7	11–24
Milk, cow's	1 cup	244	12	5

* See Fruit Exchange List, page 770, for amounts of fruit to provide 10 gm carbohydrate.

Glucose is the most useful sugar for reinforcing beverages because it requires no digestive action, fairly large amounts of it are acceptable, it dissolves readily, and commercial grades of it are very inexpensive. Maltose is sometimes used in infant feeding.

The procedures for starch cookery, including breakfast cereals, sauces thickened with starch or flour, and the preparation of batters and doughs are described in Chapters 46 and 54.

PROBLEMS AND REVIEW

1. What is the ultimate source of all carbohydrate? What are the important differences between the three classes of carbohydrates?

2. Almost half of the calories in the daily diet are derived from carbohydrate. Under what circumstances would you expect to find a higher intake of carbohydrate?

3. The chief function of carbohydrate is to supply energy. Describe in detail the steps which are necessary before the starch of a slice of bread can be utilized to supply this energy.

4. What is the form of carbohydrate circulating in the blood? What is its normal concentration?

5. If carbohydrate is eaten in excess of the body's daily requirement for energy, what happens to it?

6. Cellulose is an indigestible carbohydrate. Of what practical importance is it in the diet?

7. *Problem.* Calculate the carbohydrate content of:

> 60 gm of bread
> 120 gm of potato
> 150 gm of orange

8. *Problem.* Calculate the carbohydrate and caloric content of your diet for one day. What percentage of your calories were derived from carbohydrate? What percentage of your calories were derived from: cereal foods and breadstuffs; cakes, pies, and other pastries; sugars, candy, carbonated beverages?

9. *Problem.* Calculate the fiber content of your diet. List changes you could make in your diet to double the fiber content without increasing your total caloric intake.

10. What reasons can you give for reducing the intake of sugars and sweets? What legitimate role do they have in the diet?

CHAPTER 6 /

Fats and Fatlike Substances

Fats and fatlike substances are almost as widely distributed in nature as are the carbohydrates, and as a concentrated source of energy they supply roughly two-fifths of the calories in the American diet.

Composition. Fats, like carbohydrates, are organic compounds composed of carbon, hydrogen, and oxygen; some fatlike substances may also contain a few molecules of other elements. They differ from carbohydrates in that they contain much less oxygen and much greater proportions of carbon and hydrogen.

Classification. The term "lipid" includes true fats and also other fatlike substances which are related by reason of physical and chemical properties. Four types of lipids are of importance in nutrition:

1. *Neutral fats* or true fats are organic esters of 1 molecule glycerol, $C_3H_5(OH)_3$, and 3 molecules fatty acids. These fats constitute 98 to 99 per cent of food and body fats. *triglycerides*

2. *Phospholipids* are organic esters of fatty acids, but also include phosphoric acid and usually a nitrogenous base. *Lecithin,* the most widely distributed of these compounds, and *cephalin* are found in all cell protoplasm— brain, nerve, liver, kidney, muscle, heart, egg yolk, and so on. Sphingomyelin *supports nerve fiber*

3. *Derived fats* include free fatty acids and glycerides from which one or two of the fatty acids have been removed by hydrolysis.

4. *Sterols* are organic compounds containing a multiple ring structure. They are not chemically related to fats. From a nutritional point of view, cholesterol and ergosterol are the most important members of this group. Cholesterol is the only sterol occurring as such in the animal body. Ergosterol and cholesterol are important as precursors of vitamin D.

Fatty acids. Many fatty acids are found in food and body fats. Butter, for example, contains at least 29 different fatty acids.[30] Some of the fatty acids contain as few as 4 carbon atoms (butyric acid) and some as many as 24 carbon atoms all hooked to each other in chainlike fashion. The fatty acids in foods are straight carbon chains with an even number of carbon atoms.

Fatty acids are "saturated" or "unsaturated." Those which are saturated have no double bonds between the carbon atoms; that is, they contain as much hydrogen as the carbon atoms are capable of holding. The most commonly occurring saturated fatty acids are myristic, palmitic, and stearic acids. Unsaturated fatty acids are those in which one or more double bonds occur between the carbon atoms so that they are capable of holding more hydrogen atoms. The most common of all food and tissue acids is oleic acid ($C_{18}H_{34}O_2$); it differs from stearic acid ($C_{18}H_{36}O_2$) only in that it contains one double bond—that is, two less hydrogen atoms. Two unsaturated fatty acids, linoleic acid and linolenic acid, also contain the same number of carbon atoms as stearic acid but two and three double bonds respectively.

Characteristics of fats. Fats are insoluble in water although they dissolve readily in ether, chloroform, and other organic liquids. They are capable of forming emulsions with liquids, a property which is utilized, for example, in the preparation of salad dressings such as mayonnaise. Emulsification is a prerequisite for the digestion and absorption of fats and their transportation.

The nature of a fat—its hardness, melting point, and flavor—is determined by the kinds of fatty acids which are present. Food and tissue fats contain varying proportions of both saturated and unsaturated acids. Unprocessed vegetable fats such as olive and peanut oils are composed largely of the unsaturated oleic acid, while corn, soybean, and cottonseed oils contain predominantly linoleic acid. The hardness of a fat and its melting point increase as the proportion of the long-chain saturated fatty acids increases; thus, beef and mutton tallow contain significant amounts of the long-chain saturated stearic acid. Even solid fats such as lard and butter contain oleic acid as the single largest constituent, but with greater proportions of saturated fatty acids than do the oils.

The fat of each species is distinctive. Herbivora have harder fats than carnivora, and land animals have harder fat than fish. The diet of the animal profoundly influences the nature of its body fat. Pigs can be so fed that their fat is soft and relatively high in linoleic acid, or their diet may be such that a firm fat of low linoleic acid content is produced.

Liquid fats may be converted to solid fats by adding hydrogen to the double bonds of the unsaturated fatty acids; this process, known as *hydrogenation,* is widely used in the manufacture of many cooking fats and margarine. The amount of linoleic acid originally present in the oil is decreased in proportion to the extent of hydrogenation. As a rule, not all of the double bonds are saturated so that variable amounts of linoleic acid may still be present.

Saponification refers to the formation of a soap of fatty acid and a cation. In the alkaline medium of the small intestine, a free fatty acid may combine with calcium to form an insoluble compound which is excreted from the small intestine. In certain pathologic conditions in which fat absorption is diminished—sprue, for example—this may be of some nutritional significance.

Excessive heating of fats leads to breakdown of the glycerol, producing a pungent compound which is especially irritating to the gastrointestinal mucosa.

With exposure to air some fats become rancid and unpalatable. The resulting products may produce nausea and vomiting. Antioxidants are incorporated into many commercial food fats to counteract this tendency.

Functions. Lipids are distributed in all body cells and tissues. The body is provided with a complex system of enzymes and hormones for their digestion and metabolism, attesting to the fact that fats are essential and normal components of body functioning.

Fats are the most concentrated source of energy, and in America they provide a third, more or less, of the body's energy needs. Since each gram of fat burned in the body will yield 9 calories, it is evident that fats are more than twice as concentrated a form of energy as carbohydrates and proteins. An individual with a relatively high caloric requirement would find it necessary to consume a somewhat bulky diet if he depended upon carbohydrates to provide substantially all of his energy needs.

The high density and low solubility of fats make them an ideal form in which to store energy for the body's needs. In fact, carbohydrates and amino acids which are not promptly utilized by the tissues are rapidly synthesized into fats and stored as adipose tissue. The conversion is a continuous process in the normal individual. It is not restricted to the accumulation of adipose tissue in the person who has an excessive intake of calories.

In addition to providing energy, fats serve as (1) padding around the organs, holding them in place and absorbing the shocks to which they might otherwise be subjected; (2) protection for the nerves; (3) insulators for the body, thus avoiding rapid changes of body temperature by excessive heat loss from its surface; (4) sparers of body proteins, since a sufficient amount of carbohydrates and fats furnishes the energy needed to carry on the work of the body; (5) carriers of the fat-soluble vitamins; (6) lubricants of the gastrointestinal tract; and (7) depressors of gastric secretion, thus delaying the emptying of the stomach and retarding the appearance of hunger.

Fats contribute importantly to the palatability of the diet. The distinctive flavors of many fruits and vegetables depend upon minute quantities of certain volatile oils, many of which are lost when these foods are cooked. The culinary achievements of the home would not be possible without a variety of fats as basic ingredients. Butter and margarine enhance the acceptability of bread as well as adding flavor to many cooked foods.

Phospholipids. Brain and nervous tissue are especially rich in phospholipids, but all cells contain minute amounts of these lipids. Unlike neutral fats, they have a strong affinity for water, and thus they facilitate the passage of fats in and out of the cells. They probably play a role in the absorption of fats from the intestine and in the transport of fats from the liver. They constitute an important fraction of the blood lipids.

Essential fatty acids. The omission of highly unsaturated fatty acids—linoleic, linolenic, and arachidonic—from the diet of animals leads to failure in growth and reproduction, dermatitis, and faulty utilization and deposition of fats. Hansen [31] has observed in certain types of infantile eczema that the inclusion of these acids not only led to improvement of the skin of many of these patients but also led to greater gains in weight (see Fig. 6-1). He has pointed out that the linoleic acid content of human milk is three to four times as high as that of cow's milk.

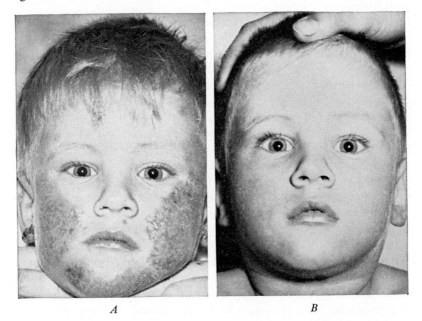

A   B

Fig. 6-1. Child, 2½ years, showing (*A*) eczema present since 2 months of age; (*B*) condition 1 month after fresh lard was added to the diet. (*Courtesy, Dr. A. E. Hansen, Galveston, Texas.*)

The metabolism of the essential fatty acids is not understood, although some experimental work suggests a role in the transport of cholesterol. Of the three, linoleic acid is of nutritional interest since it is the only one which the body apparently cannot synthesize.

Digestion and absorption. There is no digestion of fat in the mouth and very little in the stomach. The stomach, however, is important because its churning action reduces the size of the particles and because it acts as a reservoir so that fats do not reach the intestine too rapidly. Finely divided fats such as cream and egg yolk may be broken up by gastric lipase, but the action is not important.

When fat enters the duodenum a hormone, *cholecystokinin,* is produced in the intestinal wall and carried by the blood stream to the gallbladder so as to cause its contraction. Bile, secreted by the liver and stored in the gallbladder, is forced by this contraction into the common duct and thence into the small intestine. Bile stimulates the motility of the gastrointestinal tract, emulsifies the fats to provide a great increase in their surface area, and helps to provide the alkaline reaction necessary for the action of the lipase. Pancreatic lipase, also known as steapsin, is a powerful enzyme which hydrolyzes the minute fat droplets to fatty acids and glycerol. Hydrolysis is a graduated process in which one fatty acid is probably split off at the time leaving di- and monoglycerides.

Being effective wetting agents, bile and phospholipids provide the means whereby the insoluble fats are held in solution for their absorption. The products of fat hydrolysis are recombined to a considerable degree in the intestinal mucosa as neutral fats. In addition to these synthesized fats, the products entering the lymph circulation include free fatty acids, mono- and diglycerides, small amounts of fats which have not been hydrolyzed at all, phospholipids, and cholesterol esters. The water-soluble short-chain fatty acids and glycerol are carried directly to the liver by the portal circulation.

Digestibility of fats. As a rule, 93 to 98 per cent of the commonly used fats are digested and absorbed. An important requirement for the digestion and absorption of fats is that they must be liquid at body temperature. The fats containing short-chain fatty acids and unsaturated fatty acids have lower melting points than those composed of the long-chain and saturated fatty acids. Butter, for example, with a melting point of 75° F, is more completely absorbed than a hard fat such as beef fat which melts at 95° to 105° F. The occurrence in foods of triglycerides containing only the saturated fatty acids is small. Adults apparently metabolize all food fats quite well, but infants and aged persons show a selective absorption of shorter-chain fatty acids when the diet contains mixed fats.

That fats remain in the stomach longer than other nutrients is usually advantageous, for it prevents the early return of hunger and increases the *satiety value* of small meals. Glucose absorption proceeds gradually for several hours and excessive gastrointestinal motility is avoided.

Fried foods are digested more slowly because food particles coated with fat must be broken up before they can be acted upon by the enzymes. When the frying temperature is too low foods may absorb an excess of fat, and when the temperature is too high the decomposition products of glycerol may be formed. In either case digestive upsets may occur, but foods fried at the proper temperatures do not cause such digestive difficulties.

Mineral oils, which are not true fats, are not absorbed from the intestine. The presence of mineral oil in the gastrointestinal tract interferes with the absorption of the fat-soluble vitamins, and there is no justification for the use of this oil with foods as in salad dressing; as a medication, mineral oil should be used with caution and never at mealtime.

Metabolism. Lipids enter the systemic circulation from the lymph circulation. Some of the fat is withdrawn by the tissues, some remains in the fat depots, and some is withdrawn by the liver (see Fig. 6-2). In the blood circulation the lipids include triglycerides, cholesterol esters, free fatty acids, and phospholipids. Because they are insoluble in water they are carried in the blood in association with proteins, these complexes being known as *lipoproteins.*

The glycerol fraction of triglycerides is utilized as carbohydrate; about 10 per cent of the fat molecule is thus a source of available glucose. Free fatty acids may be rapidly broken down to provide energy for the tissues. The breakdown of the fatty acid occurs by removing a two-carbon fragment (acetate) at a time. Coenzyme A, a complex molecule containing pantothenic acid, a B-complex vitamin, is essential for this breakdown. The acetate is further oxidized by the tissues to yield energy, carbon dioxide, and water.

Adipose tissue, far from being an inert substance, continually contributes to the energy needs of the tissues and is, in turn, replenished by the synthesis

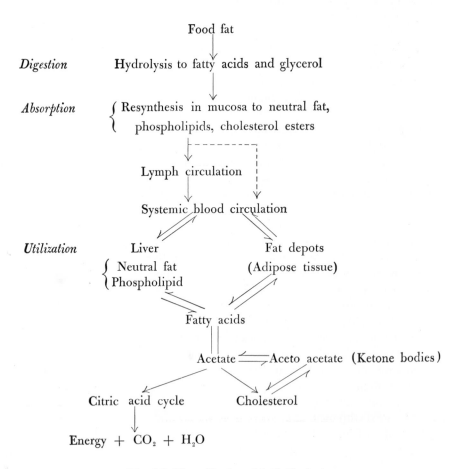

Fig. 6-2. The utilization of fat in the body.

of fats within the body. As in the breakdown of fatty acids, acetate (with coenzyme A) is also the building unit for new fats. Carbohydrates, fats, and, to a lesser degree, amino acids yield acetate and thus all three dietary constituents contribute to fat synthesis. If the caloric intake equals the body requirement, the adipose tissue formed from metabolism of the nutrients is burned between meals and no extra fat is left to accumulate in the tissues. If the caloric intake exceeds the need, some of the adipose tissue which is formed will not be burned; it will, consequently, add to one's weight.

The liver is the major organ for fat utilization. It brings about the conversion of fats to phospholipids but requires the presence of choline in order to do this. In the absence of choline, fatty deposits will accumulate within the liver. Methionine, one of the essential amino acids, and inositol can also prevent these fatty deposits; and the three substances are referred to as *lipotropic factors.*

In health the breakdown and synthesis of fatty acids proceed without any significant accumulation of intermediate products. The liver continually releases the four-carbon fragment, acetoacetate, but the tissues of the body utilize it so efficiently that it does not accumulate in the blood. In certain situations, the liver produces an excess of acetoacetate and it, together with its products acetone and beta-hydroxybutyric acid, cannot be utilized at a sufficiently rapid rate by the tissues. The blood concentration of these products increases (ketonemia) and excretion of the ketone (or acetone) bodies in the urine (ketonuria) takes place. Being fairly strong acids, acetone bodies in excess produce acidosis. Ketosis may occur (1) whenever the level of the carbohydrate in the diet is very low and the level of fat is high, as in the ketogenic diet; (2) whenever the dietary level of carbohydrate is very low and the amount of body fat being metabolized is high, as in severe and poorly controlled reduction regimens; and (3) whenever there is a disturbance in carbohydrate metabolism, as in uncontrolled diabetes mellitus (Chap. 33). In each instance, the body is making an attempt to meet its energy needs by increased oxidation of fat when carbohydrate is not available; however, the attempt is only partially successful because there is a limit to the rate of oxidation by the peripheral tissues.

Daily allowances. From a physiologic point of view, wide variations of fat intake are compatible with good health. People of the Orient consume fat accounting for only 10 per cent of their caloric intake, while in the United States fat represents more than 40 per cent of the caloric intake. The recommendation is widely made that at least 25 per cent of the energy should be provided in the form of fat, but the evidence for this is lacking. To limit the fat intake to 25 per cent of the calories is not easy in terms of foods available in the United States, and "there is as yet no proven nutritional or health reason for suggesting that its attainment is a desirable goal." *

* Gortner, W. A., ed.: *The Role of Dietary Fat in Human Health*, Pub. 575, Food and Nutrition Board, National Research Council, 1958, p. 17.

Sources of fat. The dietary survey of households in the United States [1] showed that an average of 155 gm of fat per person was daily available for consumption, accounting for 44 per cent of the available calories. This average value does not represent actual intake which will vary widely from individual to individual and from region to region depending upon cooking practices and plate waste. The data in the following table derived from this study serve, however, to illustrate the important sources of fat in the American diet and to describe the nature of these fats.

SOURCES OF FAT, HOUSEHOLDS IN THE UNITED STATES, 1955 *

(Average per person per day)

| | | | AMOUNT OF FATTY ACIDS | | |
| | AMOUNT OF FAT | | Saturated | Oleic | Linoleic |
FOOD GROUP	gm	per cent	gm	gm	gm
Invisible fats					
Beef, veal, lamb	22.1	14.2	11.0	8.8	0.4
Pork, excl. bacon,					
salt pork	15.1	9.7	6.0	7.6	1.5
Poultry, fish	4.4	2.9	1.2	1.6	0.8
Milk, cream, ice					
cream, cheese	28.0	18.0	18.5	7.6	1.0
Eggs	5.6	3.6	2.0	2.5	0.4
Baked goods, nuts,					
fruits, vegetables	18.0	11.8	3.6	9.0	3.6
Visible fats					
Bacon, salt pork	13.4	8.6	5.4	6.7	1.3
Lard	9.2	5.9	3.7	4.6	0.9
Other shortening	9.0	5.8	2.2	5.8	0.7
Oils, salad dressing	9.3	6.0	1.9	2.8	4.6
Margarine	10.4	6.7	2.6	6.4	0.8
Butter	10.6	6.8	7.0	2.9	0.4
Total	155.1	100.0	65.1	66.3	16.4
Per cent of total calories	43.6		18.3	18.6	4.5

* Adapted from Tables 1 and 2 in *Food Consumption and Dietary Levels of Households in the United States,* Agricultural Research Service, U.S. Department of Agriculture, Washington, D.C., 1957, pp. 15, 16.

Roughly three-fifths of the fat available was provided from the so-called invisible sources. It is of some interest to note that each of the six groupings of visible fats contributed approximately the same amount of fat. Saturated fatty acids accounted for 65 gm of the total fat, oleic acid for 66 gm, and linoleic acid for 16 gm.

Of the three polyunsaturated fatty acids, only linoleic acid occurs abundantly in certain foods. Linolenic acid occurs in very small amounts in foods of plant origin but it cannot substitute fully for linoleic acid in the body. Animal, but not plant, fats contain small amounts of arachidonic acid. However, the liver is able to synthesize arachidonic acid when the supply of linoleic acid is sufficient. The linoleic acid content of the American diet appears to be sufficiently generous, but the consistent omission of oils might lower the intake of an individual below desirable levels.

From the table it may be seen that oils and salad dressings were the outstanding contributors to the linoleic acid intake. The miscellaneous grouping "baked goods, nuts, fruits, vegetables" owes its relatively high level of this essential fatty acid to the use of oils in some of the baked foods and to the contribution of nuts. Outstanding sources of linoleic acid include seed oils—safflower, corn, sunflower, soybean, sesame, and cottonseed. Peanut oil is somewhat lower in its linoleic acid content, while olive oil is a relatively poor source. Of animal fats, chicken fat compares with peanut oil, and pork fat may contain 10 to 20 per cent linoleic acid by weight depending upon the diet of the animal. Beef and mutton tallow, butter, coconut oil, and cacao butter are not good sources of this essential fatty acid. (See also Fig. 36-1.)

Margarine is fortified with 15,000 I.U. vitamin A and compares nutritionally with butter. Hydrogenated fats are comparable with natural fats of similar firmness in their utilization by the body.

CHOLESTEROL

A tremendous number of investigations relating to the role of fat in the occurrence of atherosclerosis and the incidence of cardiovascular diseases have been reported in the medical literature. Cholesterol is an important constituent of the deposits which are found in the arterial walls. In humans the simplest approach has been to study the effect of various kinds and amounts of fat on the blood cholesterol level in normal individuals as well as those with cardiovascular disease. Investigators recognize certain limitations in such an approach, but to many lay persons dietary cholesterol is often looked upon as something to be avoided at all costs. It is important, therefore, that the nurse and dietitian have some understanding of the role of cholesterol in normal metabolism.

Functions. Cholesterol is found in all animal tissues, being more abundant in brain and nervous tissue, the adrenal cortex, and the liver. Although the wide distribution and relatively high concentrations in actively functioning tissues of the body indicate fundamental roles, the mechanisms are poorly understood at the present time. Cholesterol and its degradation products are important constituents of bile. It serves as a precursor for vitamin D, and the exposure of the skin to sunlight results in the conversion of cholesterol to the active vitamin. Structurally, cholesterol is also related to the sex hormones and the adrenocortical hormones, and possibly it serves as a starting point for the formation of some of these substances.

Dietary sources and synthesis. The body obtains its cholesterol from dietary sources and from synthesis within the body. The exogenous or dietary sources include egg yolk—the richest source, liver, kidney, brains, sweetbreads, and fish roe with smaller amounts from the fat of whole milk, cheese, cream, ice cream, and meat. Individuals who eat no eggs or organ meats may ingest as little as 200–300 mg per day; if they also use skim milk and no butter, the intake is further reduced to less than 100 mg daily. Those who eat one or more eggs a day and who use organ meats at regular intervals may have an intake of 1000 mg or more. A table of cholesterol values may be consulted in the Appendix (see p. 780).

By far the most important source of cholesterol to the body is that synthesized chiefly by the liver, although the adrenal cortex, skin, and intestinal wall also possess this ability. The manufacture of cholesterol proceeds at a rapid rate with acetic acid serving as the direct precursor. It will be remembered that the two-carbon acetate grouping is available to the body from fats, carbohydrates, and amino acids which are being metabolized. The rate of synthesis keeps pace with body need; more or less will be produced depending upon the dietary intake in relation to need. Obviously, it is a fallacy for healthy individuals to restrict their intake of eggs, organ meats, and dairy products in the hope that they will thereby reduce the cholesterol metabolism; in fact, such dietary changes have been shown to have no effect on the level of cholesterol in the blood. Moreover, the omission of such foods removes important sources of protein, iron, and the B-complex vitamins so that nutrition may be adversely affected.

Metabolism. Cholesterol is readily absorbed into the lymphatic circulation and is carried to the liver. This organ not only synthesizes cholesterol as needed, it also regulates the level in the blood by removing the excess. Cholesterol is oxidized in the liver to bile acids or may be disposed of without change in the bile which is excreted into the small intestine.

The concentration of cholesterol is quite variable in the blood serum, values of 80 to 300 mg per 100 ml being cited for healthy individuals. About two-thirds of this is in ester formation chiefly with unsaturated fatty acids. Being insoluble in an aqueous medium, cholesterol, like fats, is carried in the blood in combination with protein as lipoprotein.

Cholesterol metabolism is regulated by a number of hormones, including those of the thyroid, estrogens, pancreas, adrenal, and pituitary. Subnormal activity of the thyroid gland results in a high serum cholesterol level, while in hyperthyroidism the cholesterol levels are low. Blood cholesterol levels are increased in uncontrolled diabetes mellitus, nephrosis, and xanthomatosis. Gallstones are composed chiefly of cholesterol.

In experimental animals numerous dietary factors have been shown to affect blood cholesterol levels, namely, protein, lipotropic factors (choline, methionine), vitamin B_{12}, biotin, and pantothenic acid. While the dietary level of cholesterol is without effect,[32] the quantity and nature of the dietary fat may be of some importance. For example, under certain conditions, a high fat intake in which there is a significant proportion of saturated fatty acids has led to an increase in serum cholesterol levels, while a high-fat intake in which the fats were in the form of unsaturated oils actually led to a decrease of the serum cholesterol. It is too early to predict what modifications of fat, either quantitative or qualitative, may prove to be most beneficial.

PROBLEMS AND REVIEW

1. True fats contain carbon, hydrogen, and oxygen. How do they differ from carbohydrate?

2. Palmitic, oleic, and stearic acid are the fatty acids most frequently found in foods. Which of these limits the digestibility of fats? Why is this so?

3. An unsaturated fatty acid does not contain enough hydrogen to combine with all the free carbon atoms. How does this affect the hardness of a fat? Give several examples of unsaturated fatty acids.

4. What is a hydrogenated fat? Give some examples. How does it compare in nutritive value with the fat from which it was made?

5. Phospholipids, like proteins, are essential constituents of all cells. How do they differ from neutral fats? Why are they so important? What are some good food sources?

6. What is meant by an essential fatty acid? Name two. In what way may essential fatty acid deficiency manifest itself?

7. Name eight functions of fat in the body.

8. What effect will the inclusion of fatty foods such as fried potatoes and pork chops have on the digestion of the meal as a whole?

9. *Problem.* Prepare an outline which shows the digestion, absorption, and metabolism of fats.

10. What amounts of fat are desirable in the daily diet? Name six plant and six animal sources of fats.

11. List some possible results of an excessive intake of fats; of a very low fat intake.

12. *Problem.* Calculate the fat content of:

> 125 gm white bread
> 30 gm white bread with 5 gm butter
> 200 gm milk

13. *Problem.* Calculate your own fat intake for one day. Which of the foods you ate are good sources of linoleic acid? What percentage of the total calories in your diet was derived from fat?

14. What is cholesterol? What are some of the possible roles of cholesterol in the body?

15. How does the body obtain its supply of cholesterol?

16. A patient tells you he has not been eating eggs and butter and has been drinking no milk because he read in a magazine that cholesterol was harmful. How would you meet this situation?

CHAPTER 7 /

Energy Metabolism

The energy derived from food is used to perform the involuntary and voluntary work of the body, to maintain body temperature, and to synthesize new body constituents. In the United States, a caloric intake in excess of the body's energy requirement is so frequent that obesity has become a major health problem. In some parts of the world, however, there is never quite enough food to provide adequately for the energy needs of all of the people so that a high incidence of undernutrition results. A deficit of energy foods leads rapidly to low morale and diminished ability to do work. When plans are made for the rehabilitation of starving populations, it is not surprising, then, that the first emphasis is placed on providing an adequate source of calories.

Energy metabolism. The physicist defines energy as the capacity for doing work. The sun is the original source of all energy. Plants, through the action of chlorophyll with sunlight, store energy as carbohydrate, which in turn becomes available to animals and man. Potential energy is found in the foods we eat, just as potential energy is found in coal and in many other forms of fuel.

A fundamental law in physics, namely, the *law of conservation of energy,* states that energy can be neither created nor destroyed. The workings of the human body are no exception to this law. If we could keep a careful record which included the intake of food, the excretion of materials through the skin, kidney, lungs, and bowels, the heat produced in the body, and the work performed, we would find that an accurate balance exists between the energy intake and output.

No matter how slight movement may be, some fuel is required by the body. The body is frequently likened to an engine. However, when an engine stops, its use of fuel likewise stops; but with the body, as long as life goes on, there is always a need for fuel. The pulsations of the heart, the rhythmic breathing, the work of the glands in the body, and the maintenance of muscle tone are accomplished by the oxidation of foodstuffs. The maintenance of a constant body temperature is vital. The voluntary activities of daily living impose additional fuel needs. The digestion, absorption, and assimilation of

78

food eaten to satisfy the energy needs of these several activities require further caloric allowances.

FUEL VALUES OF FOODS

Methods of measurement. The energy exchanges of the body are expressed in terms of the calorie which is a heat unit. By definition, 1 *calorie* is the amount of heat required to raise the temperature of 1 kg of water 1° C. This is the large Calorie, or kilocalorie, and is 1000 times as large as the small calorie which is the unit used in physics. In nutrition literature the kilocalorie is used exclusively, and this fact is generally understood whether the word is written with a capital "C" or a small "c."

The fuel value of foods may be readily determined in the laboratory by means of an apparatus known as a bomb calorimeter illustrated in Figure 7-1. The heat given off by the burning of a weighed sample of food is dissipated into a known weight of water in which the rise in temperature can be accurately measured. From the change in the temperature of the water, one can calculate the energy value of the food by applying the definition for a calorie.

Physiologic fuel factors. The caloric values of foods burned in the bomb calorimeter are somewhat higher than those realized in the body. First of all, certain small losses occur in digestion for all three nutrients. For the typical mixed American diet, 98 per cent of the carbohydrate, 95 per cent of the fat, and 92 per cent of the protein are digested and absorbed. The carbohydrates and fats which are absorbed are entirely oxidized in the body as they are in the bomb calorimeter. In the case of proteins, however, the end products of metabolism are partly eliminated as urea and other organic nitrogen compounds which are combustible. In other words, the body loses part of the potential energy value of protein so that the net value is less than that measured by the calorimeter. On the basis of these corrections, the "physiologic fuel factors" proposed by Atwater are:

> 1 gm of pure protein will yield 4 calories
> 1 gm of pure fat will yield 9 calories
> 1 gm of pure carbohydrate will yield 4 calories

Specific fuel factors. Each food has a specific coefficient of digestibility, and thus the fuel value likewise would be specific for each given food. For example, the coefficient of digestibility for the protein in milk, eggs, and meat is 97 per cent, but for the protein of whole ground corn meal it is only 60 per cent; the coefficient of digestibility for the carbohydrate of wheat is 98 per cent when white flour (70–74 per cent extraction) is used, but is 90 per cent when whole-wheat flour (97–100 per cent extraction) is used. The errors introduced by the variations in digestibility are small for the typical mixed American diet, and for any calculations the student is likely to make Atwater's physiologic fuel values are sufficiently reliable.

Whenever the diet differs markedly from the typical diet on which Atwater based his data, considerable error is introduced with the use of average fuel values. For example, the caloric value of a diet which is predominant in cereal foods would be overestimated. This can be a serious problem when it involves suitable allocation of food to populations where the food supply is short. The Nutrition Division of FAO [33] has made a study of specific factors applicable to foods and has proposed a table for estimating calories based on these specific factors rather than on the average values. The tables of food composition used in the United States employ the specific fuel factors, although the physiologic factors—4, 9, 4—are convenient for dietary approximations.

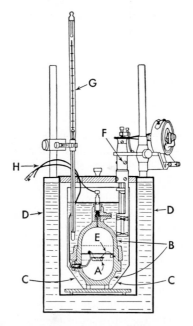

Fig. 7-1. Diagram of bomb calorimeter with bomb in position. (*Courtesy, the Emerson Apparatus Company, Boston, Mass.*)

    A. Platinum dish holding weighed food sample
    B. Bomb filled with pure oxygen enclosing food sample
    C. Can holding water of known weight in which the bomb is submerged
    D. Outer double-walled insulating jacket
    E. Fuse, which is ignited by an electric current
    F. Motor-driven water stirrer
    G. Thermometer calibrated to $\frac{1}{1000}°$ C
    H. Electric wires to send current through fuse

MEASUREMENT OF ENERGY EXCHANGE IN THE BODY

Direct and indirect calorimetry. The amount of heat produced by the body may be measured by *direct calorimetry*. By this method the individual is placed in a specially constructed room or large insulated chamber called a "respiration calorimeter." The heat given off by his body is determined by noting the volume and change in temperature of water flowing through coils in the walls of the chamber. The heat lost by the vaporization of water from the lungs is also taken into account. Some of the calorimeters which have been used in research studies have been large enough to permit study of energy metabolism with the body at rest, or with various kinds of activity. While these calorimeters have served as a basis for present-day knowledge of energy metabolism, they are costly to construct and maintain and require painstaking attention from skilled technicians.

A much simpler technique for measuring energy exchange is by *indirect calorimetry* (see Fig. 7-2). By this method the fuel exchange of the body is determined by measuring the oxygen utilization, since oxygen will be consumed in proportion to the amount of glucose or fat which is being oxidized. The caloric equivalent of 1 liter of oxygen depends on the proportion of glucose or fat which is being oxidized at any given moment, but under the conditions of the basal metabolism test 1 liter of oxygen is equivalent to 4.825 calories.

Basal metabolism test. The amount of energy required to carry on the involuntary work of the body and to maintain the body temperature is known as the basal metabolic rate, abbreviated BMR. About one-third of this energy is used to maintain the functional activities of the various organs such as the heart, kidneys, and lungs, whereas the remaining two-thirds of this energy will be needed for oxidation in the resting tissues, especially in the maintenance of muscle tone. The test consists in measuring the amount of oxygen consumed in a given length of time, usually 6 to 8 minutes; the carbon dioxide which is produced may, or may not, be measured depending upon the procedure being used. Several important factors may lead to results in the test which are not indicative of the basal metabolism. Therefore, the standard conditions for the test have been set up as follows. The patient must be:

1. In the postabsorptive state (12 to 16 hours after the last meal) to eliminate the influence of food. The test is usually performed in the morning before breakfast.

2. Reclining and relaxed but awake. Sleep, on the one hand, reduces the metabolism by about 10 per cent, while vigorous exercise, on the other hand, rapidly increases the rate of oxidation.

3. Free from emotional upsets or fear of the test itself. An increased pulse rate may suggest such effects.

4. In a comfortable room environment. Shivering rapidly increases the amount of oxidation in the tissues.

5. Afebrile. For each degree F rise in body temperature above normal, the metabolism is increased about 7 per cent. Thus, an individual with a temperature of 102.6° F will show an increase in the metabolic rate by 28 per cent.

Under the above conditions an individual is considered to have a normal metabolic rate if his metabolism comes within 10 to 15 per cent of the recognized standards.

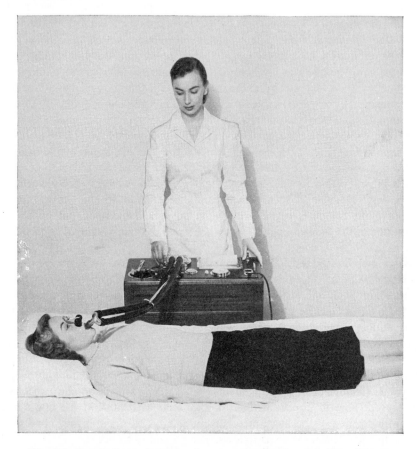

Fig. 7-2. Respiration calorimeter for measuring basal metabolism. (*Courtesy, the Sanborn Company, Cambridge, Mass.*)

Factors influencing the basal metabolic rate. The adult basal metabolic rate is approximately 1 calorie per kg body weight per hour or 1350 to 1700 calories daily for women and men, respectively. For most people, the basal metabolism accounts for the largest proportion of the total energy requirement. The rate of basal metabolism is affected by size, shape, and weight of an individual, body composition, age, rate of growth, the activity of the endocrine glands, and the state of nutrition.

Size, shape, and weight. Heat is continuously lost through the skin by radiation. Since the heat loss is proportional to the skin surface, the basal heat production is directly proportional to the surface area. A tall, thin person has a greater surface area than an individual of the same weight who is short and fat and the former therefore will have a higher basal metabolism.

Body composition. The rate of heat production is dependent upon the amount of active protoplasmic tissue. Again, a tall, thin person with little deposits of fat tissue is expected to have a higher rate of basal metabolism than the short, stout individual of the same weight who has larger amounts of inactive adipose tissue. Athletes show about 5 per cent higher basal metabolism than nonathletic individuals. The metabolic rate of women is 6 to 10 per cent lower than that of men, a fact generally ascribed to more highly developed muscles and less inactive adipose tissue in men.

Age. The basal metabolism during rapid growth is at a high level. The younger the individual, the higher his basal metabolism per unit of body weight, since much energy is stored for growth. The period when the basal metabolism reaches its highest level is between the ages of 1 and 2 years. A gradual decline occurs from 2 to 5 years with a more rapid decline (except for a slight rise at adolescence) until adult age is reached. After maturity is reached, there is a gradual decline in the metabolic rate with each decade.

Influence of the endocrine glands. The thyroid gland in particular exerts a marked influence on the energy requirements. If the thyroid gland is overactive (hyperthyroidism), the metabolism will sometimes be speeded up as much as 100 per cent; if the activity of the gland is decreased (hypothyroidism), the metabolism may be reduced by 30 to 40 per cent. Disturbances of the pituitary gland may also modify the metabolic rate. The excretion of epinephrine increases the metabolic rate temporarily.

Effect of state of nutrition. An individual who has been chronically undernourished is likely to have a lower basal metabolic rate. Analyses of metabolism in "naturally occurring" starvation and of experimental starvation "indicate that the oxidative rate of the active tissues deviates little, if at all, from the metabolic rate of the active mass under normal conditions. The observed decrease in basal metabolism is almost completely accounted for by the decrease in mass of active tissues." *

Depending upon the circumstances, undernourished children may have an increase or a decrease of the basal metabolic rate. Underweight school children sometimes show an increased rate because of the high percentage of active lean tissues as compared with very little inactive adipose tissue. When undernutrition is severe, the destruction of body tissues is likely to lower the rate.

Effect of pregnancy. During the last trimester of pregnancy the basal metabolism increases from 15 to 25 per cent. This increase can be accounted for almost entirely by the increase in weight of the woman and the high rate of metabolism of the fetus.

* Review: "The Metabolic Rate in Semistarvation," *Nutrition Rev.*, **6:**311, 1948.

Factors influencing the total energy requirement. Superimposed upon the energy expenditure for maintaining the involuntary activities of the body are such factors as voluntary muscular activity, the effect of food, and the maintenance of the body temperature.

Effect of muscular activity. Next to the basal metabolism, activity accounts for the largest energy expenditure; in fact, for some persons who are vigorously active, the energy needs for activity may exceed those for the basal metabolism. Sedentary work, which includes office work, bookkeeping, typing, teaching, etc., calls for less energy than more active and strenuous occupations such as nursing, homemaking, or gardening. A still greater amount of energy is required by those individuals who do hard manual labor such as ditch digging, shifting freight, and lumbering. The energy expenditure for many activities has been measured in adults and children,[34,35] and the data serve as a guide in setting standards for various groups of people. A few examples are given below of the number of calories expended in 1 hour by a woman weighing 120 pounds. These figures include the basal allowance.

	Calories per hour
Awake lying still (basal rate)	56
Sitting quietly	72
Typing rapidly	102
Dishwashing	104
Sweeping the floor	122
Walking slowly (2.6 miles per hour)	145
Walking moderately fast (3.75 miles per hour)	217
Swimming	362

If an exact record of activity for a given 24-hour period were kept it would be possible with data such as the above to estimate the daily caloric requirement of an adult. However, such calculations are time consuming and give, at best, only rough approximations since individuals vary widely in the efficiency of their work and in their muscle tone.

The figures above illustrate the value of exercise in weight control, for it is quite evident that the student who sits quietly watching television, for example, is expending only half as many calories as one who is walking leisurely, and only one-fifth as many calories as one who swims for an hour.

Not infrequently the question is raised as to the reason for the differing caloric needs of two people of the same build and body weight who are doing the same kind of work. The energy needs will be greater for the person who wastes many motions in the performance of a piece of work, who works under greater muscle tension, or who finds it difficult to relax completely even when at rest.

Effect of mental effort. Nervous tissue accounts for about 2 per cent of the body weight and the energy expenditure of the body is not appreciably increased even with intense mental effort such as that expended in writing examinations. Some students may become tense and restless in the solving of problems, but the increased energy expenditure in such a situation is not primarily the result of mental work.

Effect of food. A certain amount of work is expended in the digestion of food, its absorption, its transfer to the tissues, and its utilization. The increased heat production as the result of the ingestion of food is known as the *specific dynamic action.* Protein when eaten alone has been shown to increase the metabolic rate by 30 per cent, while carbohydrates and fats will produce much smaller increases in metabolism. On the basis of the mixed diets which are usually eaten, the specific dynamic action is approximately 6 per cent of the energy requirement.[36]

Maintenance of body temperature. Under normal conditions the temperature of the body is controlled by the amount of blood which is brought to the skin. When the surrounding temperature is low, most of the heat is lost by radiation and conduction; but when the environmental temperature is high, the body heat is lost chiefly through evaporation. It is a well-known fact that more heat is lost by evaporation when the air is dry than when it is humid.

During cold weather, man avoids excessive heat losses from his body by the use of suitable clothing and the heating of his home or place of work. Moreover, body heat is conserved if there is a layer of adipose tissue under the skin. The subcutaneous fat serves to keep heat in the body rather than allowing it to be dissipated through the skin—an advantage in cold weather, but a disadvantage in warm weather.

When the body is subjected to extreme cold, the body temperature is maintained by an increase in involuntary and often by voluntary activity. The blood vessels constrict so that there is less blood reaching the skin surface; the muscles become tense; and shivering follows. These involuntary activities result in a considerable increase in the metabolic rate. As anyone knows who has been exposed to a cold winter day, one is not likely to stand still. In addition, then, to the increased energy expenditure occasioned by the involuntary activities, the individual increases his voluntary activity.

Effect of growth. The building of new tissue represents a storage of energy in one form or another; for example, every gram of protein in body tissue represents about 4 calories. When growth is rapid, as during the first year of life, the energy allowance must be high. In fact, the caloric need is greater per unit of body weight at this time than at any other time in life. In pregnancy, likewise, the energy needs are increased to cover the building of new tissue. These needs are discussed in more detail in Chapters 17, 18, and 19.

CALORIC ALLOWANCES

Daily allowances. The Recommended Dietary Allowances [2] for calories take into account sex, body size, age, climate, and activity. They are based on the maintenance of optimum body weight or a suitable rate of growth, and must be adjusted upward or downward to meet individual needs. The allowances are a rough guide in dietary planning for groups; they may vary widely for any given individual. The bases for these allowances are described below.

Reference standard. The recommended allowances are stated in terms of the reference man and woman. The man and woman are in good health, 25 years of age, live in an environment with a mean annual temperature of 20° C (68° F), and weigh 70 kg (154 lb) and 58 kg (128 lb), respectively. They lead a moderately active, healthy life, including moderate outdoor recreation. The man is described as one who might be working as a painter, a delivery man, an outdoor salesman, or in light industry. Under these conditions the caloric allowance for the man is 3200. The reference woman might be a homemaker and mother, or a saleswoman, or a bench worker in a factory. She would need about 2300 calories.

Adjustment for body size. Caloric allowances should be based on the desirable weight for height and health (see Appendix, pp. 781–85). The following table gives the allowances for individuals whose weight differs from that of the reference man and woman.

CALORIC ALLOWANCES FOR INDIVIDUALS OF VARIOUS BODY WEIGHTS AND AGE *

(At mean environmental temperature of 20° C and assuming moderate physical activity)

DESIRABLE WEIGHT		CALORIC ALLOWANCES FOR MEN			CALORIC ALLOWANCES FOR WOMEN		
Kilograms	Pounds	25 years	45 years	65 years	25 years	45 years	65 years
40	88				1750	1650	1400
45	99				1900	1800	1500
50	110	2500	2350	1950	2050	1950	1600
55	121	2700	2550	2150	2200	2050	1750
58 †	128				2300	2200	1800
60	132	2850	2700	2250	2350	2200	1850
65	143	3000	2800	2350	2500	2350	2000
70 **	154	3200	3000	2550	2600	2450	2050
75	165	3400	3200	2700	2750	2600	2150
80	176	3550	3350	2800			
85	187	3700	3500	2900			

* Food and Nutrition Board: *Recommended Dietary Allowances.* Pub. 589, National Academy of Sciences—National Research Council, Washington, D.C., 1958, p. 4.
† Reference woman weighs 58 kg.
** Reference man weighs 70 kg.

Adjustment for age. The allowances are stated for the midpoint of each decade and thus the allowance at 25 years includes the period from 20 to 30 years, and so on. Between 30 and 50 years the caloric allowances are reduced 3 per cent for each decade; from 50 to 70 years they are decreased 7.5 per cent for each decade, and from 70 to 80 years a further decrease of 10 per cent is made. These corrections have been applied to individuals of 45 and 65 years in the table on page 86.

Adjustment for climate. Suitable clothing, well-heated buildings, heated means of transportation, and limited outdoor exposure of most Americans result in no increased caloric requirements during cold weather. Likewise, air conditioning in summer minimizes, for some people, the decrease in caloric allowances one might expect in warm summer weather. When, however, there is exposure to different temperatures the calories should be increased by 5 per cent for the first 10° below the standard (20° C), and further increased by 3 per cent for each additional 10° decrease. Further increases may be necessary for people who spend most of their time out of doors during extremely cold weather. When the environmental temperature is consistently above 20° C, the caloric allowances are decreased in the same manner as they are increased for the colder environments.

Adjustments for activity. Today the average work week is 35 to 40 hours; sleep may account for 50 to 60 hours; eating and travel to and from work may consume 20 hours, more or less; and leisure time may amount to 50 or 60 hours in a given week. The leisure activities may range from reading, watching television, movies, or stamp collecting, on the one hand, to such vigorous activities as tennis, gardening, golf, and swimming, on the other hand. Obviously, to set up a caloric allowance in terms of one's activity at work alone is to ignore a large part of one's day.

The recommended allowances are set up in terms of the general average of the population, but individuals will differ widely. Only rarely will these allowances need to be increased by more than 25 per cent for the healthy adult. For many Americans who are sedentary in their occupations and who are also inactive in their leisure, the allowances are too high.

The best guide to the adequacy of the caloric allowances lies in the maintenance of desirable weight. Individuals should be encouraged to weigh themselves at regular intervals. Thus, the insidious but undesirable increases in body weight over desirable levels may be checked by appropriate reduction in the intake of energy-rich foods. Likewise, suitable rates of growth may be maintained. The dangers of excessive weight gain, or of underweight, are discussed in Chapter 27.

Selecting foods for energy. The inclusion of minimum amounts of each of the Four Food Groups provides energy at approximately basal levels for the adult (see Fig. 7-3). To complete the caloric requirement, any foods desired may be selected. More foods from the bread-cereals group will not only increase the caloric intake at low cost, but will enhance the protein, iron, and B-complex vitamin level of the diet. The selection of additional foods from the other three groups will increase the caloric level of the diet in varying degree and provide further nutritional benefits in protein, minerals, and vitamins.

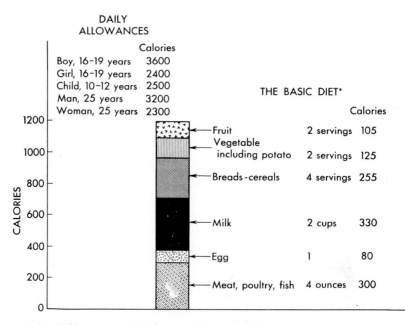

DAILY
ALLOWANCES

	Calories
Boy, 16–19 years	3600
Girl, 16–19 years	2400
Child, 10–12 years	2500
Man, 25 years	3200
Woman, 25 years	2300

THE BASIC DIET*

		Calories
Fruit	2 servings	105
Vegetable including potato	2 servings	125
Breads-cereals	4 servings	255
Milk	2 cups	330
Egg	1	80
Meat, poultry, fish	4 ounces	300

* See Table on page 178 for complete calculations.

Fig. 7-3. The Basic Diet provides approximately half of the energy requirement of the teenage girl and the woman of 25 years. The energy requirement for various categories is easily met by increasing the intake of foods in the Basic Diet and by the addition of fats and sugars.

Fats and sugars are concentrated sources of energy, and may be used to rapidly increase the caloric level of the diet. They have a legitimate place in the diet, but it must be borne in mind that fats (except butter and fortified margarine) and sugars do not contain protein, minerals, and vitamins. When they constitute a large proportion of the total calories in the diet, there is danger that other nutrient needs will not be met. Too many Americans select diets in which fats and sugars provide one-third or more of the calories. This is an important area for nutrition education.

PROBLEMS AND REVIEW

1. Define or explain what is meant by: calorie; basal metabolism; bomb calorimeter; respiratory calorimeter.

2. *Problem.* On the basis of protein, fat, and carbohydrate composition, calculate the energy value of:

> 240 gm milk
> 160 gm orange
> 20 gm dry oatmeal

3. *Problem.* Calculate the number of grams required of each of the following foods to furnish 100 calories: butter, milk, cheese, egg, potato, apple, banana, orange, sugar, bread, and lean beef.

4. The use of Atwater's physiologic fuel values is not desirable for calculating the caloric value of a diet composed chiefly of cereal foods. Why?

5. The basal metabolism is the rate of oxidation occurring in the body at rest. What are the standard conditions for performing the test? What factors might make the basal metabolism of two adult individuals of the same age vary? How does age itself affect basal metabolism?

6. *Problem.* Each liter of oxygen consumed by an individual on a mixed diet is equal to about 4.8 calories. What is the basal caloric need per 24 hours of a nurse who consumed 2 liters oxygen during a 10-minute test?

7. Explain how the following factors affect the total energy requirement of an individual: muscular activity; food; climate; clothing; growth; muscle tension; endocrine secretions. Which usually has the greatest effect?

8. *Problem.* Calculate the caloric value of your own meals for 1 day. How does this compare with your estimated requirement?

9. *Problem.* What proportion of your own caloric requirement is provided by the basic diet, page 88? What is the most economical way in which you can complete your requirement of energy using this basic diet?

10. Why would you expect the caloric requirement of many poor people to be higher during cold weather than that of people in better economic circumstances?

11. What is the best indication of adequate caloric intake?

CHAPTER 8 /

Mineral Elements

Elementary composition of the body. Water, proteins, and fats account for 96 per cent of the body weight. Thus, the four predominating chemical elements are: oxygen, 65 per cent; carbon, 18 per cent; hydrogen, 10 per cent; and nitrogen, 3 per cent. The remaining 4 per cent of the body weight is made up of the elements usually designated as minerals.

Most of the minerals are present in organic compounds such as hemoglobin, phosphoproteins, or thyroxine. Some, however, occur as inorganic compounds—sodium chloride, for example. Minerals, then, may be defined as those elements which remain largely as ash when plant or animal tissues are burned. The following table lists the mineral elements together with their

MINERAL COMPOSITION OF THE BODY *

	AMOUNT IN THE BODY			AMOUNT IN THE BODY	
	per cent	PER 70 KILOGRAMS grams		per cent	PER 70 KILOGRAMS grams
			Trace Elements		
Calcium	1.5–2.2	1050–1540	Manganese	0.0003	0.21
Phosphorus	0.8–1.2	560– 840	Copper	0.00015	0.105
Potassium	0.35	245	Iodine	0.00004	0.024
Sulfur	0.25	175	Cobalt		
Sodium	0.15	105	Zinc		
Chlorine	0.15	105	Fluorine		
Magnesium	0.05	35			
Iron	0.004	2.8			

* Calculations are on the basis of elementary composition of the body as stated by Sherman, H. C.: *Chemistry of Food and Nutrition,* 8th ed., The Macmillan Company, New York, 1952, p. 227.

approximate proportions in the body. Traces of aluminum, arsenic, nickel, silicon, molybdenum, and selenium are also present in body tissues. Some of these may have definite functions while others may be present merely as contaminants.

90

Functions. Minerals enter to a greater or lesser degree into the structure of all body tissues. The hard skeletal structures are largely composed of them, but it is equally important to realize that the nuclei of soft tissues such as nerve and muscle cells contain mineral matter.

Of vital importance is the part played by minerals in regulation of the body's functions. The contraction of muscles, the irritability of nerves, the control of water balance, the maintenance of acid-base equilibrium, and the utilization of foodstuffs are but a few of their numerous functions.

The amount of an element present gives no clue to its importance in body functions. It will be shown, for example, that a few milligrams of an element such as iodine can make a critical difference in the health of an individual.

Mineral elements are interrelated to each other and to the organic compounds in their functioning. Thus, sodium, potassium, calcium, phosphorus, and chlorine are all essential constituents of body fluids; the response of the muscle fiber, for example, depends upon not one but all of these elements being present in the correct concentrations. Likewise, calcium, magnesium, phosphorus, and others are bone constituents; a deficiency of one element will obviously affect the functioning of the others. Iron, copper, and cobalt function in an interrelated manner together with protein, vitamin B_{12}, and other nutrients for the synthesis of hemoglobin and the red blood cells.

The problem of optimum mineral intake. For the normal adult a state of equilibrium is usually desirable with respect to the minerals; that is, the intake should equal the amount which is excreted. The minerals are eliminated by various routes; namely, the kidney, the bowel, and the skin. Some are excreted by all three routes while others may be lost primarily from the kidney or the intestine. About one-fourth of the solid material of urine consists of minerals, and approximately one-tenth of the solid material of feces is mineral matter.

During growth, pregnancy, and lactation it is necessary that the intake of certain minerals be sufficient to allow for the building of new tissue, or in other words, that a state of positive balance exist.

Many minerals are essential for good nutrition; but if calcium, iron, and iodine are provided in adequate amounts, there is scant likelihood that dietary deficiency of other minerals will occur. Special consideration will then be given to these three minerals with a brief discussion of the other equally important but seldom deficient minerals.

In the selection of foods one should keep four points in mind: (1) the richness of the mineral in the food; (2) how much of the particular food is to be used; (3) whether the food has lost some of its minerals through refinement or cooking processes; and (4) whether the food contains the mineral in an available form.

CALCIUM

Functions. Calcium is by far the most abundant mineral element in the body. It is also the mineral most likely to be low in the American dietary. In the body about 99 per cent of this mineral occurs in the bones and teeth in the form of a complex salt composed of calcium phosphate and calcium carbonate embedded in an organic matrix of protein. Structurally, calcium in combination with other minerals gives rigidity to the skeleton.

Bones are also a storehouse for calcium, the ends of the bones being espe-

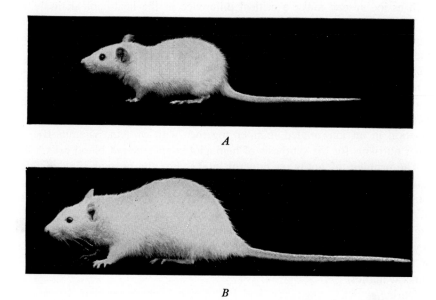

A

B

Fig. 8-1. (*A*) Insufficient calcium in an otherwise adequate diet. (*B*) Sufficient calcium added to make the diet adequate. Litter mates of the same sex, 22 weeks old. Weight of smaller, 91 gm; of larger, 219 gm. (*Courtesy, Bureau of Home Economics, U.S. Department of Agriculture.*)

cially rich in needlelike crystals of calcium salts called *trabeculae* if the diet has been adequate. The calcium is continuously removed from the bones to maintain the blood concentration; it is likewise being continuously replaced and the calcium is said to be in dynamic equilibrium.

Only 1 per cent of the body calcium is found in the blood, other body fluids, and soft tissues. Its presence in proper proportions with sodium, potassium, and magnesium is necessary in the fluids which bathe the tissues and which are responsible for contraction of muscle fibers; the rhythm of the heartbeat is dependent upon this fluid medium. Calcium is one of several factors in blood coagulation, in the normal response to nervous stimuli, in cell permeability, and in the activation of some enzymes.

Sherman has shown that a generous intake of calcium leads to greater vitality and size of experimental animals, and that this improvement results in a longer prime of life (see Fig. 8-1). It is reasonable to suppose that such benefits will accrue to human beings as well if the calcium intake is optimum.

Utilization. Calcium is absorbed only from the small intestine, most of the absorption occurring in the upper part of the intestine (see Fig. 8-2). The

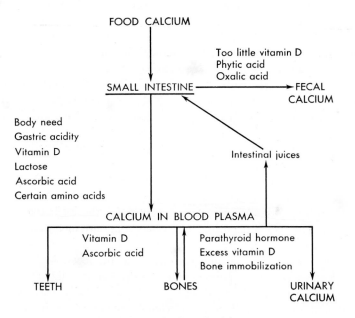

Fig. 8-2. Utilization of calcium.

amount of calcium absorption is most directly influenced by the body need. During growth and in pregnancy, the absorption is much greater than it is in adult life. The proportion which is absorbed is usually 20 to 40 per cent, more or less, of the dietary intake. However, if the body need is great and the dietary level is low the percentage which is absorbed will be much greater than if the body need is less or the dietary level is liberal. Such a mechanism helps to make the best use of calcium in a limited food supply. The body has the ability to adjust to varying levels of calcium intake, although such adjustments usually require a period of time.

Calcium salts are more soluble in acid solution, and thus the acid reaction of the gastric juice favorably influences absorption. Vitamin D is concerned with the optimum absorption of calcium, especially in children. Likewise, lactose, certain amino acids, and ascorbic acid favor the absorption of calcium.

On the other hand, oxalic acid, phytic acid, an excessive intake of fat, poor digestion of fat, and excessive fiber may interfere with the absorption of calcium. Oxalic acid is an organic acid occurring in such foods as spinach, beet greens, chard, cocoa, and rhubarb. It combines with calcium to form an insoluble salt which cannot be absorbed. While spinach, for example, contains an appreciable amount of calcium, the combination with oxalic acid renders the calcium unavailable. However, the inclusion of spinach in the diet does not adversely affect the calcium utilization of other foods.[37] Cocoa, in the amounts used by humans, has no adverse effect on calcium utilization.

Phytic acid occurs especially in the bran layer of cereal grains. Like oxalic acid, it combines with calcium to form an insoluble salt. The relatively small consumption of whole-grain cereals together with the liberal intake of calcium and vitamin D in the United States makes this factor of limited importance.

Calcium may combine with fats to form insoluble calcium soaps. When fats are poorly absorbed as in sprue (see p. 437), for example, the amount of calcium absorbed may be so small that bone changes are sometimes observed in the patient.

Calcium is transported throughout the body by means of the blood circulation. The parathyroid hormone maintains a constant blood calcium concentration of 9–11 mg per 100 ml. When the blood calcium is reduced, calcium is mobilized from the bone; when the blood level is increased, calcium is excreted by the kidney. Vitamin D is essential for the anchorage of calcium in the bones. The rate of deposit is high when bones are increasing both in size and in hardness.

As a rule, most of the calcium is excreted in the feces. Much of the fecal calcium is the unabsorbed portion from foods, but the digestive juices also contribute some calcium to the fecal excretion. Urinary calcium excretion may vary considerably in different individuals, but is relatively constant for a given person from day to day.

Daily allowances. The diet should provide sufficient calcium for optimum growth in children and to prevent negative calcium balance in the adult. The recommended allowance of calcium for the adult is 0.8 gm.[2] Adults can adjust favorably to widely varying levels of calcium intake, and in the absence of stress the requirement may be quite low.[38] It is well to encourage a liberal intake, however, because of wide individual differences in need.

For the first 9 years 1.0 gm calcium is recommended daily. Children 10 to 12 years should have 1.2 gm, boys 13 to 19 years need 1.4 gm, and girls 13 to 19 years need 1.3 gm. For pregnant women 1.5 gm calcium is allowed daily, while the allowance for lactation is 2.0 gm.

Food sources of calcium. The calcium content of typical foods is shown in the table on page 95, while the calcium contribution of the basic diet pattern is charted in Figure 8-3. Milk is the outstanding source of calcium in the diet; without it, a satisfactory intake of calcium is extremely difficult.

Whole or skimmed, homogenized or nonhomogenized, plain or chocolate-flavored, sweet or sour milks are equally good. For the adult 2 to 3 cups milk daily and for the child 3 to 4 cups daily will ensure adequate calcium intake. Cheddar cheese is an excellent source of calcium. Cottage cheese and ice cream are good sources but will not adequately substitute for milk. The dairy products, excluding butter, account for three-fourths of the calcium in the American dietary.

CALCIUM CONTENT OF SOME TYPICAL FOODS

	HOUSEHOLD MEASURE	CALCIUM mg	PER CENT OF ADULT DAILY ALLOWANCE *
Milk, fresh	1 cup	285	36
Milk, nonfat dry	3 tablespoons	285	36
Collards, cooked	½ cup	236	29
Cheese, American process	1 ounce	214	27
Turnip greens, cooked	½ cup	188	24
Salmon, pink, canned	3 ounces	159 †	20
Mustard greens, cooked	½ cup	154	19
Kale, cooked	½ cup	124	16
Clams or oysters	½ cup	113	14
Ice cream	⅛ quart	87	11
Broccoli, cooked	½ cup	98	12
Shrimp	3 ounces	98	12
Cottage cheese	3 ounces	78	10
Molasses, medium dark	1 tablespoon	44	6
Egg, whole	1 medium	27	3
Cabbage, raw, shredded	½ cup	23	3
Carrots, cooked	½ cup	19	2
Bread, 4 per cent nonfat dry milk	1 slice	19	2

* Recommended Dietary Allowance of calcium for the adult is 800 mg.
† Includes bones packed with salmon.

All of the foods other than dairy products when considered together contribute not more than 0.2 to 0.3 gm calcium daily. Certain green leafy vegetables such as mustard greens, turnip greens, kale, and collards are important sources of calcium when they are eaten frequently. Canned salmon with the bones, clams, oysters, and shrimp are likewise good sources, but they are not eaten with frequency. Meats and cereal grains are poor sources. The use of nonfat dry milk in bread enhances the calcium value of the diet. Calcium is also an optional enrichment ingredient in flours and breads.

Various calcium salts such as calcium gluconate, lactate, carbonate, and sulfate are sometimes prescribed by a physician to supplement the dietary intake, especially when milk cannot be taken for one reason or another. Calcium in organic compounds and in inorganic salts is well utilized, but it must be remembered that the substitution of salts for milk as a source of calcium

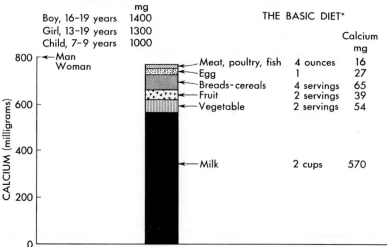

DAILY
ALLOWANCES

	mg	THE BASIC DIET*
Boy, 16–19 years	1400	
Girl, 13–19 years	1300	
Child, 7–9 years	1000	

Calcium
mg

			Calcium mg
Meat, poultry, fish	4 ounces		16
Egg	1		27
Breads-cereals	4 servings		65
Fruit	2 servings		39
Vegetable	2 servings		54
Milk	2 cups		570

CALCIUM (milligrams)

800 Man / Woman
600
400
200
0

* See page 178 for complete calculations.

Fig. 8-3. The milk group provides almost three-fourths of the calcium allowance for the adult. The addition of 1 to 3 cups milk ensures sufficient calcium during growth, in pregnancy, and during lactation.

deprives the diet of important amounts of riboflavin, protein, and other milk nutrients.

Effect of calcium deficiency. Suboptimal intakes of calcium may result in retarded calcification of bones and teeth in the young. Acute deficiency of calcium is not usually seen unless there is a concurrent lack of phosphorus and vitamin D. Such deficiency leads to stunted growth and rickets, as evidenced by bowing of the legs, enlargement of the ankles and wrists, and a hollow chest (see p. 124).

It is a misconception that adults are not subject to calcium deficiency. The gradual drainage from the bones to replace calcium ions which are lost from the body daily may not be detected by x-rays until 10 to 40 per cent of the calcium has been removed. Calcium deficiency leads to thin, fragile bones which break easily, and which heal with difficulty. Osteomalacia and osteoporosis may result from deficiencies of calcium and vitamin D. See page 126 for a more detailed discussion of osteomalacia.

Hypercalcemia. In recent years several reports have been published concerning the milk-alkali syndrome.[39] This condition is characterized by an excess of calcium in the blood and the soft tissues, by vomiting, gastrointestinal bleeding, and high blood pressure. It occurs occasionally in patients who have peptic ulcers and who have used excessive alkali therapy in conjunction with large amounts of milk over a period of years. It does not occur in the absence of alkali therapy even though large amounts of milk are taken, nor does it occur when nonabsorbable antacids are used in ulcer therapy.

Hypercalcemia may also occur in young children who are given an excess of vitamin D. Gastrointestinal upsets are noted, and growth is retarded. The condition is corrected by the removal of vitamin D.

PHOSPHORUS

Phosphorus ranks next to calcium in the total amount of mineral present in the body and constitutes about one-fourth of all body minerals. Approximately 80 per cent of the phosphorus is combined in bone structures with calcium, while the remainder is in the soft tissues and fluids of the body.

Phosphorus probably has more functions than any other mineral element. It is necessary for (1) building normal bones and teeth together with other minerals, (2) maintenance of the buffer system, (3) transport of fatty acids, (4) metabolism of fats and carbohydrates, (5) vitamin-enzyme systems, (6) muscle energy metabolism.

A diet consisting of natural foods and containing enough protein and calcium will also contain enough phosphorus. The adult requires about 1.2 gm phosphorus, while the infant, the child, and the pregnant or lactating woman should receive equal amounts of calcium and phosphorus. Thus, the pregnant woman whose calcium allowance is 1.5 gm should also receive 1.5 gm phosphorus.

Phosphorus occurs in combination with protein as phosphoproteins in the casein of milk, and as nucleoproteins in egg yolk; as phospholipids; and as phosphoric esters of carbohydrate. Excellent food sources are milk, cheese, egg yolk, meat, fish, and fowl. While whole-grain cereals are high in phosphorus, much of the phytin phosphorus is not utilized if the vitamin-D level of the diet is inadequate.[40] Vegetables and fruits are rather low in their phosphorus content.

IRON

The amount of iron present in the adult body is about 3 to 5 gm. Of this a little more than half is in the circulating hemoglobin, and about 10 per cent is in the myoglobin of the muscle. The rest is stored in the liver, bone marrow, spleen, and kidneys.

Functions. Iron is essential for the oxidative processes in the body. It is a constituent of hemoglobin, a complex substance composed of the protein, globin, and an organic iron compound, heme. Hemoglobin combines with oxygen in the lungs to form oxyhemoglobin and is carried to the tissues by the blood circulation. The oxygen is released from the hemoglobin in the tissues. On its return to the lungs hemoglobin serves as a vehicle to carry some of the carbon dioxide.

Iron is an equally essential component of myoglobin, an iron-protein compound which temporarily stores oxygen in the muscles. In fact, iron is present in all body cells. Several enzymes contain iron as a part of the molecule.

Utilization. Since iron is more soluble in the acid medium, most of the absorption takes place from the duodenum and upper jejunum. Ferrous iron is more readily absorbed than ferric iron. Reducing agents such as ascorbic acid and vitamin E aid in changing ferric iron to the ferrous state.

The rate of iron absorption is regulated by the body's need for iron (see Fig. 8-4). According to one theory, iron combines with *apoferritin,* a protein in the intestinal wall, to form *ferritin,* an iron-protein compound. When the apoferritin is saturated no more iron will be held. The iron is released from this protein compound into the plasma as required, leaving apoferritin to combine with additional iron from the intestinal contents. Approximately 10 per cent of the dietary iron is normally absorbed, but Moore [41] observed that absorption might range from 45 to 64 per cent in anemic individuals.

Iron in the plasma is bound to a specific protein from which it may be removed for the synthesis of hemoglobin in the bone marrow, for the synthesis of enzymes, or stored for later use. Minute traces of copper are necessary for the construction of the hemoglobin molecule, although the copper itself is not a part of the structure.

The body exercises amazing economy in the use of iron. When the red blood cell has fulfilled its life cycle of perhaps 100 days or a little less, the worn-out cell is broken down by the liver or spleen so that the iron may be saved for new hemoglobin. It has been estimated that 27–28 mg iron may be thus released daily and used over again.[42]

Minute amounts of iron are excreted daily in the urine, feces, sweat, hair, and desquamation of skin. The daily loss of iron in male adults is about 0.5 to 1.5 mg. Menstrual losses in women account for an additional loss of 0.5 to 2.0 mg. It should be noted that these losses do not include the unabsorbed iron in the feces.

Daily allowances. Dietary iron is required for: (1) replacement of small daily losses in all individuals; (2) an expanding blood volume and increasing amounts of hemoglobin in growing children; (3) replacement of varying losses through menstruation; (4) development of the fetus and to avoid anemia in the pregnant or lactating woman; and (5) a reserve of iron which is available when blood loss may occur from any cause whatsoever.

The recommended allowance of iron for men and women is 10 and 12 mg, respectively.[2] The diet of children should contain 7 to 10 mg during the first 9 years, and thereafter 12 to 15 mg for the preadolescent and adolescent years. During pregnancy and lactation, the allowance should be increased to 15 mg.

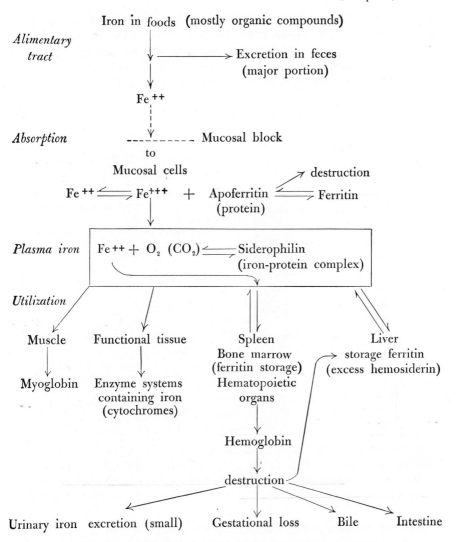

Fig. 8-4. Diagram showing the utilization of iron by the body.

Food sources of iron. From the basic diet pattern and from Figure 8-5, it will be seen that three of the Four Food Groups contribute significant and approximately equal amounts of iron. Milk, cheese, and ice cream are poor sources of iron, a fact which explains why iron-rich foods are introduced early into the infant's diet.

All varieties of liver are excellent sources of the blood-regenerating factors. Other organ meats, lean meats, shellfish, and egg yolk are good sources. Certain fruits such as peaches, apricots, prunes, grapes, and raisins are good sources if they are eaten fairly often. Green leafy vegetables, whole-grain and enriched cereals and breads, legumes, and dark molasses are also significant sources. The widespread enrichment of cereals and flours has been a decided factor in the improvement of the iron intake in recent years.

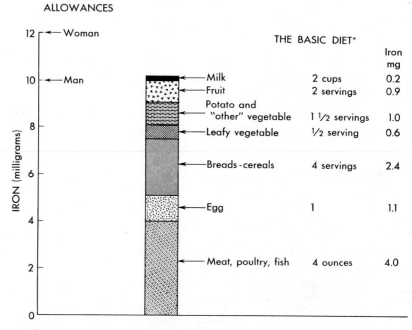

* See page 178 for complete calculations.

Fig. 8-5. The Four Food Groups of the Basic Diet fulfill the iron allowance for the man. Additional whole-grain or enriched cereals and breads are inexpensive ways to increase the intake. Note the contribution of the meat group and of a half serving of dark green leafy vegetable.

Effect of deficiency. An inadequate dietary intake of iron by growing children, by adolescent girls, or by women, especially during pregnancy and in lactation, will produce iron-deficiency anemia. If the pregnant woman has an insufficient intake of iron, the infant in turn will have a relatively low store of iron so that anemia develops early during the first year of life.

Iron-deficiency anemia may also occur even though the iron intake is normally adequate if excessive blood loss occurs or if there is faulty absorption because of gastric anacidity, intestinal disease, or diarrhea. The iron loss from blood donors is appreciable and may also lead to anemia unless appropriate measures are taken to replace iron as it is lost. A detailed discussion of anemias will be found in Chapter 38.

IODINE

Endemic goiter appears commonly in areas such as the states around the Great Lakes, the Pacific Northwest, Switzerland, Central American countries, mountainous areas of South America, New Zealand, and the Himalayas. The soil and water are so low in iodine that people living in these areas are unable to get sufficient iodine intake. Endemic goiter is not a major problem in the United States today because of the widespread prophylactic measures which have been taken in the last 40 years; but it, together with its sequel cretinism, is a serious menace in many countries of the world and constitutes a major concern of the World Health Organization.

Occurrence and function of iodine. Of the iodine in the adult body, variously estimated from 25 to 50 mg, about 5 to 20 mg are found in the thyroid gland. This represents a concentration about 2500 times as great as that in any other tissue. It is also distributed in the skin, muscles, bones, liver, blood, and other tissues.

The only known function of iodine is as a constituent of thyroxine, a hormone which regulates energy metabolism. Iodine absorbed from the gastrointestinal tract as the iodide ion is rapidly withdrawn from the circulation by the thyroid gland and is immediately incorporated into the amino acid tyrosine to form thyroxine. The hormone, in turn, is stored in a protein combination, thyroglobulin, in the thyroid gland. According to body need, it is released from the thyroglobulin into the circulation where it is again held in loose combination with protein. This protein-bound iodine increases or decreases with thyroid activity, so that the determination of its level in the blood plasma is often used to measure the functioning of the thyroid.

When thyroxine is used by the tissues, iodine is released into the circulation. About one-third of the iodine is again incorporated into new thyroxine, while the remainder is excreted in the urine. When the intake of iodine is inadequate, the stores are gradually depleted, and the thyroid gland enlarges in an attempt to produce the necessary amounts of thyroxine.

Requirement. The exact requirement for iodine has not been established, but on the basis of daily urinary losses an average allowance of 150 to 300 *0.15 —0.3 mg.* mcg is believed to be ample. Some investigators cite significantly lower levels. Since the thyroid gland stores iodine, larger amounts can be administered at intervals as in the studies of Marine and Kimball in which potassium iodide tablets were given during two periods of the year.[43]

Sources. People living in coastal areas who eat salt-water fish and shellfish regularly as well as locally produced foods may ingest enough iodine for their needs. However, foods cannot be relied upon for their iodine content since they may have been produced on iodine-poor soil. Iodized salt is the method of choice for supplying sufficient iodine intake because it is a universally used dietary item, the addition of iodine does not affect the flavor, and it is inexpensive. The concentration of iodide used in the United States is 1 part sodium or potassium iodide per 10,000 parts (0.01 per cent) of salt. Since the usual daily intake of salt is about 5 to 15 gm, the iodine intake would be 380 to 1140 mg.

At the present time, not more than half of the salt sold in the United States is iodized. It would appear that emphasis is again in order if an increase in goiter incidence is to be averted. The use of other sources of iodine is essential for patients receiving sodium-restricted diets. Amounts of iodine in excess of 1000 mcg daily have not been shown to be harmful.[44] Such amounts would be extremely unlikely except through medicinal sources.

Effects of deficiency. Iodine is the only nutrient for which a deficiency in the soil is known to have an adverse effect on human nutrition. The public health consequences of a lack of iodine in the food supply are endemic goiter, cretinism, increased incidence of thyrotoxicosis and of thyroid cancer.[45] Simple, or endemic, goiter is an enlargement of the thyroid gland, but with no other abnormal physical findings. The basal metabolism remains normal. The deficiency is more prevalent in females than in males, and is more frequent during adolescence and in pregnancy.

The studies of Marine and Kimball[43] on schoolgirls in Akron, Ohio, showed the importance of sufficient iodine intake in a striking manner. Over a period of 2½ years they found 495 cases of goiter among 2305 girls who received no supplementary iodine, but only 5 cases among 2190 girls who received sodium iodide.

The most urgent reason for stressing iodine as a preventive measure is not the goiter itself but the cretinism which is its ultimate sequel in areas severely deficient in iodine. Cretinism occurs in the infant when the pregnant woman is so severely depleted that she cannot supply iodine for the development of the fetus. Cretinism is characterized by a low basal metabolism, muscular flabbiness and weakness, dryness of the skin, arrest of skeletal development, and severe mental retardation. Desiccated thyroid given early enough to the infant results in marked improvement of physical development; mental retardation may be less severe, but any damage which has occurred to the central nervous system cannot be reversed. Endemic cretinism is rare or nonexistent in the United States today.[46]

Goitrogens. Certain substances in foods are known to interfere with the use of thyroxine and will produce goiters, at least in experimental animals, even though the iodine intake would normally be adequate. Such goitrogens are present in rutabagas,[47] peanuts—especially in the red skin,[48] and seeds of the *Brassica* family (cabbage, Brussels sprouts, cauliflower). The substances are inactivated by cooking, and there is currently no evidence that goiters in endemic regions are caused by them.

FLUORINE

Fluorine is a normal constituent of the body found primarily in the bones and teeth. Up to 3 mg fluorine are excreted daily by the kidneys and sweat glands, but excessive amounts may be deposited in the skeleton and teeth. Small amounts of fluorine bring about striking reductions in tooth decay.

If the drinking water contains fluorine somewhat in excess of 1.5 parts per 1,000,000 (1.5 ppm), mottling of the teeth occurs especially in the permanent teeth of children at the time of eruption. Instead of a lustrous appearance, the enamel of the teeth becomes dull and unglazed with some pitting. When the fluorine concentration of the water is greater than 2.5 ppm, the incidence increases, and the mottled areas of the teeth may become stained a dark brown. Such mottling is of common occurrence in certain areas of Texas and Colorado where the drinking water contains the higher concentrations of fluorine.

For some time it had been noted that mottled teeth were strikingly free of decay. For example, there were only 236 decayed, missing, and filled teeth per 100 children in Galesburg, Illinois, where the fluorine content of the water was 1.9 ppm. On the other hand, there were 1037 decayed, missing, and filled teeth per 100 children in Michigan City, Indiana, where the fluorine content of the water was only 1 ppm.[49]

The fluoridation of water is now an accepted public health measure in almost 4000 communities throughout the country. A concentration of fluorine of 1 ppm greatly reduces the incidence of dental caries, but does not lead to mottling of the teeth. The teeth of young children are benefited more than those of older children. It is doubtful whether there is a favorable effect on the teeth of adults.

Foods as well as water contain varying amounts of fluorine, milk, eggs, and fish being particularly important. The daily diet will provide 0.3 to 0.5 mg, while 6 glasses of water containing 1 ppm will provide an additional 1.2 mg. The amounts used in water and obtained from the diet are not great enough to produce toxic manifestations. Occasionally, the spray used for fruit trees has been a potential source of toxic amounts of fluorine. However, regulations of the Food and Drug Administration now restrict the concentrations within safe limits.

OTHER TRACE ELEMENTS

A number of trace elements are essential for the functioning of numerous enzymes. In some instances the trace elements are integral components of enzymes (metalloenzymes), and cannot be removed without inactivating the enzymes. In others, the mineral elements are held in loose combination with the enzymes (metal enzyme complex) but are not a constituent of the enzyme molecule; the trace elements thus exert catalytic activity.

Deficiencies of iron, iodine, and fluorine have been discussed. Dietary deficiencies of the other trace elements in human beings are virtually unknown since any reasonably good diet provides intakes in excess of body needs. One possible exception is the anemia which appears occasionally in infants fed an exclusive milk diet for many months and requires copper as well as iron for its correction.

Toxicities for some of the trace elements have been described in animals, but rarely for humans except by accidental contamination such as lead poisoning, an occupational hazard. There is no basis for the belief held by some that aluminum cooking vessels may be harmful.[50]

An outline of the nutritional roles of manganese, copper, cobalt, zinc, and molybdenum is presented on page 110. No functions have yet been ascribed to aluminum, arsenic, boron, lead, nickel, or silicon.

SODIUM, CHLORIDE, POTASSIUM, MAGNESIUM, AND SULFUR

Sodium. Practically all of the sodium of the body is found in the extracellular fluid; that is, in the blood plasma and in the fluid which bathes the tissues. It does not cross the cell membrane to any great extent. Sodium functions in the regulation of acid-base equilibrium, the maintenance of osmotic pressure and of water balance, muscle contraction, and nervous irritability.

Sodium is very readily absorbed from the small intestine, but the body content is kept within narrow limits since the kidney excretes any excess chiefly as sodium chloride or sodium phosphate. When the sodium intake is restricted, the kidney conserves body sodium by excreting very little. The amount of sodium which is excreted by the kidney is controlled by the adrenal cortical hormone. A deficiency of this hormone, as in Addison's disease, leads to an excessive loss of sodium in the urine; on the other hand, excessive therapy with the hormone may lead to sodium retention and accompanying edema. Estrogenic hormones also promote sodium retention, and this fact helps to explain the retention of water by some women before menstruation begins and during pregnancy.

Sodium is also lost from the body in the feces and from the skin, the latter loss being very considerable when one is perspiring profusely. Thus, additional intakes of sodium chloride may be necessary during hot weather until one becomes accustomed to the weather conditions.

The daily diet contains 2 to 6 gm or more of sodium, which is a liberal allowance under normal conditions. In fact, the requirement is probably considerably less except during acclimatization to extremely hot weather. Table salt is the chief source of sodium, but many foods are also high in sodium.

Among these are milk, cheese, meat, eggs, and some vegetables. A relatively high intake of sodium has not been shown to be harmful in health, since the body readily rids itself of any excess. In certain conditions such as cardiac failure and nephritis, sodium may be retained in the body, with the result that water is also held. Sodium-restricted diets (see Chap. 36) are widely used for these conditions.

Sodium deficiency is seen when there has been severe diarrhea, when the intake has been unduly restricted during hot weather, and in adrenal cortical insufficiency. It is characterized by poor appetite, abdominal and leg cramps, and disturbances in the acid-base balance.

Chlorine. Unlike sodium, the chloride ion readily crosses cell membranes and is found both within the cells and in the extracellular fluid. It occurs in the inorganic form as sodium chloride in extracellular fluid and as potassium chloride within the cell. It is one of the important acid elements for the regulation of acid-base balance, and it helps to maintain the osmotic pressure relationships in the body. Chlorine is a constituent of the acid in the stomach.

Like sodium, chlorine is readily absorbed and is excreted in relation to the intake. Much of the chlorine of the daily diet comes from table salt, the chlorine intake being approximately 3 to 9 gm from all sources including natural foods. Dietary deficiency is unlikely, but in prolonged vomiting chloride loss may become serious and replacement is necessary.

Potassium. Unlike sodium, potassium occurs primarily within the cell, muscle and red blood cells containing most of it. Potassium is essential, together with other mineral elements, in the contraction of muscle, regular heart rhythm, the conduction of the nerve impulse, and the maintenance of fluid balance. The daily intake of potassium ranges from 1.5 to 6.0 gm. Potassium is widely distributed in foods, meats containing especially liberal amounts (see Table 6, p. 776).

Dietary deficiency of potassium does not occur because of its generous distribution in foods. However, potassium deficiency may occur following prolonged failure to eat, and in certain pathologic conditions such as severe diarrhea, diabetic acidosis, excessive therapy with adrenocorticotropic hormone, tumors of the adrenal gland, and following surgery or injury accompanied by failure to eat. The deficiency is characterized by muscle weakness, loss of appetite, nausea and occasional vomiting, abdominal distention, nervous irritability, apathy, drowsiness, mental confusion, and irregular heart rhythm.

Potassium levels of the blood may increase to harmful levels in adrenal cortical deficiency (Addison's disease) and in renal failure. In these situations potassium is not excreted adequately and the action of the heart is adversely affected.

Magnesium. About 70 per cent of body magnesium is found in the bones in the form of phosphates and carbonates, but there are 100 to 200 times as much calcium as magnesium in bones. Muscles, on the other hand, contain about three times as much magnesium as calcium. Together with sodium, potassium, and calcium, magnesium functions in the regulation of cardiac, skeletal, muscle, and nervous tissues. Some of the enzymes concerned with carbohydrate metabolism are activated by magnesium.

Deficiency of magnesium in experimental animals leads to increased nervous irritability, rapid heartbeat, dilatation of the blood vessels, cessation of growth, severe kidney damage, and eventual death. No dietary deficiency has been described for man since this mineral is distributed in common food sources such as cereal grains, nuts, legumes, meat, milk, and fruit. The average daily diet provides about 300 mg magnesium. Magnesium deficiency symptoms have been described in chronic alcoholism with hepatic cirrhosis, severe renal disease, and following the extended administration of parenteral fluids without magnesium.

Sulfur. All body cells contain sulfur chiefly as a constituent of two amino acids—cystine and methionine. Cystine is important in skin, hair, and nails. Glutathione is an important sulfur-containing compound which functions in the biologic system of oxidation. Sulfur is also found in melanin pigments of skin and hair; in insulin, a hormone; in cartilage; and in numerous other body compounds. A diet adequate in protein will supply sufficient sulfur. Proteins contain roughly 1 per cent sulfur, this amount varying with the amount of sulfur-containing amino acids.

ACID-BASE BALANCE

One of the very important functions of minerals is to aid in the maintenance of the acid-base balance of the body. The acid-base condition is ultimately influenced by the food we eat.

The reaction of foods. Sodium, potassium, calcium, and magnesium are elements which in body fluids are cations; that is, they carry excess positive charges because they have lost electrons. Phosphorus (as phosphate), sulfur (as sulfate), and chlorine (as chloride) are elements which are anions; that is, they carry excess negative charges because they have accepted electrons. If there is an excess of cations remaining in the body on metabolism of a food, that food is said to produce an "alkaline ash" and the excess cations will allow the body to retain more bicarbonate ions, which will produce an alkaline reaction. Vegetables, fruits, milk, and some nuts will yield excess cations and lead to an alkaline state. On the other hand, meat, fish, poultry, eggs, cheese, cereals, and some nuts when metabolized yield an excess of anions that are not removed from the body immediately. These foods are said to produce an "acid ash." The excess anions carrying a negative charge must be balanced approximately with some cations. This yields an acid reaction because less bicarbonate, which also carries a negative charge, can exist in the body. The excess bicarbonate ions form carbonic acid increasing the acidity. Fats, sugar, and starches contain no mineral elements and are metabolized quickly to form water and carbon dioxide, which is rapidly removed from the body. These foods, therefore, do not form excess cations or anions which would disturb the neutrality regulation.

Although lemons, oranges, and certain other fruits contain some free organic acids which give them the taste of an acid (sour), they yield an alkaline ash because the body quickly oxidizes the anions of the acid to carbon dioxide and water and leaves excess cations which are removed more slowly from the body. Plums, cranberries, and prunes contain aromatic organic acids that are not metabolized in the body, and therefore they increase the acidity of the body fluids.

The alkalinity or acidity of a food can be stated in terms of the amount of normal acid or alkali to which it is equivalent. Commonly used foods have been classified as yielding an acid ash or an alkaline ash (see p. 533).

The regulation of body neutrality. The reaction of the body fluids is expressed by the term pH, which is a notation to indicate changes in the hydrogen concentration in the fluid. In an aqueous solution at room temperature where the concentration of the hydrogen ions (H^+) and hydroxyl ions (OH^-) are equal, the pH is designated as 7 and the solution is said to be neutral. An alkaline reaction is expressed as a pH higher than 7, and an acid reaction by a pH lower than 7. The pH of the blood in health is in the narrow range of 7.3 to 7.5; in other words, the blood is slightly alkaline. If the pH of the blood goes much below 7.3 an acidosis exists, while a pH above 7.5 indicates alkalosis.

The narrow range of pH in the body is maintained by the following mechanisms:

1. The presence of certain mixtures, called buffers, minimizes the change in pH when hydrogen ions are increased in the body fluids. They consist of weak acids in the presence of their sodium or potassium salts. The carbonic acid-bicarbonate (H_2CO_3-HCO_3^-) is one important buffer of the blood in maintaining the neutrality. The ease and speed with which the body can get rid of carbon dioxide obtained from this buffer mixture constitute one of the first lines of defense. The plasma bicarbonate is an indicator of the alkaline reserve of the body. Serious disturbances may occur if the alkaline reserve is depleted to a low level. Proteins, including hemoglobin in the blood, and phosphates also form important buffer mixtures.

2. Besides its buffer action hemoglobin aids in the transport of carbon dioxide in two ways which prevent great changes in reaction. The acid strength of hemoglobin is decreased when oxyhemoglobin loses oxygen whereby an extra amount of carbon dioxide can be transported without any change of reaction (isohydric transport). Hemoglobin can also transport a limited amount of carbon dioxide by forming a carbamate, which releases most of

(*Text continued on p. 111.*)

SUMMARY OF THE MINERALS

MINERAL	FUNCTIONS IN THE BODY	METABOLISM	FOOD SOURCES	DAILY ALLOWANCES
Calcium	Builds bones and teeth Muscle contraction Normal heart rhythm Nerve irritability Activation of some enzymes Most abundant mineral element in the body	*Absorption:* according to body need; aided by vitamin D, ascorbic acid, lactose; oxalic acid and phytic acid interfere *Utilization* regulated by parathyroid hormone and vitamin D *Storage* in bone trabeculae *Excretion:* feces, chiefly *Deficiency:* retarded bone and tooth mineralization; fragile bones; stunted growth; rickets; osteomalacia; osteoporosis	*Best* Milk Hard cheese Greens: turnip, collards, kale, mustard *Good* Ice cream Cottage cheese Broccoli Oysters, shrimp Salmon, clams	Children: 1.0 to 1.2 gm Teenagers: 1.3 to 1.4 gm Adults: 0.8 gm Pregnancy: 1.5 gm Lactation: 2.0 gm
Iron	Constituent of hemoglobin, myoglobin, and oxidative enzymes Present in all body cells	*Absorption:* according to body need; aided by gastric acidity, ascorbic acid *Utilization:* copper is essential; iron from worn-out cells used over again *Storage* in liver, bone marrow, spleen, kidneys *Excretion:* minute amounts in urine, sweat; most of fecal iron is unabsorbed iron from the diet *Deficiency:* reduced hemoglobin level—anemia	*Best* Liver *Good* Meat, egg yolk Enriched bread and cereals Peaches, apricots, prunes, raisins Dark green vegetables Molasses Legumes	Children: 7 to 15 mg Men: 10 mg Women: 12 mg Pregnancy: 15 mg Lactation: 15 mg
Iodine	Constituent of thyroxine which regulates rate of energy exchange	*Storage:* thyroid gland *Excretion:* in urine *Deficiency:* simple goiter with enlarged thyroid; cretinism—very rare in United States	Iodized salt is best protection Sea foods and foods grown in nongoitrous regions	Adults: 0.15 to 0.30 mg

Mineral	Functions	Metabolism	Food Sources	Daily Requirement
Phosphorus	Builds bones and teeth Buffer salts Metabolism of fat and carbohydrate Activates some enzymes Transport of fatty acids *BSF EF*	*Absorption:* aided by vitamin D; about ⅓ lost in feces *Utilization:* about 80 per cent in bones *Excretion:* in urine *Deficiency:* poor mineralization of bones; poor growth; rickets	Milk; cheese Egg yolk Meat, fish, fowl Legumes; nuts Whole-grain cereals	Children: 1.0 gm Adults: 1.2 gm Pregnancy: 1.5 gm
Potassium	Intracellular fluid balance Regular heart rhythm Regulates nervous and muscular irritability *F H I*	*Excretion:* urine, perspiration *Deficiency:* not of dietary lack, but occurs following starvation, diabetic acidosis, adrenal tumors; muscle weakness, nausea, tachycardia, glycogen depletion	Meat, fish, fowl Cereals Fruits; vegetables	Diet adequate in protein, calcium, and iron contains enough potassium
Sodium	Regulates osmotic pressure Buffer salts Maintains water balance Regulates muscle and nerve irritability *P S W I*	*Absorption:* readily absorbed *Excretion:* parallels intake; controlled by adrenal cortical hormone; chiefly by kidneys; losses in perspiration high in warm weather *Deficiency:* nausea, diarrhea, muscular cramps	Table salt Meat, fish, fowl Milk Eggs Sodium compounds such as baking soda and baking powder	Probably about 0.5 gm; diet contains 2–6 gm or more
Chlorine	Regulates osmotic pressure Constituent of gastric juice Acid-base balance *P G A*	Readily absorbed Excretion in urine parallels intake Prolonged vomiting may lead to deficiency	Table salt Meat Milk Eggs	Probably about 0.5 gm Daily diet contains 3–9 gm
Sulfur	Constituent of hair and nails, insulin, glutathione, cartilage, and melanin	Excess eliminated in urine as sulfates	Eggs Cheese; milk Meat Nuts; legumes	Diet adequate in protein will contain enough sulfur
Magnesium	Constituent of bones, teeth Activates enzymes in carbohydrate metabolism Muscle and nerve irritability *B C L*	Dietary deficiency not known in man Deficiency observed in alcoholism with cirrhosis; severe renal disease	Cereals; nuts Legumes Meat Milk	Daily diet provides ample—about 300 mg

SUMMARY OF THE MINERALS

MINERAL	FUNCTIONS IN THE BODY	METABOLISM	FOOD SOURCES	DAILY ALLOWANCES
Manganese	Thyroxine formation Formation of urea Related to lipotropic activity of choline Essential for utilization of thiamine, and metabolism of carbohydrate	Liver is most active organ of metabolism Absorption is limited; elimination chiefly by intestine	Whole-grain cereals Legumes Meat, fish, fowl Green leafy vegetables	About 0.3 mg per kg
Copper	Absorption and metabolism of iron; normal hemoglobin synthesis Oxidation of fatty acids Oxidation of tyrosine to melanin pigments Metabolism of ascorbic acid	Stored in liver and central nervous system Excreted by bile into intestine Deficiency leads to retarded hemoglobin production; occurs rarely Abnormal storage in Wilson's disease	Liver, oysters Meat, fish Nuts, legumes Whole-grain cereals	About 2 mg
Zinc	Effects transfer of carbon dioxide from tissues to lungs Constituent of digestive enzyme for hydrolysis of proteins	Found in liver, muscles, bones, and organs Excreted chiefly from intestine	Widely distributed Oysters; sea food Liver Wheat germ Yeast	About 0.3 mg per kg or less Usual intake is 10–15 mg
Cobalt	Structural component of vitamin B_{12}	Readily absorbed Little body storage Excreted in urine Diet must contain vitamin B_{12} since body cannot synthesize it		Not known
Molybdenum	Conversion of purines to uric acid			Not known

this carbon dioxide from the hemoglobin complex at the lung as the hemoglobin takes up oxygen.

3. The final adjustment to keep the body fluids within narrow pH limits is made by the kidney. The kidney is able to secrete an acid urine (pH as low as 4.5; average normal pH 6.0) and also can synthesize the ammonium ion with a positive charge which is excreted in place of other cations (sodium and potassium) which can be returned to the blood to carry more carbon dioxide as a bicarbonate ion.

Because the body makes these adjustments in the regulation of body neutrality, the reaction of the diet is of no practical significance in health. Those who become concerned about the relative acidity or alkalinity of foods have often been misled by false advertising claims of the food quack.

PROBLEMS AND REVIEW

1. Calcium and phosphorus are the two minerals occurring in largest amounts in the body. What other minerals are to be found in the body? Which of these require special planning in the diet? Under what conditions is it unnecessary to calculate allowances for the others?

2. Almost all of the calcium and phosphorus in the body are found in the bones and teeth. Name three other functions of calcium; of phosphorus. What factors affect the utilization of these minerals?

3. In selecting food for its mineral content one must consider the availability of the mineral, the amount present in the food, the frequency with which the food is used, and possible losses during cookery. How does milk rate in each of these respects?

4. *Problem.* Plan a diet for yourself which contains sufficient calcium without the use of milk or cheese. List the amounts of food and calculate the calcium content.

5. Many adults believe that their needs for calcium are low because their bones and teeth are fully developed. Explain why this reasoning is wrong.

6. While phosphorus is as important in the diet as calcium, there have been no dietary allowances listed by the Food and Nutrition Board. Why is such listing unnecessary?

7. Iron is necessary for the formation of blood and muscle hemoglobin. What factors affect the construction of hemoglobin in the body?

8. Iron is essentially a one-way substance. What does this mean? How does this fact affect the daily requirement for iron?

9. *Problem.* Calculate your daily intake of iron for 2 days. List the four outstanding sources for each day.

10. Iodine is a necessary constituent of thyroxine which regulates energy metabolism. What happens if iodine intake is inadequate?

11. Give three ways in which iodine intake can be made more adequate. Which is the most reliable?

12. Fluorine appears to be important in the prevention of tooth decay. How can fluorine intake be increased? What are the dangers of excessive fluorine intake?

13. What are the functions of copper, sulfur, sodium, potassium, magnesium, and chlorine in the body? How are these elements provided?

14. Sodium, potassium, calcium, and magnesium are the important basic elements in the diet. In which foods do these elements predominate?

15. Phosphorus, chlorine, and sulfur are the important acidic elements in the diet. In which foods do these elements predominate?

16. Acid-tasting fruits, except for cranberries and plums, are actually basic in reaction. How do you explain this?

17. The reaction of the blood and body tissues is in the narrow range of pH 7.3 to 7.5. How is this reaction maintained in the body? What happens if a diet which is acid in reaction is eaten? How does the urine give a clue to the reaction of a diet?

CHAPTER 9

The Fat-Soluble Vitamins

INTRODUCTION TO THE STUDY OF THE VITAMINS

The story of the vitamins—their discovery, their positive functions in maintaining health, and their usefulness in healing deficiency diseases—is fascinating and deserving of considerable study. Popular interest was early aroused by the discovery of the role of vitamins in preventing such severe deficiency diseases as scurvy, pellagra, beriberi, and others. It is now known that vitamins function primarily in enzyme systems which facilitate the metabolism of amino acids, fats, and carbohydrates. Those who understand the functions of vitamins do not minimize their importance in relation to the utilization of food. However, it is important that no one be misled into believing that vitamins are "cure-alls" for disease.

A brief discussion of the discovery of vitamins has been presented in Chapter 2. The properties of vitamins, their functions in metabolism, their distribution in foods, and the effects of deficiency will be discussed in the sections below.

Definition and nomenclature. The term "vitamine" was first coined by the Polish chemist, Funk, who believed that the water-soluble antiberiberi substance he was describing was a "vital amine." The final "e" was soon dropped, but *vitamins* is the name given to a group of potent organic compounds other than protein, carbohydrate, and fat which occur in minute quantities in foods and which are essential for some specific body functions of maintenance and growth. Many of them cannot be synthesized, at least in adequate amounts, by the body and must be obtained from the diet.

Early classifications listed two groups of vitamins, namely, those which are water soluble and those which are fat soluble. This classification has been generally accepted, but it is arbitrary inasmuch as the vitamins within each group are not necessarily similar nor always related to one another in their properties, functions, or distribution. Vitamins were first named for their curative properties or were given a convenient letter designation. Today, chemically descriptive names are now used for many of the vitamins; letter designations are still applied in some instances.

The B complex is a group of vitamins, each having distinct physical and chemical properties and functions. Consequently, one must use specific nomenclature for each member of the complex if there is to be clear differentiation.

Measurement. Before the chemical nature of vitamins was discovered, their potency could be measured only by their ability to promote growth or to cure a deficiency when test doses were fed experimental animals such as rats, guinea pigs, pigeons, and chicks. Such measurement is known as "bioassay," and has been expressed in terms of units. Vitamins A and D are still measured in international units (I.U.). Other vitamins, formerly measured in units, are now measured by chemical assay in milligrams (mg) or micrograms (mcg), 1 milligram being equal to 1000 micrograms or gamma (γ). Still other vitamins are measured by their ability to promote growth of microorganisms; this is known as microbiologic assay.

Selection of foods for vitamin content. In selecting the foods to furnish vitamins in the diet it is well to keep in mind the following points: (1) under normal circumstances it is better to use common food sources than concentrates, because foods furnish other essential factors as well; (2) it is important to determine how often any given food will be used in the dietary; (3) the amount of food which would ordinarily be used must be ascertained; (4) the effects of processing and preparation of foods on the vitamin retention must be clearly understood; and (5) economic factors such as availability and cost must be considered. For example, 100 gm of parsley furnish about 8200 I.U. of vitamin A, whereas 100 gm of milk supply only 160 I.U. of vitamin A. Parsley, as a garnish, will have limited use, while 1 pint of milk a day, essential in an adequate diet, furnishes about 10 per cent of the day's needs for vitamin A. Potatoes cooked in their skins or baked may be a significant source of ascorbic acid; but left over mashed potatoes cannot be relied upon for this easily destroyed vitamin.

Vitamin supplementation of the diet. In the discussion which follows it will become evident that any diet which is selected on the basis of the Four Food Groups will provide a substantial amount of the necessary vitamins. When further food selections are made at least in part from these food groups to complete the caloric requirement, the recommended allowances for the vitamins are easily met or exceeded. Vitamin pills and other forms of concentrates are, therefore, not necessary in the diets of healthy persons. As a matter of fact, the water-soluble vitamins in excess of body needs will be excreted in the urine. Vitamin A, being fat soluble, is stored in appreciable amounts in the liver; other fat-soluble vitamins are stored to a lesser degree.

Vitamin-D supplementation for infants, growing children, pregnant or lactating women is an important exception to the above statements. Vitamin supplementation is essential during emotional or physical illness when an individual may be restricted in the quality or quantity of food which can be eaten, or when absorption may be impaired. The need for such supplementation will be noted in the discussion of therapeutic diets; for example, in certain allergies, or in long-continued use of low-residue diets.

When it is known that a diet is seriously deficient in vitamins through ignorance or poor eating habits, a physician may recommend vitamin supplements to correct such dietary deficiencies. However, such supplementation should never replace efforts toward the correction of the factors leading to the dietary inadequacy.

VITAMIN A

Vitamin A was the first fat-soluble vitamin to be discovered. It was soon found to be in some way related to chlorophyll, the green coloring matter of plants, and by 1932 carotene, which occurs abundantly in yellow vegetables and in thin dark-green leaves, had been shown to be the *precursor,* or mother substance, of vitamin A.

Chemistry and characteristics. Vitamin A in its pure form is a pale yellow crystalline compound with a chemical formula of $C_{20}H_{29}OH$. Vitamin A occurs naturally only in the animal kingdom, but it has been synthesized and is now available commercially. It is soluble in fat but insoluble in water, and it is relatively stable to heat and to acids and alkalies. However, it is easily oxidized.

The ultimate source of all vitamin A is in the carotenes which are synthesized by plants. Animals in turn, and man as well, convert a considerable proportion of the carotene of the foods they eat into vitamin A. The carotenes are dark red crystalline compounds and are known as the "provitamins" or precursors of vitamin A. Alpha-, beta-, and gamma-carotene, and possibly cryptoxanthin are of nutritional significance. Each molecule of beta-carotene $(C_{40}H_{56})$ yields 2 molecules of vitamin A, while each molecule of the other three carotenes yields on hydrolysis only 1 molecule of vitamin A.

Measurement. Vitamin A is measured in international units, 1 unit being defined by the World Health Organization as the vitamin-A activity of 0.344 mcg of pure vitamin-A acetate (0.300 mcg crystalline vitamin-A alcohol) or 0.600 mcg pure beta-carotene. The U.S.P. (*United States Pharmacopoeia*) unit is identical with the international unit.

The vitamin-A concentration in foods and in body tissues may be determined by chemical methods or by the determination of growth rates when a given amount of the substance being tested is fed to rats.

Physiology. Vitamin A is more rapidly absorbed than like amounts of carotene, but the absorption of both is facilitated in the presence of fats. Bile is necessary for the absorption of carotene, but it apparently is not required by vitamin A. Like fats, vitamin A is absorbed largely into the lacteals and enters the general circulation by way of the thoracic duct.

Any factors which limit fat absorption are likely to minimize absorption of vitamin A as well. Liquid petrolatum taken immediately before or after meals interferes with the absorption of carotene, and therefore mineral oil should be used only with a doctor's prescription. Carotene is especially subject to oxidation in the intestinal tract. The presence of vitamin E helps to prevent this destruction.

The body possesses a great capacity for storing vitamin A, about 95 per cent of storage deposits being held in the liver. Small amounts are also to be found in the kidneys, lungs, and occasionally in the fatty tissues. The reserves in the liver are relatively small at birth but increase gradually with age if the diet has been good. The conversion of the precursor carotene to vitamin A occurs primarily in the walls of the small intestine, and perhaps to a lesser degree in the liver.

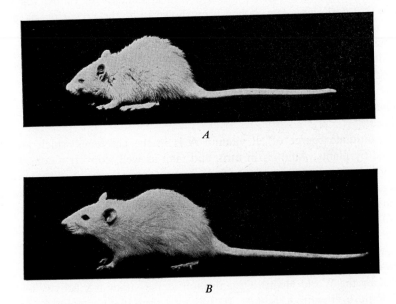

Fig. 9-1. Effect of vitamin A on growth and health. (*A*) Diet adequate except for vitamin A. (*B*) Vitamin A added to the same diet. Litter mates of the same sex, 11 weeks old. Weight of smaller, 56 gm; of larger, 123 gm. Note infected eye, rough fur, and lack of vigor in smaller rat. (*Courtesy, Bureau of Home Economics, U.S. Department of Agriculture.*)

Functions. All vitamins are necessary for growth. Consequently, no single vitamin can be termed the "growth" vitamin (see Fig. 9-1). Vitamin A seems to be especially important for skeletal growth and for normal tooth structure. It is needed for a somewhat different purpose than vitamin D, which is also essential for normal skeletal development. From work on experimental animals, it is apparent that normal reproduction and lactation cannot take place without vitamin A.

The most clearly established function of vitamin A is that related to the maintenance of normal vision in dim light. The mode of action is that of combining vitamin A with a protein to form visual purple (rhodopsin), an essential constituent of the retina of the eye. The visual purple absorbs light and is decomposed to *retinene* (vitamin A aldehyde) and a protein. The protein and retinene may recombine partially to form rhodopsin again. However, some of the vitamin A is lost so that a fresh supply is essential if complete and rapid regeneration is to take place.

Vitamin A is also essential for the integrity of the epithelium, especially that of the mucous membranes which line the eyes, the mouth and related glands, and the gastrointestinal, respiratory, and genitourinary tracts.

Daily allowances. The Recommended Dietary Allowances [2] have been set at levels which provide approximately double the minimal requirements. These allowances also assume that two-thirds of the vitamin will be supplied by the carotenes and one-third will be available from the preformed vitamin. The adult allowance has been set at 5000 I.U.; if the only dietary source is the provitamin, 6000 I.U. would be desirable, but 3000 I.U. would suffice if available from the preformed vitamin.[2]

A greater amount of vitamin A is needed per unit of body weight in children than in adults. Infants should receive 1500 I.U. daily, while the allowances for older children increase gradually to 5000 I.U. by the adolescent age. In pregnancy and lactation the allowances are 6000 I.U. and 8000 I.U., respectively.

Food sources. Only animal foods contain vitamin A as such, fish-liver oils being outstanding. These oils are generally not classed with common foods, but milk, butter, fortified margarines, whole-milk cheeses, liver, and egg yolk contain vitamin A. Milk from cows which have been eating green foliage usually contains more vitamin A than that from cows which have been eating dried fodder.

The principal source of vitamin A in the diet is likely to be from the carotenes which are widespread in those plant foods which have high green or yellow colorings. There is a direct correlation between the greenness of a leaf and its carotene content. Dark green leaves are rich in carotene, but the pale leaves, in lettuce and cabbage for example, are insignificant sources. Abundant sources of carotene are found in foods such as:

Green leafy vegetables—spinach, turnip tops, chard, beet greens
Green stem vegetables—asparagus, broccoli
Yellow vegetables—carrots, sweet potatoes, winter squash, pumpkin
Yellow fruits—apricots, peaches, cantaloupe

The vitamin-A contribution of the Four Food Groups is indicated in Figure 9-2. It should be noted that the meat group contributes only when liver is included every week to 10 days. One egg provides about one-tenth of the daily allowance.

Retention of food values. Since vitamin A is stable to the usual cooking temperatures, only slight losses are likely to occur in food preparation in the home. A long, slow cooking is more destructive than short, rapid cooking. Stirring of foods increases the rate of oxidation somewhat. The wilting of vegetables or dehydration of foods results in considerable losses. Canned and frozen foods retain maximal values for 9 months or longer. Vitamin-A activity is quickly lost in rancid fats.

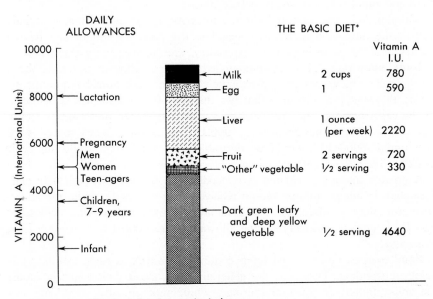

* See page 178 for complete calculations.

Fig. 9-2. The Four Food Groups of the Basic Diet provide a liberal allowance of vitamin A for all categories of persons. Note the contribution made by dark green leafy and deep yellow vegetables, and 1 ounce liver each week. Breads, cereals, and white potato do not provide vitamin A.

Effects of vitamin-A deficiency. In the United States vitamin-A deficiency resulting from faulty diet is not of frequent occurrence. The exact incidence of mild deficiency states is not known since it is difficult to establish a specific etiology for such conditions as night blindness. The severe manifestations of vitamin-A deficiency, xerophthalmia and keratomalacia, are not seen in this country, but are not infrequent, even today, in India and other countries of the Orient where grossly inadequate diets are the rule.

Vitamin-A deficiency may result from faulty absorption and metabolism such as chronic diarrhea as in sprue and colitis, liver disease, abnormal fat metabolism as in pancreatic dysfunction, or incomplete absorption because of the use of liquid petrolatum. Depending upon the reserves in the liver, vitamin-A deficiency may not be manifested for weeks or months.

Night blindness. One of the earliest signs of vitamin-A deficiency is night blindness, or nyctalopia (see Fig. 9-3). This is a condition in which the individual is unable to see well in dim light, especially on coming into darkness from a bright light as in entering a darkened theater. Drivers who are easily blinded (glare blindness) by the headlights of other automobiles and who consequently see road markers, pedestrians, etc., with difficulty constitute a special traffic hazard. Nyctalopia occurs when there is insufficient vitamin A to bring about prompt and complete regeneration of visual purple from visual yellow. Dark-adaptation tests with a biophotometer, blood carotene and vitamin-A levels, and a substantiating dietary history are useful in establishing a diagnosis of vitamin-A deficiency. Other causes of night blindness must be ruled out. If a therapeutic dose of vitamin A does not bring about relief of night blindness after a few weeks trial, it may be assumed that the condition is not a vitamin-A deficiency.

Epithelial changes. An inadequate supply of vitamin A may lead to definite changes in the epithelial tissues throughout the body: *keratinization,* or a noticeable shrinking, hardening, and progressive degeneration of the cells occurs, which increases the susceptibility to severe infections of the eye, the nasal passages, the sinuses, middle ear, lungs, and genitourinary tract. While sufficient vitamin A is essential for the maintenance of the normal epithelium, it should be remembered that increased amounts of this vitamin do not confer additional protective benefits to the epithelium; thus, the use of large doses of vitamin A as an "anti-infective" substance is unwarranted.

Skin changes in severe vitamin-A deficiency have been described, but it is doubtful that there is such a relationship to skin conditions observed in this country. In severe deficiency the skin becomes rough, dry, and scaly. The keratinized epithelium plugs the sebaceous glands so that goose-pimplelike follicles appear first along the upper forearms and thighs, and then spread along the shoulders, back, abdomen, and buttocks.

Epithelial changes in the eye. The epithelium of the eye may be so profoundly affected during vitamin-A deficiency that the condition finally becomes irreversible. The first mild symptoms of epithelial changes in the eye are sensitivity to bright light (photophobia), itching, burning, and sometimes inflammation of the lids. The eyes and the eyelids become dry and inflamed owing to impairment of the lacrymal glands whose function it is to secrete fluid to keep the surfaces moist and wash away bacteria and other foreign agents. *Xerophthalmia* is the most serious disturbance in the eye and occurs only after deficiency has been severe and prolonged. The cornea becomes dry and then inflamed and edematous. This is later followed by cloudiness and infection which leads to ulceration. The absence of the usual eye secretions provides a favorable medium for infection. The final stages of the disease,

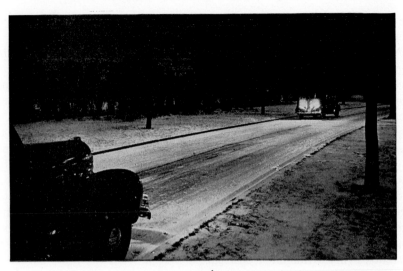

A

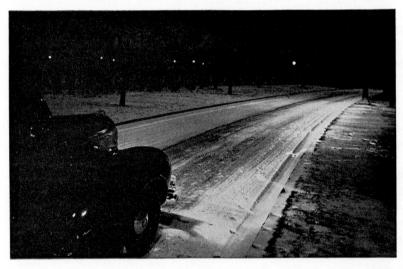

B

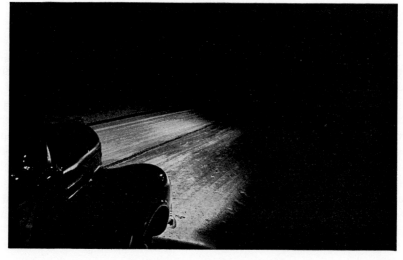

C

Fig. 9-3. Night blindness. (*A*) Safe driving at night depends, in part, on the ability of one's eyes to adjust to the glare of lights. (*B*) Properly focused headlights of an approaching automobile do not impede a good view of the road when the eye has an adequate supply of vitamin A. (*C*) The edge of the road and distances far ahead cannot be seen immediately after meeting an automobile when there is insufficient vitamin A available to the eye. (*Courtesy, The Upjohn Company, Kalamazoo, Mich.*)

keratomalacia, is a softening of the cornea with permanent blindness resulting.

Prevention and treatment. The recommended allowances for vitamin A fully protect against the evidences of vitamin-A deficiency when the absorption and metabolism are normal. Once the deficiency has appeared, therapy consists in (1) correcting the diet so that it again becomes normal, (2) removing or curing any condition which interferes with effective utilization of food, and (3) prescribing therapeutic doses of vitamin concentrates—often 25,000 to 50,000 I.U. daily for a period of time.

Toxicity of vitamin A. Therapeutic doses of vitamin A in excess of 50,000 I.U. over prolonged periods may be toxic. The symptoms of *hypervitaminosis* are observed more frequently in children than in adults. In one case reported in the literature, a 2-year-old child had been given by his mother, through error, 2 teaspoonfuls of percomorph oil with viosterol daily.[51] The symptoms of toxicity include loss of appetite, failure to grow, drying and cracking of the skin, loss of hair, swelling and pain of the long bones, enlargement of the liver and spleen, and bone fragility. When the vitamin A is discontinued, recovery takes place. Nevertheless, it is important to realize that concentrates of vitamin A must be given in carefully controlled dosages.

VITAMIN D

Cod-liver oil has been recommended as a remedy for rickets ever since the Middle Ages but does not appear to have been used with any consistency until the present century. During World War I, Doctors Hess and Unger noted the effect of cod-liver oil in protecting Negro children in New York City against rickets. Then in 1919 Mellanby found that the skeletal structure of puppies was influenced by some fat-soluble substance in food. McCollum, Steenbock, and Drummond simultaneously reported that cod-liver oil in which vitamin A had been destroyed still retained its antirachitic properties, and hence it was shown that vitamin A was not the antirachitic factor. Steenbock and Hess in 1924 independently found that foods which had been exposed to ultraviolet rays possessed antirachitic properties. Pure vitamin D was isolated in crystalline form in 1930 and was called calciferol ($C_{28}H_{43}OH$).

Chemistry and characteristics. Vitamin D is in reality a group of chemically distinct sterol compounds possessing antirachitic properties, but it is customary to speak of the group as though it were one vitamin. The vitamins are produced by irradiating a precursor or provitamin D with ultraviolet light; in other words, substances like ergosterol are exposed to ultraviolet light to form calciferol. Of the 10 or more forms of this vitamin which are known, only 2 are of nutritional interest: (1) vitamin D_2 (activated ergosterol, calciferol, viosterol)—ergosterol being the chief vitamin-D precursor found in plants; and (2) vitamin D_3 (activated 7-dehydrocholesterol)—the chief form occurring in fish-liver oils. Vitamin D_3 is believed to be the substance developed in the skin on exposure to ultraviolet light from sunshine or from a machine. Pure vitamins D are white, odorless crystals which are soluble in fats and in fat solvents. They are insoluble in water, and they are stable to heat, acids, alkalies, and oxidation.

Measurement. One international unit (I.U.) of vitamin D is the activity of 0.025 mcg of pure crystalline vitamin D. The I.U. and U.S.P. unit are identical.

Rachitic rats are the standard test animals for measuring the potency of vitamin D in materials. Young rats from mothers having a deficient supply of vitamin D are kept on a rachitogenic diet so that no calcification occurs in the ends of the long bones. When a test material is fed, its value as a source of vitamin D is measured by the amount which must be fed for 7 to 10 days to produce a good calcium line (line test) in the ends of the long bones. Standard cod-liver oil is fed to a similar group of animals and is used as a basis of comparison. No satisfactory chemical or microbiologic assay is yet available.

Physiology. Vitamin D from the dietary or from concentrates is absorbed from the intestine together with the fats. Bile salts appear to be necessary for absorption. Man can synthesize provitamin D_3 in the body, and activation takes place in the skin on exposure to ultraviolet light. Vitamin D_3 from the skin or vitamin D_2 absorbed from the intestine is stored primarily in the liver, although some is also found in the skin, brain, lungs, spleen, and bones. The body conserves its stores of vitamin D carefully.

Function. While the exact manner in which vitamin D works is not known, it has been established that it regulates the absorption and anchorage of calcium and phosphorus. Vitamin D presumably renders the intestinal membranes more permeable to calcium salts so that absorption is facilitated.[52] It also regulates the level of the enzyme *alkaline phosphatase* in the serum; this enzyme is believed to be concerned with the deposition of calcium phosphate in the bones and teeth. While optimal intake of vitamin D does not decrease the daily need for calcium, the vitamin does assist in the maximal utilization of the calcium.

Daily allowances. Whenever new skeletal tissue is being built, there is a definite increase in the need for vitamin D. This is especially marked in premature infants, in twins, and in infants who are underdeveloped. For infants, growing and adolescent children, and pregnant and lactating women, 400 I.U. of vitamin D are recommended.[2] This allowance is also believed to be satisfactory for premature infants.

The daily diet furnishes such a very small amount of vitamin D that it must be assumed either that the need for it in adults is low, or that the requirements are met by exposure to sunlight. For persons who work at night, or invalids, elderly persons, and others who may not be exposed to sunlight, an intake of 400 I.U. of vitamin D may be desirable.

Sources. Natural foods are poor sources of vitamin D, although small amounts are present in egg yolk, liver, and fish such as herring, sardines, tuna, and salmon. Milk may be fortified by adding concentrates of vitamin D. Almost all evaporated milk and much of the fresh whole milk is now fortified, the level being 400 I.U. per quart. Milk is an especially suitable source of vitamin D since it contains the calcium and phosphorus whose absorption it facilitates and because it is an important food consumed by growing children. Fortification of other foods does not appear to be necessary nor desirable.

Fish-liver oils (cod, halibut, percomorph, and others) provide the most potent source of the vitamin and should be included daily for growing children and pregnant and lactating women if fortified milk is not used. The concentration of vitamin D in these oils is indicated in the labeling of these products, and should be carefully noted in prescribing and dosing in order that excess may be avoided.

Sunlight cannot always be depended upon to supply the body with adequate ultraviolet rays to manufacture vitamin D, because these rays are so easily strained out by dust, smoke, fog, clothing, and ordinary window glass—all of which act as barriers to prevent the rays from reaching the skin.

Hypervitaminosis D. The tolerance for vitamin D varies widely. As little as 1800 I.U. over a long period of time may be mildly toxic to children,[53] while massive doses of 100,000 I.U. may be necessary and tolerated by those rare individuals who have refractory rickets. Generally speaking, daily doses of 20,000 to 50,000 I.U. may be toxic for children when continued for weeks or months, while intakes of 100,000 I.U. for similar periods may be expected to have adverse effects for adults. The amount of calcium in the diet, the exposure to ultraviolet light, and the endocrine secretions may influence the toxicity. The symptoms of toxicity are first manifest as nausea, diarrhea, weight loss, polyuria, and nocturia. Fatigue, renal damage, and calcification of the soft tissues such as the heart, blood vessels, bronchi, stomach, and tubules of the kidney occur later.

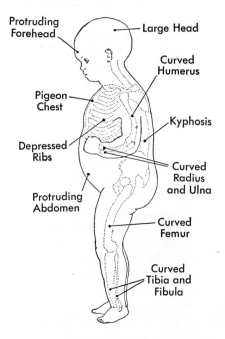

Fig. 9-4. The symptoms of rickets. (Harris, L. J.: *Vitamins,* 3rd ed. The Cambridge University Press, New York, 1938.)

Effects of vitamin-D deficiency. A deficiency of vitamin D leads to inadequate absorption of calcium and phosphorus from the intestinal tract and to faulty mineralization of bone and tooth structures. The inability of the soft bones to withstand the stress of weight results in skeletal malformations.

Rickets. Infantile rickets is rarely seen in the United States because of the widespread use of fortified milk or of fish-liver oils in prophylaxis. When such preventive measures are not taken, rickets is more prevalent in northern regions than in warm, sunny climates. It is more likely to develop in dark, overcrowded sections of large cities where the ultraviolet rays of sunshine, especially in the winter months, cannot penetrate through the fog, smoke, and soot. Poverty and ignorance may account for failure to obtain enough vitamin D from concentrates, fortified milk, or from skin exposure. Dark-skinned children are more susceptible to rickets than those of the white race.

Early rickets is difficult to diagnose, but fully developed cases present the following characteristic signs and symptoms (see Figs. 9-4 and 9-5):

1. Delayed closure of the fontanelles, softening of the skull (craniotabes),

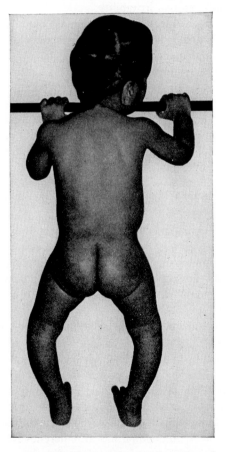

Fig. 9-5. Early skeletal deformities of rickets often persist throughout life. Bow-legs that curve laterally, as shown here, indicate that the weakened bones have bent after the second year, as the result of standing. (*Courtesy, Dr. Rosa Lee Nemir, professor of pediatrics, New York University—Bellevue Medical Center, and* The Vitamin Manual, *published by The Upjohn Company.*)

and bulging or bossing of the forehead, giving the head a boxlike appearance

2. Soft fragile bones leading to widening of the ends of the long bones; bowing of the legs; enlargement of the costochondral junction with rows of knobs or beads forming the *rachitic rosary;* projection of the sternum as in "pigeon breast"; narrowing of the pelvis; spinal curvature

3. Enlargement of wrist, knee (knock knees), and ankle joints

4. Poorly developed muscles; lack of muscle tone—pot belly—being the result of weakness of abdominal muscles; weakness, with delayed walking

5. Restlessness and nervous irritability

6. High serum phosphatase; lowered inorganic blood phosphorus

Rickets is treated by giving relatively large amounts of vitamin-D concentrates, the dosage being prescribed by the physician.

Tetany. "Tetany is a syndrome manifested by a sharp flexion of the wrists and ankle joints, muscle twitchings, cramps, and convulsions. It is due to abnormal calcium phosphorus metabolism." * Tetany may result from insufficient dietary calcium or vitamin D, from failure of absorption of calcium or vitamin D, or from a disturbance of the parathyroid gland. The physician prescribes calcium salts to control the acute spasms, a diet liberal in calcium, and vitamin-D concentrates.

Dental caries. A deficiency of vitamin D may lead to delayed dentition and to malformation of the teeth. There may be a predisposition to dental caries. It has been shown that children who have received an abundance of milk, eggs, meat, vegetables, and fruits and who have consistently had liberal intakes of vitamin D have fewer carious lesions than do children on suboptimal intakes.[54] Thus, protection against dental caries would seem to depend, at least in part, on adequate intakes and utilization of calcium, phosphorus, and vitamin D. The influence of fluoride has been discussed in Chapter 8 and that of carbohydrate in Chapter 5.

Osteomalacia, frequently referred to as "adult rickets," represents a failure of the process of calcification to keep up with the rest of the metabolic processes. It is caused by simple vitamin-D lack and calcium inadequacy. It occurs in the Orient especially in pregnant or lactating women who subsist on meager cereal diets and who are indoors most of the time.

Osteomalacia may also occur when there is interference with fat absorption and is occasionally seen in this country. A third type of this disease resembles resistant rickets in that the individual has an inherent resistance to vitamin D so that normal metabolism does not take place.[55]

The following changes take place in osteomalacia:

1. A softening of the bones, which may be so severe that the bones of the legs, spine, thorax, and pelvis bend into deformities

2. Pain of the rheumatic type in bones of the legs and lower part of the back

* Sebrell, W. H.: "Preventive Medicine," in *Handbook of Nutrition.* American Medical Association, Chicago, 1943, p. 473.

3. General weakness with difficulty in walking; there is especial difficulty in climbing stairs, and a waddling gait is frequent

4. Spontaneous multiple fractures

Since general malnutrition is no doubt present, osteomalacia is treated with a high-protein, high-calorie diet and therapeutic doses of vitamin D.

VITAMIN E

Discovery. Evans and Bishop established the fact that a fat-soluble factor was necessary for reproduction in rats. They showed that absence of vitamin E, or the antisterility factor, as it was designated, led to irreparable damage of the germinal epithelium in male rats, while female rats which had diets deficient in vitamin E were unable to carry their young to term. In severe deficiency the fetus dies and is resorbed completely. In the female the damage is not permanent; that is, normal reproduction could again take place if the diet were once more made adequate in this factor.

Chemistry and characteristics. Vitamin-E activity is exhibited by four or more compounds of related chemical structure: they are alpha-, beta-, gamma-, and delta-tocopherol. Vitamin E is related to the sex hormones chemically. Alpha-tocopherol ($C_{29}H_{50}O_2$) is the compound possessing the greatest vitamin-E activity.

High temperatures and acids do not affect the stability of vitamin E, but oxidation does take place readily in the presence of lead and iron salts or in rancid fats. Decomposition occurs in ultraviolet light. Vitamin E itself acts as an antioxidant.

Measurement. The activity of vitamin E is expressed in milligrams, using alpha-tocopherol as a standard. It is measured by its ability to prevent resorption of the fetus in pregnant rats under standard conditions.

Physiology. Vitamin E is not stored in the liver as are the other fat-soluble vitamins, but fatty tissues store small amounts of the vitamin. Adult males fed a diet containing only 2 mg d-alpha-tocopherol daily showed a progressive decline in the level of plasma tocopherol for the first 14 months and a more gradual decline thereafter; the rate of hemolysis of red blood cells increased.[56] Defective absorption of fat may reduce the tissue levels of tocopherol.

Functions. The functions of vitamin E in the human have not yet been clearly established. Perhaps one of the most interesting discoveries with respect to vitamin E is its antioxidant properties; by accepting oxygen it is able to minimize oxidation of carotene and of vitamin A in the intestine and thus it can effectively "stretch" the intake of vitamin A. Vitamin E apparently has the ability to protect red blood cells from hemolysis by such agents as hydrogen peroxide.

In rats, at least, vitamin E has been shown to promote the effectiveness of linoleic acid in preventing or curing essential fatty acid deficiency.[57] Another practical discovery has been the increased milk and butterfat production by cows on a liberal intake of alpha-tocopherol.[58] Vitamin E seems to be essential for the nuclei of cells and apparently is necessary in some way for the utilization of the sex hormones, cholesterol, and vitamin D.

Daily allowances. The requirement for vitamin E in human beings is not known. The adult consumption has been estimated to be about 14 mg of d-alpha-tocopherol daily.[59]

Sources. Oils of the wheat germ, cottonseed, rice germ, and the germs of other seeds are potent sources of vitamin E. Appreciable concentrations are present in green leafy vegetables, nuts, and legumes, with a small amount in eggs and meat.

Effect of deficiency. It is unlikely that deficiency of vitamin E occurs in the human. The therapeutic effectiveness of vitamin E in the prevention of abortion, in certain menstrual disorders, in the improvement of lactation, in muscular dystrophy, or in cardiovascular diseases has not been substantiated.

VITAMIN K

The existence of vitamin K was first suggested by Dr. Dam of Copenhagen, who in 1935 found that a "Koagulations Vitamin" was necessary to prevent fatal hemorrhages in chicks by promoting normal blood clotting.

Chemistry and characteristics. Vitamin K refers to a group of substances of similar biologic activity. Vitamin K_1 ($C_{31}H_{46}O_2$) was isolated from alfalfa, and vitamin K_2 from putrefied fish meal. Vitamin-K activity is possessed by a number of other compounds, of which *menadione,* a bright-yellow, fat-soluble compound, is three times as potent as the vitamin itself. Vitamin K is fat soluble, and its activity is easily destroyed by irradiation.

Measurement. The activity of test materials is measured in terms of milligrams or micrograms by its ability to prevent hemorrhage in young chicks. Menadione is used as the standard for measuring vitamin-K potency.

Physiology and function. Vitamin K is necessary for the formation of prothrombin, a constituent of normal blood. Prothrombin in turn is required for the production of thrombin before fibrin can be formed so that the blood can clot. The mechanism with which vitamin K works is not known, although it has been shown that impaired hepatic function leads to failure to utilize vitamin K in the formation of prothrombin. Bile salts are necessary for absorption from the intestine. The body stores only a limited amount of vitamin K, most of it being in the liver.

Daily allowances. The exact daily requirement of vitamin K is not known, but it appears that 1 to 2 mg will satisfy the daily needs. Deficiency in man is not generally a dietary problem.

Sources. Green leaves of plants such as alfalfa, spinach, cabbage, kale, and cauliflower are excellent sources of vitamin K, while cereals, fruits, and other vegetables are poor sources. Pork liver is also a good source of the vitamin. Bacterial action in the intestine is responsible for the manufacture of vitamin K in the body.

Effect of a deficiency. A lowered prothrombin content of the blood and increased tendency to bleeding result from a deficiency of vitamin K. It may occur in newborn infants since the intestinal synthesis of vitamin K is not established for a week or so following birth. As a result the infant may be susceptible to hemorrhagic disease. In infants so affected hemorrhage, especially of the brain, may prove fatal unless prompt therapy is initiated. Vascular damage observed primarily in the central nervous system of stillborn infants has been attributed by some to vitamin-K lack. As a protective measure, vitamin K is often given to the mother during the last month of pregnancy as well as just before delivery, the daily allowance usually being 1 mg.

Deficiency may occur in adults because of failure to synthesize, or absorb vitamin K or inability to synthesize prothrombin. Oral therapy with sulfa drugs or antibiotics interferes with the synthesis of the vitamin in the intestine—a factor of some importance when surgery is contemplated. In obstructive jaundice and lesions of the biliary tract, bile is not present in the intestinal tract to effect absorption of vitamin K. Severe diarrhea, as in sprue, celiac disease, and ulcerative colitis, may so interfere with absorption of vitamin K that the tendency to hemorrhage as well as to other deficiency symptoms is increased. In extensive liver damage there may be lowered prothrombin production because the liver is unable to effect synthesis from vitamin K even though absorption is adequate. Whenever there is insufficient bile present for absorption, menadione is prescribed together with bile salts. Parenteral administration may be necessary when intestinal disease interferes with absorption. Vitamin K is not effective when the liver is unable to synthesize prothrombin.

PROBLEMS AND REVIEW

1. The original source of all vitamin A is the carotene of plants. How is the carotene changed to vitamin A? How efficient is it?

2. A deficiency of vitamin A in the diet leads to clinical signs much sooner in young infants than in older children and adults. Why is this so? What are some signs of vitamin-A deficiency?

3. Vitamins A and D are the two fat-soluble vitamins which require particular emphasis in daily nutrition. By what means can you assure yourself of an adequate intake? Why do you not need to plan especially for vitamins E and K in your diet? When does vitamin K require particular attention?

4. Milk is the food most frequently fortified with vitamin D. Why is the fortification of milk desirable? How is it accomplished? How much milk must be taken daily by a child to assure adequate vitamin D?

5. Detectable signs of deficiency for the various fat-soluble vitamins seem to

(*Text continued on p. 132.*)

NOMENCLATURE	UNITS AND METHODS OF ASSAY	IMPORTANT SOURCES	STABILITY IN FOODS
Vitamin A provitamin A alpha-, beta-, gamma-caro- tene, crypto- xanthin antiophthalmic factor	I.U. Rat growth	*Animal* fish-liver oils liver butter, cream whole milk whole-milk cheeses egg yolk *Plant* dark green leafy vegetables yellow vegetables yellow fruits Fortified margarines	Insoluble in water Stable to heat by usual cooking methods Destroyed by oxida- tion, drying, and very high tempera- tures Fat soluble
Vitamin D vitamin D_2 calciferol, vi- osterol, acti- vated ergos- terol vitamin D_3 activated 7-dehydro- cholesterol antirachitic factor	I.U. Calcium line test on rats	Fish-liver oils Fortified milk Activated sterols Exposure to sunlight Very small amounts in butter, liver, egg yolk	Stable to heat and oxidation Fat soluble
Vitamin E alpha-, beta-, gamma-, delta-, tocopherol antisterility vitamin	mg as tocopherol Ability to pre- vent resorp- tion of fetus in rats	Plant tissues—oils of wheat germ, rice germ, cotton- seed; green leafy vegetables; nuts; legumes Animal foods are poor sources ? intestinal synthesis	Not affected by heat or acid Oxidized in rancid fats, presence of lead and iron salts, alkalies, ultraviolet light Fat soluble
Vitamin K antihemorrhagic vitamin coagulation vita- min menadione	mcg as mena- dione Clotting time of vitamin-K- depleted chicks	Green leaves such as alfalfa, spinach, cabbage Liver Synthesis in intestine	Fat soluble Unstable to alkali and light Fairly stable to heat

all fairly stable t heat

PHYSIOLOGY AND FUNCTIONS	EFFECT OF DEFICIENCY	DAILY ALLOWANCES *
Bile necessary for absorption of carotene Stored in liver Promotes growth, maintains integrity of mucosal epithelium, maintains visual acuity in dim light	Arrested growth Faulty bone and tooth development Night blindness Decreased ability to resist infection Keratinization of epithelium —mucous membranes and skin *Xerophthalmia*	Adult: 5000 I.U. Pregnancy: 6000 I.U. Lactation: 8000 I.U. Children: 1500–5000 I.U., depending on age

Synthesized in skin by activity of ultraviolet light
Stored chiefly in liver
Promotes normal skeletal and tooth development
Regulates absorption and anchorage of calcium, phosphorus
	Rickets in children
	   soft, fragile bones
	   enlarged joints
	   bowed legs
	   chest, spinal, pelvic bone deformities
	   delayed dentition
	Tetanic convulsions in infants
	Osteomalacia in adults
		Need is small for adults
		Children, pregnant or lactating women: 400 I.U.

Not stored in body to any extent
Humans
   reduces oxidation of vitamin A, carotenes
   prevents hemolysis of red blood cells
Animals
   normal reproduction
   utilization of essential fatty acids, sex hormones, cholesterol
	Clinical evidence in humans is lacking
	Sterility in male rats
	Resorption of fetus in female rats
	Muscle degeneration in rabbits, guinea pigs
		Not known

Bile necessary for absorption Formation of prothrombin Sulfa drugs and antibiotics interfere	Prolonged clotting time Hemorrhagic disease in newborn infants	Not known

* See Recommended Dietary Allowances, page 26, for complete listing.

be much less prevalent in this country than are deficiencies of a number of water-soluble factors. Give several possible explanations for this.

6. Explain the relationship which exists between vitamin A and vitamin E; vitamin D and calcium.

7. *Problem.* Calculate the percentage of your own daily requirement for vitamin A which 3 cups of milk would supply.

8. *Problem.* Calculate the vitamin A content of your own diet for 2 days. What percentage of your daily allowance is provided by sources rich in preformed vitamin A? By sources rich in the provitamin?

9. What dangers may result from indiscriminate use of vitamin-A and -D concentrates?

CHAPTER 10

The Water-Soluble Vitamins: Ascorbic Acid

Discovery. One of the most serious problems of the sailor, adventurer, and explorer several hundred years ago was the frequent occurrence of scurvy. While citrus and other fresh fruits and germinating seeds have long been known as both a preventive and a cure, the scientific foundations for the study of ascorbic acid were first initiated in 1907 when scurvy was produced experimentally in guinea pigs by Holst and Frölich in Norway. The isolation and synthesis of ascorbic acid, or vitamin C as it is also called, were accomplished in a number of laboratories after Dr. King and his co-workers at the University of Pittsburgh first effected chemical identification in 1932.

Chemistry and characteristics. Ascorbic acid, $C_6H_8O_6$, is a white, crystalline compound of relatively simple structure closely related to the monosaccharide sugars. It is stable in its dry form, but dissolves readily in water. Of all vitamins, ascorbic acid is the most easily destroyed. Vitamin activity is possessed by two forms: L-ascorbic acid (the reduced form) and L-dehydroascorbic acid (the oxidized form). The latter is easily oxidized further with complete loss of activity. The oxidation of ascorbic acid is accelerated by heat, light, alkalies, oxidative enzymes, and traces of copper and iron. Oxidation is inhibited to a marked degree in an acid reaction, and when the temperature is reduced.

Measurement. The concentration of ascorbic acid is expressed in milligrams. In foods or in body tissues it may be determined chemically, one method being based on the strong reducing action which will bring about the bleaching of a blue dye under specified conditions.

Physiology. Many animals are able to synthesize ascorbic acid from simple sugars such as glucose; but man, guinea pigs, and monkeys are dependent upon a dietary source. The blood plasma concentration of 1.0 mg per 100 ml indicates that the tissues are probably saturated with ascorbic acid, and that the body may be protected against scurvy for several months. A reduction in the daily intake is quickly reflected in lower blood plasma levels, but the concentration of the vitamin in the white blood cells is less subject to change.

133

The adrenal gland contains an especially high concentration of ascorbic acid, but other glandular tissues such as the pancreas, thymus, spleen, liver, and kidney also contain appreciable amounts. The amount of ascorbic acid held by the tissues is limited. When the tissues are saturated, the urinary excretion accounts for a large proportion of the intake; but if the tissues are depleted, a high percentage of the intake will be retained.

Functions. The most important function of ascorbic acid is the control which it exercises on the ability of cells to produce collagenous or intercellular material which holds the cells in proper relation to each other. The

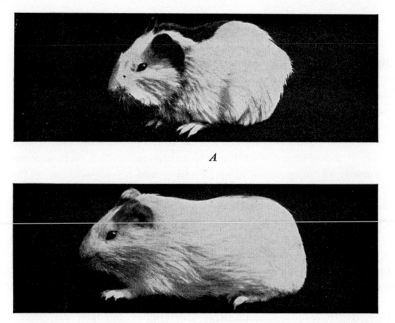

Fig. 10-1. Effect of ascorbic acid on growth and health. (*A*) Diet adequate except for ascorbic acid. (*B*) Ascorbic acid added to the same diet. Guinea pigs of the same age and sex, 22 days on the diets. The rough fur and the crouched position, due to sore joints, indicate scurvy in the smaller guinea pig. Rats do not develop scurvy. (*Courtesy, the Bureau of Home Economics, U.S. Department of Agriculture.*)

healthy development and maintenance of the capillary blood vessels, the dentine of the teeth, the bones, the cartilage, and the connective tissues are dependent upon this function (see Fig. 10-1).

Ascorbic acid facilitates the absorption of iron from the intestinal tract. The conversion of folic acid to the metabolically active form, folinic acid, requires ascorbic acid. On the basis of studies conducted on premature and young infants, vitamin C also appears to be related to the metabolism of tyrosine and phenylalanine, two amino acids.

An increase in adrenal cortical activity leads to a decreased concentration of vitamin C and of cholesterol in the adrenal gland, but to an increased output of steroid hormones. It thus appears that ascorbic acid may be involved in the synthesis of these hormones from cholesterol.

During infections such as tuberculosis, rheumatic fever, and pneumonia additional amounts of ascorbic acid are required to maintain desirable tissue levels. Undoubtedly, vitamin C is essential in providing resistance to infections, but the way in which this is accomplished is not clear.

Daily allowances. An intake of 10 to 20 mg of ascorbic acid is sufficient to protect an adult from classical scurvy. However, this represents only a fraction of that needed to maintain desirable plasma ascorbic acid levels. The standards recommended by the Food and Nutrition Board [2] provide 70 to 75 mg for the adult, 30 to 60 mg for infants and children, 75 to 100 mg for adolescents, and 100 to 150 mg during pregnancy and lactation.

Food sources. Almost all of the daily intake of ascorbic acid is obtained from the vegetable-fruit group (see Fig. 10-2). Vitamin C has been called the

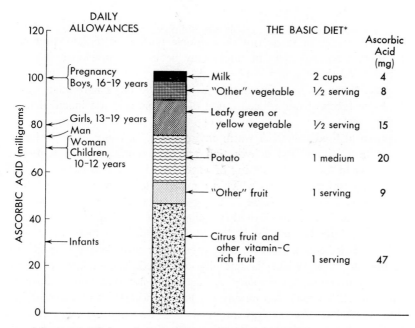

* See page 178 for calculation of ascorbic acid and other values.

Fig. 10-2. The vegetable-fruit group of the Basic Diet fulfills the recommended allowances of adults and children for ascorbic acid. Note that potatoes and leafy green vegetables contribute significant amounts.

"fresh food vitamin," since it is found in highest concentration just as the food is fresh from the plant. In general, the active parts of the plant contain appreciable amounts, while mature or resting seeds are devoid of the vitamin.

Raw, frozen, or canned citrus fruits such as oranges, grapefruit, and lemons are excellent sources of the vitamin. Orange sections including the thin white peel contain more vitamin C than an equal weight of strained juice.

Fresh strawberries, cantaloupe, pineapple, and guavas are also excellent sources. Other nonacid fresh fruits such as peaches, pears, apples, bananas, and blueberries contribute small amounts of the vitamin; when eaten in large amounts these fruits may be an important dietary source. The concentration of ascorbic acid in the nonacid canned fruits is considerably reduced.

Broccoli, Brussels sprouts, spinach, kale, green peppers, cabbage, and turnips are excellent-to-good sources even when cooked. The use of potatoes and sweet potatoes as staple food items enhances the vitamin-C intake considerably provided that preparation methods have been good.

Milk, eggs, meat, fish, and poultry are practically devoid of vitamin C as they are consumed. Human milk contains four to six times as much ascorbic acid as cow's milk, if the mother's diet has been adequate, and is able to protect the infant from scurvy. Liver contains a small amount of vitamin C, but most of this is lost during cookery.

The simplest way to ensure adequate intake of ascorbic acid is to include a serving of orange or grapefruit or a double portion of tomato, preferably at breakfast. Since a variety of juices may be used at breakfast, it is well to keep in mind that the nonacid juices do not compare with the citrus fruits in potency. When such a substitution is made, the day's allowance will be ample if two foods of fair concentration of ascorbic acid are included in the remaining meals.

Retention of food values. A warm environment, exposure to air, solubility in water, heat, alkali, and dehydration are detrimental to the retention of ascorbic acid in foods. The cutting of vegetables releases oxidative enzymes and also increases the surfaces which are exposed to leaching by water. Since the vitamin is so soluble, losses are considerable when large amounts of water are used. Vegetables should be added to a small quantity of boiling water, covered tightly, and cooked until just tender for high retention of ascorbic acid. Retention is also good when a pressure cooker is used, providing that the cookery time is carefully controlled. The practice of adding baking soda to retain green color of vegetables not only may reduce the vitamin-C level, but may also modify the flavor and texture of the vegetable. Leftover vegetables lose a large proportion of the ascorbic acid, although losses are reduced somewhat when the container is tightly covered in the refrigerator. On the other hand, citrus juices and tomatoes retain practically all of the vitamin-C value for several days.

Effect of deficiency. Early signs of vitamin-C deficiency include such vague symptoms as increased susceptibility to infection, poor wound healing, irritability, retardation of growth, and poor health in general. To establish a diagnosis is difficult, if not impossible, at this point. If the diet is practically devoid of ascorbic acid for 4 or 5 months, symptoms of scurvy begin to appear. In addition to a dietary history, the concentration of ascorbic acid in the blood plasma, the excretion in the urine, and the resistance of the capillaries to pressure such as that applied with a tourniquet are of diagnostic value.

Scurvy. The classic picture of scurvy is rarely seen in adults in the United States. The incidence is also uncommon in infants, but a gross deficiency

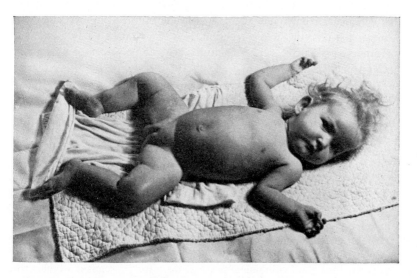

Fig. 10-3. Child in scorbutic position. (*Courtesy, Dr. Bernard S. Epstein, The Long Island Jewish Hospital, New Hyde Park, New York, and* The Vitamin Manual, *published by The Upjohn Company.*)

of ascorbic acid results in scurvy during the second 6 months of life. Infections, fevers, and hyperthyroidism may precipitate the symptoms when the intake has been inadequate. The symptoms are related to the weakening of the collagenous material.

Pain, tenderness, and swelling of the thighs and legs are frequent symptoms of infantile scurvy. The baby shows a disinclination to move and assumes a position with legs flexed for comfort (see Fig. 10-3). He is pale, irritable, and cries when handled. Loss of weight, fever, diarrhea, and vomiting are not infrequently present. If the teeth have erupted, the gums are likely to be swollen, tender, and hemorrhagic. Bone calcification is faulty because of degeneration or lack of proper development of the bone matrix. The cartilage supporting the bones is weak, and bone displacement results. The ends of the long bones and of the ribs are enlarged somewhat as in rickets, but tenderness is a distinguishing characteristic in scurvy.

Scurvy in adults results after several months of a diet devoid of ascorbic acid. The symptoms include swelling, infection, and bleeding of the gums—gingivitis; tenderness of the legs; anemia; and petechial hemorrhages. The teeth may become loose and eventually may be lost. As the disease progresses, the slightest injury produces excessive bleeding, and large hemorrhages may be seen underneath the skin. There is degeneration of the muscle structure and of the cartilage generally.

Acute scurvy responds within a few days to the administration of 100 to 200 mg ascorbic acid given in the synthetic form or as orange juice. Chronic changes which have occurred, such as bone deformities and anemia, require much longer periods for their correction.

A summary of ascorbic acid is included with three B-complex vitamins in the table on page 158.

PROBLEMS AND REVIEW

1. In what ways is ascorbic acid related to the functioning of each of these substances: iron; folic acid; cholesterol?

2. What are the clinical manifestations of a deficiency of ascorbic acid?

3. What is the effect of an intake of ascorbic acid in excess of the body's needs?

4. Why is a formula-fed baby more prone to scurvy than a breast-fed baby?

5. List the instructions you would give for the preparation and service of these foods in order that the maximum ascorbic acid would be retained: tossed green salad; buttered cabbage?

6. *Problem.* Calculate the ascorbic acid content of your own diet for 2 days. Compare your intake with the recommended allowances.

7. *Problem.* Plan food combinations for 2 days for a pregnant woman who is allergic to citrus fruits and tomatoes and who requires 100 mg ascorbic acid.

8. *Problem.* Calculate the amounts of each of the following foods necessary to furnish 25 mg of ascorbic acid: orange juice; tomato juice; sweet potato; cabbage; grapefruit; endive; strawberries; cantaloupe; apple; lettuce.

9. *Problem.* From current market prices, calculate the cost of the ascorbic acid from each of the foods listed in Problem 8. Arrange these costs in a bar graph.

CHAPTER 11

The Water-Soluble Vitamins:
The Vitamin-B Complex

In areas of the world where polished rice is a staple food, beriberi, a serious disease affecting the nerves, has been known for generations. Takaki, a Japanese medical officer, studied the high incidence of the disease among men of the Japanese navy during the years 1878–1883. Among 276 men serving on one sailing vessel he found 169 cases of beriberi at the end of 9 months, but only 14 cases occurred among a similar number of men on a second vessel who had received more meat, milk, and vegetables in their diet. Takaki believed this difference was related to the protein content of the diet.

About 15 years later (1897) Eijkman, a Dutch physician in the East Indies, noted that illness in fowls which ate scraps of hospital food was similar to beriberi seen in humans. He subsequently conducted a series of experiments which led to the first clear demonstration of a nutritional deficiency disease. He theorized that the starch of polished rice was toxic to the nerves, but that the outer layers of the rice kernel were protective. Another Dutch physician, Grijns, interpreted the findings as a deficiency of an essential substance in the diet.

A number of chemists demonstrated the effects of extracts from rice. Funk in 1911 coined the term *vitamine* for the substance which he found to be effective in preventing beriberi. McCollum and Davis applied the term *water-soluble B* to the concentrates which cured beriberi.

The water-soluble vitamin B described by Funk and others was soon discovered to be not a single substance but a group of compounds which we now designate as the vitamin-B complex. It was found that a growth-promoting factor more stable to heat remained after the antiberiberi factor was destroyed; to this substance which proved to be a water-soluble yellow pigment was given the name "vitamin G." Still further research proved vitamin G to be a mixture of riboflavin and niacin. There are 15 or more factors in the complex, many of which have been obtained in their pure form.

The complete role of the B-complex vitamins is far from clear, but it is certain that they are essential for metabolic changes which take place in all

139

cells. Many of these vitamins are known to combine with specific proteins to function as parts of the various oxidative enzyme systems which are concerned with the breakdown of carbohydrate, protein, and fat in the body. Thus, they are interrelated and are intimately involved in the mechanisms which release energy, carbon dioxide, and water as the end products of metabolism.

The student should become thoroughly familiar with the properties, functions, daily allowances, and factors in dietary planning with respect to thiamine, riboflavin, and niacin, since she will be expected to consider them in the planning and preparation of both normal and therapeutic diets. Other B-complex vitamins are equally necessary in human nutrition but will, in all likelihood, be supplied in sufficient quantities under normal conditions if the three above-named vitamins are provided in adequate amounts. The properties, functions, food sources, probable requirements, and effects of deficiency of other B-complex vitamins are presented in outline form on pages 152–57.

THIAMINE

Discovery. Crystalline vitamin B_1 was isolated from rice bran by Jansen and Donath in Holland in 1926. The synthesis and structure were accomplished in 1936 by Dr. R. R. Williams who had worked for a quarter of a century on studies of beriberi and on the factor in rice polishings which brought about cure of the disease. Noting the presence of sulfur in the molecule, the vitamin was named thiamine.

Chemistry and characteristics. Thiamine is available commercially as thiamine hydrochloride, $C_{12}H_{17}N_4OSCl.HCl$, in a crystalline white powder. It has a faint yeastlike odor and a salty nutlike taste, and is readily soluble in water. The vitamin is stable in its dry form, and heating in solutions at $120°$ C in an acid medium has little destructive effect. On the other hand, cooking foods in neutral or alkaline reaction is very destructive.

Measurement. Thiamine is now measured in milligrams or micrograms. It is determined by chemical or microbiologic methods, but in the past it was measured by using pigeons, rats, or chicks as assay animals.

Physiology. Thiamine is readily absorbed in aqueous solutions from both the small and large intestine, and is then carried to the liver by the portal circulation. In the liver, as well as in all living cells, it normally combines with phosphate to form a coenzyme, *cocarboxylase*. It may be stored in the liver in this form, or it may combine further with magnesium and specific proteins to become active enzymes known as *carboxylases*.

Liver, heart, kidney, muscles, and brain are richer in thiamine than the blood which contains only traces. During a period of deficiency the thiamine is lost rapidly from these tissues, the muscles losing the reserves first while the brain clings most tenaciously to its supply. At no time are the stores sufficiently great to last for more than a few weeks, and hence a day-to-day supply is essential in the diet.

Any excess of thiamine is quickly excreted in the urine, and to some extent in the perspiration. The body reserves of thiamine may be estimated by measuring the urinary excretion of thiamine following a test dose.

Function. As a component of the enzyme carboxylase, thiamine functions in the release of energy from the metabolism of carbohydrate. One of the intermediate products of glucose breakdown in the body is pyruvic acid, a three-carbon keto acid. Carboxylase effects the removal of the carboxyl group from this acid to produce acetate. Other ketonic acids are similarly decarboxylated by specific carboxylases, of which thiamine is a component.

As a result of the role in energy metabolism, thiamine is related to the maintenance of a normal appetite, to the normal muscle tone of the gastrointestinal tract, and to a healthy nervous system.

Daily allowances. The thiamine requirement is related to the level of carbohydrate in the diet, and for practical purposes may be expressed in terms of the caloric intake. The minimum requirement is 0.2–0.3 mg per 1000 calories, while the recommended allowance [2] is 0.5 mg of thiamine per 1000 calories. Such a margin of safety is desirable since the body has little reserve, which may be rapidly depleted by febrile diseases or surgery.

The daily allowance for the reference man is 1.6 mg and for the reference woman, 1.2 mg. An allowance of at least 1 mg is provided for adults even when the caloric intake may be under 2000. For pregnant and lactating women the allowance is 1.3 and 1.7 mg, respectively. Infants should receive 0.4–0.5 mg daily, while children are allowed 0.7 to 1.3 mg.

Fat and protein exert a thiamine-sparing effect, so that diets with liberal allowances of these nutrients will require somewhat less thiamine for metabolism than will a high-carbohydrate diet of equal caloric value.

Sources. Grain products alone provide about one-third of the thiamine of the daily diet in the United States and constitute the most important single source in the diet. Because such a small proportion of cereal foods is of the whole-grain variety, the cereal and flour enrichment program has been of special significance in improving the dietary level of thiamine during the last two decades.

Meats, poultry, and fish as a group supply about one-fourth of the daily intake of thiamine. Lean pork—fresh and cured—is especially high in its thiamine concentration; its frequent inclusion in the diet thus makes it a highly significant source. Liver, dry beans and peas, soybeans, and peanuts are also excellent sources. The thiamine in egg, a fair source, is concentrated in the yolk.

Although the concentration of thiamine in vegetables and fruits is low, the quantities of these foods eaten may be such that important contributions are made to the daily total. Milk is likewise a fair source because of the amounts which are taken in the daily diet and because milk is not subjected to treatment other than pasteurization, which does not materially reduce the thiamine level.

The thiamine level of the basic diet is illustrated in Figure 11-1.

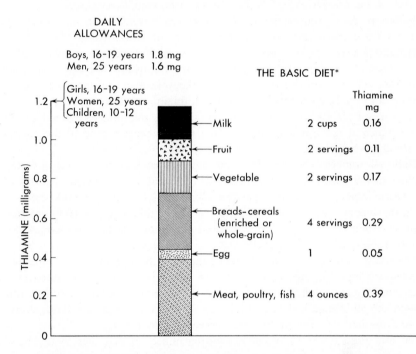

DAILY
ALLOWANCES

Boys, 16-19 years 1.8 mg
Men, 25 years   1.6 mg

THE BASIC DIET*

		Thiamine mg
←Milk	2 cups	0.16
←Fruit	2 servings	0.11
←Vegetable	2 servings	0.17
←Breads–cereals (enriched or whole-grain)	4 servings	0.29
←Egg	1	0.05
←Meat, poultry, fish	4 ounces	0.39

Girls, 16-19 years
Women, 25 years
Children, 10-12 years

THIAMINE (milligrams)

* See page 178 for complete calculations.

Fig. 11-1. Foods from each of the Four Food Groups of the Basic Diet contribute to the daily intake of thiamine.

Retention of food values. Appreciable losses of thiamine in foods through cookery may occur as a result of (1) the solubility of this vitamin in water, (2) the ready destruction in the presence of alkali, (3) high temperatures, and (4) the prolonged exposure to heat. Thiamine loss during cooking varies widely under different conditions, and no general rule can be stated which would cover the losses with the several methods of cookery.

Cooked breakfast cereals keep most of their thiamine since the water is retained and cookery takes place at moderate temperatures. Baking of bread results in a 15 to 20 per cent loss.

About 25 to 50 per cent of the thiamine may be lost in meat cookery. The smaller loss pertains to meats which have been broiled or roasted, while the larger loss is in effect when meats are cooked in liquid which is discarded. If the drippings and the liquid in which meat is cooked are eaten, the thiamine content of meat is about 75 per cent of the initial value.

Thiamine losses in vegetable cookery may be considerable if large amounts of water are used and later discarded, and if alkali is added to retain green color. Those principles of preparation which are essential for the retention of ascorbic acid (see p. 136) serve well for maximum thiamine content.

Effect of deficiency. There is meager evidence that even mild deficiency is prevalent in the United States. Beriberi has been seen only on rare occasions and is not a public health problem. Chronic alcoholism may lead to thiamine deficiency because the individual who drinks excessively eats very poorly as a rule.

Beriberi is still observed in the Orient although less commonly. High-carbohydrate diets of rice and wheat will consistently result in beriberi when the thiamine intake is less than 0.2 mg per 1000 calories. The effectiveness of rice enrichment was demonstrated in the Philippines by Williams.[60]

Thiamine deficiency may occur following gastrointestinal disturbances such as diarrhea and vomiting, or subsequent to febrile diseases or surgery when the dietary intake has been poor.

Diagnosis. The symptoms of mild deficiency are so vague that a diagnosis of thiamine lack is difficult. Some of the laboratory tests may be helpful but not necessarily conclusive. For example, an elevated level of pyruvic acid in the blood, especially after exercise and the administration of a standard amount of glucose, together with a low concentration of thiamine in the urine are suggestive of deficiency. If such tests are further substantiated with a dietary history of thiamine lack plus the appearance of peripheral neuritis and disorders in the cardiovascular system, thiamine deficiency seems apparent.

Mild thiamine deficiency. The individual who is deprived of small amounts of thiamine daily builds up an increasing deficiency state which may be characterized by fatigue, lack of interest in his affairs, emotional instability, irritability, depression, anger and fear, and loss of appetite, weight, and strength. As the deficiency becomes more marked, the patient may complain of indigestion, constipation, headaches, insomnia, and tachycardia after moderate exertion. There appears a feeling of heaviness and weakness in the legs which may be followed by cramping of the calf muscles and burning and numbness of the feet—an indication of the development of peripheral neuritis. The predominant symptoms thus concern the cardiovascular system, and the peripheral nervous system.

Beriberi. When thiamine deficiency has been prolonged and severe, it progresses from the mild symptoms described above to the incapacitating and often fatal beriberi. There is "wet" beriberi in which the chief manifestations are edema and cardiac failure, and "dry" beriberi with its multiple neuritic symptoms being outstanding. Not infrequently cardiac symptoms may predominate and failure of the heart becomes imminent. The disease is characterized by the following symptoms:

1. Gastrointestinal disturbances resulting primarily from impairment of the motor processes throughout the gastrointestinal tract.

2. Muscular weakness or paralysis of the lower limbs caused by multiple neuritic conditions. The weakness affects first the foot, then the muscles of the calf, and then the thigh. The upper extremities are also affected in severe cases. The muscle degeneration may be so pronounced that coordination is impossible and a characteristic gait is present. The pain in the extremities at this stage is usually severe. The extent of muscular atrophy may be masked by edema in wet beriberi.

3. The heart becomes enlarged, and tachycardia, dyspnea, and palpitation occur on exertion. In the acute or pernicious type of beriberi, acute cardiac failure may be fatal before the seriousness of the disease has been fully appreciated.

4. Emaciation accompanies both dry and wet beriberi, but in the latter the edema may be so marked that the extent of malnourishment is not readily evident.

Treatment. Because beriberi is a complex vitamin-deficiency disease, patients make the greatest improvement when B-complex vitamins rather than thiamine alone are prescribed. In addition to the B-complex concentrates it is customary to prescribe a diet which is high in protein and in calories (p. 373).

RIBOFLAVIN

Discovery. As early as 1879 a pigment which possessed a yellow-green fluorescence had been discovered in milk. Other workers later obtained it from such widely varying sources as liver, yeast, heart, and egg white. The pigments which possess these fluorescent properties were designated as "flavins."

In 1932 a yellow enzyme necessary for cell respiration was isolated from yeast by Warburg and Christian, who also discovered that a protein and the pigment component were the two factors in the enzyme. It then remained for Kuhn and his co-workers in 1935 to report on the synthesis of riboflavin and to note the relation of its activity to the green fluorescence, thereby establishing the fact that lactoflavin and the vitamin were one and the same thing. Riboflavin is the preferred name for this vitamin although the terms "vitamin B_2," "lactoflavin," and "vitamin G" are still seen in the literature.

Chemistry and characteristics. Riboflavin was so named because of the similarity of part of its structure to that of the sugar ribose, and its relation to the general group of flavins. Its chemical formula is $C_{17}H_{20}N_4O_6$. In its pure state, this vitamin is a bitter-tasting, orange-yellow, odorless compound in which the crystals are needle-shaped. It dissolves sparingly in water to give a characteristic greenish-yellow fluorescence. It is quickly decomposed by ultraviolet rays and visible light. This vitamin is stable to heat, to oxidizing agents, and to acids; but it is sensitive to the effects of alkali, although to a lesser degree than is thiamine.

Measurement. Riboflavin is measured in terms of milligrams or micrograms. Chemical or microbiologic methods are both used extensively.

Physiology. Riboflavin is present in the free state in foods, or in combination with phosphate, or with protein and phosphate. It is utilized in either form. The body guards carefully its stores of riboflavin so that even in severe deficiency as much as one-third of the normal amount has been found to be present in the liver, kidney, and heart of experimental animals. There may be some synthesis of riboflavin in the gastrointestinal tract, but how much absorption and utilization of the synthesized vitamin takes place is not known. Apparently the flavin content of the body tissues cannot be increased beyond a certain point, since the urinary excretion increases markedly if a great elevation of the intake occurs. On the other hand, a decided reduction in the supply leads to restriction or even curtailment of the urinary excretion.

Functions. Riboflavin functions in a number of important enzyme systems. By means of these enzymes hydrogen is transferred from a variety of substances and later released to oxygen, with water as an end product. Thus, riboflavin is an essential link in the metabolism of amino acids, fatty acids, and carbohydrates; it serves in the utilization of food for energy and also in the synthesis of body substances. It is small wonder that the body clings so tenaciously to its supply of riboflavin.

Daily allowances. The minimum requirement of riboflavin is about 0.6–0.75 mg per day, but the Recommended Dietary Allowance [2] of 1.8 mg and 1.5 mg for men and women, respectively, provides a factor of safety. These allowances are based on body weight, and are computed by multiplying the protein allowance by the factor 0.025.

During pregnancy and lactation the allowance is increased to 2.0 mg and 2.5 mg, respectively. Infants are allowed 0.5 to 0.8 mg, children 1.0 to 1.8 mg, and adolescent boys and girls 1.9 to 2.5 mg.

Increased requirements for riboflavin occur whenever there is augmented metabolism as in pregnancy and lactation, during growth, hyperthyroidism, fevers, stress of injury or illness, diarrhea, and vomiting. Achlorhydria may precipitate deficiency because the vitamin is so quickly destroyed in an alkaline medium.

Food sources. The concentration of riboflavin in many foodstuffs is not high. Among the very best sources are milk—fresh, canned, or dried—and one of the by-products of milk, powdered whey. Cheese is also a good source, but some of the riboflavin is lost in the removal of the whey. Dairy products, excluding butter, provide almost half of the riboflavin available for consumption in the United States.

Liver, kidney, and heart contain considerable quantities of riboflavin, while other meats, eggs, and green leafy vegetables contain smaller, but, nevertheless, important amounts.

It is noteworthy that cereals which are such excellent sources of thiamine are poor sources of riboflavin. During germination the riboflavin content of the grains increases strikingly. Enrichment of cereals and flours has added significant amounts of riboflavin to the diet.

Fruits, roots, and tubers are poor sources of riboflavin, and fats and oils are practically devoid of the vitamin. (See Fig. 11-2.)

Retention of food values. Pasteurization, irradiation for vitamin D, evaporation, or drying of milk account for not more than 10 to 20 per cent loss of the riboflavin content of milk. On the other hand, this vitamin's sensitivity to light may mean a considerable loss of potency if milk is allowed to stand exposed to light for any length of time. As much as three-fourths of the riboflavin may be lost by exposure of a bottle of milk for 3½ hours to direct sunlight.

Because riboflavin is so sparingly soluble, the usual cooking procedures or freezing of vegetables do not contribute markedly to destruction of the vitamin. The use of sodium bicarbonate is deleterious. Meats which have been boiled, roasted, or braised retain more than three-fourths of the riboflavin,

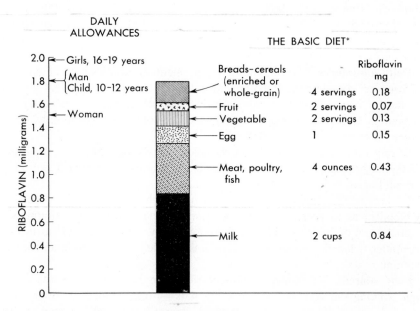

* See page 178 for complete calculations.

Fig. 11-2. Milk is the most important single source of riboflavin. The meat group, especially liver, also contributes significant amounts.

while most of the remainder can be accounted for in the drippings. Canned meats appear to retain most of the vitamin even when stored for periods of 10 months at 99° F.

Effect of deficiency. Ariboflavinosis is believed to be one of the most common of deficiency diseases. It is rare that an individual seeks medical advice for it alone, but it may accompany other deficiencies especially of the B complex.

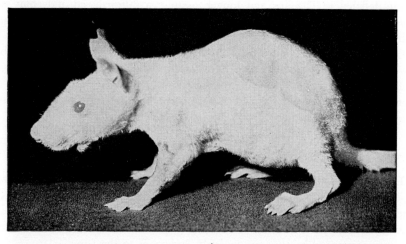

A

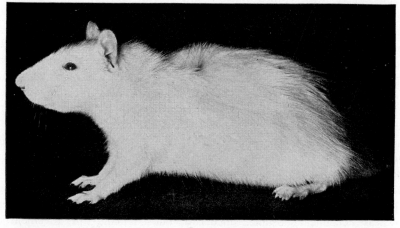

B

Fig. 11-3. (*A*) A deficiency of riboflavin affects growth and produces changes in the skin and eyes. (*B*) The inclusion of adequate riboflavin is necessary for normal growth, healthy skin, and normal vision. (*Courtesy, the Upjohn Company, Kalamazoo, Mich.*)

Symptoms. In 1939 Sebrell and Butler studied a group of women whom they placed upon a diet extremely low in riboflavin. This diet in the course of 94 to 130 days led to the development of definite symptoms such as "cracks in the skin at the corners of the mouth (cheilosis), a greasy eruption of the skin, changes in the tongue and keratitis caused by an invasion of the cornea by blood vessels." * Glossitis caused by riboflavin deficiency may become apparent in pellagrins after therapy has corrected the acute manifestations of niacin deficiency. The lips and tongue assume a purplish-red and shiny appearance in contrast to the scarlet color seen in niacin deficiency. The mouth becomes increasingly sore.

Ocular manifestations are believed to be among the earliest signs of riboflavin deficiency. The eyes become sensitive to light and easily fatigued. There is also blurring of the vision, itching, watering, and soreness of the eyes. An increased number of capillaries develop in the cornea, and the eye becomes "bloodshot" in appearance.

NIACIN (NICOTINIC ACID)

Early studies. Pellagra, which means rough skin, is a disease which was described in Italy in 1771. In the early part of this century it was one of the leading causes of mental illness and of death in this country. Its causes had been variously ascribed to toxic substances present in corn, infections from microorganisms, or toxicity produced by exposure to the sun.

Goldberger, of the United States Public Health Service, who was assigned to study the problem of pellagra in the South, early noted that the disease was almost always associated with poverty and ignorance, and that hospital attendants who worked with the patients never contracted the disease. In 1915 he performed a classic experiment on 12 prisoners who were promised release in return for their cooperation in eating a diet representative of the poorer classes in the southern states. The diet consisted of sweet potatoes, corn bread, cabbage, rice, collards, fried mush, brown gravy, corn grits, sirup, sugar, biscuits, and black coffee. After a few weeks the prisoners developed headache, stomach-ache, and general weakness, and in about 5 months the typical dermatitis of pellagra appeared. Goldberger then suggested the existence of a pellagra-preventing (P-P) factor and related it to the B vitamins.

Identification of the vitamin. Goldberger in 1922 concluded that blacktongue in dogs was similar to pellagra in humans. Nicotinic acid had been known as a chemical substance since 1867 but it remained for Elvehjem and his co-workers in 1937 to discover its effectiveness as a curative agent for blacktongue in dogs. Following this discovery, Smith, Spies, and others were soon making reports of dramatic clinical improvement in pellagrous patients who had been given nicotinic acid. The term "niacin" was suggested by Cowgill to avoid association with the nicotine of tobacco.

Chemistry and characteristics. Niacin, which is $C_6H_5O_2N$, occurs in white, needlelike, bitter tasting crystals. It is moderately soluble in hot water but only slightly soluble in cold water. It is very stable to alkali, acid, heat, light,

* Sebrell, W. H., and Butler, R. E.: "Riboflavin Deficiency in Man," *Pub. Health Rep.,* **54:**2121, 1939.

and oxidation; even boiling and autoclaving do not decrease its potency. It is available commercially as niacinamide.

Measurement. Niacin is measured in terms of milligrams. It may be determined in food and other materials by microbiologic assay or by chemical methods.

Physiology. Niacin is readily absorbed from the small intestine. Some reserves are found in the body, but, as with the other B-complex vitamins, the amount appears to be rather limited so that a day-to-day supply is essential. Any excess of niacin which may be present is excreted in the urine in several forms so that it is somewhat difficult to account for all of it. In deficiency such as pellagra, the end products in the urine diminish markedly or are absent.

Tryptophan, one of the essential amino acids, is a precursor of niacin so that a diet which contains liberal amounts of tryptophan will provide enough niacin even though the diet itself may be low in preformed niacin. Vitamin B_6 is essential for this conversion. The experimental production of pellagra can be brought about only by diets which are low in both niacin and tryptophan.

Function. All living organisms require niacin. It is a functional component of two coenzymes: coenzyme I and coenzyme II. Niacin acts in a manner similar to riboflavin; that is, the enzymes of which niacin is a constituent transfer hydrogen from the various intermediate breakdown products of the glucose molecule to riboflavin. Thus, together with thiamine and riboflavin, niacin is one of the essential components of enzymes for effecting release of energy in the body.

Daily allowances. Now that the quantitative tryptophan-niacin relationship is known, it is possible to define niacin requirements somewhat more precisely. Horwitt [61] has concluded that a minimum of 4.4 mg niacin equivalents per 1000 calories will protect against symptoms of pellagra. The recommended allowance [2] is based on a 50 per cent factor of safety, that is 6.6 mg per 1000 calories. Thus, the allowance for the reference man is 21 mg and for the reference woman is 17 mg. In pregnancy and lactation the allowances should be increased proportionate with the caloric intake.

As with other B-complex vitamins, the niacin requirements are increased whenever metabolism is accelerated—growth, pregnancy, lactation, fevers, hyperthyroidism, stress of surgery or injury.

Sources. Foods must be considered (1) for their preformed niacin and (2) for the niacin available by conversion from the tryptophan. Poultry, meats, and fish constitute the most important single food group insofar as preformed niacin is concerned. Organ meats are somewhat superior to muscle tissue. Brewers' yeast, peanuts, and peanut butter are among the richest sources of niacin, but they are not ordinarily consumed in sufficient amounts to greatly affect the dietary level.

Whole grains are fair sources of niacin, but the milling leads to a loss of 80 to 90 per cent of the niacin value. The enrichment of corn products in many southern states has been effective since this cereal is such a staple in the diet of many families.

Potatoes, legumes, and some green leafy vegetables contain fair amounts of preformed niacin, while most fruits and vegetables are poor sources.

Tryptophan constitutes approximately 1 per cent of the protein content of a diet in which complete protein foods predominate. Thus, an intake of 60 gm protein contributes 0.6 gm or 600 mg tryptophan. Since about 60 mg tryptophan are equivalent to 1 mg niacin, such a diet would provide 10 mg niacin in addition to the preformed niacin of the diet. Any reasonably good diet will contain 500 to 1000 mg tryptophan, equal to 8 to 17 mg niacin.

The preformed niacin contribution of the Four Food Groups may be seen in Figure 11-4.

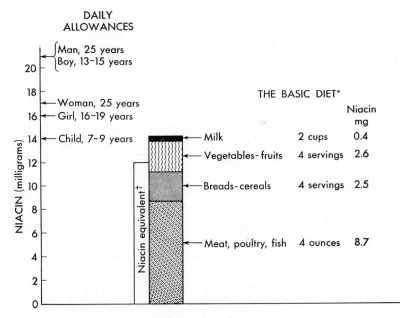

* See page 178 for complete calculations.
† Tryptophan content of the Basic Diet is estimated to be 720 mg, equivalent to an additional 12 mg niacin.

Fig. 11-4. The meat group contributes most of the niacin in the Basic Diet. Milk and eggs contain only traces of niacin but are excellent sources of tryptophan.

Retention of food values. The cookery of foods does not result in serious losses of niacin, except insofar as part of the soluble vitamin may be discarded in cooking waters which are not used. The application of principles for the retention of ascorbic acid and thiamine which have been discussed earlier will result in maximum retention of niacin as well.

Effect of deficiency. Pellagra appears after months of dietary deprivation.

The phenomenal decrease in the incidence of pellagra in the United States may be attributed to several factors including the enrichment program which is mandatory in some states, the concerted efforts in nutrition education, and the improvement in income. Pellagra is still a public health problem in some countries such as Spain, Yugoslavia, and certain areas of Africa.

Symptoms and clinical findings. Pellagra involves the gastrointestinal tract, the skin, and the nervous system. While no two cases of pellagra are exactly alike, the following symptoms are characteristic.

1. Early signs include fatigue, listlessness, headache, backache, loss of weight, loss of appetite, and general poor health.

2. Sore tongue, mouth, and throat, with glossitis extending throughout the gastrointestinal tract are present. The tongue and lips become abnormally red in color. The mouth becomes so sore that it is difficult to eat and swallow.

3. A deficiency of hydrochloric acid with a resultant anemia similar to pernicious anemia may be found.

4. Nausea and vomiting are followed by severe diarrhea.

5. A characteristic symmetrical dermatitis especially on the exposed sur-

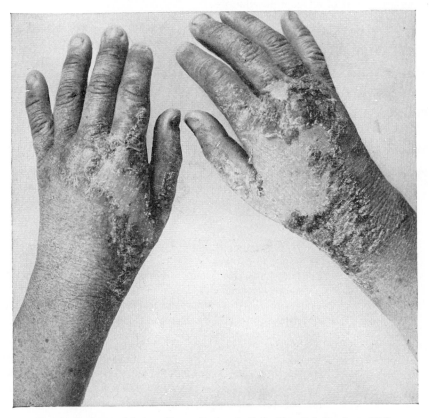

Fig. 11-5. Dermatitis in pellagra. Patient in Duke Hospital, Durham, N.C.

faces of the body—hands, forearms, elbows, feet, legs, knees, and neck—appears (see Fig. 11-5). The dermatitis is sharply separated from the surrounding normal skin. At first the skin becomes red, somewhat swollen, and tender, resembling a mild sunburn; if the condition is untreated, the skin becomes rough, cracked, and scaly, and may become ulcerated. Sunshine and exposure to heat aggravate the dermatitis.

6. Neurologic symptoms which include confusion, dizziness, poor memory, and irritability, and leading to hallucinations, delusions of persecution, and dementia are noted as severity increases.

The classic "D's" are the final stages of the diseases—dermatitis, diarrhea, dementia, and death.

Treatment and prophylaxis. Niacinamide is given in therapeutic doses, many times in excess of the Recommended Dietary Allowances. With such therapy it is possible to progress rapidly from an all-fluid diet to a soft diet. The High-protein Diets described on pages 373, 374, and 375 are indicated. Obviously, prophylaxis must include careful and persistent education in dietary improvement, emphasis on enrichment programs, and efforts to improve the economic status of affected populations.

VITAMIN B$_6$ GROUP

Nomenclature	Three active forms: pyridoxine (plant products); pyridoxal and pyridoxamine (animal products)
Properties	$C_8H_{11}O_3N$ (pyridoxine); white, crystalline, odorless, bitter tasting Water soluble; destroyed by ultraviolet light and heat
Measurement	Biologic or microbiologic; mg or mcg
Physiology and function	Pyridoxal is biologically active form. Pyridoxal phosphate is prosthetic group for enzymes which participate in degradation and interconversion of amino acids:

    a) Remove carbon dioxide (decarboxylation) from amino acids

    b) Transfer amino group (transamination) from one substance to another

    c) Transfer sulfur groups (transsulfuration) from one substance to another

Aids in conversion of tryptophan to niacin

Participates in metabolism of essential fatty acids

Deficiency	Has not been observed in adults from dietary deficiency alone. Produced experimentally by administering an antagonist, desoxypyridoxine. Symptoms include: depression; sleepiness; loss of appetite, nausea, vomiting; seborrheic dermatitis; soreness of lips and tongue; conjunctivitis; peripheral neuritis

Observed in infants receiving a formula deficient in vitamin B_6: [62]
impaired growth; hypochromic anemia; convulsions

Large urinary excretion of xanthurenic acid following test doses
of tryptophan indicates deficiency

Requirement   Estimated to be about 1–2 mg

Therapeutic   Prophylaxis for tubercular patients receiving large doses of
uses   isoniazid. Peripheral neuritis occurs with frequency in such
patients because isoniazid is apparently a vitamin B_6 antagonist

May be of some value in toxemias of pregnancy

Sources   Wheat germ, meat, liver, kidney, whole-grain cereals, soybeans,
peanuts, corn; small amounts in milk and green vegetables

PANTOTHENIC ACID

Nomenclature   Name from Greek word means "from everywhere"

Properties $C_9H_{17}NO_5$; commercially available as calcium pantothenate, a
white, odorless, slightly bitter compound

Water soluble; easily destroyed by dry heat and alkali

Stable in neutral solutions; nontoxic

Measurement   Microbiologic; mg or gm

Physiology and   Probably synthesized by intestinal bacteria
function   Utilization depends on presence of biotin and folacin

Component of coenzyme A (CoA), which participates in:

    a) Synthesis or breakdown of fatty acids through addition or
removal of a two-carbon fragment from carbon chain

    b) Synthesis of cholesterol, phospholipids, steroid hormones

    c) Oxidation of pyruvic acid

    d) Synthesis of porphyrins for hemoglobin

Deficiency   Not observed with natural diet. Feeding antagonist produces
these symptoms: loss of appetite, nausea, indigestion, abdominal pain; sullenness, mental depression; peripheral neuritis
—pains in arms and legs; repeated infections; fainting sensations, rapid pulse, lowered blood pressure; disturbed electrolyte and water balance

Requirement   Not known. Diet of 2500 calories provides about 10 mg which
is believed to be adequate

Therapeutic   Does not correct graying of hair in human beings
uses   "Burning foot" syndrome corrected in prisoners with multiple
B-complex deficiencies during World War II [63]

Needs probably increased during stress of severe illness, injury,
or following antibiotic therapy

Sources   Almost universally present in plant and animal tissue
                     Liver, kidney, yeast, egg yolk, peanuts, whole-grain cereals, lean
                        beef, skim milk, potatoes, tomatoes, broccoli, salmon
                     Loss of 50 per cent in milling of flour; 33 per cent lost in meat
                        cookery

BIOTIN

Nomenclature   Vitamin H, coenzyme R, anti-egg-white-injury factor

Properties $C_{10}H_{16}O_3N_2S$
                     Soluble in water; susceptible to oxidation and to alkali in the
                        free form; less labile in bound form
                     Stable to heat and acid

Measurement   Microbiologic; mcg

Physiology and   One of the most potent vitamins known
function   Synthesized in intestine; antibiotics interfere with synthesis;
                        avidin, a protein in raw egg white, combines with biotin in
                        intestine to prevent absorption
                     Functions not clearly understood; probably participates in
                        pyruvate metabolism, fixation of carbon dioxide, and in
                        deamination of certain amino acids

Deficiency   Unlikely in man
                     Experimental deficiency produced in man by use of high egg-
                        white intake (200 gm dried egg white daily);[64] dermatitis of
                        arms, legs; nervousness; anorexia; anemia, ashen pallor
                     In rats: spectacle eye; falling out of hair; loss of weight; loss of
                        muscular control

Requirement   Not known; probably 150–300 mcg daily
                     Intestinal synthesis may meet needs

Sources   Minute quantities widely distributed in foods
                     Liver, kidney, pancreas, molasses, milk, yeast, egg yolk

VITAMIN B$_{12}$

Nomenclature   Cobalamin; cyanocobalamin; antipernicious anemia factor; Cas-
                        tle's extrinsic factor

Properties $C_{63}H_{84}O_{14}N_{14}PCo$; only known cobalt-containing substance es-
                        sential for life
                     Deep red needle crystals; slightly soluble in water
                     Stable to heat in aqueous solutions; inactivated in alkaline or
                        strongly acid solutions or by light
                     Obtained as by-product in fermentations which produce anti-
                        biotics such as Aureomycin, streptomycin

Measurement	Microbiologic or chemical assay; mcg
Physiology and function	Absorption depends on presence of Castle's *intrinsic factor* in the stomach
	Microbial synthesis occurs in intestine, especially in ruminants; probably little if any synthesis in human intestinal tract
	Involved in purine metabolism and synthesis of nucleic acid and nucleoproteins
	Essential for maturation of red blood cells in bone marrow
	Metabolism of nervous tissue
	Metabolism of methionine; transfer of labile methyl groups; has lipotropic action
Deficiency	Pernicious anemia (see Chap. 38); following gastrectomy
Requirement	Not known; probably about 1–2 mcg
Therapeutic uses	Injections at intervals of a month or less for treating pernicious anemia
Sources	Occurs in minute concentrations chiefly in animal tissues; practically absent in higher plant forms
	Liver and kidney contain 40–50 mcg per 100 gm
	Milk, eggs, cheese, muscle meats contain 1–5 mcg per 100 gm
	Amply provided by small daily intakes of animal protein

FOLIC ACID GROUP

Nomenclature	Folacin or pteroylglutamic acid (PGA); tri- and hepta-pteroylglutamates are also active
	Folinic acid; citrovorum factor; leucovorin: biologically active form of folic acid
Properties	$C_{19}H_{19}N_7O_6$; contains pteridine, para-aminobenzoic acid, glutamic acid molecules
	Bright yellow crystals slightly soluble in water
	Easily oxidized in acid medium and in sunlight
	Not toxic except in massive doses
Measurement	Biologic, microbiologic, colorimetric, or fluorometric assay; mcg or mg
Physiology and function	Excreted in both urine and feces in excess of dietary levels; indicates bacterial synthesis occurs in intestine
	Free and conjugate forms are interchangeable
	Folic acid is transformed into biologically active folinic acid by ascorbic acid
	Participates in synthesis of purines and pyrimidines and of nucleoproteins; thus necessary for regeneration of blood cells
	Biosynthesis of methyl groups
	Related to metabolism of glutamic acid, tyrosine, phenylalanine

Deficiency	Not likely in man from dietary defects, but may occur secondary to disease; sprue, megaloblastic anemias of infancy, pregnancy In animals: anemia, leukopenia (reduced white blood cells), glossitis, diarrhea, poor feathering (in chicks)
Requirement	Not known; probably 0.1 to 0.2 mg daily
Therapeutic uses	Sprue, macrocytic anemias of infancy, pregnancy
Sources	Widespread in foods, both in free and conjugate forms Liver, kidney, yeast, deep green leafy vegetables are good sources; lean beef, veal, wheat cereal foods are fair; root vegetables, dairy foods, pork, light green vegetables are low Appreciable loss occurs in foods stored at room temperature and during cookery

CHOLINE

Properties	$C_5H_{15}NO_2$ Colorless, highly soluble, bitter tasting Stable in acid solution; decomposed in strong alkali Toxic in amounts of 15 to 70 gm
Measurement	gm or mg
Physiology and function	Synthesized by the body from methionine; is probably not a true vitamin Present in almost all cells as constituent of phospholipids: lecithin, cephalin, sphingomyelin Provides labile methyl ($—CH_3$) group which can be transferred from one substance to another (transmethylation) Interrelated with methionine, vitamin B_{12}, and folic acid in prevention of fatty livers Involved in transmission of nerve impulses through production of acetylcholine
Deficiency	Not known in man In animals: hemorrhagic degeneration of kidneys, adrenals, heart, lungs, eyes; cirrhosis; slipped tendon disease in chicks
Requirement	250–600 mg in average diet is ample Methionine exerts sparing effect
Sources	Egg yolk, best; liver, brain, kidney, heart, sweetbreads, tongue; milk, meat, nuts, cereals, vegetables, fruits

INOSITOL

Properties	$C_6H_{12}O_6$; water-soluble; sweet taste Not toxic

Physiology	Significance in human nutrition not established
	Possesses lipotropic activity
Deficiency	Not reported in man
	In animals: loss of hair, failure of lactation and growth, reproductive failure
Sources	Fruits, milk, meat, nuts, whole grains, yeast, vegetables

PARA-AMINOBENZOIC ACID

Nomenclature	Abbreviated PABA
Properties	$NH_2C_6H_4COOH$
	Colorless crystalline compound slightly soluble in water
	Stable in dilute acids and alkalies
	Easily oxidized
Physiology	Component of folic acid
	Prevents gray hair in rats and mice, but has no value in restoring natural color of gray hair in humans
Deficiency	Not observed in man
Requirement	Its need is questioned in animal nutrition
Therapeutic uses	Effective in treatment of typhus fever, Rocky Mountain spotted fever
Sources	Yeast, liver, molasses, rice bran, wheat germ

ANTIVITAMINS

"An antivitamin may be defined as any substance that interferes with the synthesis or metabolism of a vitamin as, for example, by (a) inactivation or chemical destruction, (b) irreversible combination, or (c) competitive inhibition." *

Bacteria are known to require certain vitamins for their growth. Thus, there is great interest in finding compounds which will interfere with the synthesis or metabolism of vitamins by pathogenic bacteria and will thus prove to be effective therapeutic agents. Sulfa drugs and antibiotics have been found to be substances which interfere with the growth of intestinal flora.

Nutrition workers are obviously interested in the possible effects of such antivitamins. In the first place, the use of chemotherapeutic agents may impose a vitamin deficiency not only in the bacteria which are being combated but also in the patient who is being treated. In the second place, interfering

* Wright, L. D.: "The Significance of the Anti-Vitamins in Nutrition," *J. Am. Dietet. A.,* **23:**289, 1947.

SUMMARY OF FOUR

NOMENCLATURE	UNITS AND METHODS OF ASSAY	IMPORTANT SOURCES	STABILITY IN FOODS
Ascorbic acid vitamin C antiscorbutic vitamin	mg Chemical	Citrus fruits Tomatoes Strawberries Cantaloupe Cabbage Broccoli Kale Potatoes	Highly soluble in water Most easily destroyed of all vitamins—heat, air, alkali, enzymes Acid inhibits destruction Copper accelerates destruction

Thiamine
vitamin B₁
antiberiberi
vitamin
	mg or mcg
	
	Chemical
	Microbiologic
		Pork
		Liver, other organs
		Brewers' yeast
		Wheat germ
		Whole-grain cereals and
		  breads
		Enriched cereals, breads
		Soybeans, legumes,
		  peanuts
		Milk
			Stable in slightly acid
			solution
			Quickly destroyed by
			heat in neutral or alka-
			line solution
			Sulfite quickly destroys
			it
			Highly soluble in water

Riboflavin vitamin B₂ (formerly: lactoflavin; vitamin G)	mg or mcg Chemical Microbiologic	Milk Powdered whey Liver, kidney, heart, meats Eggs Green leafy vegetables Dried yeast Enriched foods	Quickly decomposed by light and very sensitive to alkali Relatively resistant to heat in acid Sparingly soluble in water

Niacin
nicotinic acid
niacinamide
antipellagra
vitamin
	mg
	
	Chemical
	Microbiologic
		Lean meat, fish, poultry
		Liver, kidney
		Whole-grain cereals,
		  breads
		Enriched cereals,
		  breads
		Green vegetables
		Peanuts
		Brewers' yeast
			Stable to heat and oxida-
			tion, light
			Slightly soluble in water
			Stable to acid and alkali

substances may occur naturally in foods so that the vitamin is rendered inactive. One of the earliest recognized examples of this nature is avidin, which
combines with biotin. Since extremely large quantities of raw egg white must
be eaten to supply sufficient avidin to combine with the biotin before deficiency
occurs, this does not appear to be of great practical significance. Raw fish and
clams contain an enzyme that splits thiamine so that animals eating fish as
chief articles of the diet have succumbed to thiamine deficiency. This enzyme
is destroyed by cookery so that there again appears to be little to fear in the
eating of fish, except possibly raw clams.

WATER-SOLUBLE VITAMINS

PHYSIOLOGY AND FUNCTIONS	EFFECT OF DEFICIENCY	DAILY ALLOWANCES *
Very little storage in body Greatest concentrations in most active tissues Forms and maintains inter-cellular substance Metabolism of some amino acids Facilitates absorption of iron Conversion of folic acid to folinic acid	Cutaneous hemorrhages Improper bone develop-ment Weakened cartilages Muscle degeneration Anemia Stunted growth Susceptibility to infection *Scurvy*	Adults: 70–75 mg Pregnancy: 100 mg Lactation: 150 mg Children under 10: 30–60 mg Children over 10: 75–100 mg
Possibly some synthesis in body Limited storage in body Part of enzyme system, *car-boxylase,* which removes COOH group from pyruvic acid	Lack of appetite Nervous instability Depression Fatigue Gastrointestinal atony and constipation *Beriberi,* polyneuritis, cardiac failure, edema	0.5 mg per 1000 calories Adults: 1.0–1.6 mg Children under 10: 0.4–1.1 mg Children over 10: 1.2–1.8 mg
Storage in body is limited, but body retains supplies care-fully Constituent of enzyme system —transfers hydrogen from one metabolite to another	Cracks at corners of lips (*cheilosis*) Inflammation of lips and tongue Burning and itching of eyes Photophobia Blurred vision	Adults: 1.5–1.8 mg Pregnancy: 2.0 mg Lactation: 2.5 mg Children under 10: 0.5–1.5 mg Children over 10: 1.8–2.5 mg
60 mg tryptophan equivalent to 1 mg niacin Active constituent of enzyme system—transfer of hydrogen	*Pellagra:* gastrointestinal, skin, and neurologic changes	Adults: 17–21 mg Children under 10: 6–14 mg Children over 10: 16–25 mg

* See Recommended Dietary Allowances, page 26, for complete listing.
limited storage of above.

Some compounds are closely related in structure to the vitamins but are unable to function as the active vitamin. When such compounds are fed, a vitamin deficiency may be produced which could not be effected by diet alone. The use of the antagonists for pantothenic acid and vitamin B_6 has made it possible to study the functions of these vitamins.

Dicoumarin, which has been isolated from spoiled sweet clover, produces hypoprothrombinemia in a number of species. A sufficient intake of vitamin K will counteract this action. Dicoumarin may be broken down to salicylates which again have antivitamin K properties. The administration of vitamin K during salicylate therapy decreases the tendency to prolonged bleeding but does not interfere with the usefulness of the salicylates.

PROBLEMS AND REVIEW

1. Explain how the following nutrients are interrelated:

riboflavin and niacin	tryptophan and vitamin B_6
tryptophan and niacin	folic acid and folinic acid
glucose and thiamine	cobalt and vitamin B_{12}
pyridoxine and protein	folic acid and ascorbic acid
choline and fat	

2. What is the effect on carbohydrate metabolism of a deficiency of thiamine? What are clinical signs of such deficiency?

3. What is the role of niacin in metabolism? What clinical symptoms are observed in a niacin deficiency?

4. How can you explain the fact that milk is a pellagra-preventive food even though it contains very little niacin?

5. The dietary intake of vitamins may appear to be satisfactory when compared with recommended allowances, but a physician may prescribe a vitamin supplement. Under what circumstances would you expect such a supplement to be necessary?

6. What is the possible significance of each of the following in human nutrition: folic acid; choline; biotin; pantothenic acid; pyridoxine; inositol; vitamin B_{12}; antivitamins?

7. *Problem.* Examine the label information on three packages of dry cereals. Calculate the percentage of the recommended allowances provided by 1 ounce of each cereal, using your own allowances as the basis for calculation. How do these percentages compare with those indicated on the label? Explain any differences.

8. *Problem.* Mrs. Smith has asked for your guidance in the selection, storage, and preparation of foods so that maximum nutritive value will be retained. On the basis of your information concerning the stability of vitamins, indicate briefly a set of instructions for guiding Mrs. Smith. Show how these rules apply to the preparation of a meal which includes roast beef, potatoes, green beans, cole slaw, milk, and fruit cup. Which vitamin or vitamins are especially concerned in each rule which you have laid down?

9. *Problem.* Calculate the thiamine, riboflavin, and niacin content of your own diet for 2 days. Compare your intake with the recommended allowances. If there are any deficits, show how you could correct them.

10. *Problem.* A dietary calculation showed an intake of 80 gm protein and 12 mg niacin. Calculate the total niacin equivalent of this diet.

11. *Problem.* Calculate the percentage of your own daily requirement for thiamine and riboflavin which 3 cups of milk would supply. For each of these nutrients list two foods which would serve as effective supplements to the milk in supplying your daily needs.

CHAPTER 12 /

Water

The body's need for water is second only to that for oxygen. It is possible to live for days and even weeks without food, but death is likely to follow a deprivation of water within a few days. Approximately 55–70 per cent of the total body weight is made up of water. Infants and young children have a higher percentage of water in their bodies than adults. The percentage of water in lean individuals is higher than that of obese persons.

Fluid within the cells (intracellular fluid) accounts for about three-fourths of the total body water, while the remainder is found in the circulating plasma and as interstitial fluid (lymph and fluid which bathes the tissues). The circulating plasma is about 5 per cent of the total body weight.

Functions. All the chemical changes which occur in the cells of the body take place in the presence of water. It is the medium of the body fluids, the secretions, and the excretions—blood, lymph, digestive juices, bile, perspiration, urine, and feces. Water acts as a solvent for all the products of digestion, holding them in solution and permitting them to pass through the absorbing walls of the intestinal tract into the blood stream. The blood, which is about 90 per cent water, carries nutritive elements to the cells and is the vehicle for carrying carbon dioxide to the lungs and waste nitrogenous material and salts to the kidneys. Urine consists of about 97 per cent water and holds the waste materials in solution, while bowel wastes can be eliminated only if sufficient water is present to avoid constipation.

Water is also an important lubricant, for it prevents friction between moving body parts. It regulates body temperature through evaporation from the skin and lungs.

WATER IN FOODS

	Per Cent	
Milk	87	
Eggs	75	
Meat	40–75	The higher values in rare meats
Fruits, vegetables	70–95	The higher values in low-carbohydrate foods
Cereals	8–20	
Bread	35	

Sources of water to the body. There are three sources of water to the body: (1) water as such, (2) water contained in foods, and (3) water formed by oxidation of foodstuffs in the body.

All foods, even those which are considered to be dry, contain appreciable quantities of water, as may be seen below. The average diet, including milk, contains roughly 1000 ml water.

The oxidation of nutrients by the tissues results in the release of water. For example:

$$C_6H_{12}O_6 + 6\ O_2 = 6\ H_2O + 6\ CO_2$$

The amount of water which is thus released has been estimated to be: [65]

100 gm of fat	give 107.1 gm of water
100 gm of carbohydrate	give 55.5 gm of water
100 gm of protein	give 41.3 gm of water

For an average mixed diet this will approximate 300 to 450 ml daily.

Avenues of water loss from the body. Water is lost from the body through the kidneys and skin, and to a lesser degree from the lungs and gastrointestinal tract. The rate of filtration in the normal kidney is about 125 ml per minute or approximately 180 liters daily for an adult. About 99 per cent of the water filtered is reabsorbed into the blood, while 500 to 2000 ml are excreted as urine. The volume of urine reflects to some extent the fluid intake of the individual. The urine volume decreases when perspiration is excessive, unless the fluid intake is proportionately increased.

A relatively constant amount of water is lost daily from the skin as *insensible perspiration;* that is, the water loss is not noticeable because evaporation takes place immediately. This evaporation is an important means by which the body temperature is maintained. The loss of water is proportionate to the surface area of the body. During very warm weather or considerable increase in activity, much water is lost as visible perspiration. Some athletes may lose several quarts of water during a strenuous game.

Air expired from the lungs also contains water, which may amount to 300 ml or so a day under ordinary circumstances. As one's activity increases and hence the rate of respiration increases, more water will be lost by this route.

Normally, the water lost from the gastrointestinal tract is small. The volume of water contained in the daily secretion of saliva, gastric juice, bile, pancreatic juice, and intestinal juice is roughly 7000 to 8000 ml. These fluids are poured into the alimentary tract for their respective functions, and then as digestion is completed the water from these juices is reabsorbed into the blood stream. About 100 ml of water are normally lost each day in the saliva and in the feces.

Water balance. The importance of keeping the body in fluid balance is universally recognized. The body is said to be in water balance when the available water equals that of the water excreted or lost from the body. Newburgh * has illustrated this in the following table:

NORMAL WATER BALANCE

AVAILABLE WATER	gm	EXCRETED WATER	gm
Water intake as such	1100	In urine	1000
Water in diet	900	In stool	200
Water of oxidation	200	In vapor (skin and lungs)	1000
TOTAL	2200	TOTAL	2200

The body maintains water balance precisely even though the fluid intake from day to day varies widely. The regulatory mechanisms are not fully understood, but certain regions of the hypothalamus are believed to regulate thirst just as other regions regulate the appetite. Several hormones are known to control the rate of water excretion. One of these is an antidiuretic hormone produced by the posterior portion of the pituitary gland. This hormone decreases excretion of water by the kidney by increasing the rate of reabsorption from the kidney tubules. The hormones produced by the adrenal cortex regulate the excretion of sodium and hence the excretion of water, since the body fluids are maintained with constant levels of sodium. To some extent the female sex hormones influence water excretion. It is a common finding that women show slight increases in weight just before menstruation begins, and that this weight is subsequently lost.

Abnormal loss of water occurs from prolonged vomiting, as in pernicious vomiting of pregnancy and postoperative vomiting. Hemorrhage, prolonged diarrhea, protracted fevers, excessive perspiration, and burns may bring about great losses of water from the body. A deficiency of the antidiuretic hormone leads to excessive thirst and large volumes of urine, a condition known as diabetes insipidus. A loss of 10 per cent of fluid from the body represents a serious menace to health. It may lead to poor absorption of food, elevation of body temperature, circulatory failure, and impairment of renal function.

To compensate for abnormal losses of water from the body, the intake may be increased by (1) beverages, broth, ices, etc., and (2) by parenteral fluids. When the food intake is limited, and when dehydration has occurred, the replenishment of water also requires the adjustment of electrolyte balance, a subject beyond the scope of this text.

The body, in certain pathologic conditions, may be in positive water balance; that is, the intake of fluids is greater than the excretion, and the patient is said to have *edema.* Severe disturbances of protein nutrition may lead to a

* Newburgh, L. H., and MacKinnon, F.: *The Practice of Dietetics,* The Macmillan Company, New York, 1934.

lowered concentration of the serum proteins, albumin especially, so that the normal osmotic pressure is not maintained. As a result, the tissues hold water. Circulatory and renal disturbances may likewise lead to retention of sodium and of water. Congestive heart failure, cirrhosis of the liver, nephritis, and nephrosis are examples of cardiovascular and renal disturbances in which edema may be a complication.

Daily allowances. Thirst is a good guide to water intake except during abnormal conditions when dehydration has developed. Water taken in excess will be eliminated by the kidney. An intake of 6 to 8 cups water daily is sufficient under normal conditions, but in hot weather or during strenuous activity the intake may need to be several times as great. Water with meals is not objectionable if it is not used to wash down food before it is properly masticated.

PROBLEM AND REVIEW

1. List specific functions which water performs in the body.

2. What is meant by water balance? Under what circumstances does a negative water balance occur? A positive water balance?

3. If you found yourself in a situation where the amount of water for drinking was extremely scarce, what could you do to conserve your body water as much as possible?

4. During warm weather the urine volume is sometimes reduced. How can you explain this?

5. *Problem.* Keep a record of your fluid intake for a day, including all beverages taken with meals. By referring to a table of food values, calculate the water content of all the foods you ate. About how much water would be formed in oxidation if your body metabolized 80 gm protein, 100 gm fat, 250 gm carbohydrate?

6. By what routes is the water you have ingested excreted? What are the relative amounts by each route?

CHAPTER 13 /

Digestion, Absorption, and Metabolism

Only water, monosaccharides, salts, vitamins, and a few organic compounds of low molecular weight can be utilized by the body as they are consumed. Carbohydrates must be hydrolyzed to simple sugars, proteins to amino acids, and fats to fatty acids and glycerol before the body is able to use these complex food materials. *Digestion* includes the mechanical and chemical processes whereby these nutrients are broken down into small units of structure so that absorption can take place from the intestinal wall into the blood stream. By *mechanical* means the food is finely divided and propelled along the intestinal tract, so that by *chemical* means it may be readily hydrolyzed into water-soluble products which are suitable for absorption.

A thorough understanding of the principles of nutrition is not possible without some knowledge concerning the processes of digestion, absorption, and metabolism. The breakdown of protein, fat, and carbohydrate to simpler substances and the subsequent absorption and utilization have been discussed in Chapters 4, 5, and 6. The discussion in this chapter is intended as a correlation of these facts, since no diet is made up of single purified nutrients. Many good textbooks in physiology and biochemistry are available for the student who wishes to make a more comprehensive study.

The nature of enzymes. The chemical changes which take place during digestion are brought about by the activity of hydrolyzing enzymes, namely carbohydrases, lipases, and proteases. Enzymes are catalytic agents of a protein nature which are manufactured by specialized living cells and which have the power to produce chemical changes in other substances. Most enzymes take their name from the substance upon which they act, the ending *ase* being added to the root word. For example, protease derives its name from the protein upon which it acts, and amylase (*amylum*—starch, Latin) from the starch upon which it acts.

In many cases the enzyme occurs in an inactive form, *proenzyme* or *zymogen*, within the cells which produce it. It is activated at the time of secretion or subsequent to secretion by the presence of certain materials known as coenzymes

165

"coenzymes" or "activators." The substance upon which an enzyme acts is known as the "substrate." For example:

$$\text{trypsinogen} \xrightarrow[\text{(activator)}]{\text{enterokinase}} \text{trypsin}$$
$$\text{(proenzyme)} \qquad \text{(active enzyme)}$$

$$\text{protein} + \text{water} \xrightarrow{\text{trypsin}} \text{proteoses, peptones, polypeptides}$$
$$\text{(substrate)}$$

Enzymes are highly specific substances; that is, an enzyme which splits carbohydrate cannot digest protein, nor can maltase which hydrolyzes maltose have any effect on lactose. They are extremely powerful in their action, for a small amount of some of them can accomplish the digestion of as much as 4,000,000 times its own weight of substance. Even more surprising is the fact that the enzyme acts on a substance without itself being changed or entering into the reaction. Every enzyme has a specific temperature at which it works, those in the body being most efficient at body temperature. They become quite inactive in cold temperatures, but, being protein in nature, are entirely destroyed by heat. Moisture is necessary for their activity. Some enzymes, such as pepsin, work only in an acid medium, while others,

SUMMARY OF DIGESTIVE ENZYMES

ENZYME	SECRETED BY	SUBSTRATE	PRODUCTS OF ENZYME ACTIVITY
Salivary amylase (ptyalin)	Salivary glands	Cooked starch	Dextrins and maltose
Rennin	Gastric mucosa	Milk casein	Calcium caseinate
Pepsin		Protein	Proteoses and peptones
Lipase		Emulsified fats	Fatty acids and glycerol
Trypsin	Pancreas	Protein	Proteoses, peptones, polypeptides
Chymotrypsin		Protein	Proteoses, peptones, polypeptides
Pancreatic amylase (amylopsin)		Cooked and raw starch	Dextrins and maltose
Pancreatic lipase (steapsin)		Fats	Simple glycerides, fatty acids, glycerol
Enterokinase	Intestinal mucosa	Trypsinogen	Trypsin
Peptidases (erepsin—a group of enzymes)		Peptones, polypeptides, dipeptides	Amino acids
Nuclease—a group of enzymes		Nucleic acid and derivatives	Phosphoric acid, carbohydrates, purine, and pyrimidine bases
Sucrase (invertase)		Sucrose	Glucose and fructose
Maltase		Maltose	Glucose
Lactase		Lactose	Glucose and galactose

such as trypsin, work only at a slightly alkaline reaction. The enzymes of digestion with which we are concerned here are secreted by the glands in the mouth, the stomach, the small intestines, and the pancreas. The table on page 166 summarizes them.

Digestion in the mouth. Food in the mouth is cut and ground into smaller pieces by the teeth. Mastication, especially of crisp, hard foods which require longer chewing, together with psychic factors such as sight, taste, odor, and memory of agreeable foods stimulates the flow of saliva by three pairs of salivary glands, the parotid, submaxillary, and sublingual. Saliva is made up of water, mucin, inorganic salts, and enzymes known as amylase (ptyalin), and possibly maltase, which act on starch and maltose, respectively. It is weakly acid to weakly alkaline in reaction. About 1000 to 1500 ml are secreted daily.

Saliva serves several purposes in digestion: (1) it moistens and softens the food, thus assisting in mastication; (2) the mucin lubricates and assists the food in its passage down the esophagus; (3) the amylase acts upon cooked starch and changes it to the sugar, maltose. However, there is not a great deal of chemical change brought about in the starches, owing to the limited time they remain in the mouth.

Food does not remain in the mouth long enough to become completely liquefied, but it is softer and more easily swallowed. Peristaltic constrictions occur in the walls of the esophagus which propel the mass into the cardiac region of the stomach.

Digestion in the stomach. The fundus of the stomach serves as a reservoir for food (see Fig. 13-1). As there is little movement in this part of the organ, digestion of starch which was begun in the mouth is continued here for ½ to 2 hours. If the food was chewed well so as to become thoroughly mixed with saliva, starches may be broken down to a large extent before the food becomes mixed with acid. Salivary amylase reacts best in a faintly alkaline to faintly acid medium but is quickly inactivated by strong acid such as hydrochloric acid.

Food coming into the stomach expands the stomach walls, and each addition pushes the mass preceding it forward toward the central part of the organ, where small contractions begin and run toward the pylorus. These contractions are regular and increase in strength as digestion progresses. As a result, the food is broken up still further, mixed with the gastric juice, and finally reduced to a thin souplike composition called *chyme*. The deep peristaltic wave which carries the food toward the pylorus has its beginning in the central portion of the stomach. The pyloric valve which separates the stomach from the small intestine opens from time to time to allow chyme to pass through.

The emptying time of the stomach depends upon the character, type, and amount of food eaten. Liquids begin to leave the stomach in from 15 minutes to ½ hour, a fact which explains why liquid diets do not have great satiety value. Carbohydrates, when eaten alone, leave the stomach more rapidly than do proteins. Fats check the secretion of gastric juice and retard peristaltic movement, and consequently they remain in the stomach longer than the other nutrients. Mixtures of the three nutrients remain longest in the stomach. A normal stomach should empty itself in from 4 to 6 hours. A small test meal should pass out of the stomach in from 1 to 4 hours. Longer than 7 hours' emptying time indicates impairment of tone and motility.

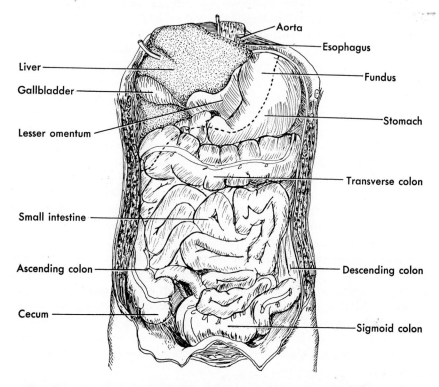

Fig. 13-1. The stomach and intestines, front view, the great omentum having been removed and the liver turned up and to the right. The dotted line shows the normal position of the anterior border of the liver. (From Kimber, D. C.; Gray, C. E.; Stackpole, C. E.; and Leavell, L. C.: *Anatomy and Physiology,* 14th ed. The Macmillan Company, New York, 1961.)

Chemical changes in the stomach are brought about by the action of the gastric juice which is secreted by cells in the middle region of the stomach. Psychic stimulation of secretion of the juice is started by the sight, odor, taste, or thought of food. Further secretion occurs as food enters the stomach. Gastric juice is made up of water, mucinlike proteins, hydrochloric acid, inorganic salts, and the enzymes rennin, pepsin, and lipase. Rennin and pepsin are secreted in their inactive forms, prorennin and pepsinogen. The *intrinsic factor* which is essential for the absorption of vitamin B_{12} is also a constituent of gastric juice. The amount of gastric juice secreted depends upon the amount and nature of the food to be digested. Gastric juice has a strong acid reaction, equivalent to 0.1 normal solution (0.4 per cent) of hydrochloric acid.

Hydrochloric acid serves several purposes in digestion: (1) it swells the protein, making it more easily acted upon by the enzymes; (2) it converts inactive pepsinogen and prorennin to active pepsin and rennin, respectively; (3) it brings about the inversion of cane sugar, making the disaccharide more easily convertible into the monosaccharide in the intestine; (4) it serves as a disinfectant, destroying some of the bacteria which enter the stomach with food; (5) it stimulates the opening of the pyloric valve in the early stages of digestion; and (6) it provides the correct reaction for the absorption of iron.

The chief digestive change in the stomach is the partial hydrolysis of proteins to proteoses and peptones through the action of a protease, pepsin. When digestion is at its height, some proteins may pass into the duodenum without being acted upon at all by pepsin and must be broken down entirely after reaching the small intestine.

Rennin is an enzyme found especially in the stomach of the infant and child. It coagulates milk, thus changing the soluble casein into insoluble calcium caseinate and preparing for its digestion by pepsin. In this way milk is kept from passing through the stomach too rapidly.

While gastric juice does contain a lipase, the action on fats in the stomach is not very important. Finely emulsified fats such as egg yolk or cream may be hydrolyzed in part to fatty acids and glycerol; the majority of fat in the diet is not acted upon until it has been emulsified by bile in the small intestine.

Digestion in the small intestine. There are two types of movement in the small intestine: (1) peristaltic waves and (2) rhythmic segmentation. Peristaltic waves carry the food mass slowly down the tract, while the segmentary wave divides the food mass into numerous segments (see Fig. 13-2). This process not only mixes the food with the juices, allowing the enzymes free access to the nutrients present, but also spreads the digested materials over a large portion of the absorbing intestinal wall. The unabsorbed contents of the small intestine begin to pass through the ileocecal valve (the valve dividing the small from the large intestine) in from 2 to $5\frac{1}{2}$ hours. From the time of eating, 9 hours or more are required for the last of a large meal to pass into the large intestine. Fiber, by reason of the pressure it exerts upon the intestinal walls, has a tendency to stimulate peristalsis, thus promoting elimination of waste material.

As chyme enters the intestine it contains partially hydrolyzed proteins, chiefly proteoses and peptones; carbohydrates in various stages of hydrolysis including incompletely digested starch, dextrins, sugars, and cellulose; and fats, a few of which are emulsified. Digestion in the small intestine is the result of the simultaneous action of bile and the enzymes secreted in the pancreatic and intestinal juices. The acid reaction of the chyme stimulates the production in the intestinal walls of a hormone, *secretin,* which is carried by the blood stream to the pancreas. Secretin in turn stimulates the cells of the pancreas to secretory activity. Since the pancreatic and bile ducts open into the intestine only a few inches beyond the pylorus, the digestive juices quickly neutralize chyme acidity and maintain the appropriate alkaline reaction for the intestinal enzymes.

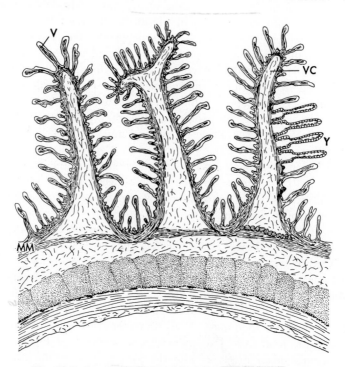

Fig. 13-2. Longitudinal section of small intestine. Three valvulae conniventes (*VC*) are shown. Many villi (*V*) are shown on the valvulae and between them. At *Y* four villi with glands between them have been diagramed. *MM:* muscularis mucosae. (From Kimber, D. C.; Gray, C. E.; Stackpole, C. E.; and Leavell, L. C.: *Anatomy and Physiology,* 14th ed. The Macmillan Company, New York, 1961.)

Pancreatic juice contains several enzymes, the chief of which are: pancreatic amylase (amylopsin), which splits both cooked and raw starch to the sugar maltose; lipase (steapsin), which splits fats to fatty acids and glycerol; and trypsin and chymotrypsin, which split proteins to proteoses, peptones, and polypeptides. The latter enzymes are secreted in their inactive forms, trypsinogen and chymotrypsinogen, by the pancreas. Trypsinogen is activated by enterokinase secreted by the intestinal mucosa, while chymotrypsinogen is activated by trypsin.

Bile is composed of bile acids, bile pigments, mucin, neutral fats, cholesterol, phosphatides, lecithin, nucleoproteins, and inorganic salts. Bile is chiefly useful in the digestion and absorption of fats. The bile salts effectively emulsify fats, thus greatly increasing the surface area so that steapsin can rapidly bring about hydrolysis to fatty acids and glycerol.

Intestinal juice (succus entericus) contains: a group of proteases, formerly thought to be a single enzyme (erepsin), which hydrolyze proteoses and peptones to polypeptides, dipeptides, and finally amino acids; three carbohydrases—(1) maltase, splitting maltose to glucose; (2) sucrase (invertase), splitting sucrose to glucose and fructose; and (3) lactase, splitting lactose to glucose and galactose; and an activator, enterokinase, which converts trypsinogen to trypsin, + intestinal lipase.

Intestinal bacteria attack cellulose in the chyme and bring about further disintegration. The intestinal bacteria are now known to be important for the synthesis of some of the vitamins needed by the body.

Functions of the large intestine. Most of the available nutrients are absorbed from the small intestine. The cecum fills slowly, and the waves which carry the mass toward the rectum, together with the antiperistaltic waves which force it back, spread the mass over the absorbing walls of the large intestine, thus giving the unabsorbed material an opportunity to pass through the walls of the large intestine. Considerable amounts of water from the digested food mass, including the digestive juices, are absorbed from the large intestine.

The emptying time of the large intestine depends upon the amount and type of food eaten. Concentrated foods leaving little residue stay a longer time in the colon than foods rich in fiber, the increase in bulk acting as a stimulus to the muscular contractions which constitute evacuation, or normal bowel movement. The feces contain not only the residues of food digestion, but also dead and live bacteria, residues from the digestive juices, and certain wastes of metabolism.

There are no enzymes of digestion in the large intestine; the secretions there show much mucin and are alkaline in recreation.

Factors affecting digestion. The term "digestibility" generally refers to the comfort or ease of digestion and to the rapidity with which food leaves the stomach rather than to the completeness of its digestion. Therefore, anything which either speeds up or slows down the emptying time of the stomach may be considered as an influencing factor in digestion.

Consistency, division, and type of food. Foods which need little if any breaking up before they are ready to be absorbed may be said to be readily digestible. For example, liquids leave the stomach rapidly and are more quickly available for absorption than are foods requiring mechanical division. Mastication plays an important part in digestion because it stimulates the flow of saliva, which softens the finely divided food and makes it accessible to the action of the enzymes which occur in the digestive juices. The amount and type of food taken at one time affect digestion. Fats digest slowly and when taken with other foods have a tendency to retard their digestion also. Of the carbohydrate foods, those rich in sugar digest quickly and completely, leaving no residue in the intestinal tract, while the starchy foods, though almost completely absorbed, pass through the tract more slowly. Foods rich in cellulose digest more slowly than those free from fiber, the cellulose itself not being digested at all. Cellulose adds bulk to the food mass, however, and stimulates its passage down the tract.

Bacterial action. Bacteria of various types inhabit the human alimentary tract shortly after birth and become so firmly established therein that they are considered almost a part of it. The types most commonly found are (1) fermentative, (2) putrefactive, and (3) bacteria of coli type. The latter exhibit characteristics of both the other types. Under normal conditions there is not much bacterial action in the stomach since the hydrochloric acid acts as a germicidal agent. However, when there is a decrease in the acid secretion, fermentative bacteria may grow rapidly, especially when excessive amounts of carbohydrate are taken.

Much fermentation of carbohydrate residues and putrefaction of protein residues occurs in the large intestine, but these reactions cause no trouble under normal conditions.

Chemical factors. There are certain chemical factors which stimulate the flow of juice in the stomach—strong acids, meat extractives, spices, etc.; others, such as fat, retard the flow.

Psychic factors. Anger, fright, or worry delays digestion by reason of their depressing effect upon the secretions. The first two emotions take immediate effect, slowing down or even stopping temporarily the process of digestion, while worry is probably responsible for a more lasting as well as more detrimental effect because it interferes with general nutrition by depressing normal appetite. On the other hand, the sight, smell, and taste of palatable food stimulate the nerves and cause a flow of juice in the mouth known as "appetite juices." These juices are actively responsible for the early appearance of gastric juice in the stomach; and while digestion in that organ will take place without the assistance of the mouth secretion, it is undoubtedly true that the latter hastens the process.

Coefficient of digestibility. While many factors may influence the comfort of digestion, the completeness of digestion is not necessarily so influenced. The coefficient of digestibility is a measure of food absorbed in relation to food consumed. For example, if the feces contain 5 per cent of the fat of the diet, the coefficient of digestibility is said to be 95 per cent. Although there are variations among foods, in general, the coefficient of digestibility for protein is 92 per cent; for fat, 95 per cent, and for carbohydrate, 98 per cent.

Absorption and metabolism of food. Almost all of the soluble nutrients are absorbed from the small intestine. Absorption is a selective process in which the end products of digestion are permitted to enter the circulation. The 4,000,000 or 5,000,000 *villi,* or tiny fingerlike projections which constitute the walls of the small intestine, together with the great length of this organ, give an enormous area from which absorption can take place. Each villus is supplied with (1) capillaries, (2) lacteals which are part of the lymphatic system, and (3) tiny muscles which contract to mechanically assist absorption. The almost continuous contractions of the intestinal wall force the blood and lymph containing the nutrients into the general circulation, while relaxation allows fresh blood and lymph to collect more nutrients.

Carbohydrates. Apparently, the monosaccharides combine with phosphoric acid in the intestinal mucosa to form a compound much more rapidly absorbed than are the sugars themselves. The absorbed carbohydrates are then carried to the liver where, through the action of insulin, they are converted to glycogen until needed. The tissues draw glucose from the circulation to meet energy needs. The liver glycogen is hydrolyzed to glucose at a rate which will maintain a constant blood sugar level of 0.1 per cent. (See also p. 60.)

Amino acids. Amino acids, like monosaccharides, are absorbed by the capillaries and carried to the liver via the portal circulation. Some investigators believe that minute quantities of soluble proteins such as peptones may also be absorbed. The amino acids may be used for tissue regeneration and synthesis, or they may be deaminized by the liver. In the latter case the ammonia is excreted as urea and the rest of the amino acid molecule is used for energy. (See also p. 41.)

Fats. A small fraction of emulsified fats may enter the lymphatics without previous hydrolysis. Most of the fats, however, must be hydrolyzed before they are ready for absorption. Fatty acids are insoluble in water, but bile salts unite with some of them to give water-soluble compounds which are readily absorbed. Other fatty acids are synthesized with glycerol, phosphoric acid, and organic base in the intestinal mucosa to form phospholipids, while still other fatty acids may be carried into the intestinal mucosa with cholesterol as esters. It is likely that the fatty acids and glycerol recombine in the intestinal mucosa to form neutral fats before absorption finally occurs.

Fats are transported from the lacteals by the lymphatics to the thoracic duct where they enter the blood circulation in the left subclavian vein. Some of the phospholipids and short-chain fatty acids are carried directly to the liver from the portal circulation. (See also p. 71.)

PROBLEM AND REVIEW

1. What is meant by the following terms: digestion; coefficient of digestibility; peristalsis; segmentation?

2. An enzyme is a catalyst produced by living cells. Name five characteristics of enzymes.

3. In what way does the chewing of food aid digestion in the stomach?

4. It is important that foods be attractively served. How does this facilitate good digestion?

5. Pepsin is a proteolytic enzyme which is secreted by the gastric mucosa as a proenzyme, pepsinogen. How is the pepsinogen activated? What is the substrate on which pepsin acts?

6. Many pediatricians permit children to have foods such as fruit and bread or crackers between meals, but advise against the use of milk for such feedings. Why would milk be more likely to interfere with the appetite for the following meal?

7. In what ways would a deficient secretion of hydrochloric acid interfere with digestion?

8. What classes of foods would be especially indicated in the diet of an individual who suffers from constipation?

9. How does fat differ from amino acids and monosaccharides in its mode of absorption and transport?

10. *Problem.* Prepare an outline which shows the steps in the digestion, absorption, and utilization of the nutrients in a meal consisting of poached egg on toast. Indicate both mechanical and chemical changes which take place, together with the enzymes involved.

UNIT III /
Dietary Planning for
Good Nutrition

CHAPTER 14 /

Meal Planning for the Family

The importance of an adequate intake of each of the nutrients in order to maintain good nutrition and health has been emphasized in preceding chapters. The next problem is the proper correlation of this information for the planning of satisfactory daily dietaries, for meal planning does not consist in a mere counting of calories or of the number of grams of protein. It is not nearly as dull as that! While it is impossible to obtain a good state of nutrition without the daily inclusion of the necessary nutrients, it is equally impractical to consider feeding from the standpoint of food essentials alone. Such factors as digestibility, safety, economy, palatability, and family customs relating to religion and nationality determine whether or not the food can be actually supplied and utilized. Dietary adequacy, meal planning in terms of family needs, and economy will be considered in this chapter. Factors affecting food acceptance, cultural food patterns, and a safe food supply are discussed in chapters which follow.

PLANNING FOR DIETARY ADEQUACY

Basic dietary pattern. A dietary pattern based on the Four Food Groups of the Daily Food Guide (p. 29) has been referred to time and again in the chapters pertaining to the nutrients. The nutritive values for foods in each of these groups are summarized in the table on page 178. The values assigned to each food group give consideration to the per capita consumption of foods in the United States. For example, the consumption of beef and pork is much higher than is that of lamb, veal, poultry, or fish; thus, the values cited for meat, poultry, fish are based on a greater weighting for beef and pork.

The basic dietary pattern provides the Recommended Dietary Allowances for the woman of 25 years for some of the nutrients, while for others the allowances are substantially met (see Fig. 14-1). Sufficient calories to maintain optimum body weight are obtained by eating larger amounts of any of the foods in the basic diet, or by adding fats, sweets, desserts, etc. Usually the foods added for a satisfactory caloric level will also contain some protein, minerals, and vitamins, but it is necessary to emphasize that an excessive use

176

of fats and sweets may jeopardize the satisfactory intake of essential nutrients.

Modification of the basic pattern. During pregnancy and lactation and during childhood the needs of protein are especially high. The basic pattern is easily adjusted by adding milk, egg, cheese, legumes, or an additional portion of meat as the individual situation may require.

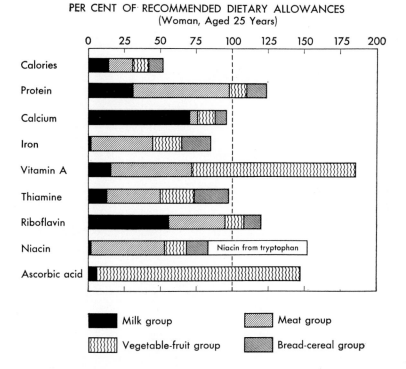

PER CENT OF RECOMMENDED DIETARY ALLOWANCES
(Woman, Aged 25 Years)

Fig. 14-1. The Four Food Groups of the Basic Diet meet, or nearly meet, the recommended allowances in all respects except calories for the woman of 25 years.

Let us suppose that an individual cannot take milk at all. By referring to the calculated values for the basic diet it quickly becomes evident that milk contributes outstandingly to the protein, calcium, and riboflavin content of the diet, and importantly to the thiamine level. Perhaps meat or eggs can be used in greater amounts to compensate for the protein of the milk, but these foods are not suitable substitutions with respect to calcium and riboflavin. Hard cheese and greens may be useful substitutes; but if they are not tolerated, it becomes evident to the student without further calculations that dietary inadequacy will result unless one resorts to supplementation.

Again, suppose that raw fruits and vegetables are omitted as in the soft diet.

NUTRITIVE VALUE OF A BASIC DIET PATTERN FOR THE ADULT IN HEALTH

(Calculated on Minimum Servings from the Four Food Groups) [1]

FOOD	MEASURE	WEIGHT gm	ENERGY calories	PROTEIN gm	FAT gm	CARBO-HYDRATE gm	MINERALS Ca mg	MINERALS Fe mg	VITAMINS A I.U.	VITAMINS Thiamine mg	VITAMINS Riboflavin mg	VITAMINS Niacin mg	VITAMINS Ascorbic Acid mg
Milk	2 cups	488	330	18	20	24	570	0.2	780	0.16	0.84	0.4	4
Meat group													
Egg	1	50	80	6	6	tr	27	1.1	590	0.05	0.15	tr	0
Meat, fish, poultry (lean)	4 ounces	120	300	33	16	tr	16	4.0	2220 [2]	0.39	0.43	8.7	tr
Vegetable-fruit group													
Leafy green or deep yellow	¼–⅓ cup [3]	50	15	1	tr	3	35	0.6	4640	0.03	0.06	0.3	15
Other vegetable	¼–⅓ cup [3]	50	20	1	tr	4	10	0.3	330	0.03	0.03	0.3	8
Potato	1 medium	122	90	3	tr	21	9	0.7	tr	0.11	0.04	1.4	20
Citrus fruit [4]	1 serving	100	45	1	tr	12	27	0.4	120	0.07	0.03	0.2	47
Other fruit	1 serving	100	60	1	tr	16	12	0.5	600	0.04	0.03	0.4	9
Bread-cereal group													
Cereal, enriched or whole-grain	½ cup	20 (dry)	75	2	tr	16	8	0.6	0	0.11	0.03	0.7	0
Bread, enriched or whole-grain	3 slices	69	180	6	3	36	57	1.8	tr	0.18	0.15	1.8	0
			1195	72	45	132	771	10.2	9280	1.17	1.80	14.2 [5]	103
Recommended Dietary Allowances													
Woman (25 years)			2300	58			800	12	5000	1.2	1.5	17	70
Man (25 years)			3200	70			800	10	5000	1.6	1.8	21	75

[1] Values for foods in the meat, vegetable-fruit, and bread-cereal groups are weighted on the basis of the approximate consumption of foods in the United States. Table 1 in the Appendix has been used for the calculations. Calories have been rounded off to the nearest 5, protein, fat, and carbohydrate to the nearest gram, and vitamin A to the nearest 10 units.

[2] An average weekly intake for meat is approximately 10 ounces beef, 9 ounces pork, 2½ ounces lamb and veal, 6 ounces poultry, 1½ ounces fish, and 1 ounce liver in this calculation. The value of vitamin A would be reduced to a trace if liver were omitted.

[3] The calculations for vegetables assume that a minimum of one full serving of leafy green or deep yellow vegetable is eaten every other day.

[4] The ascorbic acid need is met by using citrus fruit or other good source of the vitamin such as cantaloupe, strawberries, etc., in season.

[5] The protein in this diet contains about 720 mg tryptophan, equivalent to 12 mg niacin; thus, the niacin equivalent of this diet is 26.2 mg.

The use of only cooked foods may significantly lower the mineral and vitamin contributions of these classes of foods. Reference to the basic diet makes it apparent that one way to maintain the ascorbic acid intake, for example, would be to double the amount of citrus fruit juice.

Alternate basic pattern. Many basic plans could be constructed for individual needs. The basic plan on page 178 permits considerable flexibility in day-to-day choice of foods, and is applicable in any part of the United States. Nevertheless, it might be desirable to use a plan which includes greater or lesser amounts of meat, cereals and bread, milk, fruits, vegetables, etc., and still achieve nutritive adequacy. An alternate low-cost basic diet is presented in the table on page 180. This includes a selection of foods typical of the low-income groups in the southeastern states.

There are several points of interest in the low-cost plan. It will be noted that there is less milk and meat and no citrus fruit. Larger amounts of plant foods, including corn grits, corn meal, self-rising flour, cowpeas, and sweet potato, are included.

Nonfat dry milk has been used in this plan because of low cost and excellent keeping qualities in the dry state without refrigeration. This addition to the present dietary practices of low-income groups would greatly improve nutrition. Whenever whole milk or buttermilk is available, it may be substituted for the nonfat dry milk.

Egg is the only animal source of vitamin A. While the carotene is less well utilized than true vitamin A, the levels in this diet provide a wide margin of safety for the person in health.

The allowances for the B-complex vitamins are satisfactory because of the use of enriched cereal foods. If unenriched products are used, the diet would not fully meet the recommended allowances.

ACCEPTABILITY OF MEAL PLANS

In addition to the continuous application of the principles of nutrition, good menu planning calls for an understanding of family needs, careful management of time and money, and imagination. Advertisements in newspapers, the colorful illustrations and numerous suggestions for menu planning in feature articles of newspapers and women's magazines, and innumerable cookbooks are valuable aids in menu planning.

Meal patterns must fit the family. Planning meals for the family group entails a consideration of the needs of each individual. Obviously, a young child will not be allowed the wide choice of foods given to adults. The amount of food for the overweight individual will be considerably less than that for the hard-working underweight person. The adolescent child, the elderly person, the pregnant woman, or the sick individual, each has his specific needs. However, one can readily adapt the family menu to meet these needs if care is

ALTERNATE LOW-COST BASIC DIET PATTERN FOR THE ADULT IN HEALTH (SOUTHERN) [1]

FOOD	MEASURE	WEIGHT gm	ENERGY calories	PROTEIN gm	FAT gm	CARBOHYDRATE gm	MINERALS		A I.U.	VITAMINS			
							Ca mg	Fe mg		Thiamine mg	Riboflavin mg	Niacin mg	Ascorbic Acid mg
Nonfat dry milk [2]	⅜ cup	30	110	11	tr	16	390	0.2	10	0.11	0.54	0.3	2
Meat group													
Egg	1	50	80	6	6	tr	27	1.1	590	0.05	0.15	tr	0
Pork, lean and fat	2 ounces	60	215	13	17	0	6	1.7	0	0.30	0.14	2.7	—
Cowpeas or blackeye peas, cooked	1 cup	248	190	13	1	34	42	3.2	20	0.41	0.11	1.1	tr
Vegetable-fruit group													
Greens [3]	½ cup	75	25	2	tr	5	175	1.6	6140	0.05	0.18	0.9	34
Sweet potato	1 medium	147	170	2	1	39	47	1.0	11,610	0.13	0.09	0.9	25
Fruit, noncitrus	1 serving	100	60	1	tr	16	12	0.5	600	0.04	0.04	0.4	9
Bread-cereal group													
Corn grits, degermed, enriched, cooked	½ cup	121	60	2	tr	14	1	0.3	tr	0.06	0.04	0.5	0
Corn meal, degermed, enriched, dry	½ cup	72	260	6	1	57	5	2.1	210	0.32	0.19	2.6	0
Flour, enriched, self-rising	½ cup	55	190	5	1	41	150	1.6	0	0.24	0.15	1.9	0
			1360	61	27	222	855	13.3	19,180	1.71	1.63	11.3 [4]	70
Recommended Dietary Allowances													
Woman (25 years)			2300	58			800	12	5000	1.2	1.5	17	70
Man (25 years)			3200	70			800	10	5000	1.6	1.8	21	75

[1] Nutritive values have been calculated using Table 1 in the Appendix. Calories have been rounded off to the nearest 5, protein, fat, and carbohydrate to the nearest gram, and vitamin A to the nearest 10 units.

[2] Nonfat dry milk may be used in cooking or as a beverage. The liquid milk equivalent is 1⅓ cups.

[3] The average of collards, kale, mustard greens, and turnip greens has been used.

[4] The protein in this diet contributes about 610 mg tryptophan, equivalent to 10 mg niacin; thus the niacin equivalent of this diet is about 21 mg.

exercised in planning meals. For example, if steak appears on the menu for the adult members of the family, a meat patty would be suitable for the young child. A baked apple is readily prepared for the child at the same time an apple pie is being baked. The same salad can usually be used for both the overweight and underweight members of the family if the dressing is omitted for the former.

Save time in food preparation. The wise expenditure of time in the preparation of meals can mean leisure hours for the homemaker and her family. For no group is this more important than the low-income group in which the homemaker has many duties in relation to the care of the children and the home, or who, perhaps, is working to increase the family income. Time, like money, needs to be budgeted for its best use. These suggestions may help:

1. Plan meals for several days at one time.
2. Write a market order and restrict shopping to once or twice a week.
3. Shop when markets are less crowded.
4. Use simplified menus suitable for all age groups. Do not cater to every individual whim of each family member.
5. Arrange the kitchen in terms of efficient work units, keeping utensils and food supplies at point of first use.
6. Plan a work schedule for each day. In time this will show where important savings in minutes and hours can be made.

Use variety in meals. If one takes this admonition seriously, the diet is more likely to be nutritionally adequate than it would be if day after day just a few foods were used. A very common error in meal planning is that of emphasizing one type of food to the exclusion of others. A meal containing roast beef, macaroni and cheese, and custard predominates in protein, while spaghetti, potatoes, and cake in another meal would be equally bad because of the preponderance of carbohydrate. First of all, then, variety means selecting foods each day from each of the basic food groups. Thus, a breakfast of orange juice, egg, toast, butter, and milk includes foods from the Four Food Groups. The orange juice contributes ascorbic acid not found in any of the other foods, egg and milk are the chief sources of protein, egg and cereal provide most of the iron, milk is the outstanding contributor of calcium and riboflavin, and so on. Used together these foods comprise a good breakfast, but used singly some nutrients would be provided in less than desirable amounts.

Variety in meals means better acceptability; even the most avid enthusiast for steak would tire of a steady diet of steak. Variety is introduced through changes in color, texture, flavor, and methods of preparation. The first appeal to the appetite is through the eye. Attractive color combinations are important, for food must look good enough to eat. Chicken à la king, mashed potato, and cauliflower are monotonous in appearance, whereas changing the cauliflower to green peas or beans would add color appeal. Sometimes color appeal consists merely in using a garnish such as chopped parsley and paprika on fish, radish roses, green pepper rings, or some red jelly in a tiny lettuce cup. One need not restrict garnishes to the much over-worked cherry or to the wilted sprig of parsley!

Texture variation is equally important. For example, a meal made up of meat loaf, mashed potatoes, stewed squash, white bread, and baked custard would be greatly improved by changing the vegetable to one requiring some mastication and by adding a green salad and crusty rolls. Children will not eat well if all the foods in a given meal require a lot of chewing, while most adults rebel against all soft foods.

Taste appeal depends on the blending of bland and sharp flavors. Creamed onions, spicy cole slaw, pickles, and sharp cheese represent too many strongly flavored foods in a single meal; on the other hand, boiled potatoes, mashed squash, and vanilla pudding are all bland and lack interest unless contrasted with some sharper flavor. Spicy foods and marked flavors should not dominate the meal, but should provide the accent. Flavor variety precludes using the same food in two forms at one meal; for example, tomato juice and tomato salad would not be a good choice.

Even the season of the year requires some consideration, for on a cold winter day hearty soups and stews may seem especially desirable. Summer meals also require that the same nutrients be provided, but one is likely to prefer less of heavy and rich foods. One should not make the mistake, however, of serving cold foods only, or of planning salad meals which do not include protein.

Variety can be introduced by using many methods of preparation. For example, eggs may be soft cooked, poached, in omelets of various kinds, creamed, or deviled, to mention but a few methods of preparation; likewise, tomatoes may be fresh in salads, broiled, stewed, escalloped, fried green or ripe, in cream soups, in tomato juice, and so on.

Variety in meal planning is the sum total of many kinds and classes of foods served in pleasing color combinations, with a judicious mixture of soft and crisp foods, of bland and sharp flavors, and hot and cold dishes—all prepared in the best tradition of American cookery. It ensures better nutrition and enhances the interest in any meal.

Provide satiety value. A satisfying meal is one which will allay the sense of hunger until almost time for the next meal. A breakfast of orange juice and toast is digested in such a short time that a sense of hunger and fatigue quickly appears. The addition of cereal and egg will, however, postpone the appearance of these sensations.

Protein foods such as meat and eggs are high in satiety value, as are foods cooked with fat. Carbohydrate foods, fruits, vegetables, and liquids are somewhat low in their staying power. The choice of foods will then depend upon the interval between meals, long intervals demanding those of higher satiety value.

Begin with a good breakfast. Far too many people eat nothing but one or two doughnuts or a sweet roll and a cup of coffee for breakfast; many others skip breakfast entirely. Careful planning can overcome the excuses customarily given for skipping, or skimping on, breakfast.

Over a period of 6 years, a series of experiments was conducted by the Departments of Physiology and Nutrition at the State University of Iowa to determine the effectiveness of various breakfast plans on physical and mental efficiency. Seventy different subjects of various ages were used in the studies which have been reported in 20 scientific papers in professional journals. In brief, the results of these studies showed that: [66] (1) efficiency in physiologic performance, as measured by bicycle ergometer, treadmill, and maximum grip strength, decreased in late morning hours when breakfast was omitted; (2) attitude toward school work and scholastic achievement was poorer when breakfast was omitted; (3) the content of the breakfast did not determine its efficiency so long as it was nutritionally adequate; (4) a basic breakfast providing one-fourth of the daily caloric requirement and one-fourth of the daily protein allowance was superior to smaller or larger breakfasts for maintaining efficiency in the late morning hours; (5) a protein intake of 20 to 25 gm was most suitable for the maintenance of the blood glucose level during the late morning hours; and (6) the omission of breakfast was of no value in weight reduction. In fact, those who omit breakfast while on a weight reduction regimen experience greater hunger in addition to being physiologically inefficient.

TWO MENUS FOR SEDENTARY PERSONS

Orange juice	Stewed prunes
Oatmeal with sugar and milk	Poached egg on
Popovers with butter or fortified	Buttered toast
margarine	Coffee with cream and sugar
Coffee with cream and sugar	Milk for children
Milk for children	

TWO MENUS FOR MODERATELY ACTIVE PERSONS
(Adults and School-age Children)

Cantaloupe	Sliced peaches on rice flakes with cream
Shredded wheat with milk, sugar	and sugar
Ham slice with fried eggs	Griddle cakes with sirup
Whole-wheat toast with	Sausages
Butter or fortified margarine	Coffee with cream and sugar
Coffee with cream and sugar	Milk for children
Milk for children	

A change to better breakfast habits means: (1) planning simple, easy-to-prepare, but varied meals; (2) arising sufficiently early so that there is time for eating breakfast; (3) eating breakfast with the family group so that it, like other meals, has pleasant social associations.

Many combinations of foods are possible for breakfast. Breakfast should provide one-fourth of the daily nutritive needs. It may include some protein food such as egg or milk, cereal or breadstuff, or both, and a beverage. Children and teenagers should include milk for breakfast. If citrus fruit or another good source of ascorbic acid is included at breakfast, the day's allowance is assured. Cereal may be hot or cold; breads may vary from plain white enriched or whole-grain to muffins, griddle cakes, waffles, or sweet rolls, as the occasion warrants. A breakfast may be light or heavy depending upon the individual's activity and preferences.

Lunch is often neglected. Thousands of workers depend on the lunch counter in a drugstore for their lunches. All too commonly the pattern is a sandwich, a piece of pie, and a glass of carbonated beverage or a cup of coffee. Sometimes the pattern can be improved by the selection of milk, salads, and ice cream. Occasionally food choice for the worker is so limited that there is little one can do to improve the lunch pattern other than carrying a lunch. This is not feasible for the man or woman who lives in a room and has no facilities for food preparation. When the choice of foods is restricted at lunch, it is essential that basic foods (a salad, or milk, or citrus fruit, etc.) be included in morning and evening meals.

Recent years have seen a great deal of emphasis placed on hot school lunches. Undoubtedly hot food is an aid to food acceptability, but hot foods per se do not change nutritive values. A packed school lunch may be just as adequate nutritionally; but if it is much less attractive to the child, it may not be eaten.

Perhaps even more neglected than the school child and the worker are the homemaker and preschool children. Lunch may simply be a means to use leftovers or a day-to-day monotony of sandwiches or canned foods because the homemaker does not take the time for adequate preparation. Luncheons or suppers can be inexpensive, easy to prepare, tasty, and nutritionally adequate with a little foresight and planning. The following menus illustrate good luncheons, both hot and cold.

Spanish omelet
Buttered green cabbage
Fresh fruit cup
Cookie
Milk

Sandwich:
  Chopped egg, celery, mayonnaise
                    on
  Whole-wheat bread
Carrot and cucumber sticks
Potato chips
Fresh plums
Spice cup cake
Milk

Salad bowl with mixed greens, diced
  ham, cheese, tomato wedges
French dressing
Whole-wheat muffin with butter and
  jelly
Pumpkin pie
Milk

Dinner patterns are many. The chief meal of the day may be served at noon or at night, depending upon family custom. It must make up any lack which may have occurred in the other two meals. As a rule meat, fish, or fowl comprises the main dish. Potatoes or a starchy food and a green or yellow vegetable are generally served with the meat. If no salad has been included in the luncheon it should be given here. The dessert may consist of puddings, cake, ice cream, pastries, or fruit. Milk should again be given to the children. For more elaborate meals one may also include an appetizer such as a clear soup or fruit cup.

MEAL PATTERN FOR DINNER

Meat, fish, or poultry
Potato or substitute
Vegetable, green or yellow
Salad, if none at lunch
Bread, whole-grain or enriched
Butter or fortified margarine
Dessert
Beverage

SAMPLE MENU

Broiled salmon
Creamed whole potato
Fresh peas
Lettuce, grapefruit, and celery salad
French dressing
Parker House rolls
Vanilla ice cream
Coffee
Milk for children

Dinner is often a good time to balance the calories for the day. The active person may eat heartily of potatoes, rolls, desserts as well as of meat, vegetables, and milk, while the individual who needs to watch calories can eat meat, vegetables, and milk and more sparingly of the calorie-rich foods. The caloric intake each day should be such that it balances with a normal weight for one's height and body build.

Snacks are often useful. There can be no rigid rule concerning between-meal eating. Active children often benefit by having a midmorning or midafternoon snack, providing that it is of such a nature that the appetite at mealtime is not lessened. Workers in industry, nurses, students, and others experience a "lift" with a snack. This does not infer a continuous pattern of nibbling and raiding the refrigerator at any and all times.

It is the quality of the snack that is important. Concentrated sweets and carbonated beverages may contain little other than carbohydrate and may destroy mealtime appetite; but fruits, fruit juices, milk, or a sandwich depending upon the individual's activity and the interval between meals carry many valuable nutrients. Between-meal snacks, properly chosen, may actually aid some persons to maintain weight by reducing the tendency to overeating at mealtime.

ECONOMY IN DIETARY PLANNING

Food is the largest single item in the budget of most families. One can be adequately nourished at many cost levels, but to do so when the income is low requires careful planning, considerable ingenuity, and time to make the less varied diets interesting.

The amount of money required for food for any given family depends on the size of the family, the number of children and their ages, the activities of the various members, special needs for pregnancy and lactation, and possible therapeutic requirements. The cost of food is decidedly influenced by the choice of foods within each group, the amount of preparation the food has undergone before its sale, the type of market, packaging, and so on.

Master food plans. The nurse, nutritionist, and social worker frequently

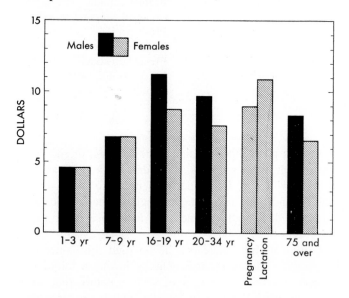

Fig. 14-2. The cost of a week's food (July, 1960) using the moderate-cost food plan (see p. 189) is shown for individuals of various ages. (Data from *Family Economics Review*, Agricultural Research Service, September, 1960.)

are called upon to help families plan for the kinds and amounts of foods for adequate nutrition. Welfare agencies also need guides to establish suitable allowances for the purchase of foods for families or for institutions. While the Four Food Groups are a guide for planning nutritionally adequate menus, they do not serve as an adequate basis for setting up a food budget. To meet these needs the Institute of Home Economics of the U.S. Department of Agriculture has constructed plans for 19 age and sex categories using 11 food groups at low, moderate, and liberal cost levels. (See Figs. 14-2 and 14-3; see also pp. 188–89 for low-cost and moderate-cost plans.)

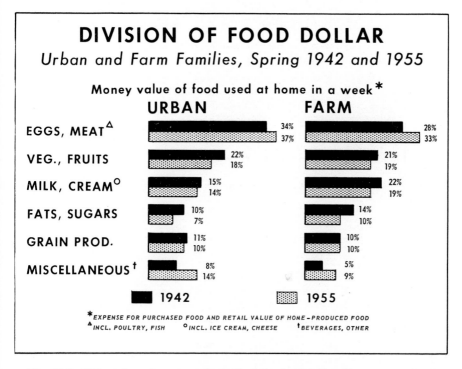

Fig. 14-3. Milk and meat groups take half of the food dollar. Note greater proportions of money spent for meat group in 1955. (*Courtesy, Agricultural Research Service, U.S. Department of Agriculture.*)

A quick examination of the food classes shows that they represent a more detailed breakdown of the Four Food Groups and also make allowance for fats and oils, and sugars and sweets. These plans have been set up on the basis of actual food buying practices at various economic levels, and are sufficiently flexible for considerable variety in menu planning. The amounts of food listed for each age category will provide the Recommended Dietary Allowances.

The low-cost plan has more flour, cereals, baked goods, potatoes, dry peas,

(*Text continued on p. 190.*)

FOOD PLAN AT LOW COST: SUGGESTED WEEKLY QUANTITIES OF FOOD (AS PURCHASED, ASSUMING AVERAGE CHOICES WITHIN GROUPS) FOR 19 SEX-AGE GROUPS *

FAMILY MEMBERS	MILK, CHEESE, ICE CREAM (qt)	MEAT, POULTRY, FISH		EGGS (no)	DRY BEANS, PEAS, NUTS		FLOUR, CEREAL, BAKED GOODS		CITRUS FRUIT, TOMATOES		DARK GREEN AND DEEP YELLOW VEGETABLES		POTATOES		OTHER VEGETABLES AND FRUIT		FATS, OILS		SUGAR, SWEETS	
	qt	lb	oz	no	lb	oz	lb	oz	lb	oz	lb	oz	lb	oz	lb	oz	lb	oz	lb	oz
Children:																				
Under 1 year	5½	1	0	5	0	0	0	12	1	8	0	2	0	8	1	0	0	1	0	2
1–3 years	5½	1	4	5	0	1	1	4	1	8	0	4	0	12	2	4	0	4	0	4
4–6 years	5½	1	8	5	0	2	2	0	1	12	0	4	1	4	3	4	0	6	0	6
7–9 years	5½	2	0	6	0	4	2	4	2	0	0	8	2	0	4	4	0	8	0	10
10–12 years	6½	2	4	6	0	6	3	0	2	4	0	8	2	8	5	0	0	8	0	12
Girls:																				
13–15 years	7	2	8	6	0	4	3	0	2	4	0	12	2	8	5	0	0	10	0	12
16–19 years	7	2	8	6	0	4	2	12	2	4	0	12	2	4	4	12	0	6	0	10
Boys:																				
13–15 years	7	2	8	6	0	6	4	4	2	8	0	12	3	4	5	4	0	12	0	12
16–19 years	7	3	4	6	0	8	5	4	2	8	0	12	4	12	5	8	0	14	0	14
Women:																				
20–34 years	3½	2	8	5	0	4	2	8	2	0	0	12	2	0	5	0	0	6	0	10
35–54 years	3½	2	8	5	0	4	2	8	2	0	0	12	1	8	4	8	0	4	0	10
55–74 years	3½	2	8	5	0	4	2	4	2	0	0	12	1	4	3	8	0	4	0	6
75 years and over	3½	2	8	5	0	4	2	0	2	0	0	12	1	4	3	0	0	4	0	6
Pregnant	7	2	8	7	0	4	2	8	3	8	1	8	2	0	5	0	0	6	0	8
Lactating	10	3	4	7	0	4	3	0	4	8	1	8	3	4	5	8	0	8	0	10
Men:																				
20–34 years	3½	3	12	6	0	6	4	4	2	4	0	12	3	4	5	8	0	12	1	0
35–54 years	3½	3	8	6	0	6	3	12	2	4	0	12	3	0	5	0	0	10	0	12
55–74 years	3½	3	4	6	0	4	3	8	2	4	0	12	2	8	4	12	0	10	0	10
75 years and over	3½	3	4	6	0	4	3	4	2	0	0	12	2	4	4	8	0	8	0	10

* Stefferud, A., ed.: Food, the Yearbook of Agriculture, 1959, U.S. Department of Agriculture, Washington, D.C., 1959, p. 582.

FOOD PLAN AT MODERATE COST: SUGGESTED WEEKLY QUANTITIES OF FOOD (AS PURCHASED, ASSUMING AVERAGE CHOICES WITHIN GROUPS) FOR 19 SEX-AGE GROUPS *

FAMILY MEMBERS	MILK, CHEESE, ICE CREAM	MEAT, POULTRY, FISH		EGGS	DRY BEANS, PEAS, NUTS		FLOUR, CEREAL, BAKED GOODS		CITRUS FRUIT, TOMATOES		DARK GREEN AND DEEP YELLOW VEGETABLES		POTATOES		OTHER VEGETABLES AND FRUIT		FATS, OILS		SUGAR, SWEETS	
	qt	lb	oz	no	lb	oz	lb	oz	lb	oz	lb	oz	lb	oz	lb	oz	lb	oz	lb	oz
Children:																				
Under 1 year	6	1	4	6	0	0	0	12	1	8	0	2	0	8	1	8	0	1	0	2
1–3 years	6	1	12	6	0	1	1	0	1	8	0	4	0	12	2	12	0	4	0	4
4–6 years	6	2	4	6	0	1	1	12	2	0	0	4	1	0	4	0	0	6	0	10
7–9 years	6	3	0	7	0	2	2	0	2	4	0	8	1	12	4	12	0	10	0	14
10–12 years	6½	4	0	7	0	4	2	12	2	8	0	12	2	4	5	8	0	10	0	14
Girls:																				
13–15 years	7	4	8	7	0	2	2	12	2	8	0	12	2	4	5	12	0	12	0	14
16–19 years	7	4	4	7	0	2	2	8	2	8	0	12	2	0	5	8	0	10	0	12
Boys:																				
13–15 years	7	4	12	7	0	4	4	0	2	12	0	12	3	0	6	0	0	14	1	0
16–19 years	7	5	8	7	0	6	5	0	3	0	0	12	4	4	6	4	1	2	1	2
Women:																				
20–34 years	3½	4	4	6	0	2	2	4	2	8	0	12	1	8	5	12	0	8	0	14
35–54 years	3½	4	4	6	0	2	2	0	2	8	0	12	1	4	5	4	0	8	0	12
55–74 years	3½	4	4	6	0	2	1	12	2	4	0	12	1	4	4	4	0	6	0	8
75 years and over	3½	3	12	6	0	2	1	12	2	4	0	12	1	0	3	12	0	6	0	8
Pregnant	7	4	4	7	0	2	2	4	3	8	1	8	1	8	5	12	0	8	0	12
Lactating	10	5	0	7	0	2	2	12	5	0	1	8	2	12	6	4	0	12	0	12
Men:																				
20–34 years	3½	5	8	7	0	4	4	0	2	12	0	12	3	0	6	8	1	0	1	4
35–54 years	3½	5	4	7	0	4	3	8	2	12	0	12	2	8	5	12	1	14	1	0
55–74 years	3½	5	0	7	0	2	3	4	2	12	0	12	2	4	5	8	0	12	0	14
75 years and over	3½	5	0	7	0	2	2	12	2	8	0	12	2	0	5	4	0	10	0	12

* Stefferud, A., ed.: Food, The Yearbook of Agriculture, 1959, U.S. Department of Agriculture, Washington, D.C., 1959, p. 584.

189

and beans. The moderate-cost and liberal plans allow more meat, eggs, fruit, and vegetables other than potatoes. All three plans include generous amounts of milk. Within each plan more or less expensive selections can be made. The moderate-cost plan will cost roughly 25 to 35 per cent more than the low-cost plan, while the liberal plan will cost an additional 10 to 20 per cent, or even more.

What's in each food group. The common foods in each of the 11 groups are given below.[67]

1. *Milk, cheese, ice cream*

    Milk—whole, skim, buttermilk, dry, evaporated, condensed.
    Cheese, ice cream.
    Quantities suggested in the food plans are in terms of quarts of milk. When using cheese or ice cream, count the quantities used as about equal to these amounts of milk:

    1 pound cheese, Cheddar type . . . . 3 quarts milk
    12 ounces cheese, cottage . . . . 1 cup milk
    4 ounces cheese, cream . . . . ¼ cup milk
    1 quart ice cream . . . . 2 cups milk

2. *Meat, poultry, fish*

    Beef, veal, lamb, pork, including bacon and salt pork; variety meats such as liver, heart, tongue; luncheon meats; poultry; fish, and shellfish.
    Assume that not more than ⅓ pound of bacon and salt pork is bought for each 5 pounds other meat, poultry, and fish.

3. *Eggs*

4. *Dry beans and peas, nuts*

    Dry beans of all kinds, dry peas, lentils; soybeans and soya products; peanuts and peanut butter; other nuts.

5. *Flour, cereals, baked goods* (whole-grain, enriched, restored)

    Flour or meal made from any grain—wheat, buckwheat, rye, corn; cereals, including ready-to-eat cereals; rice, hominy, noodles, macaroni, spaghetti; bread, cake, other baked goods.
    Amounts suggested in the master food plans are in terms of pounds of flour and cereal. Bread and other baked goods average about two-thirds flour by weight. Therefore, count 1 pound of bread and other baked goods as ⅔ pound of flour.

6. *Citrus fruit, tomatoes*

    Grapefruit, lemons, limes, oranges, tangerines, tomatoes.

7. *Dark green and deep yellow vegetables*

Broccoli, chard, collards, kale, green peppers, spinach, and other dark greens; carrots, pumpkin, yellow winter squash, sweet potatoes.

8. *Potatoes*

9. *Other vegetables and fruits*

Asparagus, beets, Brussels sprouts, cabbage, cauliflower, celery, corn, cucumbers, green Lima beans, snap beans, lettuce, okra, onions, parsnips, peas, rutabagas, sauerkraut, summer squash, turnips.
Apples, bananas, berries, cherries, dates, figs, grapes, peaches, pears, plums, prunes, raisins, rhubarb.
All other vegetables and fruits not included in other groups.

10. *Fats, oils*

Butter, margarine, mayonnaise, salad dressing, salad and cooking oil, fat drippings, lard and other shortening, suet.

11. *Sugar, sirup, preserves*

Sugar (beet and cane)—granulated, powdered, brown, maple; molasses, sirup, honey; jams, jellies, preserves.

How to use the food plans. To use these plans, four steps are required:
1. List the quantities of food required in 1 week from each food group for each member of the family. Total the amounts for the family. These totals serve as a guide for the family from week to week.
2. Plan menus for the week, keeping the amounts of the 11 food groups in mind.
3. Prepare the market order, listing the kinds and amounts of foods required for the 11 food groups.
4. Compare the amounts of foods required for the menus with the totals from the 11 food groups required by the family. If the amounts required for the menus differ widely from the suggested plan, revise the menus so that the two correspond. After practice for a few times, these plans are very easy to use.

An example of a week's menus and a market order for a family of six, using the low-cost plan is given below.* The family in this example includes a father and mother, both about 40 years of age; a boy, 16 years old; a girl, 14; a girl, 11; and a boy, 8.

* *Food for Families with School Children,* Home and Garden Bulletin No. 13, U.S. Department of Agriculture, Washington, D.C., 1960.

After listing the total amounts of foods required from each of the 11 food groups, the menus were planned for the week as follows:

SUNDAY

Grapefruit juice
Wheat griddlecakes with sirup
Milk for children

Roast shoulder of pork with stuffing
Sweet potatoes (roasted in pan
with meat)
Green beans   Coleslaw
Bread
Apple gingerbread
Milk

Poached or scrambled eggs
Cottage-fried potatoes
Apple-and-celery salad
Toast
Ice cream

MONDAY

Orange juice
Hot wheat cereal with milk
Toast
Milk for children

Egg salad sandwich
Peanut butter and shredded-lettuce
sandwich
Gingerbread
Milk

Pork pie with potatoes
(pork left from Sunday roast)
Sour beets and beet greens
Bread
Raisin-rice pudding
Milk for children

TUESDAY

Stewed prunes
Ready-to-eat cereal with milk
Toast
Milk for children

Meat turnover (ground beef)
Potato salad
Vegetable slaw: Cabbage, minced
onion, radish slices, and dressing
Peanut butter cookies
Milk

Lima bean-tomato casserole
Spinach
Corn-meal muffins
Sweet-potato custard
Milk for children

WEDNESDAY

Grapefruit juice
French toast   Sirup
Milk for children

Cheese and lettuce sandwiches
Beet and green bean salad
Graham crackers
Milk

Spaghetti with meat balls
Salad bowl:
Lettuce, celery, carrot, cabbage
French bread
Baked apple with milk

THURSDAY

Tomato juice
Hot wheat cereal with milk
Toasted rolls
Milk for children

Lima bean soup
Cottage cheese and lettuce sandwich
on raisin bread
Oatmeal cookies
Milk

Oven-fried chicken
Scalloped potatoes   Carrots
Orange, chopped prune,
and cabbage salad
Bread
Butterscotch pudding

FRIDAY

Stewed prunes
Oatmeal and milk
Toast
Milk for children

Corn and onion soup
Deviled egg sandwich, or deviled
egg salad for those at home
Celery
Bread
Orange
Milk

Baked perch fillets
Mashed potatoes
Green peas and onions
Biscuits
Hot apple pie
Milk for children

SATURDAY

Orange juice
Fried corn-meal mush with sirup
Milk for children

Cold chicken
Potato cakes   Shredded carrot salad
Pickles
Bread
Oatmeal cookies
Milk

Braised liver
Riced potatoes   5-minute cabbage
Jellied tomato and cottage cheese salad
Bread
Sliced peaches   Cookies
Milk for children

The market order for the week's menus is listed below. It coincides closely with the totals for the 11 food groups required by the family (see figures in parentheses for each food group).

Milk, cheese, ice cream   21 quarts fluid whole milk
(33 quarts)   1 13-ounce package dry skim milk (to make 4 quarts liquid)

Milk, cheese, ice cream (*Continued*)	4 14½-ounce cans evaporated milk ¾ pound Cheddar-type cheese 1½ pounds cottage cheese 3 pints ice cream
Meat, poultry, fish (16 to 17 pounds)	5–6 pounds chicken 2–2½ pounds ground beef 5½–6 pounds pork shoulder 1½ pounds liver 2 pounds frozen perch fillets
Eggs	3 dozen
Dry beans and peas, nuts (2 pounds)	1 pound lima beans 1 pound peanut butter
Grain products (20 to 21 pounds)	12 loaves bread (4 whole wheat, 5 enriched, 1 rye, 1 French, 1 raisin) ¾ pound rolled oats 1 pound wheat cereal ½ pound ready-to-eat cereal 4–6 pounds enriched flour 1 pound enriched corn meal 1 pound enriched spaghetti ¼ pound rice 2 boxes graham crackers 1 pound pancake mix 1 14-ounce package gingerbread mix 1 box soda crackers
Citrus fruits, tomatoes (13 to 14 pounds)	3½ pounds oranges 2 6-ounce cans frozen concentrated orange juice 1 46-ounce can grapefruit juice 2 No. 2 cans tomatoes 1 46-ounce can tomato juice
Dark green and deep yellow vegetables (3½ to 4 pounds)	2½ pounds carrots 1½ pounds spinach 3–4 pounds sweet potatoes
Potatoes	16–17 pounds potatoes
Other vegetables and fruits (28 to 30 pounds)	2 pounds beets 1 large head cabbage 1 large bunch celery 1 No. 2 can corn 2 medium heads lettuce 1½ pounds onions 2 No. 2 cans peas 1 bunch radishes

2 pounds green snap beans
5 pounds apples
1 No. 2½ can peaches
1½ pounds prunes
¼ pound raisins

Fats, oils
(about 3½ pounds)

2 pounds butter or margarine
1 pint salad oil
1–1½ pounds lard or shortening

Sugar, sweets
(about 4½ pounds)

3 pounds sugar
1 pound brown sugar
¼ pint molasses

Some ways to effect economy. Unfortunately, many people in all income groups do not know how to plan a budget, or what constitutes economy in food purchases. Many homemakers are employed outside the home so that only a small amount of time can be spent on food preparation. The limited budget is often spent on prepared foods high in cost, but making a low contribution to nutrition of the family. Appreciable savings can often be effected if the suggestions listed below are observed.

General recommendations. 1. Plan meals for several days at one time.

2. Watch for weekly sales and take advantage of them in menu planning.

3. Use a market list. Resist the temptation to purchase many luxury foods now available in any good market. Be prepared to make substitutions when other foods of equal nutritive value are cheaper.

4. Purchase goods on a cash-and-carry basis. Supermarkets, as a rule, offer foods at lower cost than small independent markets.

5. Read labels on cans and packages. Know what the specifications mean. Compare weights and costs of various brands.

6. Buy in larger quantities if price per unit is less, if there is space to store the food properly, and if the food can be used before it spoils.

7. Provide storage conditions which maintain the wholesomeness and nutritive value of food.

8. To minimize table waste, cook food for maximum palatability, and serve it attractively in the size portions which are likely to be eaten.

9. Cook just enough food for each meal, especially with respect to vegetables. Leftovers deteriorate in nutritive value and sometimes are not eaten. If food is left over, plan for its use, usually within 24 hours.

10. Eat meals at home or carry lunch whenever possible. Food eaten in restaurants or at lunch counters generally costs more than twice as much as similar food prepared at home.

Milk group. 1. Buy half-gallon containers of fresh milk if easily stored and quickly used. Milk purchased in a supermarket may be slightly less expensive than milk delivered to the door.

2. Use nonfat dry milk for cooking and baking.

3. Use reconstituted nonfat dry milk for a beverage, especially for weight watchers. It may be mixed half and half with whole milk for acceptability by the entire family.

4. Use homogenized, evaporated, or top milk instead of cream in coffee and on cereals.

5. Use chilled, whipped evaporated milk or whipped nonfat milk in place of whipped cream.

6. Use domestic rather than imported varieties of cheese.

7. In terms of nutritive values received, cream, cream cheese, and ice cream are the more expensive dairy items.

Meat group. 1. Consider the cost per serving. Large amounts of bone, gristle, and fat in a piece of meat may increase the cost per serving of lean meat. For example, 1 pound short ribs will serve two persons; 1 pound round pot roast will serve four persons.

2. Liver, kidney, and heart are good buys; pork and lamb liver are less expensive than calves' liver and just as nutritious.

3. Stretch the amount of meat by using stews, casserole dishes, creamed dishes, and meat loaves.

4. Pork, veal, and occasionally lamb may be better buys than beef.

5. Fresh, canned, and frozen fish are less expensive than meat, as a rule. Select grade of canned fish according to use; for example, salmon loaf requires less fancy grade than salmon salad.

6. Poultry, while having a high percentage of waste, may be economical at certain seasons.

7. Eggs, peanut butter, dry peas and beans may be used occasionally in place of meat when the latter is expensive. One egg, 1 ounce cheese, 2 table-spoons peanut butter, or ½ cup cooked beans or peas is equal in protein value to 1 ounce meat.

8. Compare the cost of various sizes of eggs; in late summer small eggs may be a best buy, while at other times large eggs may cost only a few cents more per dozen than medium-size eggs.

9. Grade-B eggs are usually a best buy for cooking purposes.

10. Buy brown eggs if they are cheaper; their nutritive value is the same as that of white eggs.

Vegetable-fruit group. 1. Use raw vegetables and fruits for salads and desserts for maximum nutritive value. Eat whole oranges in preference to using the juice.

2. Select fruits and vegetables in season, and locally available. Cabbage and carrots are generally inexpensive.

3. Compare cost of fresh, canned, frozen, and dried foods. For example, fresh peas (2 servings per pound) may be more expensive than frozen peas (4 servings per package). Canned peas may be cheaper or more expensive.

4. Select foods in relation to use; for example, broken pieces of canned fruit are cheaper than whole fruit and will serve just as well in salads and fruit cups.

5. Minimize waste in preparation. For example, cook potatoes in their skins or pare them thinly; use outer leaves of lettuce or cabbage.

6. Remember that fresh fruits and vegetables are perishable. Buy only what can be refrigerated and used promptly.

7. Raise foods in a garden whenever possible. Many farm families and those living in small communities and in the suburbs of cities could lower food costs by raising more fruits and vegetables. Gardening is not only kind to the budget, but it can become a satisfying hobby.

Bread-cereal group. 1. Select enriched, whole-grain, or restored cereals and breads; this includes enriched macaroni, spaghetti, noodles, etc.

2. Day-old bread is usually a good buy.

3. Use cooked breakfast cereals often.

4. Use large packages of cereals in place of the individual portion variety packages. Sugar-coated cereals are especially expensive, as are also some cereals which are advertised as containing exceptional nutritive values.

5. Prepare sweet breads, cakes, cookies, pastries at home if time permits.

6. Use breads and cereals generously in casserole dishes with cheese, milk, eggs when meats are too expensive.

7. Use dry bread crumbs for coating meat loaf, for topping casseroles, for croutons, Melba toast, etc.

Fats, sweets, and snack foods. 1. Fortified margarine is a good buy.

2. Sugar, vegetable oils, and cooking fats are inexpensive sources of calories. They do not provide other nutrients in appreciable amounts.

3. Use sparingly such snack items as popcorn, pretzels, potato chips, pickles, relishes, carbonated beverages, candy.

PROBLEMS AND REVIEW

This family group may be used for one or more of the following projects:

Father: 25 pounds underweight; works in a factory; carries lunch to work; age 36 years

Mother: pregnant (seventh month); age 32 years; does all her own housework

Boy: 10 years; in school; very active; comes home at noon for lunch

Girl: 3 years

1. *Problem.* Tabulate the daily nutritional requirements of each member of the family by referring to the table of recommended allowances.

2. *Problem.* Using the moderate-cost food plan, tabulate the amounts of foods from each food group for the entire family.

3. *Problem.* Plan menus for a week on the basis of the moderate cost plan.

4. *Problem.* Prepare a market list for the menus, being sure that the market order and the food allowances from the 11 food groups correspond.

5. *Problem.* Determine the cost of the market order using current prices in the local market.

6. Name five ways in which each of the following foods may be used in meals: eggs, milk, American cheese, potatoes, apples, carrots, beef. Consult any good cookbook or popular magazine for ideas.

7. Select a series of menus from any popular magazine. Check them in terms of nutritive adequacy and note good examples of each of the points in menu planning outlined in this chapter.

8. Visit a local food market to observe food quality. Compare the cost of similar food items in several markets.

CHAPTER 15

Factors Influencing Food Habits and Their Modification

Just as "You can lead a horse to water, but you cannot make him drink," so the presentation of well-prepared, highly nutritious food to people does not mean that they will eat it. The subject of food acceptance is an exceedingly complex one, concerning which numerous articles based on physiologic, psychologic, and cultural approaches are appearing continuously in professional journals and books. The improvement of an individual's state of nutrition can be effected only when one understands the factors which influence his choice of food as well as the nutrient requirements for an adequate diet.

Man is not completely rational in his acceptance or rejection of food. Indeed, few aspects of living are as likely to be emotionally charged as those associated with food. Manufacturers, for example, who develop new food products know that they must plan skillful advertising campaigns to gain acceptance of their products. Large sums of money are spent by them on so-called motivation research. An analysis of much food advertising shows that it is planned to appeal to the emotions rather than to the intellect.

To understand fully the factors which determine food acceptance requires the multidisciplinary approach of the anthropologist, psychologist and psychiatrist, educator, social worker, and nutritionist. It is beyond the scope of a single chapter, such as this, to provide the depth of understanding of all factors influencing food acceptance. The objectives of the discussion which follows are (1) to create for the reader an awareness of the complexity of factors which determine food acceptance; (2) to provide some basis for understanding that the same food may have quite different meanings to different individuals; (3) to develop attitudes of respect and tolerance for individuals who may have food habits differing widely from those of others; and (4) to provide some guides for helping people to improve their food habits.

PHYSIOLOGIC BASES FOR FOOD ACCEPTANCE

Hunger. Probably several mechanisms serve to explain hunger. Physiologic studies have established that contractions of the empty stomach are governed by the hypothalamus, and that hunger sensations are associated with a drop in the blood sugar level. Anliker and Mayer [68] have developed the *glucostatic* theory to explain the sensations of hunger. According to this theory, the difference between the level of the glucose in arterial and venous blood (called delta glucose, designated Δ-glucose) determines whether one experiences sensations of hunger or satiety. The hypothalamus contains a so-called "feeding" center and a "satiety" center. Following the eating of a meal, the Δ-glucose is relatively large so that the glucose receptors in the hypothalamus cause a cessation of hunger. On the other hand, when some time has elapsed since the last meal, the difference between the arterial and venous glucose is small; when this occurs, there is a stimulation of the feeding center, the hunger contractions of the stomach result, and eating ensues.

Starving people will usually, but not always, accept anything edible which will fill the stomach. This might even be that which would normally be quite repellent. It is also true that people may refuse food for the relief of acute hunger when religious or cultural taboos are strongly entrenched.

Man does not choose by instinct that which is best for him. In different environments, he eats what is available and sometimes learns through experience that some foods may be better for him than others. This method of trial and error, at best, is time consuming and may, in the meantime, jeopardize one's state of health. It could also lead to gross misconceptions concerning foods. Quite obviously the scientific planning of diets, rather than guidance by hunger and instinct, is the only sound basis for being sure that physiologic needs are being met.

Sensations produced by food. The palatability of food is a composite of taste, smell, texture, and temperature. It is further conditioned by the surroundings in which food is consumed.

Sweet, sour, salty, and bitter are terms used to describe the sensations which result when foods placed in the mouth produce specific stimuli to the taste buds on the tongue. The sense of taste is more highly developed in some individuals than in others; foods may be too salty for one individual and just right for another; or they may be too sweet for one, but not quite sweet enough for another. Some persons can detect slight differences in taste, others cannot. The number of taste buds varies not only from individual to individual, but also from age to age. Later in life the taste buds diminish in number, and this fact may explain, in part, why adults prefer spiced and tart foods while children voluntarily select bland or sweet foods.

Taste and smell of foods are directly linked. If one were to hold the nose while eating a piece of fruit, much of the enjoyment would be lost. As a matter of fact, odor is the most important component of flavor and an individual would derive limited pleasure from food if the tongue were the sole source of the sensations. The stimulation of the olfactory organs is brought about by certain volatile oils. Foods may be accepted because of their aromas, or they may be rejected because of their repulsive odors. No doubt, the odors of certain cheeses, for example, are the determinants in their acceptance by some and their rejection by others.

The sense of touch is highly developed in the tongue. Temperature, pain, and variations in texture or "feel" are experienced. Steaming hot foods are necessary to enjoyment by some, but children usually prefer foods which are lukewarm. A choice of ice cream may be influenced as much by its texture—smooth, creamy, and velvety, or crystalline and grainy—as by its other flavor qualities. Children may reject foods which are slippery such as baked custard or a gelatin dessert only later to learn to enjoy this texture sensation. The stringiness of certain vegetables, the stickiness of some mashed potatoes, the greasiness of fried foods may be important factors in rejection.

SOCIAL AND EMOTIONAL FACTORS INFLUENCE FOOD ACCEPTANCE

Role of culture. Montagu,[69] Lee,[70] and many other writers have pointed out that what, how, when, and where one eats are largely determined by one's culture. Food habits may have existed among a given ethnic group for centuries, and such a heritage may account for great conservatism in accepting change. These patterns reflect the social organization of the people, including their economy, religion, beliefs about the health properties of food, and their attitudes toward the various members of the family. The emotional reactions to the consumption of certain foods may be so deeply rooted that effecting acceptance of them is almost impossible.

A few comparisons of American cultural patterns with those of other parts of the world may serve to illustrate some of the problems of effecting change in food habits. In America advances in agriculture, technology, and transportation have combined to make it possible to provide a variety of foods literally undreamed of even 50 years ago. Mass communication media daily place before the public the values of new foods, using an appeal that is as often emotional as it is geared to nutritional benefits. Great emphasis is placed on providing variety in meal planning; yet Americans, too, rebel against variety if it includes at one time too many foods with which they are unfamiliar. In other cultures, bread is literally the "staff of life" to some people, rice is to others, and corn to still others; the availability of these foods represents life itself and is, in no sense, thought of in terms of a monotonous diet. In America today, the cereal grains do not occupy the important place in the diet which they held half a century ago.

Meal patterns, themselves, are dictated by culture. For many Americans, breakfast is a hearty meal which can be well rationalized on the basis of physiologic need; the European, however, is more accustomed to a light breakfast—perhaps bread or a roll without butter, and coffee—and finds it difficult to consume a meal he considers to be heavy. The farmer may prefer to have dinner at noon, while the urban worker, away from home all day, has his biggest meal in the evening. Recreation, itself, may modify one's meal patterns—witness the trend to frozen TV dinners and meals frequently eaten in front of the television set!

Today, as never before, people all over the world are eager to accept that which is new. Even food habits of long-standing origin can be changed providing that new innovations are worked into existing patterns as a means of enrichment rather than attempting to eliminate entrenched food habits. More detailed description of the food habits of several ethnic groups is included in the following chapter.

Social values of food. "To break bread" together has been from time immemorial an act of friendship. One provides food for friends during a visit in the home; one likewise extends friendship to the stranger by inviting him to share food. The food served to guests is the best that one can afford and the table appointments are as beautiful as one can make them. Important family events are joyously celebrated with meals: the wedding breakfast or reception; birthday parties; Christmas dinner; a Fourth of July picnic. To eat together, whatever the occasion, is to provide friendly relaxation and conversation. The loneliness of eating by oneself, day after day, is not appreciated by those who have never tried it.

Eating together also has connotations of status. Throughout history one's place at the table has been governed by his social standing. To be placed "above the salt" at a medieval banquet, to sit at the "head" table at a banquet today, and to be invited to eat at the Captain's table while on board ship are marks of social distinction. In some societies women are considered to be inferior to men, and must wait to eat until the men and boys have finished the meal. In other authoritarian situations, children may not be permitted to eat until the father has had his meal; in such a society, the father is always served the choicest foods. Many bonds of business or of politics are cemented at the businessmen's luncheons or the political dinners.

Prestige, it would appear, may be ensured when one serves foods which are costly, difficult to obtain, distinctive in flavor, or time consuming in preparation. Caviar, lobster, filet mignon, champagne, flaming crepes suzette are examples of such prestige foods. In the nineteenth century, the purchase of white sugar and white flour conveyed the idea that one could afford to buy that which was refined and therefore "better." Is the purchase today of the more costly breads prepared from hand-ground meals an expression of status with respect to one's supposed knowledge of nutrition, or to one's ability to buy or bake that bread which is distinctive from the more commonly available loaf?

Some foods are looked down upon by many people as lacking status; thus, a delicious stew, or ground meat, or fish—no matter how good they may be—

are considered by some to be food for the poor. However, these attitudes also are subject to change. Tourists to seacoast cities now seek out restaurants which specialize in sea foods, and may be willing to spend considerable amounts of money for a specialty. Teenagers are likely to look upon the hamburger as a food fit for the gods!

Some people delight in being epicures or gourmets. They derive a certain satisfaction from adventurous eating of food which is unusual, or which might be, in fact, unacceptable to most people—rattlesnake meat, for example. Others make a specialty of dining at unusual or expensive restaurants, or in becoming known for their abilities to prepare complex, unusual dishes.

Religious and moral values attributed to foods. Almost all religions place some regulations on the use of foods (see Fig. 15-1). The association of a food with religion may give some clue to its importance in daily living. In the Middle East, bread becomes a symbol in the religious ceremonies of the people; to the Indians of Mexico, corn, the staple food, is invested with religious significance.

Certain foods are forbidden by religious regulation. Pork is forbidden to the Orthodox Jews and to the Islamites. Buddhists are vegetarians; they will eat no flesh of any animal, and many of them also refrain from eating eggs and milk.

Fasting is common to most, if not all, religions. On fast days one food may be substituted for another or foods may be abstained from altogether. A substitute food, such as fish for meat, is likely to be associated with denying oneself, and so when one wishes enjoyment, he doesn't choose to eat fish!

Moral attributes—"good" and "bad"—are often ascribed to foods. A child may be told to eat liver even if he doesn't like it because it is "good" for him; he may also be told not to eat candy, which he likes, because it is "bad" for him. Or he might be told that he may have candy if he eats his liver!

Food is often used as a reward, punishment, or as a means of bribery. Thus, if a child has behaved well he is often rewarded with a prized food—candy, ice cream, cake; but if he has behaved badly he may be punished by being deprived of a food such as dessert. Adults, too, may reward themselves after a strenuous day or a trying experience by eating a special food or an expensive meal, often saying as they do so: "I certainly earned this today!" The family may feel a sense of reward, as well as the expression of a mother's love, when they sit down to a meal of their favorite foods; they may feel punished and unloved when the meal includes foods which they dislike.

Age and sex influence food choices. Too often foods are categorized as being suitable for a given age group, or as more suitable for one sex than the other. Peanut butter, jelly, and milk are looked upon as foods for children, but olives and coffee are appropriate for adults! Teenagers adopt current fashions in foods: the hot dog, hamburger, pizza, ice cream with many sauces and toppings. Women are said to prefer light foods such as soufflés, salads, fruits, and vegetables, while filling meals such as meat, potatoes, and pie represent the more usual choice of men.

Emotional outlets provided by food. Eating provides gratification for life stresses: the difficult examination in school; the homely adolescent who has no date to take her to the movies; the quarrel with a friend; the frustration

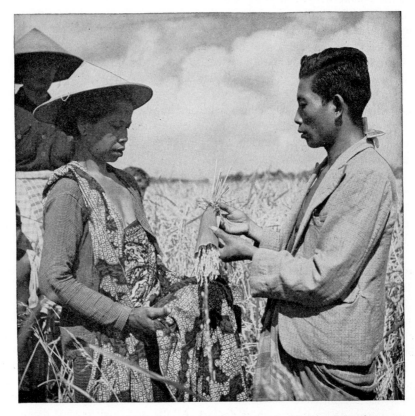

Fig. 15-1. Food and religion are closely associated. After traditional prayers to Goddess of Rice and offerings of palm leaves, sugar cane, and dried cluón leaves, the village priest cuts the first ten crop heads and bundles them together. This is called Mantenan, or the wedding-of-the-crops ceremony. Here the priest is seen handing over the bunch of paddy to the farmer's wife in Katen Village, Java. (*Courtesy, Official United Nations Photo, Department of Public Information.*)

and loneliness of having no friends; the profound grief at the death of a dear one; and countless others.

Food is a symbol of security to many. Milk, the first food of the infant, may be associated with the security of the infant held lovingly in his mother's arms. A person may be away from home, or may be ill, and looks upon milk as expressing the comfort and security of the home; or, milk might be refused because the individual drinking it experiences a feeling of dependence which he does not want to admit, and so he says he doesn't "want to be treated like a baby."

Food may be used as a weapon. An insecure child may refuse to eat food so that his mother will be concerned about him. The ill and the lonely may impose dietary demands upon those caring for them in an effort to gain as much attention as possible.

Illness modifies food acceptance. The patient's acceptance of food is governed by all of the factors discussed above. In addition, inactivity, the disease process itself and its influence on the appetite, anxiety, the strange surroundings of a hospital, modified diets, and other factors may interfere with food acceptance. A more complete discussion is presented in Chapter 23.

EFFECTING CHANGE IN FOOD HABITS

Food habits develop early. Eating is one of life's first experiences. The newborn infant rapidly adapts to breast or bottle feeding and soon associates feeding with security and comfort, or in rare instances with pain. His acceptance of new foods will be determined by his readiness in terms of his physical development and by the environment in which these foods are provided. The food habits of a lifetime are formed during infancy and childhood, and efforts of the mother to provide nutritious foods with due consideration for the mental and emotional development of the child will be richly rewarded (see Fig. 15-2). Food habits, good or bad, become more firmly established with each year that passes, and become less amenable to change. Practical suggestions for the establishment of good food habits throughout childhood are included in the chapters on infant and child feeding (see Chaps. 18, 19).

Determining the need for change. The first step in bringing about a change in food habits quite obviously is to find out just what the needs of the individual or group may be. The need for improvement in food habits may be grossly apparent in an individual who has physical evidences of malnutrition. In others, modified diets are prescribed by a physician as the sole or supportive therapy in disease. For still others, the desirability for dietary improvement is in terms of achieving optimum health as well as the prevention of the deficiency states.

When instructing the healthy or the ill, the dietitian or nurse needs first to determine the present and previous patterns of eating. Having obtained a reliable dietary history, she must interpret this pattern in terms of the adequate diet for the given individual. She must avoid the tendency to judge a diet as being inadequate simply because it doesn't conform to a specific food pattern which she, in her limited experience, may think is the only correct way of eating. Numerous widely varying food patterns provide the essential nutrients for health. Nor must she fall into a second error by assuming that a state of deficiency exists because the daily intake of one or more nutrients is below the Recommended Dietary Allowances. She must remember that these allowances were established to provide for the nutritional needs of individuals varying widely within each age group. The dietary history, then, becomes one of the many tools which the physician might use in making a diagnosis; it also becomes, when properly used, a means whereby satisfactory meals in the hospital setting and nutrition education can be planned so that individuals are more likely to enjoy optimum nutrition.

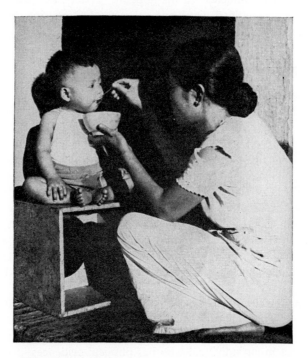

Fig. 15-2. Attitudes towards food are developed early in life. (*Photograph from Indo-China; courtesy, Food and Agriculture Organization and the French Government.*)

Motivation. Few people are motivated to change their food habits simply because they are told that foods are good for them or that they will be healthy. Any attempts to modify food acceptance must be directed to finding what goals are important to the individual or group. When these goals are known, the individual must then be brought to see that what he eats may have an effect on his achievement of these goals.

Mothers are believed to be the group who can bring about significant improvements in food habits. A pregnant woman is desirous of doing what is best for the baby, and when prospective fathers can be involved, the strengthening of desirable food habits is further enhanced. Mothers serve as an example by their own food habits, they provide the food for the family, and they continue to be motivated in terms of doing what is best for each member. When they are given guidance in their management of the feeding of infants and preschool children, subsequent feeding problems are likely to be few. Montagu has stated that emphasis on the family meal is a "contribution to better nutrition, a better family and social relationships." *

Teenagers scorn suggestions that they must eat certain foods to be healthy. However, the training table for the team is evidence of the adolescent boy's acceptance of correct diet as a means of achieving physical strength and athletic prowess. The adolescent girl desires a slim figure, clear skin, beautiful hair, and pep to take part in school and social activities; but, on the other hand, she probably does not want to become too muscular or too tall.

The improvement of health itself is sometimes a motivating factor to the person who has experienced illness. Such a person if obese, for example, may willingly accept the dietary restriction; but for another obese person the goal which serves to motivate her may be a slender figure so that she can wear the current fashions. Return to one's home, or to work or school, or to avoid pain or recurrent illness may be the goals of the patient. When illness strikes the older person, motivation to change the habits of a lifetime is not easy.

Avenues of action. From the foregoing discussion two facts stand out, namely, that numerous influences determine food habits; and, as a consequence, the pathways of effecting change must be many. Education in nutrition implies that one's food habits have been changed in the desired direction. For example, it is not enough for the adolescent to know that a quart of milk is essential in his diet; he must follow through by actually consuming the milk each day!

Nutrition education appropriately belongs in the elementary and secondary school. Suitable references pertaining to the teaching of nutrition in the school may be noted in the Appendix. The school lunch probably has a more far-reaching effect on food habits than many people realize (see p. 273). In a less formal way, nutrition education has a place in many programs for youth—4-H clubs, Girl Scouts, Boy Scouts, and others.

Many opportunities exist within the community for extending nutrition education: mothers' clubs and other women's organizations, parent-teacher associations, prenatal clinics, well-baby clinics, and others. Official and voluntary public health agencies employ numerous programs and many techniques

* Montagu, M. F. A.: "Nature, Nurture, and Nutrition," *Am. J. Clin. Nutrition,* **5:**243, 1957.

to bring about change in food habits. Further discussion concerning community nutrition is presented in Chapter 22.

The media of communication must not be overlooked. Reliable information on food economy, recipes utilizing plentiful foods and giving emphasis to wider use of unusual foods, suggestions for menu planning, and authentic articles on good nutrition for various age categories may be found in many newspapers and magazines. Local libraries may be helpful if their selection includes up-to-date books and pamphlets which have been prepared by professionally qualified dietitians and nutritionists. Radio and television, through programs and through advertising, are powerful media for influencing the attitudes and actions of people. In all of these media, one must be able to distinguish between factual information supported by research on the one hand, and faddism and quackery with its emotional appeal on the other.

The nurse and dietitian are more directly concerned with effecting change in the food habits of the patient. Concrete suggestions for dietary instruction are presented in the introductory unit to the study of diet therapy (see p. 333).

REVIEW

1. How do you feel about food? List insofar as you are able the meanings which you clearly associate with foods. List the foods you especially like; those you especially dislike. Can you give any specific reason for placing the food in one category or another?

2. Note for one day the comments made by people around you about food. Do any of these fall within the physiologic or psychologic categories discussed in this chapter? Do they give you any clue concerning readiness to change food habits?

3. A patient in a hospital who needs a high-protein diet has been served meat but says he cannot eat it because it is a fast day for him. How would you handle this?

4. How can you explain the fact that some patients adjust very readily to diets which contain no added salt, but that others find it almost impossible to do so?

5. Suppose you were trying to introduce nonfat dry milk to a group of people who were entirely unfamiliar with it. How would you go about gaining acceptance?

CHAPTER 16 /

Cultural Food Patterns in the United States

Travel and study provide understanding. Each year hundreds of thousands of Americans travel from one part of the United States to another or to practically every part of the globe. Most of them will be adventurous and eager to try the favorite dishes of a given locality; many of them may later prepare certain typical dishes in their homes, and thus the American cuisine, at its best, becomes truly cosmopolitan. Some persons find the study of foreign food patterns to be a fascinating and rewarding hobby, for knowledge of a people's dietary habits leads to better understanding of its culture. One can find an almost limitless array of articles in journals and books, including cookbooks, for a lifetime of browsing and reading.

Perhaps an especially significant group of world travelers are the students who spend a year or longer in one country or another. Those who come to the United States from various countries of Europe are able to make adjustments quite readily since the foods to which they are accustomed are everywhere available. On the other hand, students from the Far East and from tropical climates often require a longer period of adjustment. Fruits and vegetables with which they are familiar may not be available in the northern markets, so they need to acquire new tastes. Many of these students, used to highly seasoned dishes, may describe American dishes as "having no flavor" or "bland"; others are vegetarians and find the typical American meal does not provide enough of the plant protein foods to which they are accustomed. The fact that the majority of these students do adapt their dietary regimens readily to the usual foods served in public dining rooms attests to the ability of people to change their food habits when the motivation is sufficiently great. Be that as it may, one recognizes the important role of the cultural food patterns when one experiences the enjoyment these students show at being able to entertain their American faculty and friends at a meal typical of their country. And so, through student interchange of ideas, a bridge of understanding is provided between various cultures.

Dietary planning for various ethnic groups. The nurse and the dietitian come in contact with people from many ethnic origins. Today, in America, most of the population are those whose forebears have been here for many generations. They have come not only to accept but also to enjoy the abundance and endless variety of foods available. The pressures of advertising, the nutrition education in the classroom and through the school lunch program, and the frequency with which people today eat in restaurants have done much to unify the food patterns. Many people, however, continue to relish favorite dishes associated with holidays and religious customs even though their food habits as a whole can no longer be described in the light of those prevailing in the country of their origin. In a given hospital or home it may be quite important to make allowance for the inclusion of such dishes in menu plans in order to gain the fullest acceptance of the meals.

Relatively speaking, only a small number of the people living in the United States have been born in another land or climate, and have experienced at first hand the cultural environment of the land of their origin. Such a group of people, for example, are the Puerto Ricans who have come in considerable numbers especially to the eastern cities, and who encounter the multiple problems of employment and income, inability to speak English, and inability to make satisfactory substitutions for the foods which they used in abundance while in Puerto Rico. For such groups of people, the dietitian or nurse must be thoroughly conversant with the native food habits so that she can make the best recommendations for adjustment in this country.

So vast a study as that of cultural food patterns can be only touched upon in this chapter. The discussion which follows is limited to those patterns which fairly frequently may pose problems to the dietitian or nurse as she works with patients and their families either in the hospital or within the home. The list of references in the Appendix, page 810, should be consulted for further guidance.

The physical development of any people depends upon the available supply of energy foods, protein, minerals, and vitamins. Food the world over supplies these nutrients, although the agriculture and technologic development of a country may be such that the supply is inadequate to meet fully the needs of the population. It is important for the health worker to recognize that widely varying patterns may provide the essentials of good nutrition and that she should learn to build upon the desirable characteristics of any given diet. She needs to remember that people who are ill, or who have had little education, or who are economically underprivileged, are less readily motivated to effect change in their existing food habits.

REGIONAL FOOD PATTERNS OF THE UNITED STATES

Perhaps nowhere in the world can one find so great a variety of foods and methods of preparation as in the United States. The dietary patterns are an amalgamation of the foods native to the region and the habits and customs handed down by generations of foreign-born. The foods vary from the wheat of the North Central plains to the rice of Louisiana, the potatoes of Maine to the citrus fruits of Florida, the dairy products of Minnesota and Wisconsin to the beef of the western ranges, the fish of the seacoast to the fruits of the Far West. One might associate baked beans with New England, chile con carne with the Southwest, and fried chicken with the South, but today these dishes are served everywhere in the United States. Advances in technology and modes of transportation bring foods within days—or even hours—from all parts of the country to our American homes, especially those in metropolitan areas.

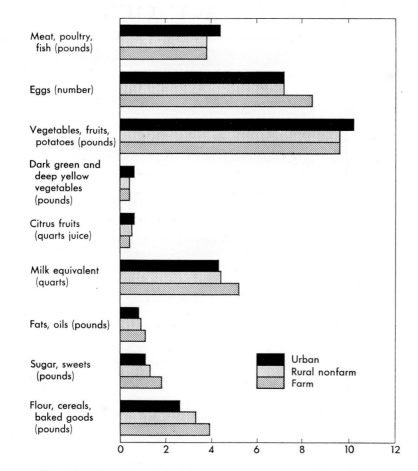

Fig. 16-1. Quantities of food eaten per person per week by urban, rural nonfarm, and farm families. (*Data from Agricultural Research Service, ARS 62-6, U.S. Department of Agriculture.*)

A dietary survey conducted by the United States Department of Agriculture in 1955 [1] has brought out that the greatest variations in food consumption in the United States occur between rural and urban families, regardless of region. Farm families were found to consume greater quantities of energy-rich foods such as grain products, sugars, sweets, and fats, presumably because their work increases their energy requirement over that of city dwellers. Farm families also consumed more milk and eggs but somewhat less meat, fruits, and vegetables than city families. These differences are readily apparent in Figures 16-1 and 16-2. Farm families received larger amounts of

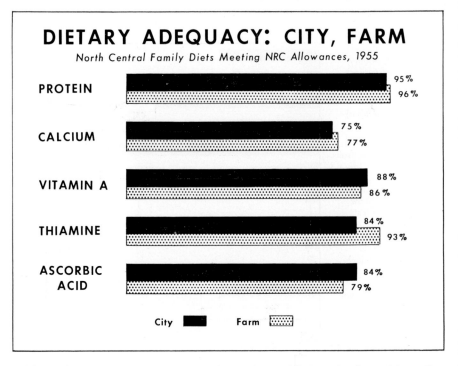

DIETARY ADEQUACY: CITY, FARM

North Central Family Diets Meeting NRC Allowances, 1955

PROTEIN — 95% City, 96% Farm

CALCIUM — 75% City, 77% Farm

VITAMIN A — 88% City, 86% Farm

THIAMINE — 84% City, 93% Farm

ASCORBIC ACID — 84% City, 79% Farm

City ▮   Farm ▦

Fig. 16-2. The family survey of 1955 showed fewer differences in city and farm diets than in earlier surveys. Farm diets still supply more of all nutrients except vitamin A and ascorbic acid. (*Courtesy, Agricultural Research Service, U.S. Department of Agriculture.*)

all nutrients except vitamins A and C than did city families. They consumed less beer, wine, and the like, but equal quantities of coffee, tea, and soft drinks. They ate fewer meals away from home.

Comparisons were made in this survey between the northeastern, central, southern, and western regions. While some slight differences were found to exist, they were no greater than might be found between individual families within a community, and were not as great as the variations between city and farm families of a given region. The South differed more from the other three regions than these regions differed from each other. The people of the South consumed more fats, sugars, grain products, and fresh vegetables, but somewhat less meat, milk, and processed fruits and vegetables. The effects of these differences may be seen in Figure 16-3. The Northeast was somewhat lower in thiamine than the remaining three regions owing to the lower consumption of grain products and pork. In all other nutrients the South fared least well. The most serious lack in the southern diets was in calcium because of the lower consumption of milk, and in ascorbic acid because of the less frequent use of citrus fruits and tomatoes.

While the regional differences in the amounts of food consumed from each of the food groups were not great, somewhat wider variation occurred in the selection within groups. Thus, in the South sweet potatoes and corn products are extensively used, while in the North Central region white potatoes and wheat products are the comparable items of choice. It is pertinent to list, even briefly, some of the traditional dishes and patterns of each region, for people derive a sense of well-being when such a favorite dish, even though it does not dominate the dietary, is served to them.

In addition to the baked beans and brown bread on a Saturday night, in New England one is likely to encounter such favorite dishes as codfish cakes, lobster, clam chowder, and other sea-food specialties. Pumpkin pie, squash, and turkey originated with the Pilgrim fathers.

The Pennsylvania Dutch are known for many rich foods including potato pancakes, many kinds of sausage, Philadelphia scrapple, sticky cinnamon buns, pickles and relishes ("seven sweets and seven sours"), and shoofly pie.

Fried chicken, country ham, and hot biscuits are specialties of the South. Green vegetables such as turnip tops, collards, kale, and mustard greens are well liked; they are likely to be cooked for a relatively long time with fat pork as a flavoring agent. The water in which the vegetables is boiled (pot liquor) is often consumed, thus retaining some of the minerals and vitamins which would otherwise be lost. Sweet potatoes are preferred to white potatoes, and corn is the cereal of choice, although rice and wheat are also widely used. Corn appears in such forms as corn pone, corn bread, hominy grits, spoon bread, and hush puppies—in Florida and Texas, especially.

Dairy products, meat, and eggs abound in the Middle West. Here one finds dietary patterns similar to those of Scandinavia, Germany, Poland, England, and other northern European countries.

New Orleans is noted for its fine restaurants, which show the influence of French and Creole cookery. Soups and fish dishes are often highly seasoned, while sauces are used for many meats and vegetables.

The Mexican and Spanish influences are felt in the Southwest where pinto beans, tortillas made from flour or lime-treated corn, and chili, a hot pepper,

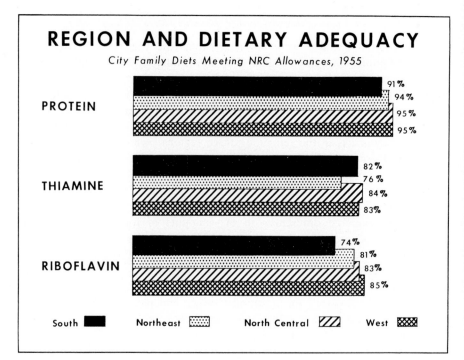

REGION AND DIETARY ADEQUACY

City Family Diets Meeting NRC Allowances, 1955

PROTEIN
91%
94%
95%
95%

THIAMINE
82%
76%
84%
83%

RIBOFLAVIN
74%
81%
83%
85%

South ▪ Northeast ░ North Central ▨ West ▩

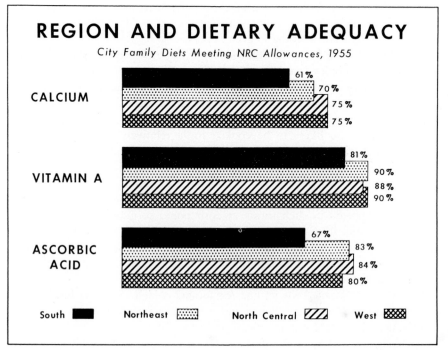

REGION AND DIETARY ADEQUACY

City Family Diets Meeting NRC Allowances, 1955

CALCIUM
61%
70%
75%
75%

VITAMIN A
81%
90%
88%
90%

ASCORBIC ACID
67%
83%
84%
80%

South ▪ Northeast ░ North Central ▨ West ▩

Fig. 16-3. Some regional differences in food consumption and dietary adequacy still exist. People of the southeastern region consumed less of all nutrients except thiamine. (*Courtesy, Agricultural Research Service, U.S. Department of Agriculture.*)

are important constituents of the diet.[71] Usually these staple food items are served with highly seasoned sauces (see Mexican dietary patterns, p. 219).

The abundance of luscious fruits and vegetables in the Far West leads to a much greater consumption of salads as main dishes as well as accompaniments of the meal. The Oriental influence is especially noted in the delicious vegetables of Japanese and Chinese cookery. Sea foods abound in great variety on the West Coast, as in the East, but the salmon of the Pacific Northwest is especially prized.

ORTHODOX JEWISH FOOD HABITS

Outstanding characteristics. The description of the dietary pattern of the Jewish people presented here is based, in large part, on a recent article by Kaufman.[72] Orthodox Jews observe dietary laws based on Biblical and rabbinical regulations. These laws pertain to the selection, preparation, and service of food. Conservative Jews nominally observe the laws but make distinctions within and without the home, while Reform Jews minimize the significance of dietary laws. Food habits of the Jewish people may also be influenced by the country of origin—for example, Russia, Poland, and Germany.

Milk and its products are never eaten in the same meal as meat. Usually two meals contain dairy products and one meal contains meat and its products.

Religious festivals include certain food restrictions. No food is cooked or heated on the Sabbath. Yom Kippur (Day of Atonement) is a 24-hour period of fasting from food or drink. For 7 days during the Passover, only unleavened bread and cakes may be used (Exod. 12:15–20; 13:3–10; 23:15). Only utensils and dishes which have made no contact with leavened foods may be used during this time.

The diet is generally rich in pastries, cake, many preserves, and relishes. Breads, cereals, legumes, fish, dairy products are used abundantly. Encouragement should be given to the inclusion of more fruits and vegetables.

Typical foods and their uses

Milk group

Milk, cottage and cream cheese, sour cream used abundantly. Milk and its products may not be used at same meal as meat (Exod. 23:19; 34:26; Deut. 14:21). Milk may not be taken until 6 hours after eating meat. Separate dishes and utensils must be used for milk and meat dishes

Meat group

ALLOWED FOODS:

All quadruped animals that chew the cud and divide the hoof (Lev. 11:1–3; Deut. 14:3–8): cattle, deer, goats, sheep. Organs of these animals may be used

Animals must be killed in prescribed manner for minimum pain to animal, and for maximum blood drainage

Meat must be *kosher,* that is, drained of blood (Gen. 9:4; Lev. 3:17; 17:10–14; Deut. 12:23–27). Meat is soaked in cold water, thoroughly salted, allowed to drain, washed in three waters

Poultry: chicken, duck, goose, pheasant, turkey. Chicken is common for Sabbath eve meal

Fish with fins and scales (Lev. 11:9; Deut. 14:9–10): cod, haddock, halibut, salmon, trout, tuna, whitefish, etc.

Eggs. Fish and eggs may be eaten at both meat and milk meals

Dried beans, peas, lentils in many soups

Corned beef, smoked meats, herring, *lox* (smoked, salted salmon) are well liked

Cholent: casserole of beef, potatoes, and dried beans. Served on Sabbath

Gefillte fish: chopped, highly seasoned fish

Kishke: beef casings stuffed with rich filling and roasted

Knishes: pastry filled with ground meat

Kreplach: noodle dough filled with ground meat or cheese filling

PROHIBITED FOODS:

Animals which do not chew the cud or divide the hoof (Lev. 11:4–8): pork

Diseased animals or animals dying a natural death (Deut. 14:21)

Birds of prey (Lev. 11:13–19; Deut. 14:11–18)

Fish without fins or scales (Lev. 11:10–12): eels, shellfish such as oysters, crab, lobster

Hindquarters of meat, unless part of thigh with Sinew of Jacob (Gen. 32:33) is removed

Vegetable-fruit group

All kinds used without restriction

Cucumber, lettuce, tomato very frequently used

Cabbage, potatoes, and root vegetables are often cooked with the meat

Borsch: soup with meat stock and egg, or without meat stock and with sour cream; includes beets, spinach, cabbage

Dried fruits are used in many pastries

Bread-cereals group

All kinds used without restriction. Rye bread (pumpernickel), white seed rolls; noodles and other egg and flour mixtures.

Bagel: doughnut-shaped hard yeast roll
Blintzes: thin rolled pancakes filled with cottage cheese, ground beef, or fruit mixture; served with sour cream
Bulke: light yeast roll
Challah: braided loaf or light white bread
Farfel: noodle dough grated for soup
Kasha: buckwheat groats served as cooked cereal or as potato substitute
Kloese: dumplings, usually in chicken soup
Latkes: pancakes

Other foods

Unsalted butter preferred
Chicken fat or vegetable oils for cooking
Rich pastries are common
Cheese cake
Kuchen: coffee cake of many varieties
Leckach: honey cake for Rosh Hashana (New Year)
Strudel: thin pastry with fruit, nut filling
Teiglach: small pieces of dough cooked in honey, with nuts
Sponge cake and macaroons at Passover
Many preserves, pickled cucumbers, pickled green tomatoes, relishes
Many foods are highly salted

PUERTO RICAN FOOD HABITS

Outstanding characteristics. Most of the Puerto Ricans now living in the eastern states have come recently from the island and are therefore accustomed to the foods of that tropical climate. Many of these foods may not be available in the northern cities to which they have come. Because of unfamiliarity with the English language, expensive imported foods are often bought in stores managed by other Puerto Ricans. Some familiarity with the American supermarket would help these people to obtain similar, if not identical, foods more in keeping with their limited income. Nurses and dietitians who work with these people can be of considerable assistance if they are familiar with the typical dietary pattern of the Puerto Rican as described by Torres.[73]

Rice, legumes, and *viandas* (starchy vegetables) are basic to all diets. Dried codfish (*bacalao*) and milk are used as the income permits. Meat is well liked but it is too expensive except for the well-to-do. Fruits on the island are abundant and provide ample ascorbic acid; green vegetables are also abundant. Neither fruits nor vegetables are eaten as much as they should be. The diet is high in carbohydrate and fat. Increased amounts of protein, vitamin A, and ascorbic acid should be provided.

A typical breakfast for the very poor consists of *café con leche* with or without bread; oatmeal and egg are included when income permits. Lunch in the rural areas is a plateful of viandas with codfish and oil; rice and stewed beans might be used in the city. Dinner in urban and rural areas consists of rice and beans, and viandas or bread. Between-meal eating is frequent.

Families with a more liberal income add meat to the daily meals. Chicken, pork, and beef are well liked. Desserts are not always used, but fruits cooked in syrup are especially well liked.

Typical foods and their uses

Milk group

Milk is well liked but low-income groups cannot afford it. Nonfat milk solids well accepted; people must be shown how to use it

Most of the milk is used in strong coffee (*café con leche*); 2–5 ounces milk per cup. May drink this several times a day

Cocoa and chocolate used widely

Meat group

Chicken, pork especially well liked. Seldom used by low-income groups, but liberally by the prosperous

Chicken often cooked with rice (*arroz con pollo*)

Codfish used frequently; served with viandas

Legumes (*granos*): chick peas, kidney beans, navy beans, dried peas, pigeon peas, and other varieties. Stewed and dressed with sauce (*sofrito*). About 3–4 ounces legumes eaten daily

Vegetable-fruit group

Viandas (starchy vegetables): green bananas and green plantain most common; white sweet potatoes; ripe plantain; white *ñame;* white *tanier;* breadfruit in some parts of the island; yautia; cassava, occasionally. Viandas are boiled and served hot with oil, vinegar, and some codfish—often as a one-dish meal in rural areas

Beets and eggplant most commonly used vegetables

Carrots, green beans, okra, and tomatoes in small amounts

Some spinach and chard but insufficient succulent vegetables eaten

Yellow squash (*calabaza*) used in soups or fritters. Yellow sweet potato is little used

Fruits usually eaten between meals rather than at meals. Include: acerola (richest known source of vitamin C), cashew nut fruit, grapefruit, guava, mango, orange, papaya, pineapple

Preference often shown for imported canned peaches, pears, apples, fruit cocktail

In the United States, potatoes and sweet potatoes may be used instead of tropical viandas. Citrus fruits should be stressed

Bread-cereals group

Rice (*arroz*) used once or twice daily by all (7 ounces per capita daily). Enriched by Puerto Rican law. May be boiled with lard added or may be combined with legumes, chopped pork sausages, dry codfish, or chicken
Corn-meal mush made with water or milk is popular
Oatmeal may be cooked in thin gruel for breakfast
Corn meal may substitute for rice, and may be eaten with beans and codfish
Wheat bread, noodles, spaghetti are widely used. Cream of Wheat and other cereals imported by the well-to-do
In the United States suggest whole-grain and enriched cereals and potatoes for some of the rice

Other foods and seasonings

Sofrito: sauce made of tomatoes, onion, garlic, thyme, and other herbs, salt pork, green pepper, and fat. This is basis for much of cooking
Annato: yellow coloring used with rice
Lard, oil, salt pork, or ham butts used in cooking. Lard is used on bread
Sugar in large amounts in coffee, cocoa, chocolate; molasses
Coffee (Mocha, never a blend) is very strong; consider American coffee to be very weak and dislike it. Coffee usually served with hot milk
Carbonated beverages are being used more frequently

MEXICAN FOOD HABITS

Outstanding characteristics. The chief foods of the Mexicans are dried beans, chili peppers, and corn, but wheat is gradually replacing corn (see Fig. 16-4). Many families eat one good meal daily at noon, such as lentil-noodle vegetable soup, while breakfast and supper consist of a sweet coffee or sometimes milk and tortillas.[74] Calcium, riboflavin, and ascorbic acid intakes are low; the quantity and quality of the protein are also low. Greater emphasis should be placed on the use of whole-grain or enriched cereals and flours, milk, eggs, and vegetables.

Typical foods and their uses

Milk group

Very little milk is used; some evaporated milk for infant feeding

Meat group

Beef and chicken well liked; meat used only two or three times weekly
Eggs: two or three times a week
Fish: infrequently

Pinto or calico beans used daily by some; two or three times a week by others

Chile con carne: beef with garlic seasoning, beans, chili peppers

Enchiladas: tortilla filled with cheese, onion, shredded lettuce, and rolled

Taco: tortilla filled with seasoned ground meat, lettuce, and served with chili sauce

Tamales: seasoned ground meat placed on masa, wrapped in corn husks, steamed, and served with chili sauce

Vegetable-fruit group

Corn: fresh or canned; *chicos,* corn steamed while green and dried on the cob; *posole,* similar to hominy

Chili peppers: fresh, canned, or frozen are good source of ascorbic acid

Beets, cabbage, many tropical greens, peas, potatoes, pumpkin, squash, string beans, sweet potatoes, turnips

Bananas used frequently. *Chayotes* (cactuslike fruit), oranges

Bread-cereals group

Corn is staple cereal with wheat gradually replacing it. Rice, macaroni, spaghetti. Some yeast bread; sweet rolls very popular

Atole: corn-meal gruel

Masa: dried corn which has been heated and soaked in lime water, washed,

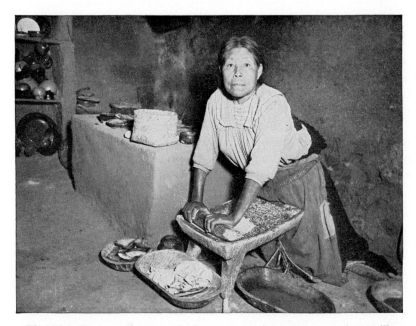

Fig. 16-4. Tarascan woman grinding corn on the metate to make tortillas. (*Courtesy, E. Tejada and Department of Public Information, Food and Agriculture Organization.*)

and ground while wet into puttylike dough; contains appreciable amounts of calcium

Tortilla: thin, unleavened cakes baked on hot griddle, using masa; wheat now replacing lime-treated corn

Other foods and seasonings

Ground red chili powder is essential to most dishes; garlic and onion very common; salt in abundance

Cinnamon, coriander, lemon juice, mint, nutmeg, oregano, parsley, saffron

Butter rarely used

Coffee with much sugar used in large amounts

Sugar and sweets in large amounts

ITALIAN FOOD HABITS

Outstanding characteristics. The favorite foods for the Italian diet are readily available, and the nurse or dietitian should experience no difficulty in adapting the diet of a given locality to the Italian pattern. Cantoni [75] has recently summarized the prevailing pattern for Italian people in the United States.

Pastas, available in a great variety of shapes, are an important staple of the Italian diet. They are prepared from durum wheat of high-gluten content. Crusty white bread is widely used. The Italians use fruits, vegetables, and cheese liberally, and should be encouraged in continuing to do so. Milk is not as widely used as it should be, although cheese will substitute in part. Dietary instruction should include emphasis on the use of enriched flour for bread and pastas.

The typical breakfast consists of fruit, Italian bread with butter, and coffee with hot milk and sugar. The main meal of the day comes at noon if all members of the family are at home, but will come in the evening when some members are away from home all day. The main meal may consist of broth with noodles, meat or chicken or pasta with sauce, vegetables, green salad, bread without butter, fruit, and coffee with milk. The evening meal (or lunch) includes a substantial soup as a main dish, Italian bread, coffee with milk and sugar, sometimes cold cuts or cheese or salad, and sometimes wine.

Typical foods and their uses

Milk group

Goat milk is preferred. Most adults drink milk with coffee or chocolate; dislike plain milk

American cheese disliked. Prefer expensive Italian cheeses: *Mozzarella* and *Ricotta* for cooking and with bread; *Parmesan* and *Romano* for grating; *Gorgonzola*

Meat group

Chicken: roast; baked with oil, garlic, salt, pepper; *cacciatora,* browned in oil, simmered in wine, tomato sauce

Lamb

Pork: roasted or fried sausages; baked or fried chops

Veal: cutlets, *scallopine* or with tomato sauce

Cold cuts: *coppa* (highly peppered), *mortadella* (bologna), *prosciutto* (cured ham), salami

Meats often browned in salt pork or oil and simmered in a sauce with combinations of celery, garlic, onion, parsley, green pepper, tomato purée, wine; meat balls; meat loaf. Smaller quantities of meat eaten than by Americans

Fish, canned: anchovies, sardines, tuna. Fish sauces (anchovy, clam, tuna) for spaghetti on fast days

Chick peas, kidney beans, lentils, split peas in soups. *Pastafasiole:* bean soup. *Minestrone:* substantial soup of vegetables, chick peas, pasta

Frittata: omelet with eggs, cheese, bread crumbs, seasonings

Vegetable-fruit group

Favorite vegetables: artichoke, asparagus, broccoli, eggplant, escarole, peppers, squash (zucchini and others), string beans, tomatoes in sauce

Cooked in water, drained, dressed with olive oil or oil and vinegar or lemon juice

Insalata: salad of greens; may be mixed with celery, onions, green peppers, tomatoes. Dressed with olive oil, vinegar (often wine vinegar), garlic, pepper, salt

Fruits are well liked and eaten abundantly when available: apricots, cherries, dates, figs, grapes, melons, peaches, plums, quinces

Bread-cereals group

White crusty bread forms substantial part of meal. Made of high-protein flour, water, yeast, salt, and little if any fat. Flour not likely to be enriched except where state law requires it

Pasta: includes macaroni, spaghetti, noodles in many forms and shapes. Used two to three times a week. Spaghetti is usual pasta of southern Italy, but rice, corn meal, and noodles are more common in northern Italy

Pastasciutta: pasta with gravy or sauce

Noodle doughs filled with meat, vegetable, or cheese mixtures: *cannelloni, lasagne, manicotti, ravioli, tortellini*

Polenta: thick corn-meal mush served plain, or in casserole with sausages, tomato sauce, grated cheese

Risotto alla Milanese: rice cooked in broth, flavored with Parmesan cheese, onion, mushroom, saffron, wine

Other foods and seasonings

Butter, olive oil, salt pork. Oil in cooking; preference for olive oil

Pies and pastry used more in America than in Italy

Cannoli: filled pastries

Farfalleti dolci: dough mixtures fried in fat
Torta: cake
Zabaglione: soft custard with egg yolks, white wine, sugar
Tutti-fruitti ice creams
Seasonings: basil, celery, garlic, nutmeg, onion, oregano, parsley, pepper, green pepper, hot peppers, rosemary, saffron, tomato purée, wine

DIETARY PATTERNS OF THE NEAR EAST— ARMENIA, GREECE, SYRIA, TURKEY

Typical foods and their uses

Milk group

Cow's, goat's, or sheep's milk; fermented preferred to sweet (yoghurt)
Soft and hard cheeses

Meat group

Lamb is preferred; also mutton, goat, beef, pork, poultry
Fish: fresh, salted, or smoked; octopus, squid, shellfish, roe
Eggs
Beans, peas, and lentils
Nuts may be used with wheat and rice in place of meat; pignolias, pistachios
Ground or cut meat often cooked with wheat or rice, or in stews with cereal grains and vegetables. For example:
Breast of lamb stuffed with rice, currants
Squash stuffed with chopped meat, onions, rice, parsley
Cabbage rolls with ground meat, rice, and baked in meat stock; served with lemon juice
Barbecued meats on special occasions; skewered meats are broiled
Shashlik: mutton or lamb marinated in garlic, oil, vinegar; roasted on skewers with tomato and onion slices

Vegetable-fruit group

Eggplant, greens, onions, peppers, tomatoes; also cabbage, cauliflower, cucumbers, okra, potatoes, zucchini
Vegetables cooked with olive oil and served hot or cold; cooked in meat or fish stews; stuffed with wheat, meat, nuts, beans; salads with olive oil, vinegar
Grapes, lemons, oranges; also apricots, cherries, dates, figs, melons, peaches, pears, plums, quinces, raisins. Fresh fruits widely used in season; fruit compotes

Bread-cereals group

Bread is staff of life; used at every meal. Baked on griddles in round, flat loaves
Cracked whole wheat (*bourglour*) and rice used as starchy food, or with vegetables, or with meat (*pilavi*)
Corn in *polenta*

Other foods and seasonings

Olive oil and seed oils used in cooking. Butter is not much used
Nuts (hazel, pignolia, pistachio) used for snacks, in desserts, pastries
Paklava: pastry with nuts and honey
Black olives
Herbs, honey, sugar, lemon juice, seeds of caraway, pumpkin, and sesame
Apricot candy, Turkish paste
Wine, coffee

DIETARY PATTERNS OF THE CHINESE

Typical foods and their uses

Milk group

Milk and cheese are well liked but need to be emphasized

Meat group

Pork, lamb, chicken, duck, fish and shellfish, eggs, and soybeans. Organ meats
including brain and spinal cord, blood, and bone are used
Egg rolls: shrimp or meat and vegetable filling rolled in thin dough, and fried
in deep fat
Egg foo yung: combination of eggs, chopped chicken, mushrooms, scallions,
celery, bean sprouts cooked similar to an omelet
Sweet and pungent pork: pork cubes coated with batter and fried in oil; then
simmered in a sauce of green pepper, cubed pineapple, molasses, brown sugar,
vinegar, and seasonings
Chow mein: veal, chicken, shrimp, with celery, mushrooms, water chestnuts,
bamboo shoots, in sauce; served with soy sauce. A popular dish made for American tastes

Vegetable-fruit group

Cabbage, cucumbers, many greens, mushrooms, bamboo shoots, soybean
sprouts, sweet potatoes
Vegetables are thinly sliced or chopped; cooked in a little oil for a short time
before water is added to seal in flavor, preserve crispness, and fresh green color.
Any juice remaining is served with the vegetable

Bread-cereals group

Rice is staple food served with every meal
Wheat and millet are widely used

Other foods and seasonings

Lard, soy, sesame, and peanut oils used in cooking
Soy sauce present in almost every meal contributes to high salt intake

Almonds, ginger, sesame seeds for flavoring
Tea is beverage of choice

PROBLEMS AND REVIEW

1. What factors must be kept in mind in teaching normal nutrition to people whose food habits differ widely from our own?

2. What technologic advances of the twentieth century have tended to eliminate regional differences in food patterns of the United States?

3. *Problem.* Select any one ethnic group and plan menus for one day including recipes for special dishes.

4. *Problem.* Special problems may be worked out in correlation with diet therapy. For example, plan a diet for a Puerto Rican child with diabetes; a Mexican man who has peptic ulcers; an Italian woman who has nephritis.

5. *Problem.* Make a survey of the ethnic groups represented in the class. List favorite dishes for each of these ethnic groups. Discuss the nutritive values of these dishes. What foods require emphasis in the patterns of these ethnic groups?

UNIT IV /
Special Nutritional Needs
Throughout the Life Cycle

CHAPTER 17 /

Nutrition During Pregnancy and Lactation

Every baby should have the right to begin life with a healthy, well-formed body free of defects, and to receive the advantages of his mother's milk. Every mother should be able to provide for the optimum development of the fetus, should remain in good health throughout pregnancy, and should encounter no unusual difficulties in the periods of labor, the puerperium, and lactation.

Remarkable progress has been made toward lowering the death rate of children under 1 year of age. In spite of this, the mortality during the newborn period constitutes the third leading cause of death in this country.[76] Such a fact does not take into account the losses through stillbirth and miscarriage, nor does it consider the incidence of prematurity when the infant survives, and the unnecessary illness of many mothers during and following pregnancy. Most tragic of all is the malformed child who survives but who is physically and mentally so damaged that a healthy, happy, normal life is impossible. These obstetric and pediatric problems constitute a major challenge in public health.

Significance of nutrition. Pregnancy is a period of great anabolic activity when the most rapid rate of growth known to medicine takes place. Popular opinion has long held that the fetus develops at the expense of the mother. This idea is fallacious, however, and the infant as well as the mother will suffer the effects of a poor prenatal diet. The nutritional needs during pregnancy include the normal requirements of the mother, those of the developing fetus, including also the uterus and the placenta, and the building up of reserves in preparation for labor and for lactation.

The *perinatal concept* [77] is now used to describe the nutritional needs of the fetus. It assumes that the mother is in a good nutritional state prior to conception, and that this status will be maintained throughout pregnancy, labor, and the period after birth. Evidence for the important role of nutrition in governing the outcome of pregnancy has been accumulated by animal experimentation, through careful balance studies on selected individuals, by surveys on large numbers of pregnant women, and by examination of the

228

health records of various population groups during periods of severe stress such as war. While the results of such studies are not always in full agreement, the findings all substantiate the essential role of good nutrition prior to and during pregnancy.

Prematernal nutrition. Fewer complications in pregnancy, fewer premature births, and healthier babies result when the mother is well nourished prior to conception. Tompkins [78] has pointed out that the woman who is underweight at the time she becomes pregnant has the greatest probability of premature labor and toxemia. He found a strikingly high incidence of prematurity in infants born of mothers who were both underweight and anemic.

World War II afforded ample opportunity to study nutritional problems including those of pregnancy. Stearns [79] has discussed the reasons for the more serious effects in pregnant women of Leningrad as compared with those of Holland. During October 1944 to May 1945, the food rations in Holland were severely restricted so that pregnant women early in 1945 had less than 1000 calories and 30 to 40 gm protein available. The pregnant women had reasonably adequate nutrition prior to this time. The babies conceived before and born during the hunger period were shorter and lighter than those born before this time, this being a direct result of the mother's diet during the latter half of pregnancy. There was no increase in the rate of stillbirths, prematurity, and malformations, but the rate of conception fell off markedly during the hunger period.

The siege of Leningrad resulted in a very serious food situation especially between August, 1941, and February, 1942. During 1942 the birth rate fell off markedly, the stillbirth rate was twice as high, and the incidence of prematurity had increased 41 per cent. The infants had low vitality and poor resistance to infection, and did not suckle well, thus suggesting that the mother's bodies were not able to supply the necessary nutrients. The less favorable results in Leningrad as compared with those of Holland were attributed to the chronic undernutrition of women prior to the siege.

Animal studies [80] have shown that severe congenital malformations involving the skeleton, the central nervous, cardiovascular, excretory, and other systems can be produced in the fetus when the mother is given diets markedly deficient in one or another nutrient such as vitamin A or riboflavin. The deficiencies imposed upon animals, however, are far more severe than those seen in human beings and one cannot make direct application of these findings to congenital malformations in human beings.

Many women do not enter pregnancy in a satisfactory state of nutrition. At the present time, one-fourth of all first pregnancies occur in teen-age girls. The earlier marriage age means that many young women enter upon pregnancy before their own bodies are fully developed. Teen-age girls are known to have the least satisfactory diet of any age category. They succumb readily to social pressures, are overly concerned about slender figures, and indulge in food jags. The intake of sweets, carbonated beverages, and a wide array of snack foods may be excessively high, while milk, vegetables, fruits, and eggs are often shunned. Discovering ways to guide the adolescent girl into more satisfactory eating patterns provides a real challenge to the nutrition educator.

Prenatal nutrition. Burke and her co-workers [81] studied 216 pregnant women over an extended period during which the women were examined and their diets analyzed. The diets were rated as excellent if they contained 100 per cent of the optimal standards for each of the nutrients. Ratings of good, fair, poor, and very poor were given to diets containing 80, 60, 50, and less than 50 per cent respectively of the optimal levels for the food constituents.

These studies of Burke and her associates indicate that a woman who has a poor or a very poor diet during pregnancy will in all probability have a poor infant; that is, prematurity, congenital defects, and stillborn infants occurred almost entirely in this group. On the other hand, the women who had good-to-excellent diets almost invariably bore infants in good physical condition. Inadequate nutrition during pregnancy resulted in relatively greater harm to the fetus than to the mother. It is of further interest that no cases of eclampsia were noted in those women receiving excellent or good diets, whereas 50 per cent of those receiving poor or very poor diets developed toxemia of varying degrees of severity.

The Vanderbilt cooperative study of 2338 pregnant white women of low income showed the effects of weight status and hemoglobin levels of the mother on the infant.[82] Underweight women (less than 85 per cent of standard) produced smaller babies, prematurity occurred more frequently, and artificial feeding was more common. The overweight group (120 per cent of standard) had more stillborn children and a threefold increase in pre-eclampsia. Women who gained too much, especially during the second trimester, had more toxemia.

Low intakes of iron and ascorbic acid were correlated with lower hemoglobin levels and blood levels of vitamin C. However, during the first year of life the infants of these mothers maintained hemoglobin levels equal to those whose mothers had higher hemoglobin levels, showing that appropriate infant feeding practices can make up for the deficient infant stores of iron.

The Vanderbilt study did not fully establish nutritional deficiency as a primary causative factor in metabolic diseases of pregnancy. The investigators point out that the patient cannot be assured of freedom from complications simply through a satisfactory intake of nutrients. They did observe that diets which contained less than 50 gm protein and less than 1500 calories resulted in a greater frequency of complications of pregnancy and of the newborn, but they felt that the low levels of intake were a result of the complications rather than the cause.

Physiologic changes in pregnancy. In order that the fetus may develop satisfactorily and that the milk supply may be established, many changes controlled by hormone activity must take place in the mother's body. Vital organs including the liver, kidneys, thyroid, adrenals, pituitary, and uterus increase their activity. These changes are reflected in the composition of the blood and the urine, and the retention of nutrients.

Pregnancy may be considered in three stages: [77]

1. The pre-implantation period, about 2 weeks following conception.

2. The period during which organ formation is taking place, approximately 2 to 8 weeks.

3. The period of rapid growth of the fetus and the establishment of the maternal reserves in preparation for labor, the puerperium, and the production of milk, from the eighth week to term.

Hormonal control. Progesterone, a hormone produced by the corpus luteum, the placenta, and the adrenal cortex, prepares the inner lining of the uterus for the implantation of the fertilized ovum. Gonadotropins are especially concerned with organ formation up to about the fourth month of pregnancy, and with fetal growth. Estrogen production increases appreciably after about the one-hundredth day of gestation. Estrogen and progesterone stimulate the growth of the mammary glands and also inhibit the lactogenic function of the pituitary gland until delivery of the infant. Steroid hormones are produced in greater amounts with the result that water and sodium are more readily retained in the body.

The *placenta* is the organ to which the fetus is attached by means of the umbilical cord and by which the nutrition of the fetus is maintained. It achieves its maximum size early in gestation. Materials which are carried in solution by the maternal circulation and which can cross the semipermeable membranes are made available to the developing fetus. The placenta is rich in protein, fat, carbohydrates, minerals, vitamins, hormones, and enzymes and modifies its relative composition as pregnancy progresses according to the changing needs of the developing fetus. It is likely that a faulty placenta may well contribute to poor development of the fetus and to malformations, but nutritional factors which may lead to an imperfect placenta are not understood.

Weight gain. The gain in weight for the healthy woman entering pregnancy with normal weight is about 16 to 24 pounds. This is accounted for by the weight of the full-term baby of about 7½ pounds; increase in size of the uterus, 2 pounds; placenta and membranes, 1¼ pounds; amniotic fluid, 2 pounds; increase in breast tissue, 1½ pounds. Some increase in weight is accounted for by the increase in blood circulation which amounts to about 25 per cent, and by the tendency to retain more fluid in the tissues. Considerable stores of nitrogen and of minerals—especially calcium and phosphorus—are established in preparation for parturition and lactation.

Tompkins has emphasized that a failure to gain at a normal rate during the first 2 trimesters as well as initial underweight status increases the probability of premature labor. On the other hand, overweight at the beginning of pregnancy or an excessive rate of gain during the second and third trimester results in greater likelihood of pre-eclampsia and eclampsia. The recommended rate of gain by Tompkins is 5, 8, and 10 pounds during the first, second, and third trimesters, respectively.

Basal metabolism. During the third and fourth month of pregnancy the basal metabolism is slightly reduced, but thereafter it increases until it is as much as 25 per cent over the normal rate by the end of the term. This increase is accounted for in part by the gain in weight and also by the high metabolic activity of the fetus and the placenta. Some increase in thyroid function also occurs.

Nutritional allowances. The recommendations of the Food and Nutrition Board [2] apply to the second half of pregnancy and are based on the assumption that the woman has enjoyed good health prior to pregnancy. In many cases this is not true, and qualitative and quantitative changes must be made as soon as possible.

RECOMMENDED DAILY DIETARY ALLOWANCES, 1958 [2]

	NORMAL WOMAN *	PREGNANT WOMAN * (second half)	LACTATING WOMAN * (850 ml milk daily)
Calories	2300	2600	3300
Protein, gm	58	78	98
Calcium, gm	0.8	1.5	2.0
Iron, mg	12	15	15
Vitamin A, I.U.	5000	6000	8000
Thiamine, mg	1.2	1.3	1.7
Riboflavin, mg	1.5	2.0	2.5
Niacin, mg equivalents	17	20	19
Ascorbic acid, mg	70	100	150
Vitamin D, I.U.		400	400

* Reference woman: 25 years old; 58 kg; 163 cm; normally vigorous.

Caloric allowances. The additional need for calories is small during the first half of pregnancy, while an increase of 300 calories is estimated by the Food and Nutrition Board to be satisfactory for the second half of pregnancy. Some women who remain inactive throughout pregnancy will not require this increase, while the young, active woman may require more than this. It is the rate of gain, rather than a calculated caloric level, which should be used as the indicator for increase or decrease in caloric intake. When the woman is obese, or when the weight gain is too rapid, a moderate caloric restriction is required. The 1800 and 1500 calorie plans on page 235 will usually suffice.

Protein allowance. The foods furnishing the protein must contain a sufficient amount of all the essential amino acids to maintain the mother's tissues, provide for the building of the new tissues of the developing fetus, and supply a reserve for the losses during the puerperium and for the onset of lactation. The protein allowance is satisfactory when 20 gm protein are added to the normal daily allowance of 1 gm per kg body weight.

Mineral allowances. Some calcium and phosphorus deposition takes place early in pregnancy, but the amounts are small. The first set of teeth begins to form about the eighth week of prenatal life, and they are well formed by the end of the prenatal period. The 6-year molars which are the first permanent teeth to erupt begin to calcify just before birth. Most of the calcification of bones occurs during the last 2 months of pregnancy. If the mobile reserve of calcium is lacking in the mother, the demands of the fetus can be met, perhaps inadequately, only at severe expense to the mother. For many women it is advisable to increase the calcium intake early in pregnancy even though fetal calcification does not occur until later. The phosphorus allowance should be about equal to that for calcium, and will be readily supplied through the calcium-rich and protein-rich foods.

From 700 to 1000 mg iron must be absorbed and utilized by the mother throughout pregnancy. Of this total, about 240 mg are spared by the cessation of the menstrual flow. The remainder must be made available from the diet. A daily increase of 3 mg will provide sufficient iron except for the anemic woman who requires supplements of iron salts. The rate of iron absorption is increased threefold in the third trimester when the fetal needs are highest.

Iodine must be provided in adequate amounts to protect against the incidence of goiter in mother or infant. Iodized salt is the most practical way to ensure an adequate iodine intake. When a sodium-restricted diet is ordered, the physician may prescribe iodine supplementation since most foods cannot be counted upon for their iodine content.

McGanity and his associates [82] have stated that mineral and vitamin supplementation should be based on need as established through biochemical studies rather than routine use. In their studies they did not find any improvement of fetal or maternal health when supplements were used except in the case of iron supplementation for anemic women.

Vitamin allowances. The thiamine and niacin allowances are increased in proportion to the caloric increase, while riboflavin allowances are increased according to the higher protein level. The need for vitamin D is increased during pregnancy to facilitate the utilization of greater amounts of calcium and phosphorus. The need is met when 1 quart milk fortified with vitamin D is included daily. Ascorbic acid in its vital role in tissue structure is required in considerably increased amounts.

During the early days of life, the infant often has low blood prothrombin levels until intestinal synthesis of vitamin K is fully established. Vitamin K is sometimes given to the mother before the birth of the infant thus affording some protection, but the use of supplements during the course of pregnancy is not considered to be necessary.

Selecting the daily diet. The inclusion of a quart of milk becomes imperative in the daily diet because no other food can so readily provide the calcium, phosphorus, riboflavin, and protein (see Fig. 17-1). The milk may

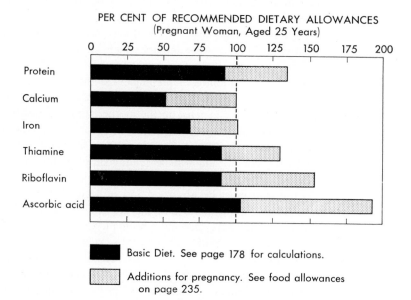

Fig. 17-1. The Basic Diet provides ample vitamin A and niacin equivalents (not shown in chart above) and almost meets the needs for protein, thiamine, and riboflavin of the pregnant woman. Calcium and iron allowances can be met only through the inclusion of additional foods from each of the Four Food Groups.

be whole or skim, fresh, evaporated, or dry, and taken as a beverage or incorporated into foods. Cheddar cheese or other hard cheese may substitute for part of the milk. Eggs, meat, fish, poultry, legumes, and peanut butter are important for their protein, iron, and B-complex vitamins. When legumes or peanut butter are used in the main dish of the meal, some complete protein food should also be included at that meal; for example, a milk dessert and milk for beverage would be satisfactory.

One of the simplest and least expensive ways to increase the ascorbic acid intake is to include 2 portions of citrus fruit daily. Vegetables, especially dark green leafy vegetables, should be emphasized for their carotene and iron contents, and for the additional bulk they give to the diet.

The following list of foods illustrates easy modifications for caloric intake, with no compromise in the nutrient levels. Each list provides the recommended daily allowances for the pregnant woman.

DIET DURING PREGNANCY

FOODS TO INCLUDE DAILY	2600 CALORIES	1800 CALORIES	1500 CALORIES
Milk	1 quart, whole	1 quart, whole	1 quart, skim
Meat, fish, or poultry—liver weekly	4 ounces	4 ounces	4 ounces
Eggs, or equivalent. One egg equals:	2	2	2
1 ounce Cheddar cheese			
1 ounce meat, fish, or poultry			
¼ cup cottage cheese			
2 tablespoons peanut butter			
½ cup cooked dried peas, beans, or soybeans			
Vegetables, including:			
Dark green leafy or deep yellow	1 serving	1 serving	1 serving
Potato	1 medium	1 medium	1 medium
Other vegetables	2 servings	2 servings	2 servings
One vegetable to be raw each day			
Fruits, including:			
Citrus	2 servings	2 servings	2 servings
Other	1 serving	1 serving	1 serving
Cereal, enriched or whole-grain	1 serving	1 serving	1 serving
Bread, enriched or whole-grain	5 slices	3 slices	3 slices
Butter or fortified margarine	2 tablespoons	1 tablespoon	1 tablespoon
Desserts, cooking fat, sugars, sweets	To meet caloric needs	None	None
Vitamin-D supplement (or use fortified milk)	400 I.U.	400 I.U.	400 I.U.
Iodized salt			

MEAL PATTERN

Breakfast
  Fruit
  Cereal—preferably whole-grain or enriched
  Milk for cereal
  Egg
  Toast or roll with butter or fortified margarine
  Hot beverage with cream and sugar, if desired

Midmorning
  Milk

Luncheon or supper
  Egg or substitute of cheese, meat, fish, fowl, or legumes
  Potato, rice, spaghetti, noodles, macaroni, or vegetable
  Green or yellow vegetable—preferably raw
  Bread—whole-grain or enriched—with butter
  Milk
  Fruit

Midafternoon
  Milk

Dinner
   Orange, grapefruit, or tomato juice—1 cup
   Meat, fish, or fowl
   Potato
   Vegetable—raw or cooked
   Bread—whole-grain or enriched—with butter
   Dessert
   Tea or coffee, if desired

Before retiring
   Milk

COMPLICATIONS OF PREGNANCY

Mild nausea and vomiting. During the first trimester, the physiologic and biochemical balances are often disturbed, possibly because of excessive hormone production. Gastrointestinal upsets, including loss of appetite, nausea, and vomiting are relatively frequent; loss of weight occasionally takes place because of inability to eat sufficient food. The development of specialized tissues may be adversely affected during this period, resulting in the greatest likelihood of miscarriage.

Mild early morning nausea may usually be overcome by the use of high-carbohydrate foods such as crackers, jelly, hard candies, and dry toast before arising. Frequent small meals rather than three large ones may be preferable. Fluids should be taken between meals rather than at mealtime. Fatty, rich foods such as pastries, desserts, fried foods, excessive seasoning, coffee in large amounts, and strongly flavored vegetables may be restricted or eliminated if the nausea persists or if the patient complains of heartburn or gastric distress.

Pernicious vomiting. When vomiting becomes severe and persistent, feeding by mouth is frequently impossible for a time. The nutritional status may be maintained partially by the use of intravenous glucose solutions, protein hydrolysates, electrolytes, and vitamins. Tube feedings may also be used. Vitamin B_6 has been effective in alleviating the symptoms in some patients.

As soon as the patient is able to eat, a high-carbohydrate, low-fat diet will usually prove to be well taken. The following outline will direct the administration of such a diet.

HIGH-CARBOHYDRATE LOW-FAT DIET
(for pernicious vomiting of pregnancy)

Characteristics and general rules:

   Give food every 2 hours during the day and once or twice during the night. Fasting aggravates the condition and feedings should not be skipped.

Since the psychologic factor is important, it is essential to consult the patient frequently as to likes and dislikes. Foods which are appealing to the appetite are more likely to be retained.

Give small portions of food at a time, restricting bulk to 100 to 200 gm per meal in severe cases. Dry foods may be more readily retained than liquid foods.

Since dehydration may occur, liquids may require emphasis; often parenteral fluids are the only way in which the liquids can be administered.

Select foods high in carbohydrate and low in fat.

Give foods that are easily digested.

Include vitamin concentrates, especially those of the B complex.

Meal plans:

The highly individual character of the diet makes it inadvisable to suggest a meal pattern. The following foods are among those best tolerated at first:

Dry toast with jelly	Baked potato
Crackers with jelly	Plain gelatin
Hard candy	Broth
Cereal with milk and sugar	Tomato juice

As the patient's condition warrants—usually after 3 or 4 days—foods may be gradually added until first a soft and then a regular diet is attained. Each addition must be made with caution. The diet must not be progressed until the patient can tolerate more food.

Foods to avoid:

Foods high in fat such as fried foods, gravies, pastries, rich desserts, whipped cream. Moderate amounts of butter and light cream are usually tolerated.

Highly seasoned foods

Strongly flavored vegetables

Constipation. The occurrence of constipation especially during the latter half of pregnancy is common. The amount of pressure exerted by the developing fetus on the digestive tract, the limitation of exercise, and insufficient bulk may be contributing factors in its causation. The normal diet outlined on page 235 provides a liberal allowance of fruits, whole-grain cereals, and vegetables, and consequently of fiber. It is also necessary to stress the importance of adequate fluid intake and of regular habits of exercise, elimination, sleep, and recreation.

Overweight. Excessive weight gain increases the incidence of toxemia, and may be avoided by careful adjustment of the caloric intake from time to time. Usually the 1800 calorie level will suffice, but the 1500 calorie level may be necessary for the woman who is quite inactive. Either of these levels requires care in planning to ensure adequate protein, mineral, and vitamin intakes. The lists on page 235 will serve as a basis for planning the meals.

Anemia. Inasmuch as the blood volume may increase as much as 25 per cent during pregnancy, it is apparent that a corresponding lowering of the hemoglobin level and red cell count will occur without a decrease in the total circulating blood elements. This state is often referred to as the "physiologic anemia of pregnancy."

On the other hand, many women experience a marked reduction in hemoglobin level and in red cell count because they do not have the necessary reserves to meet their own needs and those of the infant. The recommended increase in the iron intake is based on the needs of the woman who has adequate iron stores at the beginning of pregnancy, and is insufficient for the woman who is anemic at the time of conception. Because the anemic woman is more prone to delivering prematurely, and because her infant will not enter life with sufficient iron stores, it is essential that iron salts be prescribed to supplement the diet.

In some women the gastric acidity is reduced during pregnancy and an anemia characterized by low cell count, increase in cell size, and low hemoglobin level results. This anemia bears some resemblance to pernicious anemia (see p. 542) but is corrected by folic acid therapy, and, unlike pernicious anemia, can be cured.

Toxemia. By toxemia is meant that combination of symptoms which may include edema, hypertension, albuminuria, and, if allowed to progress, convulsions. The importance of a good diet in reducing the incidence of toxemia has already been discussed (p. 229). Some toxemias are undoubtedly occasioned by kidney or circulatory disease already present in the woman. When toxemia does occur, the dietary management must be related to the etiology as well as to the symptoms which may be present.

Of paramount importance is an adequate protein intake (85 to 100 gm or more) to alleviate the hypoproteinemia which is almost invariably present and which may be primarily responsible for the edema. The nitrogen of the amino acids used in building can be of no harm to the kidney, for it will not be excreted as long as it remains to be used in tissue construction.

Restriction of sodium is desirable for the control of edema. The concurrent need for a high-protein and high-calcium intake makes it impractical to restrict sodium as markedly as may be advocated for some heart and kidney conditions (see Chap. 36), but the general rules for the planning and preparation of low-sodium diets should be respected (p. 507). It is indeed questionable whether severe restriction of sodium is as important as an adequate intake of protein. When severe restriction is resorted to, sodium-deficient milk must be substituted for regular milk.

Overweight is often present in women with toxemia, and a reduction in the caloric intake may be advisable.

Diabetes. The diabetic woman, like the normal woman, has increased nutritive requirements during the latter half of pregnancy which must be met with an increased prescription and insulin as necessary. (See Chap. 33.) While lactation may be possible for the diabetic mother, it is usually necessary to provide supplementary feedings for the infant.

LACTATION

Nutritive requirements. McGanity and his associates [82] found that women who had high intakes of calcium, phosphorus, and riboflavin from their diets nursed their babies more frequently than did women who drank less than 3 glasses of milk daily and who had calcium supplements. When one considers the nutritive value of human milk, and that the nursing mother will produce 20 to 30 ounces each day, it becomes apparent that the requirements for protein, minerals, vitamins, and calories are even greater than they were during pregnancy. The recommended allowances for the various nutrients have been listed on page 232.

The need for protein is greatest when lactation has reached its maximum, but it is a need which should be anticipated and planned for during pregnancy. The mechanics of converting food into milk protein is only about 50 per cent efficient, and thus about 2 gm of food protein are required to produce 1 gm of milk protein. This conversion takes place when there is a suitable mixture of all of the essential amino acids, and therefore the proteins of milk, eggs, meat, poultry, fish should have priority.

Approximately 130 calories are required for each 100 ml of milk, and thus the daily production of 850 ml of milk (30 ounces) would necessitate an additional 1000 calories in the diet.

Even liberal intakes of calcium may not be successful in completely counteracting a negative calcium balance. Consequently, a high level of calcium intake and the building of considerable reserves throughout pregnancy cannot be overemphasized. The baby is born with a relatively larger reserve of iron since milk is not a good source of iron. A good allowance of iron in the mother's diet during lactation does not convey additional iron to the infant. Nevertheless iron-rich foods are essential for the mother's own health, while supplements are included early in the infant's diet.

Selecting the daily diet. The pattern of diet used during pregnancy (p. 235) may be used during lactation, provided the following additions are made: (1) one pint of milk; (2) foods as desired to provide the additional calories. Weight gain, beyond that desirable for body build should be avoided. When the baby is weaned, the mother must reduce her food intake in order that obesity may be avoided.

The choice of foods during lactation may be wide. There are no foods which require restriction, except where distress may occur in individual cases following the taking of a particular food such as strongly flavored vegetables or highly seasoned or spicy foods. Successful lactation is dependent not only upon an adequate diet, but also upon sufficient rest for the mother, freedom from anxiety, and a desire to nurse the baby.

PROBLEMS AND REVIEW

1. What evidence exists that diet is of importance in the development of the fetus and the health of the mother?

2. What physiologic changes occur during the course of pregnancy?

3. Name the hormones which are especially important in controlling the changes occurring during pregnancy? What is the effect of an excess production?

4. In what way do the nutritional practices of teen-age girls affect the outcome of pregnancy?

5. What weight increases are recommended for each trimester? What are the dangers of excess weight gain? Of underweight or insufficient weight gain?

6. What foods are especially important for their protein content in the diet during pregnancy and lactation?

7. What mineral elements require especial attention during pregnancy? What changes occur in the rate of absorption of calcium and iron?

8. Discuss the need for an increased vitamin intake. What foods would you recommend for this?

9. Mrs. A. does not like milk and is taking calcium gluconate to correct calcium deficiency. Why is this less desirable than taking milk? List ways by which she could incorporate milk into her diet.

10. What recommendations can you make to a woman with complaints of nausea, vomiting, and gastric distress?

11. What instructions are in order for the woman who complains of constipation?

12. What is meant by the "physiologic anemia of pregnancy"? What are the hazards of iron deficiency anemia? What measures are essential for its prevention and treatment?

13. A woman secretes 800 ml milk daily. What amount of protein is here represented? What allowances must be made in the diet for protein?

14. *Problem.* Plan a low-cost diet for a woman of moderate activity during the second half of pregnancy. Calculate the nutrients in this diet and compare them with the recommended allowances.

15. *Problem.* Modify the diet in Problem 14 for a woman who is lactating.

16. *Problem.* Plan a 1000 mg sodium, 100 gm protein, 2000 calorie diet for a woman during the last trimester.

CHAPTER 18 /

Nutrition During Infancy

Growth and development of the infant. During the first year the infant will grow and develop more rapidly than at any other time of life. At a weekly gain ranging from 5 to 8 ounces he will double his birth weight in the first 5 months. The weekly gain slows down to 4 to 5 ounces for the remainder of the year, and he will have tripled his birth weight by the time he is 10 to 12 months old.

The baby will increase his birth length of 20 to 22 inches by another 9 to 10 inches during the first year. At birth he has a large head in proportion to the rest of his body, but his short arms and legs will grow especially rapidly in the next 12 months.

The gastrointestinal system of the full-term infant is able to digest protein, emulsified fats, and simple carbohydrates, but starches and most fats are poorly tolerated until some months later when the digestive enzyme production is more fully developed.

The infant's body contains a much higher proportion of water than that of older children and adults, while the muscles are poorly developed and the amount of subcutaneous fat is limited. Since the skin surface area is high in proportion to the total body weight, the loss of body water and of body heat is also relatively high. The skeleton contains a high percentage of water and cartilage, and will be only gradually mineralized throughout childhood and adolescence.

The infant of a well-nourished mother has a good store of iron and a high blood hemoglobin level. The iron stores are gradually depleted in the first few months of life so that the hemoglobin concentration may eventually drop to anemic levels unless the diet is supplemented with iron-rich foods.

Several criteria may be applied to determine whether an infant is well nourished, namely: steady gain in height and weight, but some weekly fluctuations are to be expected; sleeps well, is vigorous, and happy; firm muscles and a moderate amount of subcutaneous fat are developed; teeth begin to erupt within 5 to 6 months, and from six to 12 teeth have come through by the end of the year; and elimination is normal for the type of feeding. The

241

breast-fed baby usually has two to three soft, yellow stools each day, while the formula-fed infant has one to two yellow, somewhat firmer stools.

BREAST FEEDING

Approximately 87 per cent of all mothers can supply their infants with enough milk to justify the continuation of nursing if there is proper management.[83] In this country, however, less than half of all mothers breast-feed their babies. If breast feeding is to be successful, the advantages must be sold to the mother early in pregnancy. An adequate diet, exercise, rest, and freedom from anxiety are important during the prenatal period as well as during lactation (Chap. 17). The sucking of a hungry baby stimulates the mother's breast to produce milk and should be started during the first 24–48 hours of life.

Advantages of breast feeding. Human milk is the natural food for the infant. Breast feeding gives a safe and protected feeling to the infant, and a sense of satisfaction to the mother. In lower economic groups breast-fed infants have a consistently lower mortality rate, probably because there is no problem of sanitation. As a rule, there are fewer and less serious illnesses and feeding problems among breast-fed infants; constipation also occurs less frequently. On a practical basis breast feeding eliminates preparation of a feeding; the milk is available at proper temperature; and errors in calculation and in formula preparation are avoided.

Contraindications to breast feeding. If the mother can supply less than half of the infant's needs, breast feeding usually is not practical. It must be discontinued when (1) chronic illnesses are present in the mother, such as cardiac disease, tuberculosis, severe anemia, nephritis, epilepsy, insanity, and chronic fevers; (2) another pregnancy ensues; (3) it is necessary for the mother to return to employment outside the home; or (4) the infant is weak or unable to nurse because of cleft palate or harelip. Temporary cessation is also indicated when the mother acquires an acute infection which the infant has not yet acquired; in such a situation the mother's breasts should be completely pumped at regular intervals so that the milk supply will not dwindle.

Colostrum. The clear, yellowish secretion from the breast during the first few days after delivery is not mature milk, but a substance richer in protein and in vitamin A than the milk secreted later. The levels of carbohydrate, fat, niacin, pantothenic acid, biotin, and riboflavin are low initially and reach mature milk levels by the tenth day. Both colostrum and mature milk contain the same levels of ascorbic acid.

The infant receives only 10 to 40 ml of colostrum during the first 2 to 3 days, but by the end of the first week the supply of milk will usually satisfy the full nutrient needs. While the nutritive contribution of colostrum seems to be small, the secretion apparently confers an immunity to certain infections during the first few months and aids in the development of the digestive enzymes.

Intervals of feeding. To feed the infant whenever he cries or to adhere to a rigid time schedule are equally bad, and it is now realized that the intervals of feeding may be reasonably flexible. Healthy infants will establish, after a few weeks, schedules of their own which are reasonably regular from day to day if they are fed when they indicate that they were hungry. Self-demand feeding is not successful, however, for premature infants or those who are weak and sickly.

The success of self-demand feeding depends also upon the mother's ability to determine when the child is hungry. The infant who cries at intervals much shorter than 3 hours may be underfed, may have swallowed too much air at the previous feeding, or may be crying because of other discomforts.

The very young infant may require as many as 10 or 12 feedings at first, but he soon establishes a rhythm of feeding which falls into approximately 3- to 4-hour intervals. After the second month, the night feeding usually may be discontinued. By the end of the fourth or fifth month, the infant sleeps through the night and will no longer require a feeding around 10 P.M.

Adequacy of feeding. About 2.5 ounces of human milk per pound of body weight result in satisfactory weight gain. The baby is getting enough milk if he is satisfied at the end of a 15- to 20-minute feeding, if he falls asleep promptly and sleeps quietly for several hours thereafter, and if he makes satisfactory gains from week to week. The infant should be weighed once a week in the same amount of clothing each time.

Insufficient milk intake is indicated when the infant is not satisfied at the completion of the feeding, when he is restless and fails to fall asleep quickly after nursing, when he awakens frequently if he does go to sleep, and when his gains are not satisfactory. In such cases, the physician may advise adding a supplementary food, or replacing one or more of the breast feedings with bottle feedings.

Even human milk is low in some nutrients required by the growing baby so that it is necessary to supplement the diet of the breast-fed infant according to the routine suggested on page 252.

Weaning the baby. As a rule, weaning is started during the fifth to the ninth month by substituting a cup feeding for the breast at any convenient interval. When the baby has become accustomed to this—after about 4 to 5 days—the second cup feeding is offered, and so continued in this way until the baby is entirely weaned. Weaning usually requires a period of 2 to 3 weeks. The transfer from breast to cup should be gradual.

If breast feeding must be terminated at an earlier age, it is usually necessary to substitute bottle feeding, and subsequently to proceed with weaning to the cup. Breast feeding after 9 months has no special advantages for the infant, and may lead to serious depletion of the mother.

FORMULA FEEDING

Comparison of human and cow's milk. The most widely used substitute for human milk is properly modified cow's milk. Goat's milk is used in some countries for infant feeding, and occasionally in this country when the infant is allergic to cow's milk. Milk of other mammals such as the water buffalo, llama, camel, and sheep is used in countries where such milk is available. The table below gives a comparison of human and cow's milk.

NUTRIENT VALUES FOR HUMAN AND COW'S MILK
(Values for Each 100 Grams) *

	HUMAN	COW'S		HUMAN	COW'S
Total protein, gm	1.2	3.3	Vitamin A, mcg	54	37
Fat, gm	3.8	3.8	Carotenoids, mcg	32	39
Carbohydrate, gm	7.0	4.8	Thiamine, mcg	15	42
Energy, calories	71	69	Riboflavin, mcg	47	158
Calcium, mg	34	126	Niacin, mcg	172	85
Phosphorus, mg	16	99	Ascorbic acid, mg	4.4	1.8
Iron, mg	0.21	0.13			

* *The Composition of Milks,* Publication 254, revised 1953, National Research Council, Washington, D.C.

About half of the protein in human milk is in the form of lactalbumin, which can be quickly digested, whereas only about one-fifth of the protein of cow's milk is in this form. Human milk forms fine flocculent curds, while cow's milk forms larger, tougher curds.

The full-term infant utilizes well the fat from both cow's milk and human milk. Cow's milk, however, contains a larger proportion of the volatile, short-chain fatty acids (such as butyric acid), which are somewhat more irritating than the long-chain fatty acids (such as oleic acid) found in human milk.

Human milk contains about 50 per cent more lactose than cow's milk. Both milks provide approximately 20 calories per ounce. The concentrations of calcium and phosphorus in human milk are much lower than those of cow's milk. The two milks vary widely in their vitamin content. Neither milk contains adequate levels of iron and vitamin D for the infant's needs of the first year.

Nutritional requirements. The Food and Nutrition Board has recognized that human milk is the best food for infants, and will meet the nutritive requirements early in life. Recommended allowances, summarized in the following table, have been stated in terms of nutrients provided by cow's milk and by supplements beginning with the second month of life.

RECOMMENDED ALLOWANCES FOR NORMAL INFANTS DURING THE FIRST YEAR *

NUTRIENT	2 to 6 MONTHS PER POUND BODY WEIGHT	7 to 12 MONTHS PER POUND BODY WEIGHT	HOW THE REQUIREMENT IS MET
Calories	55	45	Chiefly milk, 1½–2 oz per pound; sugar in formula; supplements in increasing amounts
Protein	1.6 gm	1.4 gm	Chiefly milk; egg yolk; meat; cereal
	Total daily need	*Total daily need*	
Calcium	600 mg	800 mg	Milk
Iron	5 mg	7 mg	Egg yolk, meat, fruits and vegetables
Vitamin A	1500 I.U.	1500 I.U.	Whole milk, fish-liver oil
Vitamin D	400 I.U.	400 I.U.	Fish-liver oil or concentrate
Thiamine	0.4 mg	0.5 mg	Milk, egg yolk, enriched cereals, fruit, meat, vegetables
Riboflavin	0.5 mg	0.8 mg	
Niacin	6 mg	7 mg	
Ascorbic acid	30 mg	30 mg	Orange or tomato juice; ascorbic acid supplement

* *Recommended Dietary Allowances—Revised 1958,* Food and Nutrition Board, National Research Council, Washington, D.C., 1958, p. 18.

Energy. The caloric requirement of the infant is high in terms of his body weight because the proportionately larger skin surface leads to large heat loss, the rapid rate of growth represents a considerable storage of energy, and the activity of the infant is great. Since the activity of the infant varies even more widely than that of the adult, the stated allowances can serve only as an approximation. Some infants who are relatively inactive might show excessive weight gains if they received the recommended energy allowances, while others who are very energetic might require more calories than the levels recommended. The healthy baby, given an appropriate formula without having it forced upon him, regulates his appetite according to his needs surprisingly well.

Protein. An allowance of 3.0 to 3.5 gm protein per kg body weight represents a level three times as high as that of the adult, and is considerably greater than that provided by human milk. Such a level provides a generous intake of all the essential amino acids, and no amino acid supplementation—for example, lysine—is necessary.[84]

Fat. Whole cow's milk contains satisfactory levels of the essential fatty acids, linoleic acid and arachidonic acid, required by the infant. Low-fat milks used for a short period of time present no problem since the infant has generous reserves of the essential fatty acids. When low-fat milks are used for a prolonged period of time, or when milk substitutes are used because of allergy, consideration must be given to the inclusion of the essential fatty acids.[85] Vegetable oils such as corn, soybean, and cottonseed oils are good sources.

Water. The daily fluid needs of the infant are approximately 2.5 ounces per pound of body weight. The water balance is more easily disturbed than that of the adult because of the large fluid losses through the skin and respiration, and because of the needs for elimination.

Minerals and vitamins. When compared with the needs of adults, all minerals and vitamins are required in proportionately greater amounts by the infant. During the first 4 months the liberal stores of iron of the healthy infant suffice for the rapidly expanding blood circulation, but thereafter special emphasis must be placed on the inclusion of iron-rich foods lest anemia result.

The dangers of toxicity of vitamins A and D must be kept in mind. Usually the concentrates prescribed are rich sources of both vitamins. The adverse effects of vitamin A are noted when very large amounts are ingested over a prolonged period of time (see p. 121), but the safe margin of intake for vitamin D is apparently narrower than was once stated. The vitamin-D needs are met with a daily intake of 400 I.U., and levels of 1500–1800 I.U. may depress growth.[86] The importance of regulation of the dosage of concentrates can scarcely be overemphasized.

Planning the formula. The type of milk, amount of milk, kind and amount of carbohydrate, and the fluid requirement must be considered in planning the formula.

Types of milk. The milk selected should be one which is suited to the infant's needs, is readily available, is inexpensive, and is safe. Fresh pasteurized, evaporated, and dried cow's milks are all used frequently. The milk is modified by dilution, homogenization, heating, or acidulation to produce a finer, smoother curd which is more readily digested by the infant.

Evaporated milk is used for a large proportion of all infant formulas because it is inexpensive, readily available, and stored without refrigeration until the can is opened. It contains fat in a finely divided form, produces a fine, soft curd, and is fortified with 400 I.U. vitamin D per tall can.

Plain or homogenized fresh milk may be used. The latter has a more finely divided fat and forms softer curds than plain milk.

Dried milk may be obtained as whole, skim, or protein milk. It does not require refrigeration, but once the can has been opened the milk powder should be kept in a cool place in a container with a tight lid. By correct dilution the milk may approximate fresh liquid milk, or it may be prepared in a more concentrated form.

Acid-milk formulas prepared from fresh or evaporated milk are occasionally prescribed. Certain advantages are claimed for these formulas: (a) the curd formed is fine and smooth; (b) less dilution is required so that infants with a small capacity may be more readily nourished; (c) the tendency to vomit is reduced; (d) the acid counteracts the neutralizing effect of cow's milk, and calcium and iron may be more completely absorbed.

Numerous commercial milk products and milk substitutes have been developed to meet particular needs of an infant. For example, dried milk may be reduced in its fat content and increased in its protein content. Infants who are allergic to milk may be nourished satisfactorily with formulas prepared from protein hydrolysates, soybeans, and meat bases. The vegetable-protein mixtures initiated in Central America [18] provide another approach for the feeding of infants with milk allergies.

Amount of milk. About 1.5 to 2 ounces of fresh whole milk per pound of body weight is suitable for the healthy infant.

Sugar. Most of the day's caloric needs are met by milk. Since cow's milk is diluted, sugar is added to complete the caloric requirement. Sucrose and corn sirup are inexpensive, easily digested, and lend themselves readily to formula preparation, although they possess the slight disadvantage of sweetness. Lactose, the sugar of milk, is expensive and is seldom used in infant feeding. Dextrinized products such as Dextri-maltose are less sweet and are sometimes prescribed.

During the first 2 weeks the amount of sugar added may be ½ ounce; thereafter, 1 ounce is sufficient until the sixth or seventh month when sugar is eliminated from the formula. As other foods are added to the diet, the sugar in the formula may be reduced or discontinued.

Liquid. A baby will usually take 2 or 3 ounces more of fluid in a single feeding than his age in months. More than 7 ounces at one feeding is usually undesirable before the infant is 7 months old. Feedings larger than 8 ounces are not needed after 6 months since the infant will be taking other foods as well. The total fluid requirement of the infant is met by offering water between feedings, and by the fruit juices.

Intervals of feeding. As with breast feeding, the number of feedings and the amount taken at each feeding should be flexible. Formula-fed infants should not, as a rule, be fed at less than 3-hour intervals since cow's milk remains for a longer time in the stomach than breast milk.

Calculation of the formula. An example of the calculation of a formula is given below.

Infant, 5 months old, weighs 14 pounds
Number of feedings . . . . 5 (assuming approximately 4-hour intervals)
Size of feedings: age in months plus 2 . . . . 5 + 2 = 7 ounces
Daily total: 5 × 7 ounces = 35 ounces
Whole milk: 14 × 1.75 ounces = 24.5 ounces

Water: $35 - 24.5 = 10.5$ ounces
Sugar: 1 ounce

This formula provides 490 calories from milk and 120 calories from sugar, or a daily intake of about 44 calories per pound of body weight. Food supplements given at this age will further increase the caloric intake. The formula contains 24.5 gm protein or about 1.7 gm protein per pound of body weight.

Technique of feeding. The feeding should always be given at body temperature. Remove the bottle from the refrigerator, and stand it in a deep saucepan full of warm water. Heat the water rapidly, and shake the bottle several times to assure that the mixture is uniformly heated. It takes only a few minutes to reach the desired temperature of 100° F. To test the temperature of the milk, invert the bottle and allow a few drops of formula to fall on the inner surface of the forearm; it is the correct temperature when the heat is barely felt.

The mother or other individual feeding the baby should sit in a comfortable chair, and should hold the infant in a semireclining position. In this way the infant is given the sense of security and love which is so important. The baby should not be propped up with his bottle.

The hole in the nipple should not be too large since the rapid taking of the formula together with the swallowing of much air will cause discomfort and perhaps regurgitation. On the other hand, a very small hole in the nipple will necessitate too long a period of feeding; a not overstrong baby may become exhausted before obtaining enough food.

The baby should not be forced to empty the bottle at each feeding. Any formula remaining in the bottle must be discarded.

If the nipple is filled with fluid, and not air, during the feeding, less air will be swallowed. Even so, it is necessary that the baby be allowed to belch. He should be held over the shoulder, or allowed to sit upright on one's lap, and patted gently on the back. This "bubbling" should be done midway and at the end of each feeding—more frequently during the early part of the feeding, if necessary.

FORMULAS FOR THE PREMATURE INFANT

Nutritive requirements. The premature infant is born with poorly developed muscle tissues, very little body fat, low stores of iron, and an inadequately mineralized skeleton. Regulation of the body temperature is difficult because of the very high surface area and the incomplete development of the sweat glands. The digestive ability is limited since the stomach can hold little food at the time, and the digestive enzymes are not sufficiently developed for satisfactory digestion and absorption of fat.

Very small infants are unable to suck, while somewhat larger infants may be overfatigued if sucking is prolonged. Feeding by medicine dropper or by gavage may be necessary.

The first need is for fluid, and in most instances, with a graduated program, the baby will be receiving his full nutritive requirements by the end of the first week to 10 days. The following allowances have been recommended for some of the nutrients:

> Calories: 55 to 60 per pound
> Protein: 2.0 to 2.7 gm per pound [87]
> Vitamin A: 2500 I.U.
> Vitamin D: 400 I.U.
> Ascorbic acid: 30–50 mg

Intervals of feeding. Since very small babies can take only limited amounts of fluid, they are preferably fed at 2-hour intervals for the first few days; thereafter, 3-hour intervals may be used.

Choice of formula. Human milk, evaporated milk, or partially skimmed milk formulas are used. Human milk, however, contains insufficient protein, calcium, and phosphorus for the rate of growth required of the premature infant; it may be fortified by using skimmed cow's milk. Under careful supervision, better gains are obtained with mixtures of partially skimmed cow's milk or evaporated milk because of the somewhat greater protein and mineral content. Feeding mixtures which may be employed are illustrated in the following table.

FEEDING MIXTURES DESIGNED TO GIVE 120 CALORIES PER KILOGRAM
(55 Calories per Pound) *

	PER KILOGRAM	PER POUND	GRAMS/KILOGRAM			PERCENTAGE OF TOTAL CALORIES		
			PROTEIN	FAT	CARBO-HYDRATE	PROTEIN	FAT	CARBO-HYDRATE
Human milk	180 ml	2½ oz	2.2	6.7	12.9	7	50	43
Evaporated milk	70 ml	1 oz	4.8	5.5	12.9	16	41	43
Carbohydrate	6 gm	3 gm						
Water to make	150 ml	2¼ oz						
Half-skim milk powder	18 gm	1 tbsp	6.0	2.2	19.4	20	16	64
Carbohydrate	11 gm	5 gm						
Water to make	150 ml	2¼ oz						

* Gordon, H. H., et al.: "Feeding of Premature Infants. A Comparison of Human and Cow's Milk," *Am. J. Dis. Child.*, 73:442, 1947.

Amount of feeding. The first feedings for the small infant should be only ½ teaspoonful at a time, with slightly larger amounts for larger babies. When it is clearly evident that the infant can tolerate the initial amount given, the feedings are increased by ½ to 1 teaspoonful. It is advisable to make increases at every other feeding rather than at every feeding.

Suggested daily program. *First 12 hours:* Nothing by mouth.

Second 12 hours: A 5 per cent solution of glucose or lactose is given at 2- to 3-hour intervals, beginning with ½-teaspoonful amounts, and increasing the feedings by ½ teaspoonful at alternate feedings.

Third 12 hours: One of the formulas listed in the table on page 249 is prepared and diluted with an equal amount of 5 per cent glucose solution. One-half-teaspoonful amounts of the diluted formula are given at the first feeding. This is alternated with the glucose solution throughout the next 12 hours. The amount of formula is increased at alternate intervals.

Fourth 12 hours: Feedings of the formula are now given every 2 to 3 hours, the amount being increased at alternate intervals as tolerated.

Third day and thereafter: By the fourth or fifth day most babies can take the formula in the full concentration outlined above, and by the end of a week to 10 days they can take the fully prescribed amounts of formula to meet their nutritive needs. One should not increase both the concentration and volume at any single feeding. The formula must be adjusted every few days to correspond to the baby's weight.

Ascorbic acid in gradually increasing amounts up to 50 mg is given by the end of the second or third week. Orange juice is not given until the baby is several weeks to 1 or 2 months old.

The infant should receive 400 I.U. of vitamin D daily by the end of the second or third week, preferably as a water-soluble preparation.

PREPARATION OF THE FORMULA

Equipment needed. The usual equipment includes:

Bottles, 8 oz graduated, of heat-resistant glass; wide-mouth bottles are easier to clean; provide one for each feeding plus 2 or 3 extra for water and orange juice
Nipples, one for each feeding, plus extra for orange juice and water
Bottle caps, glass, metal, plastic, or paper
Bottle sterilizer or large kettle with wire rack to hold bottles
Saucepan or pitcher with pouring lip, 2–3 quart size, for mixing formula
Standard measuring cup with pouring lip, graduated in ounces
Standard measuring spoons
Long-handled spoon
Funnel
Bottle brush with stiff bristles and long handle
Tongs are convenient
Jar for used nipples

Fine strainer
Can opener if evaporated milk is used

Care of equipment. Before starting to make the formula the hands should be scrubbed thoroughly and the work area should be scrupulously clean. Persons with a skin disease should not be permitted to prepare feedings.

Immediately after each feeding rinse the bottle and nipple with cold water. Fill the bottle with cold water and allow to stand. Scrub all bottles at one time with detergent and water, using a long-handled brush which will reach into the corners of the bottles. Rinse bottles thoroughly in warm water. Scrub nipples inside and out with water and rinse. Test each nipple to be sure that the hole has not become plugged.

Terminal sterilization. Measure the required amount of sugar, leveling off the spoon with a knife, and put into a large pitcher or saucepan. Add measured amounts of milk and water and mix well. Pour formula into bottles according to the amount required for each feeding. Put nipples on bottles and test the flow of milk. Cover loosely with nipple covers.

Place bottles on rack in sterilizer. Include one or two extra bottles of drinking water. Pour water into the sterilizer until water comes halfway up on the bottles.

Cover the sterilizer. Bring water to a boil and continue boiling gently for 15 minutes. Remove sterilizer from heat and let stand until bottles are cool enough to handle. Press nipple covers down firmly. Cool bottles to room temperature and then place in the refrigerator.

Standard clean technique. Place clean bottles upside down in the wire rack. Lower rack into pot containing 2 inches of water. Place nipples in jar with metal top in which holes have been punched. Place bottle caps, nipples, funnel, and strainer in sterilizer with the bottles. Cover the pot and allow to boil for 3 to 5 minutes after steam begins to escape in appreciable amounts.

Mixing the formula. Into the saucepan measure the required amount of sugar with a tablespoon, leveling off the top with a knife. Measure the specified amount of water with a measuring cup and add to the sugar. Allow a little extra water to take care of the loss in evaporation—usually ½ to 1 ounce. Invert the milk bottle several times to ensure uniform mixture, and hold it under running water before removing the cap. After wiping the cap, add the amount of milk specified in the formula prescription to the water and sugar. Mix well and boil for 3 minutes, stirring constantly. Allow to cool for a few minutes, stirring from time to time to keep scum from forming.

Filling the bottles. Lift the sterilized bottles from the pot without touching the mouth of the bottle. Insert the funnel into the neck of the bottle, and put the strainer in place over the funnel. Pour the exact amount of milk required for each feeding into the hot bottles. Place a nipple on each bottle, being careful not to touch the part which goes into the baby's mouth. Cover nipple with metal or glass cap. Cool the bottles rapidly under running water, using care to avoid contamination of nipples with the water. Store in the refrigerator until needed.

Evaporated-milk formula. Evaporated milk may be substituted for fresh cow's milk if properly diluted. For example, if the formula calls for 20 ounces of fresh cow's milk and 10 ounces of water, one would use 10 ounces of evaporated milk and 20 ounces of water. Before the can of milk is opened, the top should be scrubbed with soapy water and rinsed well with hot water. The procedure for preparation of the formula is the same as that for fresh-milk formulas.

Dried-milk formulas. If a dried-milk product is used, measure the required amount of water into a saucepan. Then measure the dried milk with a dry tablespoon, leveling each spoonful with a knife. Sprinkle the dry powder on the surface of the water and beat thoroughly with the egg beater until well mixed. Add sugar, mix well, and then proceed as for fresh-milk formulas, using either terminal sterilization or clean technique.

Acid-milk formulas. The use of lactic acid or lactic acid-producing bacteria to acidify milk produces a milk having a fine curd. Lactic acid is diluted by adding 6 ml of 85 per cent U.S.P. lactic acid to 1 ounce of boiled water. The diluted solution is poured slowly with constant stirring into 1 quart milk which has been boiled and cooled. The necessary amount of sugar is then mixed with the acid milk. No further heating or dilution is necessary. There are several brands of dried acid milk on the market which may be substituted for the acid milk prepared at home.

SUPPLEMENTARY FOODS DURING THE FIRST YEAR

From the second week of life it is necessary to supplement both breast and formula feedings so that the optimum level of nutrients may be obtained throughout the first year of growth. The infant also learns to take liquid, then semiliquid, and finally semisolid and solid foods.

Introduction of new foods. A number of practical suggestions are offered for the introduction of new foods.

1. Introduce only one new food at a time. Allow the infant to become familiar with that food before trying to give another.

2. Give very small amounts of any new food—teaspoonfuls or even less—at the beginning.

3. Use a very thin consistency when starting solid foods. Gradually the consistency is made more solid as the infant learns how to use his tongue in propelling the food back. A small spoon is put into the baby's mouth so that the food is placed on the middle of the tongue and swallowing is more readily accomplished. The fact that a baby spits out his first feedings of

solid food may indicate that he hasn't yet learned the tongue movements rather than that he doesn't like the food.

4. Never force an infant to eat more of a food than he takes willingly.

5. If, after several trials, it is apparent that a baby has an acute dislike for a food, omit that item for a week or two and then try it again. If the dislike persists it is better to forget about that food for a while and substitute another.

6. Food should be slightly seasoned with salt. Other seasonings are avoided.

7. Use foods of smooth consistency at first—strained fruits, vegetables, and meats.

8. When the baby is able to chew, gradually substitute finely chopped fruits and vegetables for puréed foods—usually at 8 to 9 months.

9. Infants may object to taking some foods by themselves but will take them willingly if they are mixed with another food. For example, egg may be mixed with formula, cereal, or vegetable; again, vegetables may sometimes be made into a soup with a little milk until the baby becomes accustomed to the new flavor.

10. Variety in choice of foods is important. The baby, like older persons, may tire of the repetition of certain foods, especially cereals and vegetables.

11. The mother or anyone feeding the infant must be careful to avoid showing in any way a dislike for a food which is being given.

Sequence of additions. No uniformity of opinion exists concerning the time and sequence at which supplements are added. Some pediatricians introduce cereals, egg yolk, strained meats, fruits, and vegetables very early. In many infants the swallowing reflex is not fully established until the third or fourth month, and too early feeding, especially if forced, could lead to resistance and rebellion later on. The outline on page 254 for feeding during the first year is typical of many.

Vitamins. Cod-liver oil, concentrated fish oils such as percomorph or haliver oil, or water-miscible preparations of vitamin D are started during the second or third week of life. A teaspoonful of one preparation may be required to provide the necessary amount of vitamin D, while only a few drops of a concentrate may suffice. Since vitamin D and the vitamin A also present in most preparations are both toxic, great care must be taken to see that the exact dosages prescribed are used.

Supplements for ascorbic acid are usually begun during the second or third week of life. One teaspoonful of strained orange juice (fresh, canned, or frozen) is diluted with an equal amount of boiled water and given at first. The amount is gradually increased until the baby is taking 3 ounces of juice a day by the age of 3 months. Grapefruit or tomato juice may be used, but the latter must be given in twice as great amounts to provide equivalent vitamin C. The mother must be cautioned not to boil the juices.

SUGGESTED OUTLINE FOR FEEDING NORMAL BABIES DURING THE FIRST YEAR *

HOUR	FOOD	1–2 WEEKS	1 MONTH	2 MONTHS	3 MONTHS	4 MONTHS
6 A.M.	Formula †	2½–3 oz	3–4 oz	4–5 oz	5–6 oz	6 oz
8 A.M.	Orange juice ‡ Cod-liver oil §	1–2 tsp ¼ tsp	1 oz ½ tsp	3 oz ¾ tsp	3 oz 1 tsp	3 oz 1 tsp
10 A.M.	Formula Cereal	2½–3 oz	3–4 oz	4–5 oz	5–6 oz ¼–2 tbsp	6 oz 1–2 tbsp
2 P.M.	Formula Egg yolk	2½–3 oz	3–4 oz	4–5 oz	5–6 oz	6 oz ¼–2 tsp
6 P.M.	Formula Cereal	2½–3 oz	3–4 oz	4–5 oz	5–6 oz	6 oz 1–2 tbsp
10 P.M.	Formula	2½–3 oz	3–4 oz	4–5 oz	5–6 oz	6 oz
2 A.M.	Formula	2½–3 oz	3–4 oz	4–5 oz	Discontinued	

HOUR	FOOD	5 MONTHS	6 MONTHS	7–9 MONTHS	10–12 MONTHS
6 A.M.	Formula †	6–7 oz	7–8 oz	8 oz	6 A.M. Orange juice, 3 oz
8 A.M.	Orange juice ‡ Cod-liver oil §	3 oz 1 tsp	3 oz 1 tsp	3 oz 1 tsp	Zwieback, ½ piece
					Breakfast, 7:30 A.M.
10 A.M.	Formula Cereal	6–7 oz 2–3 tbsp	7–8 oz 2–4 tbsp	8 oz 2–4 tbsp	Cereal, 2–5 tbsp Milk, 8 oz Chopped fruit,
2 P.M.	Formula Egg yolk Meat Vegetable Potato	6–7 oz ½–1 yolk ¼–2 tbsp	7–8 oz 1 yolk 2–3 tbsp	8 oz 1 yolk *or* ½–2 tbsp 2–4 tbsp ½–2 tbsp	1–2 tbsp Cod-liver oil, 1 tsp Dinner, 11:30–12 Meat, ½–1 oz, *or* Egg, 1 whole
6 P.M.	Formula Cereal Fruit Zwieback	6–7 oz 2–3 tbsp	7–8 oz 2–4 tbsp ¼–2 tbsp	8 oz 2–4 tbsp 2–4 tbsp ½ piece	Potato, 2–4 tbsp Chopped vege- table, 2–4 tbsp Milk, 8 oz
10 P.M.	Formula	6–7 oz	Discontinued		Supper, 5:30 P.M. Cereal or potato, 2–5 tbsp Milk, 8 oz Chopped fruit, 1–2 tbsp Toast or zwieback

* The feeding intervals, amounts of food, and age at which supplements are given are subject to individual variation.

† Formula or breast feeding; plain milk after 7 to 9 months.

‡ Tomato juice may be used in double these quantities.

§ Percomorph oil or other concentrate may be substituted, the number of drops being prescribed by the physician.

Some pediatricians give 25 mg ascorbic acid in $\frac{1}{2}$ ounce of water from the first week of life, and defer the giving of orange juice until about 1 month of age or later.

Cereal foods. Cereals are often the first semisolid foods given to the baby, at approximately 2 to 4 months. Specially formulated dry infant cereal foods possess the distinct advantage of enrichment with iron, thus bolstering the iron intake when body reserves have reached a low point. These cereal foods are mixed with a portion of the warm formula to the desired consistency.

Cooked cereals given to the rest of the family may also be used for the baby if they have been thoroughly cooked, are well strained, and are diluted with part of the formula. Cooking directions appear on the containers in which the cereal is purchased.

Crisp toast, zwieback, and graham crackers may be given when the teeth begin to appear, about 5 to 8 months.

Egg yolk. The rich source of iron and of B-complex vitamins, as well as vitamin A, are reasons favoring the introduction of egg yolk at the third to the fifth month. Hard-cooked egg yolk (see p. 687 for method of preparation) may be mashed with a fork and mixed with part of the formula, cereal, or vegetable. Only $\frac{1}{4}$-teaspoonful amounts should be given initially since some infants may be allergic to the egg protein. Soft custard is also a suitable way in which to introduce the egg yolk. Egg white, which leads to allergic manifestations more frequently, is not given until the infant is 8 to 10 months old, and then is introduced very cautiously.

Fruits. Ripe banana and strained orange or grapefruit juice are the only raw fruits permitted during the first year. Cooked or canned prunes, pears, applesauce, peaches, and apricots are the fruits with which an infant first becomes acquainted, usually by the third to fourth month. These fruits are strained for the first few months they are offered, but they may be chopped by the end of the first year. Most babies accept fruits very well.

Vegetables. Strained carrots, green beans, spinach, squash, peas, asparagus, and tomatoes are all suitable for the infant from the fourth month or earlier. They are conveniently purchased in small cans, or the vegetables may be cooked at home until very soft, lightly seasoned with salt, and pressed through a sieve. (See vegetable preparation, p. 704.) The first feeding of less than 1 teaspoon is gradually increased to 3–4 tablespoons daily by the end of the year. Chopped vegetables are substituted for strained vegetables at 10 to 12 months. Baked or mashed potato may be included occasionally by the seventh month.

Meats. Canned strained baby meats may be used as early as the second month, although they are more usually introduced at the fifth to the seventh month. When the baby is accustomed to strained meats and meat soups, he may be given ground meat including beef, lamb, lean pork, thoroughly boned fish, chicken, and liver. The baby who is teething often enjoys a piece of crisp bacon.

Other foods. In some areas such as the Southwest, a variety of beans are widely used. They are a good source of protein, iron, and B-complex vitamins, and may be cooked and sieved for the infant. The infant may be given simple puddings toward the end of the first year. It is desirable that the amounts of sugar used in the preparation of fruits and puddings be kept small so that the infant does not develop a special craving for sweets.

ESTABLISHMENT OF GOOD FOOD HABITS

Most of the feeding problems of children begin during the first few months or years of life. Spock [88] calls attention to one of the early problems, namely, the loss of appetite and even refusal of food, as being traceable to overfeeding by the overanxious mother who has been sent home from the hospital with a formula a little too large. When the baby takes enough of the formula to satisfy him he promptly goes to sleep; the mother looks with alarm at the amount left in the bottle and, fearing the baby has not taken enough, proceeds to waken him. Although he cries in protest, she slips the nipple into his mouth and stirs it vigorously in an attempt to get him to suck. Spock says that the rapidly increasing appetite at this time helps the baby to catch up with his formula before the mother has taken away his appetite entirely. If the mother is instructed in the proper care and handling of the feeding as well as other problems of infancy during her stay in the hospital, it is possible that many objectionable situations may be avoided.

Toward the end of the first year and during the second year the baby will show a marked drop in appetite. He starts to refuse foods he formerly liked, and he may eat much less than he did. This is occasioned in part by the growing individuality and the negativistic attitude which appear at this age; it is also explained by the slower growth rate at the end of the first year and during the next few years. If the mother would have the baby retain good food habits, she will permit the baby to adjust the amounts of food he will take. It may be necessary to omit certain formerly liked items of food for a while or to serve them in an entirely new manner.

One of the most harmful practices is that of trying to make the feeding pattern of a baby and his physical development correspond exactly to a textbook description or to match or surpass the accomplishments of a neighbor's child. Each baby is an individual; some learn slowly and others rapidly; some are more active than others, and so on. The fact that one baby may eat vegetables well at 4 months of age is no indication that another baby will not make equal progress even though he learns to eat vegetables in only small amounts at 6 to 7 months! Likewise, some babies will happily adjust from bottle to cup at 9 months while others may not do so until they are almost a year old. Parents and others who are responsible for the feeding of children should remember this individuality and the need for flexibility concerning the intervals of feeding, the amounts of food that may be taken, the age at which new foods are given, and the response which may be expected.

The attitude of the parents has much to do with the establishment of good eating habits. Learning to eat food that is different in texture and flavor, trying to hold a cup and bring it to the mouth without spilling, or putting food onto a spoon and eating it are new and interesting experiences for the baby. He may wish to handle the food to see what it feels like, or he may prefer to use his fingers in eating. Then again, he may delight in throwing the food about him or onto the floor. The mother must be very patient at these times lest she be tempted to say "Don't do that!" and thus create antagonisms in the child. Equally harmful is the overattentive attitude in which the mother or other bystander laughs at the "cute" tricks of the baby, thus encouraging repetition of the action. The best way to overcome an undesirable practice before it becomes habit is to ignore, by look, word, or deed, such action on the part of the child. Approval, given at the right time, will quickly teach a baby to repeat favorable behavior.

Learning to like new foods may depend on the manner in which they are started. (See suggestions on p. 252.) It is best to introduce new foods at the beginning of the feeding when the baby's appetite is still on edge. One cannot overemphasize the importance of gradually accustoming the baby to new tastes with no attempt at using force or bribery. The parent must avoid showing any concern when a food is not taken but should be ready to praise when a new food has been taken well. The very smooth strained foods should not be continued too long since it may be difficult to adjust the baby to chopped or coarser foods.

Even babies react to the general atmosphere about them. They must be comfortable if they are to enjoy their food. They will eat better if the mother is unhurried, calm, and pleasant but not overtalkative.

PROBLEMS AND REVIEW

1. For what reasons is breast feeding preferred to artificial feeding? Under what circumstances would it be contraindicated?

2. Even though human milk is the ideal food for infants, it does not always provide adequate amounts of ascorbic acid and is especially low in vitamin D. How are the infant's needs for these vitamins met?

3. Weaning should be a gradual transition from the breast to the bottle or cup. When is it usually started? What procedure will ensure satisfactory weaning?

4. Cow's milk is the best substitute for human milk. In what respects does cow's milk differ from human milk?

5. Fresh, evaporated, and dried milks may be used for the preparation of formulas. What advantages may be claimed for each type of milk?

6. Human milk and whole cow's milk both contain about 20 calories per ounce. Why is water added to the cow's milk formula for the young infant? How is the caloric level of 20 calories per ounce maintained?

7. The normal rate of gain during the first half year is 5 to 8 ounces. What explanation may be given for a 4-month-old baby who has shown only 6 ounces gain in 4 weeks?

8. *Problem.* Calculate a formula for an infant 4 months of age who weighs 12 pounds. Describe in detail how you would instruct a mother in the preparation of this formula. What changes would be necessary if you were using evaporated milk? Dried milk? Include directions for terminal sterilization of the formula. Why is this preferred to clean technique?

9. Supplements must be added to the infant's formula at various intervals throughout the first year in order to supply the necessary nutrients and to accustom the infant to a solid diet. What supplementary foods are usually included, and at what age is it advisable to start each? What nutrients are especially important in each of these?

10. What recommendations could you give to a mother who is beginning the use of supplementary foods for her infant so that satisfactory food habits are established?

11. Egg white is customarily omitted from the young infant's diet. Why?

12. *Problem.* Outline the day's diet for an infant of 7 months. Include a calculation of the formula.

13. *Problem.* How do the nutritive requirements of premature infants differ from those born at full term? Describe a feeding program during the first week of life for a premature infant who weighs 3½ pounds.

14. What recommendations could you give for the preparation of a formula when no refrigeration is available?

CHAPTER 19 /

Nutrition of Children and Teenagers

The child's nutritional needs differ in several important respects from those of the adult. The first of these is the rather large requirement for growth, so that practically every food eaten must carry some protein, minerals, and vitamins. Secondly, the activities of children of all ages are proportionately higher so that the daily caloric allowances per unit of body weight must be increased. Thirdly, the selection of foods often requires some modification, especially for young children, in terms of ability to chew and digestibility. Finally, childhood represents a period of rapidly changing attitudes and emotional development when food habits can be most favorably channeled.

Growth and development. The term *growth* refers to an increase in size because of cell multiplication, while the term *development* denotes an increase in the complexity of function. Both growth and development are modified by heredity, diet, and environment—social, economic, housing, and others.

The rate of growth during fetal life and the first year is not equaled at any later time in life. The infant gains 8 to 10 pounds during the second year, thus quadrupling his birth weight. Thereafter, the yearly gains are approximately 4 to 7 pounds up to the preadolescent period. For a year or two before and during adolescence an accelerated rate of growth again takes place. The maximum gain in weight and in height occurs in girls at 11 to 13 years and in boys at 13 to 15 years. Girls are taller and heavier than boys at 11 to 12 years, but thereafter the boys catch up with and exceed the girls. Weight gain is generally more rapid in the fall and early winter, while the greatest gains in height usually occur in the late winter and spring.

The number, size, and composition of the bones change from birth to maturity. The skeleton has usually reached its full size at 17 years in girls, and at 20 years in boys. The water content of the bones gradually diminishes as the mineralization increases. For several years following the attainment of full size, bone mineralization continues, providing that the diet remains good. This helps to ensure bones less liable to injury under physical stress, and is also a distinct advantage to the girl in preparation for motherhood.

Criteria of good nutritional status. A full assessment of the nutritional status of a child can be made only by specialists qualified to give comprehensive physical and dental examinations; to make biochemical studies of the blood and urine; and to evaluate patterns of growth as by the Wetzel grid, measurements of body size, x-rays of the bones, and many others. However, certain physical and behavioral characteristics may be noted by the mother, teacher, or nurse which would indicate that some children should be studied more carefully with respect to the adequacy of their nutrition. The well-nourished child may be expected to exhibit these characteristics:

sense of well-being: alert; interested in activities usual for the age; vigorous; happy
vitality: endurance during activity; quick recovery from fatigue; looks rested; does not fall asleep in school; sleeps well at night
weight: normal for height, age, and body build (see tables pp. 781–84)
posture: erect; arms and legs straight; abdomen pulled in; chest out
teeth: straight, without crowding in well-shaped jaw
skin: smooth, slightly moist; healthy glow; reddish-pink mucous membranes
eyes: clear, bright; no circles of fatigue around them
hair: lustrous; healthy scalp
muscles: well-developed; firm
nervous control: good attention span for his age; gets along well with others; does not cry easily; not irritable and restless

Are children well nourished? Studies on nutritional status were conducted from 1947 to 1958 by more than 200 investigators in 39 states on approximately 4000 children 5 to 12 years old, and an equal number of adolescents 13 to 20 years old.[89] (See Fig. 19-1.) At all ages the nutrient intakes by boys were somewhat better than by girls. Elementary school children more nearly met the recommended allowances than did teenagers. In fact, no segment of the population established as poor a nutrient intake as did the adolescent girl.

Up to the age of 12 years, boys and girls had mean intakes of all nutrients in excess of the recommended allowances,[2] except that the calcium intake was slightly low for the girls. For boys of 13 to 20 years, mean intakes of all nutrients except vitamin C were more than adequate. The mean intakes of girls, 13 years and over, equaled or exceeded the recommended allowances only for vitamin A, riboflavin, and niacin. The intakes of calcium, ascorbic acid, and thiamine were seriously inadequate, while the intake of protein was moderately low. Regional differences and the effects of income were noted in the studies. The investigators emphasized that intakes of nutrients below recommended allowances are not necessarily indicative of poor nutritional status in children since it is well recognized that the allowances provide a generous margin of safety for most people.

In terms of health, the over-all nutritional status of the child in the United States may be characterized as good. Children today are taller and heavier than they were 50 years ago. One does not see many obviously malnourished

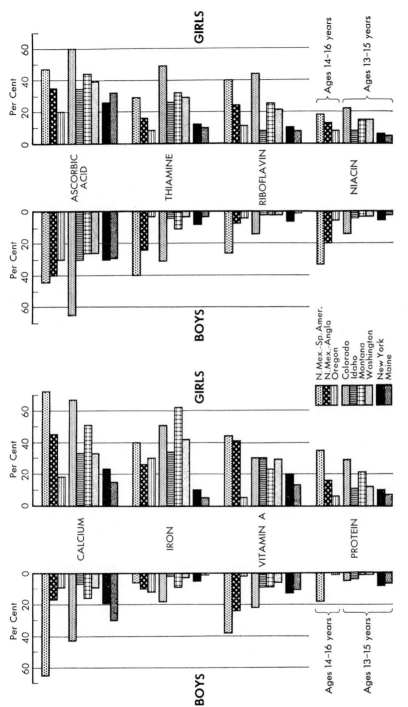

Fig. 19-1. Percentage of boys and girls 13 to 16 years of age in six western and two northeastern states who ate less than two-thirds the recommended amounts of mentioned nutrients. (*Courtesy, California Agricultural Experiment Station.*)

children. Nevertheless, individual children in all communities, for one reason or another, do not have the full benefits of good nutrition. In the cooperative studies cited above, some correlation was found between the dietary intake and blood levels of ascorbic acid and vitamin A, and between the dietary protein and iron, and the blood hemoglobin levels. They also found some skin and eye changes, such as inflammation of the eyes and reddened gums, to be associated with low vitamin-A and -C levels of the blood.

Failure to maintain normal weight is a frequently recurring problem. The cooperative studies indicated that overweight and underweight occurred with equal frequency in boys and girls prior to adolescence. During adolescence, girls were more often overweight and boys were more frequently underweight, the degree of overweight or thinness increasing with age. Studies on overweight girls have shown that the caloric intake, surprisingly, is not as great as that of girls of normal weight; however, the activity of the overweight girls has been less.[90,91]

Dental decay is probably the most prevalent disease in the country, although no agreement has been established concerning the role of heredity and specific dietary and other environmental factors.

Stresses of various kinds may have an adverse effect on nutrition. The incidence of tuberculosis is higher than it should be in the adolescent years and in early adulthood, and is believed to occur more frequently in those who have had inadequate diets, especially with respect to protein and calcium. A large proportion of infants are born to young women who have not yet completed their own body growth and maturation. The stress of pregnancy can have serious effects on the girl who has had a poor intake of protein, calcium, and iron during the preceding years. Johnston [92] has called attention to the frequency with which slipping of the upper femoral epiphysis takes place in rapidly growing adolescent girls.

Common dietary errors. The mean intakes of nutrients by children of all ages do not give any indication of the numbers who receive less than the recommended levels. Ascorbic acid, calcium, iron, and vitamin A are the nutrients which are most frequently provided in less than recommended amounts in the diets of children. These lacks occur with unsatisfactory intakes of milk, fruits (especially those rich in ascorbic acid), and vegetables (especially those which are green leafy or deep yellow). A number of poor dietary habits contribute to these deficiencies:

> *poor breakfasts or none at all:* lack of appetite; getting up too late; no one to prepare breakfast; monotony of breakfast foods; no protein at breakfast, meaning that the distribution of good quality protein is poor even though the day's total may be satisfactory; too little fruit, meaning that ascorbic acid often is not obtained

poor lunches: failure to participate in school lunch program; poor box lunches; spending lunch money for snacks or other items; unsatisfactory management of school lunch program with resultant poor menus, poor food preparation, excessive plate waste

snacks: account for as much as ¼ of calories without providing significant amounts of protein, minerals, and vitamins; often eaten too near to mealtime thus spoiling the appetite

overuse of milk, especially by younger children: other foods are not eaten so that the intake of iron and certain vitamins may be low

self-imposed dieting, especially by teen-age girls: caloric restriction but no consideration given to protein, minerals, and vitamins

irregular eating habits: few meals with the family group; no adult supervision in eating; children often prepare own meals without guidance

NUTRITIONAL REQUIREMENTS

The recommended allowances for children of all ages (p. 26) are proportionately higher than those for adults.

Energy. Body size, age, and activity influence the caloric requirement of the child. The very young child has a high basal metabolic rate incident to intensive cellular activity and to a proportionately high surface area. Year by year the rate of metabolism decreases, then accelerates somewhat during adolescence, after which it again declines to the adult level. The basal metabolism of boys is higher than that of girls owing to the greater muscle mass. Superimposed upon the basal metabolic rate are relatively large requirements for growth and for activity.

The requirements of individual children vary widely, and the recommended allowances can only serve as a guide. The 1- to 3-year-old needs about 1300 calories daily, the 10- to 12-year-old should have 2500 calories which is more than his mother is likely to need, and the 16- to 19-year-old boy requires 3600 calories. Boys engaged in competitive athletics or heavy labor must have considerably more calories if they are to grow satisfactorily. Macy and Hunscher [93] have shown that a deficit of as little as 10 calories per kg body weight resulted in failure to grow and depression of nitrogen retention even though the protein intake had been satisfactory.

Protein. A liberal allowance of protein is desirable throughout childhood in order to provide for increase in muscle mass, for the formation of the matrix of skeletal tissues, and for protection against infection—especially tuberculosis. The total daily protein allowance for children 7 to 12 years, for example, equals that for their parents, while adolescent boys and girls require more. Based on body weight, the allowance decreases from 3.3 gm per kg for the 1- to 3-year-old to 1.4 gm per kg for the teenager. About 12 to 15 per cent of the calories should normally be obtained from protein.

Since the requirement for essential amino acids (see p. 48) is proportionately greater for children than for adults, one-half to two-thirds of the protein should be selected from complete protein foods.

Minerals. From 1 to 9 years the recommended calcium allowance is 1.0 gm; for 10- to 12-year-olds, it is 1.2 gm; for girls and boys 13 years and over, it is 1.3 and 1.4 gm respectively. Stearns [94] has found that the greatest retention of calcium and phosphorus precedes the period of rapid growth by 2 years or more, and that liberal intakes of these minerals before the age of 10 is a distinct advantage. She has also found that children whose diets have been poor require a good diet for as long as 6 months before they can equal the calcium and phosphorus retention of children on a good diet.[95] Such a lag in retention can be a special hazard for the poorly nourished teen-age girl who becomes pregnant.

Adequacy of calcium intake is directly correlated with the intake of milk or milk foods. All nonmilk foods can be expected to yield only 0.2 gm calcium in the diet of young children, and 0.3 gm calcium in the diet of older children.

Iron. The recommended allowances of iron—from 7 to 15 mg, depending upon age—can be satisfied only when consistent emphasis is placed upon the inclusion of enriched or whole-grain cereals and breads, eggs, meats of all kinds, legumes, fruits, and green leafy vegetables. Far too often children of all ages consume minimum amounts of fruits and vegetables, thus leading to suboptimal iron intakes. Milk, which is low in iron, may be consumed in excessive amounts by some children, thus crowding out other essential foods.

Iodine. Throughout childhood, but especially during adolescence, the use of iodized salt should be encouraged because the high energy metabolism increases the activity of the thyroid gland and the corresponding likelihood of simple goiter.

Vitamins. The vitamin requirements of children have not been extensively studied. Throughout childhood and adolescence 400 I.U. vitamin D should be provided—an allowance easily met by using fortified milk or a vitamin-D concentrate. The vitamin A needs are related to body weight, and the allowance increases from 2000 I.U. at 1 to 3 years to 5000 I.U. at 16 to 19 years. Vitamin-D concentrates often contain vitamin A as well. Milk, butter or margarine, egg yolk, green leafy vegetables, and deep yellow fruits and vegetables may be counted upon to supply the need.

The allowance for ascorbic acid ranges from 35 mg for the 1- to 3-year-old to 100 mg for the 16- to 19-year-old boy. The allowances for thiamine and niacin are based on the caloric requirement, namely 0.5 mg and 6.6 mg, respectively, per 1000 calories. Riboflavin allowances are computed on the basis of 0.025 mg per gm protein intake.

DIET FOR THE PRESCHOOL CHILD

Characteristics of food acceptance. The nutritional requirements of the child cannot be satisfied apart from an understanding of behavioral changes which occur. During the second year the appetite tapers off corresponding to the slower rate of growth. Beal [96] found that healthy, well-nourished girls reduced their milk intake as early as 6 months, and returned to higher intakes at 2 to 3 years of age. Boys also reduced their milk intake at about 9 months, but started to increase their consumption between 1 and 2 years. An intake of 2 cups or less is not uncommon for a period of time. Some children's appetites improve by 5 years or earlier, but others have poor appetites well into the school years. Many mothers must be reassured that the child will remain well nourished providing that foods abundant in protein, minerals, and vitamins are offered, and that feeding does not become an issue between mother and child.

Food jags are not uncommon, especially between the ages of 2 and 4 years. The child may shun all but a few foods, such as milk or peanut butter and jelly sandwiches. Such occurrences do not last too long, if the parent does not show concern, and if the foods which constitute the child's preference at the moment are generally speaking nutritious.

The preschool child is almost constantly active. His interest is readily diverted from food. If he becomes overtired or excessively hungry, his appetite may lag a great deal.

Selection of foods. Some compensation for the reduced consumption of milk may be made by incorporating milk into foods such as simple puddings. The occasional use of flavorings such as molasses, cocoa, or the use of vegetable colors may introduce additional interest. Children may sometimes be encouraged to drink milk if they are permitted to pour the milk into a small glass or cup from a small pitcher. Cottage cheese and mild American cheese are often well liked, and help to increase the calcium and protein intake.

The ability of the child to chew should determine the texture of foods which may be given. The toddler may be given chopped vegetables and ground meat, while the 3- to 5-year-old can manage diced vegetables and minced or bite-size pieces of tender meat. Children enjoy chewing some foods such as zwieback, crackers, and strips or wedges of vegetables. Foods which are stringy such as celery, sticky such as some mashed potatoes, or slippery as custard are often disliked because the child is not familiar with the texture.[97]

Preschool children have highly developed senses of taste and smell, and, as a consequence, they prefer mildly flavored foods to those of strong flavor, or those which are spicy. Vegetables as a class of foods are frequently disliked. Most young children enjoy raw vegetables but they are unlikely to consume sufficient amounts because they become fatigued with chewing. Plain foods are generally well liked, but mixtures such as casserole dishes, creamed foods, and stews are not popular.

Fruits are well liked, and may be given raw or cooked, although melons and berries should be used with discretion if at all. Simple desserts such as milk puddings, sherbets, ice cream, plain cakes and cookies may be included.

The gastrointestinal tract of the preschool child is easily irritated by very sweet or rich foods, fried foods, excessive amounts of cellulose, or by foods inadequately chewed such as nuts. Foods of this nature may also displace dietary essentials and it is advisable to omit them in the diet of 1- to 3-year-olds, and to use them seldom for older preschool children.

The table on page 267 lists the average quantities of foods which preschool children may be expected to consume during the day and at individual meals, but healthy children often vary widely from these amounts. They will consume more at some times, but much less at others.

Snacks. Most young children with a limited capacity for food are more likely to obtain all the dietary essentials if they are fed something in the middle of the morning and the afternoon. Moreover, very active children become excessively fatigued and hungry if they are not fed between meals. Snacks should make a liberal contribution to one or more of the nutrient needs. Some which are suitable for preschool children are:

> fruit juices with little or no sugar
> milk and milk beverages
> fruit of any kind; raw vegetables
> small sandwiches; crackers with peanut butter
> molasses, oatmeal, or peanut butter cookies

Food habits. Suggestions have been made in the preceding chapter for the establishment of good food habits in the infant. In addition, the following considerations are conducive to the development of good food habits in the preschool child.

Meals should be served at regular hours in a pleasant environment. The child should be comfortably seated at a table. Deep dishes permit the child to get his food onto the fork or spoon with greater ease. A fork, such as a salad fork with blunt tines, and a small spoon can be handled comfortably. A small cup or glass should be only partially filled with liquid to minimize spilling; however, the coordination of eye, hand, and mouth is difficult and some spilling is to be expected. (See Fig. 19-2.)

Children enjoy colorful meals just as do adults. Their appetites also vary from day to day, and like adults they react strongly to portions which are too large. It is much better to serve less than the child is likely to eat and to let him ask for more.

FOODS THAT WILL MEET NEEDS OF HEALTHY CHILDREN FROM 1 TO 6 *

FOOD	APPROXIMATE QUANTITY NEEDED DAILY	AVERAGE SIZE OF SERVING FOR EACH AGE		
		1 YEAR	2 AND 3 YEARS	4 AND 5 YEARS
Milk, to drink and in or on foods	3 to 4 measuring cups	½ to 1 cup	½ to 1 cup	1 cup
Eggs	1	1	1	1
Meat, poultry, fish, cottage cheese	1 to 4 tablespoon-fuls.†	1 tablespoon-ful	2 to 3 table-spoonfuls	4 tablespoon-fuls
Potatoes, white or sweet	1 serving	2 tablespoon-fuls	3 table-spoonfuls	4 tablespoon-fuls
Other cooked vege-tables (mostly green leafy or deep yellow ones)	1 to 2 servings	2 tablespoon-fuls	3 table-spoonfuls	3 to 4 table-spoonfuls
Raw vegetables (car-rots, cabbage, to-matoes, lettuce, etc.)	1 serving	Small portion (such as, ¼ medium-sized carrot)		
Fruit for vitamin C	1 medium orange or ⅓ cup citrus fruit juice or ⅔ cup tomato juice	⅓ to ½ cup	⅓ to ½ cup	⅓ to ⅔ cup
Other fruit (apples, apricots, bananas, pears, peaches, prunes, most ber-ries, etc.)	1 serving	¼ cup	⅓ cup	½ cup
Bread, whole-grain or enriched	1½ to 3 slices	½ to 1 slice	1 slice	1 to 1½ slices
Cereal, whole-grain, enriched or re-stored	1 serving	¼ cup	⅓ cup	½ cup

Butter or fortified margarine—Spread on bread, and used to season vegetables

Fish-liver oil or vita-min-D concentrate or vitamin-D milk	400 units	(A quart of vitamin-D milk contains 400 units.)		

* Children's Bureau, U.S. Department of Health, Education, and Welfare: "Your Child from One to Six," Publication 30, revised 1956, Washington, D.C.

† One tablespoon means a level tablespoonful. A rounded tablespoonful is equal to 2 level ones.

Even favorite foods should not be served too often. Breakfasts do not need to be stereotyped. A hamburger or sandwich with an orange cut in sections to be picked up with the fingers is just as satisfactory as a juice, cereal, and egg breakfast.

Fewer difficulties are likely to be encountered if new foods are given at the beginning of the meal when the child is hungry. A food is more likely to be accepted if it is given in a form which can be easily handled, which can be chewed, and if some favorite food is also included in the same meal. The parent should assume that the child will also take some responsibility in accepting the offered food.

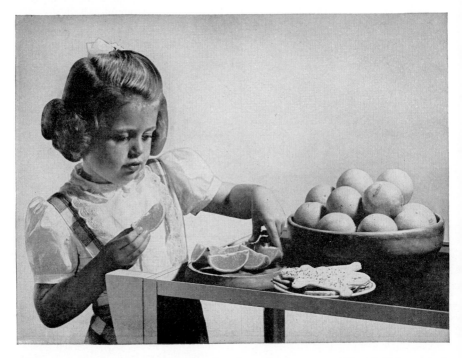

Fig. 19-2. Foods children like, offered as finger foods, can provide valuable nutrients without creating parent-child tensions. (*Courtesy, Sunkist Growers.*)

Whether or not the preschool child should eat with other members of the family or alone is a matter which each mother must determine for the child's greatest good and the family's convenience. If the father returns from work at such an hour that the evening meal must be late, if the child becomes over-excited about the family doings, or if the child is expected to live up to a code of behavior beyond his young years, it is better that he be allowed to eat before the rest of the family in a pleasant, quiet atmosphere with his mother nearby. Even so, an occasional meal with the family may be a treat for the child and parent if tension can be avoided. Since children are great imitators, they enjoy doing just as Daddy or Mother or the other children are doing.

The child may well learn early in life that he is expected to eat foods prepared for him, but this does not mean that nagging or bribery will accomplish anything. Children, like adults, enjoy attention, and they are quick to realize that food can be a powerful weapon for gaining such attention. It is therefore important to recognize that a display of concern or the use of force in getting a child to drink milk or to take any other food, can have nothing but unfavorable effects. When a child refuses to take a food, the unwanted item should be calmly removed without comment after a reasonable period of time. If the child is refusing to eat because he thereby attracts attention, the mother should make certain that the child receives his full share of affection and companionship at other than mealtimes. By so doing the child will lose interest in using food as a weapon.

DIET FOR THE SCHOOL CHILD

Characteristics of food acceptance. Elementary school children are usually better fed than preschool children or adolescents. Group acceptance is extremely important at this time, and the child needs to be able to keep up with his classmates and to have a sense of accomplishment. When the child goes to school for the first time he makes acquaintance with food patterns which may be different from those he knows at home (see Fig. 19-3). He learns that certain foods may be acceptable to the peer group, while other foods from a different cultural pattern may be looked upon with disdain; as a result he may be unwilling to accept these foods at home—good though they may be. On the other hand, within a group he is willing to try foods with which he is unacquainted and which he would not try alone.

School children have relatively few dislikes for food except possibly for vegetables, which are usually not eaten in satisfactory amounts. By the time they reach 8 to 10 years of age the appetite is usually very good. Feeding problems are more likely to result because parents are unduly concerned with behavior at mealtime which does not come up to adult standards. Most children of this age are in a hurry, and don't like to take time for meals. Breakfast, especially, is likely to be skipped.

School children may be subject to many stresses which affect the appetite. Communicable diseases occur often in this age group. They reduce the appetite on the one hand, but they increase body needs on the other. School work, class competition, and emotional stresses in getting along with many children may have adverse effects on appetite, as may also an unbalanced program of activity and rest.

Choice of foods. The table on page 271 lists the kinds and amounts of foods which may be taken in a day by healthy school children. A number of other equally satisfactory patterns could be devised for different cultural groups. A diet for adults which places emphasis first on the inclusion of protein, minerals, and vitamins is also a good one for school children. The amount of milk given to children should be greater than that for the adult. While no foods need to be forbidden to this age group, it is extremely important that high-carbohydrate and high-fat foods not be allowed to replace essential items of the diet.

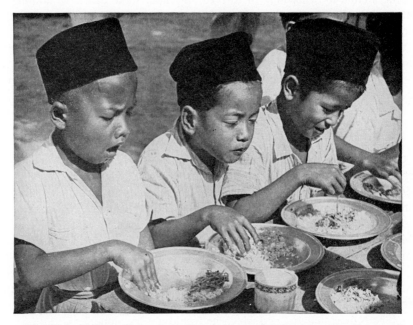

Fig. 19-3. Malaya. These boys like their meal! (*Courtesy, The Food and Agriculture Organization and the Department of Public Relations, Federation of Malaya.*)

Food habits. The suggestions concerning good food habits for preschool children also apply to school children. A good school lunch program (see p. 273) may introduce new foods in a setting where the child is anxious to conform to the group. The elementary teacher may integrate nutrition education with the total classroom experience so that good food habits are strengthened.

Since children are likely to be in a hurry, it is often wise to require that a certain time be spent at the table—say 15 or 20 minutes—so that the child will take time to eat. Children learn good manners by imitation of adults, and not by continuous correction at the table. During the elementary school years, little can be gained by overemphasis on manners. In fact, the food intake may be adversely affected.

FOODS TO MEET NUTRITIONAL NEEDS OF ELEMENTARY SCHOOL CHILDREN AND TEENAGERS

FOOD	6 TO 9 YEARS	10 TO 12 YEARS	13 TO 15 YEARS
Milk	3–4 cups	3–4 cups	4 cups or more
Eggs	1	1	1 or more
Meat, poultry, fish	2–3 ounces (small serving)	3–4 ounces (average serving)	4 ounces or more (large serving)
Dried beans, peas, or peanut butter	2 servings each week. If used as an alternate for meat, allow ½ cup cooked beans or peas or 2 tablespoons peanut butter for 1 ounce meat		
Potatoes, white or sweet (occasionally spaghetti, macaroni, rice, noodles, etc.)	1 small or ⅓ cup	1 medium or ½ cup	1 large or ¾ cup
Other cooked vegetable (green leafy or deep yellow 3 to 4 times a week)	¼ cup	⅓ cup	½ cup or more
Raw vegetable (salad greens, cabbage, celery, carrots, etc.)	¼ cup	⅓ cup	½ cup
Vitamin-C food (citrus fruit, tomato, cantaloupe, etc.)	1 medium orange or equivalent	1 medium orange or equivalent	1 large orange or equivalent
Other fruit	1 portion or more, as: 1 apple, 1 banana, 1 peach, 1 pear, ½ cup cooked fruit		
Bread, enriched or whole-grain	3 slices or more	3 slices or more	4–6 slices or more
Cereal, enriched or whole-grain	½ cup	¾ cup	1 cup or more
Butter or fortified margarine	1–2 tablespoons	2 tablespoons	3–4 tablespoons or more
Vitamin D	400 I.U. at all ages, using: fortified milk, fish-liver oil, or vitamin-D concentrate		
Additional foods	Sweets, desserts, etc. to satisfy energy needs		

DIET FOR THE TEENAGER

Characteristics of diet. Even children who have had excellent dietary patterns are likely to succumb to bizarre, unbalanced habits during adolescent years. The changes in food habits may be ascribed to the growing feeling of independence and the need to assert authority; to the influence of their associates; and to the concern about figure and skin problems or physical fitness.

Milk is often regarded by teenagers as fattening, or as a food for babies but not one appropriate for a social gathering. Tea and coffee may be selected because they represent adult choices. Snacks of all kinds are eaten—ice cream with rich sauces, pastries, candy, soft drinks, popcorn, potato chips, pretzels, hamburgers, pizza, hoagies, and others. In fact, it may seem that the boy or girl at this age eats all day long without regard for mealtimes.

Boys have a better nutrient intake than girls, probably because the volume of food they consume is bound to provide some nutrients in addition to supplying the energy needs. Moreover, their selection often tends to be in terms of sandwiches of some kind, including protein-rich foods. Girls, with much lower caloric requirements, cannot select as many foods from the empty calorie group and still remain reasonably well nourished.

Emotional stress has an adverse effect on the retention of nutrients. This has been borne out when students were taking examinations, and has been observed in young women who were especially upset about a pregnancy.[79,95] Emotional difficulties may stem from the feeling of social inadequacy, or the pressures of school work. The home may likewise be the scene of tension between child and parent, with food choices, acceptance of responsibility, use of money, dating hours, and many other factors as the source of friction.

Selection of foods. The boy and girl 13 years and over will have an excellent diet if meal planning at home and in the school lunch uses the list on page 271 as the starting point. It is no more than good common sense to include favorite foods often. After all, lettuce and tomato, cold cuts, pickles, and buns have the same nutritive value whether served as a cold plate or as a hoagie!

Milk, green leafy and deep yellow vegetables, and citrus fruits are the foods which especially require emphasis. Moderate amounts of sweets, soft drinks, coffee, and tea cannot be considered harmful, providing that they do not replace essential foods in the diet.

Food habits. Good health in general is too abstract an approach to interest the teenager. Most of them have never known anything but good health. Young[98] has suggested a number of approaches which work well with adolescents. Girls can be appealed to on the basis of a better figure, an improved complexion, and glossy hair. Boys are especially interested in physical fitness and the greater ability to compete in athletic contests. They, too, are concerned about complexion problems. Adolescents are more anxious to improve their eating habits when they are reminded that their acceptance of foods makes them a more appreciated dinner guest.

The author of this text has found that boys and girls give a surprisingly good performance when given responsibilities concerning meals at home. When they share in the planning of menus, in the purchase of foods, and in the preparation of meals, they take pride in showing their skills in shopping, or in trying a new recipe. Of course, it is good psychology to share these responsibilities as a privilege of growing up, and not as a burden imposed by the parent! In their fulfillment, with subtle guidance and praise where merited, food habits are often improved.

THE SCHOOL LUNCH PROGRAM

In 1853 the Children's Aid Society of New York opened a vocational school for the poor and served meals to those who attended. School feeding was initiated in some elementary schools in Philadelphia in 1894. After the turn of the century many schools throughout the country provided meals or hot-dish supplements to carried meals.

The school lunch program has experienced rapid growth since the 1930's when surplus commodities were first distributed following the passage of a law in 1935. Today, about 12 million children, or approximately one-third of the elementary and secondary school population, are participating in plate lunches on any given school day while an additional 12 million children have the opportunity to so participate.

National School Lunch Act. In 1946 the National School Lunch Act was enacted to provide participating schools with (1) cash assistance; (2) donation of surplus food commodities; and (3) technical assistance in the purchase and use of foods and in the management and equipment of the school lunch room.

To participate in the national program, a school must operate its own program on a nonprofit basis, must serve nutritious meals meeting standards established by the Department of Agriculture, and must provide lunches at lower cost, or free, to children who cannot afford to purchase them. The United States Department of Agriculture establishes standards and maintains general supervision of the program throughout the country. Within the states the programs are supervised by the departments of education, while in each community the program is administered through the local school officials. On the average, 56 per cent of the cost of the program is provided by the children, 22 per cent by the state, and 22 per cent by the federal government.[99]

Type A lunch. Five components are included in the Type A lunch:

1. Fluid whole milk, ½ pint, served as a beverage
2. Protein-rich food such as: 2 ounces cooked or canned lean meat, fish, poultry; 2 ounces cheese; 1 egg; ½ cup cooked dry beans or peas; 4 tablespoons peanut butter; or an equivalent of any combination of these in a main dish
3. Vegetables and fruits, at least ¾ cup, consisting of 2 or more servings. One serving of full strength juice may be counted as not more than ¼ cup of the requirement
4. Whole-grain or enriched bread, 1 slice; or muffins, corn bread, biscuits, rolls made of enriched or whole-grain flour
5. Butter or fortified margarine, 2 teaspoons, as a spread, as a seasoning, or in food preparation

The Type B lunch is no longer used. When there are no facilities for food preparation, milk may be provided under the program.

Nutritive value of Type A lunch. When foods are served in the amounts specified, and additions are made to satisfy the appetite, the Type A lunch provides, on the average, one-third of the recommended allowances for the 10- to 12-year-old child. Larger portions must be provided for older children. Since the child eats but five meals in the school each week, the contribution represents about one-fourth of his total nutritive needs.

Some care must be taken in the selection of fruits and vegetables. A vitamin C-rich food should be served daily, and a vitamin A-rich food at least twice a week. Well-managed school lunch programs seldom permit sales of soft drinks, candy, pretzels, and similar carbohydrate-rich foods because they contribute little except calories to the child's nutritional needs, and because the child's money may be used for these empty calories rather than the more nutritious foods. The American Medical Association, the American Dietetic Association, and the National Congress of Parents and Teachers have opposed the sale of candy and soft drinks within the schools.[100]

The school lunch and nutrition education. Through the feeding program the pupil is helped to develop a liking for nutritious foods, and to overcome prejudices. He is guided in food selection, and he becomes familiar with the essentials of an adequate diet. If the educational value of the school lunch is to be fully realized, the meals must not only demonstrate the principles of good planning for nutrition, they also must be considerate of cultural food patterns, palatably prepared, and attractively served.

In addition to the daily opportunities to learn by eating, the lunchroom may serve as a laboratory for many subjects studied at the elementary and secondary levels. For example, individual and group dietary evaluations might become a problem in mathematics, biology, or home economics. A tour of the kitchen and lunchroom permits the physics student to observe the nature of the equipment and to learn principles of its operation, aids the biology student in applying his understanding of microorganisms to the development of sanitary practices, and challenges the English student with timely and varied materials for a theme or the school paper. Art students may prepare posters relating to the lunch patterns or to depict practices in dining room conduct, while a social studies class may find opportunity to discuss cultural food patterns. Many opportunities exist for developing good attitudes and practices regarding social behavior and group conversation.

PROBLEMS AND REVIEW

1. What criteria, other than height and weight, may be used to determine nutritional status?

2. What average yearly gains may be expected from the end of the first year until maturity is reached? How do these vary for boys and girls?

3. Compare the protein and caloric needs of the 1- to 3-year-old; 7- to 9-year-old; 10- to 12-year-old; and 13- to 15-year-old boy with those of the adult.

4. Why would you expect the calcium, phosphorus, and iron needs to be especially high during childhood?

5. How long should vitamin-D supplementation be provided? Why?

6. In terms of food habits, what can be expected at each of these ages: 18 months to 2 years; 5 years; 7 years; 10 years; 15 years?

7. Discuss the role of cultural pressures on food habits and attitudes to food.

8. In what way may disturbances in the mother-child relationship be reflected in feeding difficulties?

9. What is meant by the Type A lunch?

10. Why is skipping breakfast a serious problem? What factors may interfere with the child's appetite for breakfast?

11. What objections may there be to the use of fried foods in the diet of preschool children? To the sale of soft drinks and candy on school premises?

12. *Problem.* Record the food intake of a child for one day, and calculate the nutritive values. Are all the nutrients provided at recommended levels? What suggestions can you make for the improvement of the diet?

13. Plan three menus for packed lunches for an 8-year-old boy. Do these lunches provide $\frac{1}{3}$ of the day's recommended allowances?

14. A mother asks you about the advisability of allowing her children to eat between meals. What suggestions can you make to her?

15. *Problem.* Plan a menu for 1 day for a family consisting of father, mother, 16-year-old boy, 13-year-old girl who tends to be overweight, 8-year-old girl, and 3-year-old boy. Indicate in table form the approximate amounts of food for each, and include any modifications in preparation which may be required.

16. *Problem.* List several ways in which you, as a school nurse, could assist in bringing about the improvement of food habits of school children.

CHAPTER 20

Nutrition after Fifty

Population changes. A baby born today can look forward to living three score and ten years. Persons who have reached the age of 65 have a life expectancy of 14 years, while those who have reached 70 years may expect another 10 years of life. About 17 million persons over 65 years now live in the United States; almost a million of these are 85 years and over.

The proportion of persons 45 years and older has been steadily increasing in the United States. While the population as a whole has approximately doubled since 1900, the number of persons 65 years and older has quadrupled. This fact has several important implications: a greater number of workers in the older age group who must be given opportunities for independence and a useful life; increased needs for social security benefits; expanded requirements for social programs for the aging—housing, health, continuing education.

Older persons are an asset to the community inasmuch as the experience they have gained should bring good judgment and efficiency. (See Fig. 20-1.) One need not look far to find examples of persons who have accomplished some of their greatest work in literature, music, politics, education, and so on after they reached the age of 70 years.

Role of nutrition. It is understandable that good nutrition throughout youth is sound insurance for health in the years of maturity. Until recent years, however, the feeding of individuals who had passed middle age was a problem more or less overlooked in nutrition research. Today it is quite clear that the health and vitality of many persons can be improved if there is a willingness to accept the information offered and to put into practice the rules governing a modified way of life, including food habits. Malnutrition occurs too frequently among older people. Many physiologic, sociologic, and psychologic problems are accentuated during these years so that special attention must be given to their solution in order that good health can be maintained.

Physiologic and nutritional changes. Aging is a process beginning with conception and ending only at death. The rate of aging varies from individual to individual, and also among the many parts of the body. The rate may be affected by heredity, by use or abuse of the body, and certainly by nutrition.

276

The basal metabolic rate gradually declines from the time maturity has been reached. This may be explained by the increasing proportion of body fat to body tissue, the lesser muscle tension, and sometimes by a diminution of thyroid activity. The decline in basal metabolism is somewhat less when it is related to the active protoplasmic tissue rather than the total body weight. Thus, a group of vigorous, healthy women of middle age were found to have a higher rate of metabolism than has been reported for other women of similar age.[101]

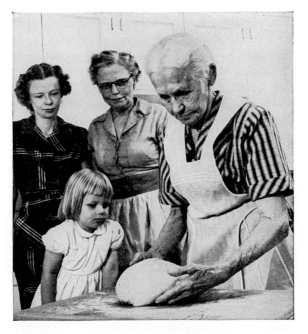

Fig. 20-1. Senior citizens enjoy the benefits of good nutrition and health. In contributing to the whole family's welfare and happiness they experience a sense of usefulness and personal worth. (*Courtesy, the Minneapolis Sunday* Tribune.)

The individual of 60 to 70 years cannot be expected to be as physically active as the person 25 years of age, but the eating habits of youth are likely to be continued into the later years. In the population as a whole the weight increases steadily throughout the years of maturity until it plateaus at the decade of 65 to 74 years.[102] Thereafter, a gradual decline takes place. However, several studies have shown that the incidence of overweight and underweight after 65 years follows the pattern of the population as a whole. Undoubtedly, obesity increases the susceptibility to the degenerative diseases of middle age, becomes an extra burden on weight-bearing joints, and increases the likelihood of accidents.

The senses of taste and smell are less acute in later life, thus interfering with the appetite for many foods. The loss of natural teeth and a seeming inability on the part of the individual to become accustomed to dentures make it difficult to chew food properly or to eat with comfort. Consequently, more and more carbohydrate-rich foods which require a minimum of chewing may be selected, leading to seriously deficient intakes of protein, minerals, and vitamins.

Digestion in later years is affected in a number of ways. A reduction of the tonus of the musculature of the stomach, small intestine, and colon leads to less motility so that the likelihood of abdominal distention from certain foods is greater, as is also the prevalence of constipation. The volume, acidity, and pepsin content of the gastric juice are often reduced, achlorhydria being observed in 35 per cent of those 65 years and older.[103] A reduction in acidity is known to have an adverse effect on the absorption of calcium and iron, and may also explain the lower vitamin-B_{12} levels of blood observed in many older persons.

Fats are often poorly tolerated because they further retard gastric evacuation, because the pancreatic production of lipase is inadequate for satisfactory hydrolysis, and because chronic biliary impairment may interfere with the flow of bile to the small intestine.

The fasting blood sugar is usually normal. Likewise, the absorption of carbohydrate from the intestinal tract seems to be unchanged, but there is a somewhat diminished utilization of carbohydrate as may be seen by higher than normal blood lactic acid and pyruvic acid levels after exercise.

Many older persons, especially men, have an elevated blood urea nitrogen and blood uric acid, indicating some deterioration of kidney circulation. The occurrence of nocturia may lead to a voluntary reduction of the intake of fluid, thereby increasing the difficulty of satisfactory waste elimination.

Blood levels of vitamin C and hemoglobin are reduced in many older persons. In part, these levels may be correlated with low intakes of vitamin C and iron. The low hemoglobin levels may also result from the poor absorption of iron when gastric acidity is reduced, or when antacid preparations are used in the treatment for ulcers.

Hormonal imbalances occur more frequently during later years. A reduction of thyroid activity is reflected in a reduced energy requirement and also may be related to the occurrence of degenerative vascular disease. In women, especially, imbalances may lead to disturbances of calcium and nitrogen metabolism and the resultant condition known as osteoporosis. Nevertheless, a high proportion of women with this bone disease have been poor milk drinkers throughout life,[104] and do seem to have the ability to utilize calcium for bone remineralization if sufficiently high calcium intakes are provided.

About 90 per cent of the deaths from heart disease, malignancies, and vascular accidents of the central nervous system occur in people over 45 years of age. The blood cholesterol is usually elevated as age increases and is believed to be associated with an increased incidence of cardiovascular disease. The kind and amount of fat in the diet, the degree of overweight, the stresses of life, and many other factors are being actively investigated with respect to their effect on the blood cholesterol. While no conclusions can be drawn at this time, it appears that maintenance of normal weight throughout life is of major importance.

Food habits. The older person tends to follow dietary patterns of his earlier years. He has been influenced by the many factors which determine food acceptance from infancy throughout life (see Chap. 15). By the time he reaches the age of 50 or 60, his pattern has become fixed and it is indeed difficult to introduce new foods or markedly changed patterns of eating.

With increasing years the individual sees and hears less well, moves more slowly, and may be troubled with chronic illness. When persons reach the age of retirement from a position, they may have a sense of not being needed either by their families or by the community. The frustrations and isolation from the people and work one loves, and the feelings of being rejected and unwanted, may be expressed by complaints against food and refusal to eat, or, on the other hand, by self-indulgence in favorite foods such as sweets.

Good food served in pleasant circumstances by people who care may indicate to the older person that someone cares for him and that he is important. Attention to holiday customs, for example, bolsters the morale and the food intake. On the contrary, food poorly prepared or carelessly served may be associated with lack of love and thus will be refused.

Older persons who live alone often have no incentive to cook. They may eat carbohydrate foods to excess because they are easy to chew, require no preparation, and are inexpensive. Milk is taken poorly by many because of erroneous ideas concerning its value for adults, its supposed constipating or gas-producing effects, and its cost. Vegetables may be considered as too difficult to chew and too expensive. Fruits are often thought to be too "acid." Many older persons labor under the mistaken notion that their food needs are small because they no longer have growth needs, and because they are inactive.

Older persons are particularly susceptible to the claims of the food faddists. Having lost some sense of well-being they are likely to be misled by claims of unscrupulous persons concerning "miracle" diets and drugs. While the foods recommended by these faddists may not in themselves be harmful, the undue emphasis placed upon them may mean that the necessary foods for nutritional adequacy are neglected and that the individual delays too long in seeking medical advice for his ills.

Economic factors. Many older persons do not have satisfactory living arrangements. Some live alone in a room with a fixed income totally inadequate in terms of today's living costs, while others are dependent upon meager welfare allowances. Facilities for food preparation are often limited. Physical handicaps and chronic ill health may interfere with marketing and with food preparation so that more and more reliance is placed upon a few packaged foods seemingly low in cost but inferior in nutritive value.

Dietary allowances. The basic needs of the healthy older person are the same as those of the younger individual.

Energy. The Recommended Dietary Allowances provide a reduction in calories of 7.5 per cent per decade from 45 to 65 years, and 10 per cent per decade after age 65; thus, the allowance for a man at 65 years is 2550 calories, whereas at 25 years for similar activity it is 3200. This assumes that the individual is one who is normally vigorous and living in a temperate climate. The maintenance of ideal weight is the final criterion as to one's optimum caloric intake.

Protein. Adults of all ages should be provided with 1 gm of protein per kg of ideal body weight. Older persons who have had poor dietary habits or illness may benefit by increased intakes.

Carbohydrate and fat. Since the caloric requirement is reduced, the carbohydrates and fats which comprise the rest of the diet must be chosen with considerable care in order that the protein, calcium, iron, and vitamins may be included in optimum amounts. It has been suggested by some that the fat intake might be reduced to 25 per cent of the total calories, and that part of this fat might well be obtained from the vegetable oils which are rich in polyunsaturated fatty acids.

Minerals and vitamins. Although the needs for minerals and vitamins are the same as for younger adults, special emphasis must be placed on the adequacy of calcium, iron, and ascorbic acid intakes since the consumption of milk, meat, green leafy vegetables, and citrus fruits is so often reduced. The B-complex vitamins are likely to be obtained in more nearly adequate amounts if enriched bread is used inasmuch as many older persons eat rather large amounts of bread.

Water and fiber. About 6 to 8 glasses fluid is as essential for the older person as it is for the younger individual. The kidneys can function more adequately when there is sufficient fluid with which to eliminate the waste solids. Water stimulates peristalsis and thus aids in combating constipation. When nocturia is a problem, the individual should be encouraged to take as much water as possible early in the day.

Many older persons select diets which are smooth in character. This together with an inadequate fluid intake leads to persistent constipation and often to the use of harmful laxatives and mineral oil. While rough fiber is not advised for older persons, the fiber of tender vegetables, fruits, and whole-grain cereals will encourage normal peristalsis.

Planning the daily diet. The basic list of foods (p. 29) should serve as a foundation for planning the diet after 50 just as it does for young adults. To this list may be added other foods as desired for the maintenance of normal weight. The following suggestions may be helpful in specific situations.

For foods easy to chew. Meat, vegetables, and fruits can be finely minced with a sharp kitchen scissors or knife, or they may be ground. In either case, food is sufficiently finely divided for ease in swallowing and rapid digestive action. These should be emphasized:

milk as a beverage
cottage or cream cheese; American cheese in sauces or casserole dishes
eggs, soft-cooked, scrambled, poached
tender meat, or poultry, finely minced or ground; flaked fish; finely diced meat in sauces often taken more readily
soft raw fruits as banana, berries; canned or cooked fruits; fruit juices
soft-cooked vegetables, diced, chopped, or mashed. Raw vegetables such as tomatoes can often be eaten if finely chopped—skin and seeds removed
cooked and dry cereals with milk
bread, crackers, and toast with hot or cold milk
desserts: diced cake with fruit sauce; fruit whips; gelatin; ice cream and ices; puddings; pie, if crust is tender and cut up

For enjoyment of meals, ease of digestion, and good rest, give heed to the following:

1. Serve colorful foods attractively on a tray if eating alone.
2. Eat leisurely in pleasant surroundings.
3. Eat four or five light meals instead of three heavier meals.
4. Include essential foods first. Sweets may be taken in moderate amounts but excess may cause discomfort and lead to overweight.
5. Eat a good breakfast to start the day right.
6. Fats may retard digestion. If there is discomfort, avoid:

fatty meats and fish
fried foods
gravies, sauces, and salad dressings
rich cakes, doughnuts, pastries, and puddings

7. Certain foods may cause distress for some people. These are most likely to be:

dried cooked beans, Brussels sprouts, cabbage, cantaloupe, cauliflower, cucumber, onions, radishes, turnips, watermelon

8. Eat the heaviest meal at noon rather than at night if sleeping is difficult.

9. Avoid tea and coffee late in the day if insomnia is a problem.

10. Drink hot milk just before going to bed.

PROBLEMS AND REVIEW

1. What changes occur with aging which may modify the digestion of foods?

2. Compare the nutritional needs of the adult of 25 years with one of 65 years.

3. What reasons can you give for the difficulty many older women experience in the healing of a bone?

4. What are the dangers of overweight in the middle aged?

5. A widow has no cooking facilities in her room and eats dinner in a restaurant. Her income is limited. What are some foods she could eat at home which require no cooking, but which would be nutritionally valuable?

6. *Problem.* Plan menus for 2 days which could be prepared with only a single gas burner available for cooking.

7. *Problem.* Using the low-cost plan on page 188 plan a week's menus for a man and woman 65 years old.

8. Consult the suggestions for effecting economy in food purchasing on page 195. Which of these might not be practical for a single person or an older couple? Why?

UNIT V /
Nutrition and Public Health

CHAPTER 21 /

Safeguarding the Food Supply

ILLNESS CAUSED BY FOOD

The ancient Egyptians realized that meat of animals which had died a natural death was unfit for human food. Greek records of many centuries ago note that the wife, daughter, and two sons of the Greek poet Euripides died after having eaten poisonous fungi by mistake. For centuries official food tasters were employed to protect kings against poisoning. That an adequate supply of food of high nutritive value is essential for health and well-being of man has been established. It is equally well recognized that food may be an occasional cause of disease.

Illness which sometimes results from the eating of food may be caused by bacterial contamination or parasitic infestation of the food, by the presence of some poisonous chemical in the food, or by sensitivity of the individual to a given food or foods. Bacterial, parasitic, or chemical contamination will be discussed here, while the subject of allergy is considered in more detail in Chapter 39.

When one considers the total population of the United States and the amount and variety of foods consumed each day, it becomes evident that the incidence of outbreaks of illness from the food supply is indeed very low. This attests, in general, to the wholesome quality of the American food supply. Food handlers from the field to the factory and retail store share the responsibility for the production of a clean, safe, and nutritious food supply. Everlasting vigilance in the maintenance of the highest standards in food production is the joint responsibility of local, state, and national public health agencies and of the food industry.

Diseases transmitted by foods. Typhoid fever, dysentery, tuberculosis, diphtheria, streptococcic sore throat, and undulant fever are some of the diseases which may be transmitted by contaminated foods and water. Some of these diseases are carried by the food from the infected animal; for example, tuberculosis and brucellosis. Today these dangers have been practically removed because of stringent regulations for the inspection of animals and the pasteurization of milk.

284

Food handlers may be responsible for the transmission of disease through the food they prepare. This may come about through carelessness with respect to washing the hands, failure to cover the nose and mouth when sneezing or coughing, handling of food by those with skin infections, and so on. During the early part of this century, typhoid fever was quite common. Drinking water which had been contaminated by excreta of infected persons was usually held responsible. Today, because of measures to safeguard water and milk supplies, especially in urban communities, typhoid fever is of rare incidence.

Foods which are improperly protected from access by insects, flies, roaches, rats, or mice are rapidly contaminated with pathogenic organisms and may cause outbreaks of illness. Failure to refrigerate promptly cooked foods and perishable meats, dairy products, and other foods provides an optimum environment for the rapid multiplication of bacteria.

Bacterial food poisoning. *Staphylococci* are the most frequent cause of food poisoning which affects the gastrointestinal tract of thousands of people, especially during the summer months. The enterotoxin produced during the growth of the staphylococci, rather than the bacteria, causes the illness within 1 to 5 hours after eating contaminated food.

Staphylococci are found in the air and occur especially in infected cuts and abrasions of the skin, boils, and pimples. They may be present in the nose and throat of food handlers. The contaminated food usually does not smell, taste, or appear to be spoiled; and only constant vigilance in maintaining high standards of food handling can reduce the occurrence of illness.

The staphylococci grow most rapidly at 50° to 120° F and are readily killed at cooking temperatures. However, the enterotoxin is destroyed only by prolonged high temperatures. Thus, the low-temperature methods of cookery used for milk and egg mixtures are not a safeguard when the toxin has already developed. This is borne out by the fact that staphylococcal food poisoning most frequently occurs with semisolid foods such as custards, cream fillings in pastries, cream puffs, cream sauces, and mayonnaise. Other foods which have been implicated in epidemics are chicken and turkey salads, croquettes, potato salad, poultry dressing, ham, ground meat, stews, and fish.

Botulism. A news story in 1959 gave an account of the death of three members of a family and the serious illness of three others following the eating of home-canned beets.[105] The presence of botulin, a toxin produced by *Clostridium botulinum,* was established as the cause of illness. The bacteria are found in soils all over the world and consequently infect the vegetables grown thereon. The spores produced by the bacillus are relatively heat resistant, and they will develop rapidly under anaerobic (without oxygen) conditions such as are found in canned foods. The toxins produced are extremely poisonous, and it has been estimated that as little as $\frac{1}{100}$ mg may prove fatal to man. The toxin must be produced in the food before it is consumed.

Foods which contain little or no acid such as meat, beans, asparagus, corn, and peas are very good media for the growth of the bacillus botulinus, while acid-containing foods such as tomatoes and certain fruits are not favorable for growth. The processing of canned vegetables in boiling water is not adequate for destruction of spores, and therefore the use of sterilization with steam under pressure should be urged for the home as well as for commercial establishments. Botulism at the present time occurs as a result of the consumption of improperly canned vegetables in the home.

Botulinus-infected foods do not necessarily taste or smell spoiled, so that home-canned vegetables should always be brought to a vigorous boil before being used since the toxin is inactivated in 6 to 10 minutes by heat at 80° C. It goes without saying that any food which shows gas production or change in color or consistency should be destroyed without even tasting it. The contents of any can which has bulging ends should likewise be discarded. It is important that such foods be burned since animals eating them will otherwise be poisoned.

Ptomaine poisoning. The designation "ptomaine poisoning" is incorrectly applied to almost any sort of illness resulting from the consumption of food. Ptomaine comes from the Greek word "ptoma" meaning dead body. True ptomaines are nitrogenous products which are formed in the later stages of food decomposition, but the foods are so obviously spoiled that people would refuse to eat them. Ptomaines have never been shown conclusively to produce illness when they are given by mouth, although their injection in experimental work has sometimes led to illness.

Parasitic infestations of food. Many animal parasites gain admission to the body by means of food. Among them are *Endamoeba histolytica,* which causes amebic dysentery, and various worms such as beef and pork tapeworm, pinworm, and Ascaris. Flies and other insects carry cysts of the ameba from feces and contaminate food and water with which they come in contact. In the United States contaminated water has been, on rare occasions, responsible for epidemic outbreaks of amebic dysentery. Food handlers who harbor the organism may be sources of amebic infection unless great care is taken regarding cleanliness of the hands.

Trichinosis is one of the most serious of worm infestations and results from eating raw or partially cooked pork infected with *Trichinella spiralis.* Autopsy reports indicate that the disease is much more common than is generally believed.

Trichinosis may be avoided by eating only those pork products which have been thoroughly cooked; this means that pork should not be eaten if the meat is pink. Pork which has been kept frozen at 0° F for 72 hours or longer is safe, because the Trichinae are destroyed at this low temperature. Government inspection of meat does not include examination for Trichinella since it is impractical to do so at the present time. The United States Public Health Service has long recommended that garbage used for hogs be cooked, and many local health authorities now require that this be done. This precaution will go a long way in reducing the Trichinella infestation of hogs.

Chemical poisons in plants and fish. Another type of poisoning occurs from the consumption of plants which contain poisonous alkaloids, such as strychnine, atropine, scopolamine, solanine, and others. Varieties of hemlock have been mistaken for parsley, horse-radish, or wild parsnip and eaten in salads or soup only to produce immediate illness which was often fatal. Monkshood, foxglove, and deadly nightshade have from time to time been mistaken for edible plants and caused violent illness.

The increased consumption of mushrooms has led to more frequent poisonings by fungi, for many people are unable to distinguish the very poisonous *Amanita* from the harmless varieties. The ingestion of one type of poisonous mushroom results in mortality of more than half of the victims. This source of poisoning can be eliminated if people will use only the commercially grown mushrooms.

The eating of certain weeds such as white snakeroot by cows produces the disease "trembles." This disease, also known as milk sickness, is transferred to man through the milk supply or through the eating of meat from the diseased animal.

The green part of sprouting potatoes contains sufficient solanine to produce pain, vomiting, jaundice, diarrhea, and prostration. Rhubarb leaves contain appreciable quantities of oxalic acid, and should not be used in place of other greens since serious illness usually results.

Mussels from the Pacific coast extending from Alaska to California contain one of the most poisonous alkaloids known.

Chemical poisoning. Lead is a particularly dangerous metal since it accumulates in the body and results in chronic illness characterized by severe anemia and changes in the kidneys and arteries, death occurring in some cases. A minute quantity of lead occurs naturally in food and is ingested daily, but whenever the daily intake is 1 mg or more the eventual accumulations may become toxic. Food may become contaminated with lead if it is exposed to dust containing lead, or if it is kept in containers in which solders, alloys, or enamel containing lead have been used. Canned foods were formerly subject to lead contamination, but the canning industry has long since devised containers which are entirely safe for food.

Cadmium, zinc, and antimony are readily soluble and will quickly produce illness if ingested. They are not used in the manufacture of utensils or cans.

Accidental poisonings have occurred when chemicals have been mistaken for powdered milk, flour, or baking powder. Some years ago in a state institution 47 deaths resulted when roach powder containing sodium fluoride was mistaken for dry milk powder and used as such.[106] In another instance boric acid was used in place of lactic acid for the preparation of infant formulas.

The coloring of pesticides green or some other color unusual to foods could prevent accidental poisonings. It goes without saying that insecticides, lye, moth balls, and numerous other poisons should be placed where small children cannot reach them.

The metals used in cooking utensils and in food containers have been a source of much controversy. Many studies have shown that glass, stainless steel, aluminum, agate, and tin are suitable containers for food since these materials are practically insoluble or, when dissolved to a slight degree, are not harmful to health. Acid foods may dissolve some of the tin from cans so that a change of flavor results from the iron underneath the tin coating, but the ingestion of these foods is not harmful. It is recommended that acid foods be transferred from the can to a covered glass container if the food is to be refrigerated after opening.

Many chemicals are added to foods intentionally to enhance some property of the food, or are present incidentally as a result of packaging, spraying, or other treatment. Chemical additives may, on occasion, be a source of food poisoning. They are discussed further on page 294.

PRESERVATION OF FOODS

Factors contributing to food spoilage. From the foregoing discussion it is apparent that the safety of foods is determined by the absence of pathogenic organisms, either bacterial or parasitic. That molds and yeasts may lead to food spoilage is well known. Foods also contain enzymes which accelerate chemical changes, thus leading to deterioration of texture, flavor, and nutritive values.

Chemical changes are brought about by contact with light, air, heat, and moisture. For example, the riboflavin content of milk is rapidly reduced if milk is left exposed to sunlight; fats may become rancid when exposed to air; water-soluble vitamins may be lost in liquids which are discarded. It is estimated that the rate of chemical change is doubled for each 18° F rise in temperature.

Food preservation, therefore, is directed toward killing microorganisms, as by heat, or rendering them inactive by dehydration or by a cold environment; and toward retardation of the rate of chemical change by inactivating enzymes, reducing temperature, avoiding exposure to light, and minimizing contact with air.

Making milk safe. Of all foods, milk is perhaps most susceptible to contamination. Pasteurization is the most effective measure which can be taken to protect the milk supply, although the inspection of the cows, barns, and milk handlers is also desirable. More than 90 per cent of all milk consumed in the United States is now pasteurized.

There are two methods for pasteurizing milk: (1) in the *holding* process milk is heated to at least 143° F and kept at that temperature for at least 30 minutes; or (2) in the *high-temperature short-time* method the milk is heated to at least 160° F and kept at that temperature for at least 15 seconds.

Milk may be sterilized by boiling it for a specified time as in the preparation of infant formulas or by heat as in the processing of evaporated milk. Pasteurization does not appreciably change the color or the flavor of milk, but sterilization deepens the color and gives to the milk a slightly caramelized flavor.

Certified milk is produced and marketed under very strict supervision of local medical boards. At the time of delivery to the consumer it must contain fewer than 10,000 bacteria per ml when raw, and less than 500 bacteria per ml when pasteurized. It is used primarily for the feeding of infants. While some of it may be sold raw, most cities now require that it be pasteurized.

As soon as possible after delivery, milk should be put in the coldest part of the refrigerator. It should be kept covered in the bottle or container in which it was pasteurized. Fresh and old milks must not be mixed, since spoilage will occur more quickly in the whole lot. Evaporated and reconstituted dry milks require the same care as fresh milk since they are subject to the same spoilage factors.

Cheese, butter, and ice cream may harbor pathogenic organisms, and the milk used for the preparation of these foods is usually handled with the same sanitary precautions, including pasteurization.

Cooking. Boiling temperature (212° F), if maintained sufficiently long for heat to completely penetrate the food, will quickly kill bacteria, but spores of bacteria such as those of the botulinus or of molds are not always destroyed. When temperatures above the boiling point—that is, with the aid of pressure cookers—are employed, these spores are also destroyed. Bacteria may not be killed when low-heat cookery is employed as in the preparation of custards, or where heat penetrates very slowly food masses such as casserole dishes and roasts. Such foods are particularly likely to cause poisoning if they have been carelessly handled prior to cookery.

Canning. According to data released by the industry, 1294 different canned products in 658 million cases were offered to consumers in 1957.[107] Nicolas Appert, a Frenchman, is credited with the first successful application of canning during Napoleon's day, while Pasteur established the role of micro-organisms in food spoilage some 50 years later.

Commercial firms now employ standard methods for canning each food. Sterilization is brought about by means of steam under pressure. No commercially canned food has been known to produce illness from microbial spoilage since the late 1920's. By means of agitation of the cans during processing, heat penetration of the can contents is accelerated and the heating time is shortened with a great improvement in flavor and in color.

High-temperature, short-time processing is a new development in canning.

Bacterial destruction is increased tenfold for each 18° F rise in temperature, while the rate of chemical changes which result in quality loss is only doubled. At temperatures of 275–350° F a product may be sterilized in a few seconds, whereas minutes or even hours were earlier required. *Aseptic* canning is an application of the high-temperature processing. The product is first sterilized in a matter of seconds, cooled, and filled aseptically into presterilized containers in a sterile atmosphere. The method has been used for fluid products such as soups, sauces, fruit juices, milk, and baby foods and appears to be applicable to other foods in small pieces. The resultant product is of better color and flavor, and retains more of the heat-labile vitamins.

Some nutritive losses, especially of heat-labile vitamins, occur during canning, but the newer techniques have reduced these losses considerably. The manner of storage is probably the major factor in nutrient retention or loss. As much as 25 per cent of ascorbic acid and thiamine may be lost from fruits and vegetables stored for a year at 80° F. Meats, likewise, lose 20 to 30 per cent of their thiamine content after 6 months storage at 70° F, but the riboflavin content is not adversely affected. Carotene losses in fruits and vegetables are small even after months of storage. Water-soluble nutrients distribute themselves evenly throughout the solids and liquid; thus, if the solids constitute two-thirds of the total, one-third of these water-soluble nutrients will be lost if the liquid is not used.

Home canning. When foods are canned in the home, a pressure canner should always be used for low-acid foods, including most vegetables, poultry, and meat, in order that bacteria and their heat-resistant spores may be destroyed. Fruits and tomatoes, being acid foods, may be safely canned at boiling temperatures. The packing of food into jars and heating for stipulated lengths of time in a water bath is preferable to the open-kettle method of packing hot food into jars without further heating.

Cold storage. Modern refrigeration has been largely responsible for the tremendous variety of foods available all over the country, in season and out. By means of it foods can be kept for long periods of time in commercial cold-storage rooms at the proper humidity, or may be transported from coast to coast without danger of loss from spoilage or freezing, or may be kept in the home refrigerator to reduce the number of trips the homemaker makes to the market.

Fruits and vegetables are kept just above the point at which they will freeze, this being in most instances 31 to 33° F. Butter and meats may be kept at much lower temperatures. Cold-storage eggs are often of better quality than so-called "fresh eggs" which have been improperly cared for.

Cool storage is being gradually extended to canned and dehydrated foods to retain optimum color, flavor, and nutritive values. Many chemical reactions occur twice as rapidly at 68° F as at 50° F and four times as rapidly at 86° F as at 50° F.

Freezing. In the quick freezing of foods, first developed as a practical method of processing some 30 years ago, bacteria are unable to grow and enzymes are inactivated. Today an almost endless variety of frozen foods is available: fruits, vegetables, juices, meats, poultry, fish, pies, cakes, cookies, rolls, stews, casserole dishes, and complete dinners. About 10 billion pounds of frozen foods were marketed in 1955 to save countless hours of preparation time for the homemaker.

Foods to be frozen must be carefully selected for quality, maturity, and highest sanitary standards. No frozen product is ever any better than the raw materials from which it was frozen. Because ready-to-eat foods involve mixtures and are subject to more handling prior to freezing, special care must be taken to enforce the most rigid sanitary practices. Some foods such as raw salad vegetables and tomatoes cannot be frozen satisfactorily because of texture changes. Fruits are softened by the freezing process.

Before freezing, vegetables are blanched to inactivate the oxidative enzymes. The darkening of fruits may be prevented by immersion in a sugar sirup or by using ascorbic acid. Foods are packaged in such a way that air is excluded as much as possible. Polyethylene bags and containers, and moisture-proof wrappings including heavy foil, heavily waxed papers, and cellophane are used. Small packages are placed in direct contact with the freezing units so that the entire mass can be quickly penetrated and rapidly frozen. Rapid freezing at temperatures as low as $-30°$ F to $-35°$ F results in minimum damage to the cell walls of the product.

For optimum retention of flavor, texture, and nutritive value, foods should be preferably stored at temperatures below $0°$ F. Ascorbic acid losses are greater than those for other nutrients. Orange juice held at $32°$ F for a year loses no more than 5 per cent of its ascorbic acid, but nonacid foods lose appreciable amounts at $0°$ F and much lesser amounts at $-10°$ F to $-20°$ F. Frozen foods should be kept for only a few days in the usual freezing compartment of a refrigerator.

Frozen foods should be used promptly upon thawing. If allowed to stand for some time subsequent to thawing, microorganisms multiply, and changes occur in consistency and flavor. Foods which have been thawed should never be frozen again because further deterioration will take place. Fruits retain the best color if they are thawed in the container before it is opened. Most vegetables are cooked by dropping the frozen vegetable directly into a small quantity of boiling water and rapidly returning it to the boiling point. Corn on the cob should be thawed before it is cooked. Meats may be cooked while still frozen or may be thawed prior to cooking; the former procedure requires a considerable increase in the cooking time.

Dehydrofreezing, a relatively new process, consists in evaporating about half the water, and then freezing the product. It has been applied particularly to fruits and vegetables. The costs of packaging, shipping, and storage are thus reduced. Water is added to reconstitute the food when it is cooked.

Freeze-drying consists in placing the frozen food under a vacuum to remove the water. The product retains its original shape, and looks and tastes very much like the fresh product when it is rehydrated. The process is quite costly and is currently used only on an experimental basis by the Quartermaster Corps of the Army.

Dehydration. Drying of foods is an effective means of avoiding spoilage since microorganisms cannot grow in the absence of water. Certain fruits such as prunes, apricots, peaches, apples, figs, dates, and raisins as well as the legumes have been dehydrated for centuries. Every market today features numerous dried foods: nonfat dry milk; quick bread, yeast bread, cake, cookie, and pudding mixes; dehydrated soups; instant coffee; instant mashed potatoes; citrus juice powders; precooked rice and beans; cereals; and many others. Dried whole eggs and egg whites are used extensively in the baking industry. Dried foods possess the special advantages of light weight and small volume, and are easily transported and stored.

Spray drying equipment for milk and eggs results in less heat damage to the product and a much more acceptable flavor. Nonfat dry milk by a new process is now a fluffy, porous product which dissolves instantly in water. Dehydration under high vacuum is now in its experimental stages and holds great promise for the drying of fruit juices without change in flavor.

Chemical preservation. Sugar is employed in high concentrations for the preparation of jams, jellies, and preserves. The water is made unavailable to the microorganisms, and hence spoilage will not occur. However, molds will grow on the surface of these foods if sterility is not maintained. Sodium chloride and vinegar are also good preservative agents as employed in brining and pickling.

The number of chemicals which may be used for preservation is now strictly limited by government regulations. Benzoic acid or sodium benzoate may be used up to a concentration of 0.1 per cent if labels specifically indicate its use. Sulfur dioxide may be used in the drying of apples to lessen darkening. Meats may be cured with smoke which contains phenols. Older methods of curing meat employed considerable amounts of salt so that preservation was possible at ordinary room temperature. Recent processes employ less salt and more uniform though shorter curing periods, but it is important to emphasize that hams so cured are perishable and require refrigeration. Failure to refrigerate hams has caused a number of outbreaks of food poisoning in recent years. Spices such as cloves and cinnamon have been much overrated for their preservative properties, since concentrations sufficient to inhibit bacterial growth would render food inedible. See also food additives on page 294.

Antibiotics in food preservation. The uncontrolled use of antibiotics in foods or as drugs is a potential hazard to approximately 10 per cent of the population who react unfavorably to contact with them with symptoms ranging from a mild skin rash to fatal anaphylactic shock.[108] The repeated ingestion of antibiotics may produce an immunity in other individuals so that they do not respond to therapeutic doses required in the treatment of disease conditions. It is, therefore, a prime requirement that the food supply which may have had any contact with antibiotics contain no residues when eaten.

Many antibiotics are used in food production. The farmer adds antibiotics to feeds to stimulate the growth of swine and poultry, or he may employ antibiotics to prevent and treat illness in animals. Crops are sometimes sprayed with antibiotics. Since no residues of the antibiotics are present in the foods as eaten, these practices constitute no health hazard. One possible source of antibiotic residues has been milk from cows which have been treated for mastitis. Regulations of the Food and Drug Administration now specify that milk obtained for 3 days following treatment for mastitis with antibiotic drugs must not be used for human consumption.

The shelf life of poultry, fish, meat, ground sausage, cured ham, and vegetables can be increased two to three times when the product is treated with an antibiotic since the growth of microorganisms is thereby retarded. The Food and Drug Administration has approved the use of chlortetracycline (Aureomycin) and oxytetracycline (Terramycin) in the cooling water for dressed poultry, allowing a maximum residue of 7 ppm in the uncooked poultry. These antibiotics may also be used in the ice slush for packing raw fish and shellfish, the legal limit of residue in the uncooked fish being 5 ppm. The cooking of poultry and fish destroys all antibiotic residues at these levels. The commercial use in other foods must await further testing.

Preservation of foods by irradiation. One of the potential peacetime uses of atomic energy is in the radiation preservation (cold sterilization) of foods. Microorganisms can be destroyed by using gamma rays or high-speed electrons, both types of radiation being referred to as ionizing radiations. The unit of radiation is the "rep" (roentgen equivalent physical), one rep being defined as the absorption of 93 ergs of energy per gram of material, water being the reference substance. Irradiation does not make the food radioactive. No irradiated foods are presently available for public consumption, nor does the Food and Drug Administration permit the sale of such foods. Long-term experiments with animals must be conducted to eliminate the possibility of toxicologic and carcinogenic manifestations, although there is no evidence of such danger at present. Under carefully controlled conditions shorter tests have also been conducted on human volunteers by the Quartermaster Food and Container Institute for the Armed Forces.

Small doses of irradiation—less than 100,000 rep—will destroy the insects which may infest flour, cereals, and spices, inhibit the sprouting of potatoes and onions, delay the ripening of fruit, and destroy the Trichinae of pork. Such doses of irradiation do not have adverse effects on acceptability of the product.

At somewhat higher levels of irradiation, that is, 100,000 to 1,000,000 rep, most microorganisms are destroyed but the product is not sterile. Fruits and vegetables may be kept for a longer time; and meats, poultry, and fish may be kept under refrigeration for appreciable lengths of time without deterioration. Radiopasteurization with doses of less than 500,000 rep holds promise of market application in the not-too-distant future.

To effect sterilization, that is, complete destruction of bacteria, 4.8 to 6.0 million rep are required, the spores of *Clostridium botulinum* being especially resistant. The inactivation of enzymes requires such high levels that it appears some heat treatment, such as blanching prior to radiation, is the only practical solution. At high dosages of radiation such as required for sterilization, adverse changes occur in color, flavor, and texture so that many products are no longer acceptable. Moreover, modifications of nutritive value also occur. Vitamins A and E, ascorbic acid, and thiamine are especially sensitive.

FOOD ADDITIVES

A casual inspection of the labels which appear on food packages in any American home will reveal the presence of several dozen chemicals in a reasonable variety of foods. An additive is any substance which is not normally present in the food in question and which is added, either deliberately or incidentally, in order that some quality of the food may be improved. A chemical additive is a substance for which the exact chemical nature is known. Over 550 chemicals used in food manufacture were listed in the 1956 bulletin published by the Food Protection Committee, but new ones are constantly being introduced.[109] In addition, numerous other chemicals are used for pest control and may be incidentally present in the food.

Intentional additives. Chemicals are intentionally added to foods by the processor in order to enhance some quality of a food such as texture, color, flavor, nutritive value, keeping properties to gain better consumer acceptance. The table on page 295 illustrates some of the functions of additives, and gives a few examples of chemicals together with typical foods to which they may be added. Many chemicals serve more than one function. For example, ascorbic acid might be added to prevent the darkening of a fruit, but an excess might also increase the net ascorbic acid intake.

Incidental additives. A food may contain minute traces of a chemical as a result of contact with a substance used in its production, processing, or packaging. Since its presence serves no useful purpose in the final food product, such a chemical is considered to be an incidental additive. For example, food may pick up a material from a wrapper or a container, either by dissolving it out or by abrasion from the container into the food. Detergents used for cleaning dishes or food equipment, likewise, could be such an incidental source.

Of greatest concern are the pesticides which are used in crop production in order to avoid destruction by insects, viruses, fungi, or other plant perils. Residues of some of these pesticides sometimes may be present on fruits and vegetables even after careful washing of the foods. It is self-evident that these chemicals are toxic to some forms of life or they would not have their protective properties for the crop. Just what hazard they pose for man is a fundamental question. Since the minimum lethal dose of these chemicals for various species of animals is well known and the products must be used according to specified concentrations, likelihood of acute toxicity to man is remote. More difficult to determine is the effect of build-up in the body when foods which contain such residues are eaten day after day for long periods of time—even a lifetime. Toxicologic studies on animals throughout their life cycles, including the effects on reproduction and the next generation, are continuously being conducted to minimize such hazards.

Role of the Food Protection Committee. To study the legitimate uses of chemical additives, the Food Protection Committee was established in 1950 as a permanent committee of the Food and Nutrition Board. The membership

TYPICAL USES OF SOME INTENTIONAL ADDITIVES

FUNCTION	CHEMICAL COMPOUND	EXAMPLES OF FOOD
Improve nutrition	mineral salts, vitamins	See page 315
Preservative	sodium chloride	pickles, salted meats
	sodium benzoate	dried codfish; maraschino cherries
	chlortetracycline	antibiotic dip for dressed poultry
(inhibit mold)	calcium propionate	bread, rolls
(fungistat)	sorbic acid	cheese
Antioxidant	ascorbic acid	frozen peaches
	butylated hydroxyanisole (BHA)	lard, potato chips, meat pies, cereals, crackers
	lecithin	margarine, candy
	sulfur dioxide	dried fruits
	tocopherol (vitamin E)	candy, oils
Texture	alum	firm pickles
(anticaking agents,	disodium orthophosphate	evaporated milk, cheese
retain moisture,	mono- and diglycerides	margarine, chocolate
emulsifiers, give body,	sodium alginate	cream cheese, ice cream
thickening, jelling,	pectin	jelly, French dressing
binding)		
Buffers, acids, alkalies	acetic acid	cheese, catsup, corn sirup
	sodium hydroxide	pretzel glaze
	baking powder, baking soda	See page 625
Coloring	annatto; carotene	butter, margarine
	certified food colors	baked goods, soft drinks
Flavoring (over 300	aromatic chemicals, essential	
compounds in use)	oils, spices	
	monosodium glutamate	meat, seasoning salts
Nonnutritive sweeteners	calcium and sodium	dietetic foods
	cyclamate; saccharin	
Yeast food; dough	calcium phosphate; calcium	bread
conditioner	lactate	
Whipping agent	carbon dioxide	whipped cream in pressurized can

of the committee is subject to change from time to time, but it has included specialists in biochemistry, pharmacology and toxicology, pathology, nutrition, food technology, food industry, entomology, and others who are qualified to establish criteria for the evaluation of additives on the basis of their chemical and physical properties, their toxicologic aspects when tested in several species, and their metabolic and nutritional aspects.

The Food Protection Committee acts as a clearing house for information on pesticides and intentional chemicals; it reviews the information and makes it available; it assists in the integration and promotion of research in foods; it aids regulatory agencies in the formulation of principles and standardized procedure; it aids in the dissemination of accurate information to the public. The committee cooperates closely with the Food and Drug Administration so that suitable legal controls may be enacted (see p. 298).

SAFE FOOD PRACTICES

The National Sanitation Foundation has adopted a slogan "Sanitation is a way of life." It is not difficult to formulate standards to be observed in the preparation and serving of foods both in public eating places and in the home, but it is quite another matter to educate the food handler to apply given rules intelligently. Routine medical examination of the food handler is no guarantee that the individual will remain free from disease until time for the next examination. Moreover, thorough examinations are expensive and may require time-consuming laboratory tests. However, communities should maintain adequate regulation of known carriers of disease such as typhoid, dysentery, tuberculosis, and diphtheria.

One of the best guarantees for sanitary food practices is to employ intelligent individuals with high standards of personal cleanliness who are willing to cooperate in the best sanitary procedures. In all respects, education of the food handler with regard to (1) personal cleanliness, (2) correct use of equipment with regard to sanitization, and (3) proper refrigeration of food is the best guarantee for safeguarding the food supply. Some cities provide courses for food handlers which cover these points. The following rules illustrate the application of the principles of safe food practices.

Personal hygiene. 1. Do not permit individuals with colds, sore throat, or diarrhea to handle food until they have recovered.

2. Do not permit anyone with boils, pimples, or carbuncles on hands or face to handle food or tableware.

3. Avoid sneezing or coughing near foods.

4. Always wash hands after using the toilet, scratching the head or other part of the body, or blowing the nose. Suitable hand-washing facilities, includ-

for those few who flagrantly violate the laws because of greed or ignorance. Those who violate the law may be fined, imprisoned, or both. Injunctions may be issued by the court to prevent repetition of a violation.

Adulteration and misbranding. Under the law definitions of adulteration and misbranding have been developed.

Adulteration of food has occurred if: it contains any substance injurious to health; it contains any filthy, putrid, or decomposed substance; it is prepared, handled, or stored under unsanitary conditions; diseased animals have been used in preparation; the container is made of a poisonous substance which will render the contents harmful; valuable constituents have been omitted; sub-

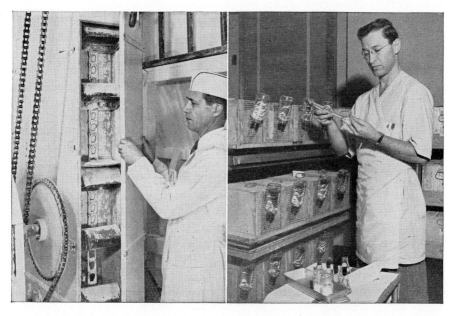

Fig. 21-1. The FDA inspector knows the interior of the elevator is a common place for insect development if flour is allowed to remain. (*Courtesy, Food and Drug Administration.*)

Fig. 21-2. An FDA biochemist checks the vitamin-D content of milk by feeding the test doses to a laboratory animal. (*Courtesy, Food and Drug Administration.*)

stitutes have been used to conceal inferiority; it contains coal-tar colors other than those permitted by law; it contains pesticide residues or additives not recognized as safe.

Misbranding has occurred if: the label is false or misleading; the food is sold under another name; imitations are not clearly indicated; the size of the container is misleading; statement of weight, measure, or count is not given or is wrong; manufacturer, packer, or distributor is not listed on the package forms; it is below standard without indication of substandard quality on the label; it fails to list nutrient information when it is supposed to be for special dietary purposes; it fails to list artificial colorings, flavorings, and preservatives.

Standards for foods. The FDA has developed standards of identity, of quality, and of fill of container. Standards of identity state what ingredients may be included in such foods as flours, breads, and rolls (see p. 619), cheese and cheese products, many canned fruits and vegetables, jams, jellies, and preserves, and many others. The standards also define the minimum and maximum amounts of various ingredients which must be present in the standard product and list permissible optional ingredients which may be used. (See Fig. 21-2.) Foods which are labeled "enriched" must contain the amounts and kinds of enrichment ingredients provided by the law (see p. 316) and no others. These standards create uniformity of product and exclude substances not included in the definition so that the consumer knows exactly what to expect when he buys the food. Except for preservatives, artificial colorings, and flavorings, the ingredients in a food for which a standard of identity has been established need not be stated on the label. The law requires that ingredients for nonstandardized foods must be indicated on the label in the order of predominance by weight if such food is offered for interstate sale.

Standards of quality define the color, tenderness, and freedom from defects of a product, while standards of fill protect against misleading containers.

Dietetic foods. The FDA has established Minimum Daily Requirements (see Appendix, p. 790) for a number of nutrients as a basis for accurate labeling. The student should not confuse these requirements with the Recommended Dietary Allowances, and should learn to read label information carefully for correct interpretation of nutrient percentages.

When a food contains vitamins or minerals in addition to those naturally present, or when it is intended for special dietary uses, it must be labeled to give specific information on the claims made for it. For example, vitamin and mineral values must be stated in percentages of the minimum daily requirements supplied by a quantity of the food which could reasonably be eaten in a day. If no minimum requirement has been established, the amount must be stated in grams or milligrams for a given amount of the food. The sodium content of foods intended for sodium-restricted diets must be indicated in milligrams per 100 gm of the food and for an average serving. The labels of foods containing artificial sweeteners must specify that the foods are intended for persons who must restrict the use of sweets. The labels for low-calorie foods must state the number of calories in a specified amount of the food, and must be significantly lower in calories than that of other similar foods.

Federal Meat Inspection Act. The Meat Inspection Act is enforced by the Bureau of Animal Husbandry and provides for inspection of all meat in interstate trade as well as of all imported and exported meats. The present law provides for (1) the inspection of animals intended for slaughter; (2) the inspection of carcasses and all meat products; (3) enforcement of sanitary regulations;

(4) guarding against the use of harmful preservatives. This inspection takes care of two-thirds of the nation's supply of beef, veal, mutton, lamb, and pork. Meat which is sound and wholesome is stamped "Inspected and Passed," while that which is unfit for human consumption is marked "Inspected and Condemned."

State and community legislation. All foods which are produced for consumption within a state or community are subject only to the laws of that state or community and do not come under the jurisdiction of the federal government. These local laws vary widely.

Milk usually is under control of state and municipal authorities only. Legislation concerning it should include adequate control of sanitation, maintenance of nutritive value, and prevention of fraud. Sanitary inspection should include examination of the cow to detect diseases such as tuberculosis and Bang's disease. High standards for cleanliness of barns, utensils, health and cleanliness of milkers, and bacterial counts of milk must be maintained. Pasteurization should be carried out for all milk.

PROBLEM AND REVIEW

1. List several ways in which bacterial diseases may be transmitted by foods.
2. What organisms are responsible for most cases of summer food poisoning?
3. Formulate several rules which might be enforced in the prevention of food-borne diseases.
4. Explain what is meant by botulism. Which types of food are most apt to contain botulinus toxin? What measures are necessary to eliminate the possibility of botulinus poisoning?
5. What is ptomaine poisoning?
6. Describe the effects of Trichinella infestation. How can it be avoided?
7. Lead and arsenic are especially poisonous to man. In what ways do they sometimes contaminate food supplies?
8. Name several plants which are poisonous to man. What type of chemical compound produces this poisoning?
9. What are the causes of food spoilage?
10. Why are commercially canned foods likely to be superior in their vitamin content to home-canned foods?
11. Which method of canning is preferable for home use? Why?
12. Discuss the uses of cold storage for various foods.
13. Why do dehydrated foods keep so well?
14. What losses of nutritive value occur in dehydration?
15. Name five chemical agents frequently used for preservation.
16. What is the object of the Food, Drug, and Cosmetic Act? Under its provisions what is meant by misbranding? By adulteration?
17. What provisions are included in the Meat Inspection Act?
18. Discuss the importance of state and community legislation.
19. *Problem.* Determine what regulations exist in your own community for the

sale of milk. List several other laws which are designed to safeguard the local food supply.

20. Examine the labels of several packages or cans of dietetic foods. What information is given? Does it comply with the law?

21. What is the nature of each of these in food preservation: irradiation; aseptic canning; dehydrofreezing; antibiotics? What advantages and disadvantages may be claimed for each?

22. Read the labels of a variety of packaged foods and list the additives. Try to determine the reason for each additive. What objections can you see to the use of additives? Would it be advisable to avoid the use of all additives? Explain your answer fully.

CHAPTER 22 /

Nutrition in the Community

The best resource of a community is its people, for it is the population which determines and controls the use of the physical resources. The people may be well educated, well fed, and in optimum health, and the community will prosper; or the people may be circumscribed by the taboos and ignorance of centuries, unable to adapt to the limitations of their environment, ill fed, and in ill health. While it is an oversimplification to say that food alone makes the difference, yet one can see that the individual, by being well fed, is helped to achieve that state of health which enables him to play a responsible role in society.

The many problems inherent in the improvement of the nutrition, and hence the health of a people, have necessitated group action in the community —local, state, national, international. Some dietitians and nurses find worthwhile careers in governmental and private agencies whose primary concern is better health through better nutrition. But all professional workers are helped to do a better job when they utilize the resources of these groups.

The term *public health nutrition* is generally understood to be concerned with those problems of nutrition which affect large numbers and which can be solved most effectively through group action. The term *community* may be used to refer to any group of people—small or large; it might be, for example, a closely knit group such as the student community, or it might be a city, state, or nation in which one lives.

The purposes of this chapter may be listed thus: (1) to enable the student to appreciate that problems of nutrition are a concern of the community; (2) to create an awareness of the many facilities which exist in official and voluntary organizations for working with these problems; and (3) to show that the cooperative efforts of professional and lay workers can give rich rewards in better health. Only a few examples of needs and programs can be given in this chapter since the numerous agencies and their activities are too diversified to permit comprehensive description.

NUTRITION PROBLEMS IN THE UNITED STATES

Defining nutritional needs. The young and the old—the healthy and the sick—the rich and the poor—people in all walks of life have needs in terms of better nutrition. No sound program of nutrition can be initiated without first establishing the need of the time in a given place. The statistics on incidence of disease and of mortality are usually valuable. Data obtained on food production, imports and exports, and income may point the way to changes in agricultural policies. The survey technique has been used widely to determine what courses of action are necessary.

A survey might be concerned with information on the food consumption of individuals and the correlation of nutrient intakes with physical and biochemical measurements of nutritional status. Surveys might likewise study the food habits, buying practices, food preparation procedures, and so on (see Fig. 22-1). Surveys of dietary intakes and nutritional status are time consuming, costly, and require the most careful planning of a public health team, in-

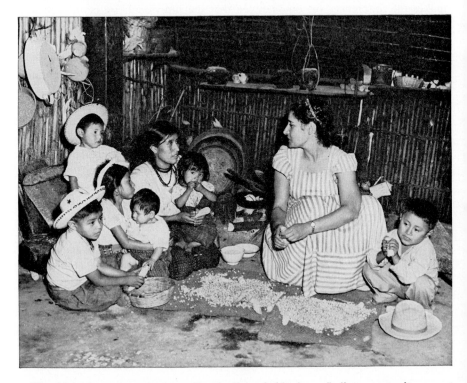

Fig. 22-1. An anthropologist studies the living habits in an Indian community as part of a nutrition survey. (*Courtesy, Pan American Sanitary Bureau, World Health Organization.*)

cluding such personnel as physicians, nurses, nutritionists, laboratory technicians, statisticians, and others. The surveys not only point out the kinds of
action which are necessary, but they also have the advantage of alerting and
interesting the individuals and the organized groups within the community
to their own problems. A number of surveys have been cited in other chapters
of this text (see pp. 8, 229, and 260).

All age groups are concerned. The earliest efforts of public health nutrition
in the United States were directed to the health and well-being of infants and
their mothers. More recently the satisfactory nutrition of the school child,
the teenager, and the aging individual has also been accepted as a responsibility
of health agencies. The specific problems of these age groups and ways to
meet their needs have been detailed in Chapters 17 to 20.

Dietary imbalances. Classic deficiency diseases are rarely seen in the United
States, but the study of the causes of dietary imbalances and their treatment
and prevention are included in the programs of health groups. Overweight
is a problem of children, young adults, and the middle aged (Chap. 27), while
underweight is also too common, predisposing the individual to infections such
as tuberculosis. Endemic goiter is still a possibility not overlooked by public
health authorities. Factors affecting food acceptance and cultural food patterns
may impose inadequacies in certain situations (Chaps. 15 and 16).

Special population groups. The nutritional and health problems of certain
groups may be seen in one part of the country and not in another. For example,
the rapid influx of Puerto Ricans to eastern cities of the United States means
that many have low incomes and are living in crowded quarters, with limited
ability to speak English, without access to familiar foods, and not knowing
how to use American foods (see p. 217). More than one million migrant
workers and their families present a complex problem to the public health
worker. They too are living in crowded, often unsanitary, conditions, with
low, uncertain incomes, and no fixed roots in any community so that their
needs are not fully appreciated.[111] The 370,000 American Indians living on
reservations have long experienced poverty, malnutrition, and disease. Only
recently, an augmented program of health services including nutrition has been
initiated by the United States Public Health Service.[112] In every large city
unemployed persons, families in which the breadwinner is absent, and many
retired persons are unable to achieve an adequate diet. All of these groups
require education and guidance in the selection of an adequate diet, assistance
in budgeting, tangible aid with surplus foods, and sometimes financial assistance.

Group feeding. Children in orphanages, schools, and camps; prisoners; the
retarded in mental institutions; the physically handicapped or invalids in
nursing homes; and the aged are captive to the dietary regimen of the place
in which they are living. The inadequate training and experience of food
service managers and personnel employed in many of these situations may

lead to poor use of money available for the purchase of foods, improper sanitary practices, nutritionally inadequate meals, poorly prepared food, and chronic malnutrition for the residents. Most institutions are eager for assistance in the improvement of food service standards.

Needs of the sick. Research pertaining to the cause of disease, programs for the prevention of disease, and the rehabilitation of the sick are continuing problems of community nutrition. That diet plays an etiologic role in cardiovascular diseases is generally accepted, although the specific factor or factors involved have not been established. The amount and nature of the dietary fat, the vitamin-B_6 intake, and the protein level of the diet are among the elements being studied in cooperative research of the United States Public Health Service, state departments of health, medical centers, and hospitals.

Suitable programs for therapeutic diets, such as diabetic, sodium-restricted, low-calorie, bland, and others, are an ever-present need. Consultant services to nursing homes and hospitals which do not have the services of qualified dietitians, the preparation of diet manuals for the use of personnel in such institutions, and in-service training programs for physicians, nurses, nutritionists, and food service supervisors are among the continuing needs related to therapeutic nutrition.

Plans for the rehabilitation of the sick and handicapped go beyond the responsibility of the nurse or dietitian in the hospital. Rehabilitation might involve a better kitchen arrangement which minimizes effort for a homemaker with a damaged heart; a camp for a diabetic child; suitable feeding equipment for a child with cerebral palsy or who is crippled; or adapting a therapeutic diet to a foreign food pattern. These and many other problems in rehabilitation occur with such frequency that research in the development of satisfactory solutions is a legitimate function of a public health agency.

Food quackery. The exploitation of the public by the food quack presents at least three dangers: the economic waste, the placement of good nutrition in jeopardy, and the hazard to health. More than half a billion dollars is spent annually by Americans for nonmedically prescribed food supplements and pills. This money is often spent by the economically depressed, people in poor health, or the aged. While the purchases are usually, in themselves, harmless, the prices paid are fantastic in terms of value received. Moreover, the misrepresentation of the nutritive value of the product and the diversion of money to buy the product often mean that a nutritionally adequate diet cannot be realized. The greatest harm comes to those who believe the claims that the food supplement can cure organic diseases such as cancer, diabetes, ulcers, and others; too often medical advice is not sought early enough.

The Food and Drug Administration has listed four myths around which current quackery is centered: [113]

Myth 1. All diseases are due to faulty diet. It is held that it is almost impossible to get an adequate diet without using a food supplement. Advertising for such supplements lists scores of diseases and may imply, or actually claim, that the supplement cures them.

Myth 2. Malnutrition is caused by soil depletion; chemical fertilizers are useless or are poisons.

The facts are that genetic make-up of the seed rather than soil composition affects the nutritive value of foods. Both chemical and organic fertilizers increase crop yields but do not improve the nutritive value per unit of weight.[15]

Myth 3. Foods are overprocessed; much of the nutritive value of foods has been lost.

The facts: While processing results in some losses, the claims are grossly exaggerated. Freezing and canning of fruits and vegetables takes place at the moment of peak nutritive values, and the product may be as good as, or better than, fresh foods which have been shipped long distances before reaching the market. Both fresh and processed foods are needed in the diet. The homemaker does not require expensive cooking equipment to retain maximum nutritive values.

Myth 4. Subclinical deficiencies are common; aches, pains, and fatigue are ascribed to a faulty diet.

The facts: Many vicissitudes of life lead to fatigue, aches, and pains. Nutritional deficiency is not common in the United States. Only qualified physicians can diagnose vitamin and mineral deficiencies.

Nine types of products being foisted upon the unwary consumer have been listed by the Food and Drug Administration: [113]

1. *"Shotgun" vitamin formulas*—usually expensive and including numerous ingredients. The Council on Foods and Nutrition of the American Medical Association [53] has indicated the need for only 12 minerals and vitamins in general-purpose food supplements.

2. *Loaded formulas*—high-potency preparations. When taken without specific medical prescription they are a waste of money; they may be toxic.

3. *"Natural" or "organic" foods*—those produced without the aid of chemical fertilizers, pesticides, etc. The foods are usually wholesome, although it may sometimes be doubted that they have been grown under the conditions claimed for them. They are expensive sources of nutrients readily available from any good diet.

4. *"Miracle" foods*—certain supplements or foods represented as cures: vitamin E for muscular dystrophy; garlic pills for high and low blood pressure; royal bee jelly for cosmetic preparations and for sexual rejuvenation; and many others.

5. *Reducing products*—drugs and food supplements. Drugs for curbing the appetite should be used only under a doctor's guidance. Food supplements are of no value in weight loss or in curbing the appetite.

6. *Mail-order products*—mail solicitation is now at an all-time high.

7. *Doorbell "doctors"*—salesmen attempt to discuss health and problems of diet.

8. *Products to reduce blood cholesterol and prevent heart disease*—to substitute such products for medical supervision is dangerous. See page 499 for full discussion.

9. *Popular books on nutrition*—many are interwoven with scientific facts, fiction, and unsound medical advice which the lay reader cannot unravel.

INTERNATIONAL PROBLEMS OF NUTRITION

The problems in nutrition facing people all over the world are not entirely unlike those which have been described in the United States, but they are greatly intensified.

Nutritional surveys. Research teams of the United States Interdepartmental Committee on Nutrition for National Defense have cooperated with local investigators of countries of the Near and Far East in conducting nutritional studies. While these studies were primarily concerned with the armed forces, they do give information pertaining to the economics of the country, the development of food technology, and the food habits of the population. Two surveys under private auspices have also been completed in Cuba and Haiti.

The most widespread deficiency observed in these surveys was that of riboflavin.[114] The signs of ariboflavinosis include angular stomatitis and nasolabial seborrhea, both of which are symptoms that cause little alarm. Whether lack of riboflavin may result in more serious impairment of human life has not yet been established.

Next to riboflavin, diets were most likely to be lacking in ascorbic acid and vitamin A. Biochemical and clinical studies showed that the nutritional status of the military forces was adversely affected by these dietary inadequacies. Comparisons with civilian populations indicated that the armed forces, in general, were better fed.

Deficiencies. In the underdeveloped countries malnutrition is not necessarily universally existent, since the food supplies vary widely from one area to another, food preparation practices and food habits may differ, and economic variability means that there are the "haves" and the "have-nots." The most vulnerable groups are infants, preschool children, pregnant and nursing women. Using mortality figures as indicative of malnutrition, Hundley[4] has cited the fact that the mortality of infants under 1 year ranges from 18 to 28 per thousand in three well-developed countries—Sweden, Switzerland, and England, while it ranges from 94 to 208 per thousand in three underdeveloped countries—Egypt, Mexico, and Brazil. For children between 1 and 4 years of age, mortality is 1.0 to 1.6 per thousand in the three well-developed countries but 16.2 to 49.7 per thousand in the underdeveloped countries. The high incidence of kwashiorkor (see p. 52) is at least partly responsible for the high mortality rate in the latter countries. Infantile protein malnutrition prevails in those countries where any of these staple foods—rice, wheat, corn, cassava, and millet—is the predominant food of the infant.

The classic deficiency diseases described in Chapters 9 to 11 remain as public health problems in some parts of the world. Even though it could be eradicated, beriberi is still prevalent in rice-eating countries of south and east Asia, especially affecting infants. Pellagra is of frequent occurrence in some eastern European countries and in Egypt, Basutoland, and Southern Rhodesia. Xerophthalmia and keratomalacia occasioned by vitamin-A deficiency account for much blindness and many infant deaths in southeast Asia and Africa. Macrocytic anemias which appear to be associated with deficiencies of vitamin B_{12} and folic acid, and microcytic anemias caused by iron deficiency are widespread. Endemic goiter is a major public health problem in Yugoslavia, Burma, Thailand, Central America, and other areas.

Food needs. Hundley cites the causes of deficiency as "agriculture, climate, economics, cultural and social patterns, transportation, communication, educational and even religion." * Of all of these, he asserts that expansion of agricultural production is the key to permanent correction of malnutrition. Asia comprises one-third of the land surface of the world, but must feed two-thirds of the world's population. India, for example, is increasing in population at the rate of 40 million per decade, but its food production is practically stationary. By contrast, Africa is a vast continent with a sparse population. It has a land area four times that of the United States; yet the population of 180 million cannot escape hunger. No country of Latin America is free of hunger; it is estimated that two-thirds of the people are ill fed, ill clothed, and ill housed. Since the world's population increases by approximately 100,000 per day, the provision somehow of more food of better quality is the basic need for two-thirds of the world's population (see Fig. 22-2).

MANY DOORS OPEN TO BETTER NUTRITION

Nature of services. In the hospital or clinic the nurse and dietitian give direct service to the individual. Some nutrition services of the community are also provided on an individual basis, especially at the city-county level. For example, such direct services are given by a visiting nurse, or a homemaker from a welfare agency, or a volunteer who delivers a hot meal to an aged person. Direct service may also be provided by a physician, nurse, or other member of a public health team which is setting up a study or a demonstration project in a given locality.

Community programs in nutrition seek to improve nutrition through re-

* Hundley, J. M.: "Malnutrition—A Global Problem," *Federation Proc.,* **18**(No. 2, Part II):78, 1959.

search, education, improvement of the food supply, and feeding. The individual reaps the rewards of activities such as these: legislation which protects the food supply; research concerning the preventive and therapeutic aspects of diet with respect to disease; methods for preserving the food supply; the development of new and better foods through food technology; a more abundant food supply because of research on plant varieties, soil conservation, pest control; education for an adequate diet—and so on.

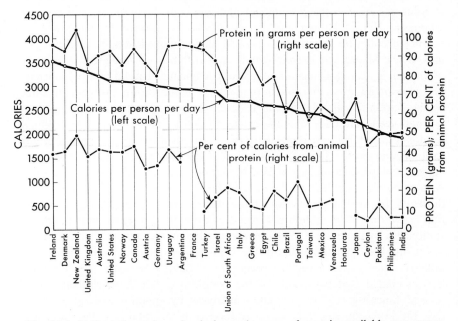

Fig. 22-2. Estimated number of calories and grams of protein available per person per day in food supplies of 30 countries. Note that those countries having the least amount of protein available also receive the lowest per cent of calories from animal protein. (With one exception, the data are for 1954 to 1956 or 1957 to 1959 and are taken from the *Statistical Yearbook of the United Nations, 1959.*)

Facilities of the community. The problems of food production and of nutrition are being met by a large number of groups which work either cooperatively or independently. The partial listings on pages 311, 312, and 313 give the student some idea of the scope of efforts being made by many groups at local, state, national, and international levels. A number of categories are included: official agencies constitute those which have been authorized by the government and which are tax supported; voluntary agencies are supported by private funds, such as the United Fund, foundations, and other means; professional organizations; and industrial groups, especially from the food industry.

Nutrition education. Perhaps the greatest single challenge in nutrition today is that of educating people to make full use of the available knowledge in the selection of the daily diet. The needs of various age categories have been emphasized throughout this text, and methods for the instruction of patients have been discussed in some detail in Chapter 23.

Nutrition education should be an integral part of the classroom instruction throughout elementary and secondary school. It should be supported by a school lunch program (see p. 273) which affords opportunity to put knowledge gained in the classroom into practice. Thus, it becomes a joint responsibility of the administration and faculty to include nutrition in the curriculum and to provide the facilities for a successful program. Many prospective teachers now include a course in nutrition in their college programs. Fully effective programs are possible only when all teachers have some preparation in this area of education, not only through college courses but also in continuing education supported by the school administration—in-service courses, conferences, etc.

Nutrition education also belongs in our industries, health agencies, clubs, and homes. Industrialists have recognized that well-organized feeding programs lead to greater efficiency, less lost time from illness and injury, and

A PARTIAL LIST OF ORGANIZATIONS AT THE LOCAL-STATE LEVEL CONCERNED DIRECTLY OR INDIRECTLY WITH NUTRITION PROBLEMS

Official

Department of Agriculture (state)
Department of Health
   food sanitation
   nutrition
Department of Welfare
Board of Education
   health education
   home economics
Extension services
Public libraries
State universities

Voluntary

Educational groups:
   private elementary and secondary
     schools
   private colleges and universities; home
     economics, medicine, nursing
   parent-teachers associations
   libraries
Social agencies: church and community
   support

Voluntary (*cont.*)

   children's aid
   family service
   Salvation Army
   settlement houses
     visiting nurse societies
   welfare
Institutions:
   children's camps, day nurseries, orphanages
   hospitals, nursing and convalescent
     homes
   homes for the aged
   correctional institutions
Professional organizations: see national
   listing
Civic groups:
   chambers of commerce
   service organizations
   women's clubs
Industry sponsored:
   health centers and hospitals
   plant cafeterias and restaurants
   demonstration programs of stores and
     utility companies

A PARTIAL LIST OF ORGANIZATIONS AT THE NATIONAL LEVEL CON-
CERNED DIRECTLY OR INDIRECTLY WITH NUTRITION PROBLEMS

Official	*Voluntary*
Department of Agriculture	American Red Cross
Agricultural Marketing Service	National Academy of Sciences—National
Food Distribution Program	Research Council
Agricultural Research Service	Food and Nutrition Board: committees
Institute of Home Economics	on food protection, dietary allow-
Bureau of Animal Husbandry	ances, amino acids, cereals, milk,
Meat Inspection Division	fats, protein malnutrition, infant nu-
Bureau of Dairy Industry	trition, and others
Bureau of Plant Industry, Soils, and	Professional societies and voluntary health
Agricultural Engineering	associations:
Federal Extension Service	American Academy of Pediatrics
Foreign Agricultural Service	American Cancer Society
Office of Experiment Stations	American Dental Association
Department of Health, Education and Wel-	American Diabetes Association
fare	American Dietetic Association
Children's Bureau	American Heart Association
Food and Drug Administration	American Home Economics Association
Office of Education	American Institute of Nutrition
Public Health Service	American Medical Association
Bureau of Medical Services: hospitals,	Council on Foods and Nutrition
Indian Health	American Nurses' Association
Bureau of State Services: special	American Public Health Association
health services (aging, diabetes,	American School Food Service Associa-
cardiovascular, tuberculosis), dental	tion
health, international health	Institute of Food Technologists
National Institutes of Health: allergy	National League for Nursing
and infection, arthritis and meta-	Foundations:
bolic, cancer, heart, mental	Milbank Memorial Fund
Department of the Interior	National Vitamin Foundation
Bureau of Commercial Fisheries	Nutrition Foundation
Bureau of Indian Affairs	Williams-Waterman Fund of the Re-
Department of State	search Corporation
International Cooperation Administra-	Industry sponsored groups:
tion	American Institute of Baking
Interdepartmental Committee on Nutrition	Cereal Institute
for National Defense (includes rep-	National Dairy Council
resentation from departments of	National Livestock and Meat Board
State; Defense; Agriculture; Health,	
Education and Welfare; and the	
Atomic Energy Commission)	

better attitudes toward work. Many industries have comprehensive health programs, including nutrition advice not only for the worker but also for his family. Nutrition education is likely to be well accepted by the woman having her first baby, because she is anxious to do her very best in ensuring her child's health. The physician, nurse, and nutritionist have an excellent opportunity at this point. Boy Scouts, Girl Scouts, 4-H clubs, and women's clubs can be effectual in the furtherance of nutrition information.

SOME INTERNATIONAL ORGANIZATIONS CONCERNED WITH
NUTRITION PROBLEMS

United Nations Specialized Agencies
  Children's Fund (UNICEF)
  Educational, Scientific and Cultural Organization (UNESCO)
  Food and Agriculture Organization (FAO)
  International Bank for Reconstruction and Development
  World Health Organization (WHO)
Church groups such as: American Friends Service Committee, Catholic Relief Services,
  Joint Jewish Distribution Committee, Lutheran World Relief, and others
CARE
Foundations: Ford, Rockefeller, and others

Among the many factors determining the success of an educational endeavor, the following should be kept in mind:

1. Nutrition education must recognize the complex social, emotional, economic, and physiologic factors which may be involved in changing food habits of long-standing origin.

2. Education must be directed to the needs of the individual. One may begin with the felt needs, but it is often necessary to bring about realization of needs not felt by the individual.

3. The individual must take an active part in the learning process.

4. Learning should proceed from the simple to the more complex concepts.

5. The individual should know where he can get reliable information. He needs to know what is not true, as well as what is true, if he is not to be misled by the food faddist and quack.

6. Every diet has something good about it, and should be used as the starting point for improvement of food habits.

7. Nutrition education involves a change in behavior—the adoption of improved food habits. Knowledge concerning the principles of nutrition cannot, of itself, be considered as nutrition education.

SOME TYPICAL ACTIVITIES IN COMMUNITY NUTRITION

Some of the groups listed in the tables on pages 311–13 are concerned primarily with problems of nutrition, while others include nutrition as one part of broader programs. Several are concerned solely with the distribution of food, others with education, still others with research, while many are more or less involved in all aspects of community nutrition. Three examples of nutrition programs within the United States have been selected for more detailed discussion: the activities of a nutrition division of a state department of health; the enrichment program which has had such far-reaching effects; and emergency feeding as a program which has not yet caught the interest of much of the population. Other programs of special importance discussed elsewhere in the text are: the development of dietary allowances and guides by the Food and Nutrition Board and the Institute of Home Economics, respectively (Chap. 3); the role of the Food Protection Committee and the Food and Drug Administration (Chap. 21); the school lunch program (Chap. 19). In addition, a brief description of three international agencies will be presented.

A typical state program. The organization of a nutrition department varies from state to state, and likewise no two states will have identical programs at any given time. A good nutrition program is tailored to the needs of the population of that state, and is thus dynamic. Nutritionists in state programs work closely with physicians, nurses, dentists, dental hygienists, social workers, administrators of institutions, food service managers, dietitians, and others. The activities listed below are representative of those included in a number of state nutrition programs:

Provide materials on nutrition information
  Analyze and interpret findings of science
  Prepare leaflets on topics such as: weight control; meal planning; infant feeding; food misinformation; recipes for use of special foods such as nonfat dry milk or for therapeutic diets; diet patterns for various cultural groups; teenagers; senior citizens
  Prepare diet manuals, food value charts, exhibits, newspaper, magazine, radio, and television releases
Consultant service to institutions: child caring, nursing homes, small hospitals, mental, homes for the aged
  Planning food service facilities
  Personnel training; budgeting; menu planning; purchasing; sanitation; preparation and service of food; therapeutic diets
Work with schools: elementary, secondary, college, medical, nursing
  Plan and conduct dietary surveys as part of research program
  Assist in developing projects such as "Better Breakfast" and weight control
  Conduct workshops for school faculty
  Assist in training programs for school lunch personnel; help to interpret educational value of school lunch
Cooperate with other health groups in rehabilitation and in chronic disease programs: cardiovascular disease, diabetes, tuberculosis, arthritis, cerebral palsy, orthopedic disabilities, mental retardation, etc.
  Preparation of materials for professional and lay instruction
  Conduct of institutes for staff education of nurses, nutritionists, physicians
Work with patients (usually on a demonstration basis with nurses)
  Clinics: child health, crippled children, cardiovascular, diabetes, prenatal, tuberculosis
  Food budgets
  Home visits

Work with other groups:
   Social and welfare agencies on dietary standards and budgets
   Public instruction
Assist in programs of research with schools of home economics, medical schools,
   departments of health, federal and private agencies

ENRICHMENT OF FOODS

Few nutritional programs have been of greater significance than the enrichment and fortification of foodstuffs. The success of this venture in public health has been brought about through the combined efforts of public and private agencies at state and national levels together with the cooperation of the food industry.

Policies for enrichment. A statement of policy for addition of nutrients to foods has been set forth by the Council on Foods of the American Medical Association and the Food and Nutrition Board.[115] The added nutrient must be one for which a need has been established in substantial parts of the population; the addition must make a significant contribution to the diet; it must be stable to normal processing and preparation procedures; it must be used in a food which has lost the nutrient during refining or which constitutes an effective vehicle (for example, flour is suitable for thiamine enrichment, and milk for vitamin-D fortification); it must be added to a food which is universally used so that it reaches everyone.

No additions of nutrients to any foods are currently required by federal law. However, when certain nutrients are added voluntarily the amounts must conform to standards established by legislation. Many states have enacted laws requiring the enrichment or fortification of certain foods; usually the regulations conform to federal standards. The term _enrichment_ designates the addition of thiamine, riboflavin, niacin, and iron to cereal foods according to federal standards of identity. _Fortification_ is used to designate the additions of vitamin A to margarine and vitamin D to milk.

Enrichment of cereals. A reduced consumption of meat and eggs together with the use of highly refined cereal foods during the 1930's was responsible for the startling fact that one-third of all diets were classed as poor, especially in B-complex vitamins and iron. In view of these findings, the Council on Food and Nutrition of the American Medical Association, the Food and Drug Administration, the National Research Council on Medicine, and the milling and baking industries through cooperative endeavor made recommendations for the enrichment of flour and bread. The program was endorsed in 1941; the enrichment of all baker's bread was mandatory in January, 1943, until wartime legislation ended in October, 1946. Since that time 28 states, including Hawaii and Puerto Rico, have enacted laws requiring the enrichment of flours and breads; at least five southern states require the enrichment of degerminated corn meal and grits; and South Carolina also requires that rice be enriched. Moreover, the industry has voluntarily enriched flours, breads, and cereal foods so that between 80 and 90 per cent of all family flour and bread are enriched.

Maximum and minimum limits for enrichment have been defined by the

FEDERAL STANDARDS OF IDENTITY FOR ENRICHED FOODS
Minimum and Maximum Levels in Milligrams per Pound

FOOD	THIAMINE	RIBOFLAVIN	NIACIN	IRON
Bread, rolls, and other baked foods	1.1–1.8	0.7–1.6	10.0–15.0	8.0–12.5
Flour *	2.0–2.5	1.2–1.5	16.0–20.0	13.0–16.5
Farina	2.0–2.5	1.2–1.5	16.0–20.0	13.0— — †
Macaroni, noodle, paste products ‡	4.0–5.0	1.7–2.2	27.0–34.0	13.0–16.5
Corn meal and grits	2.0–3.0	1.2–1.8	16.0–24.0	13.0–26.0
Rice §	2.0–4.0	1.2–2.4	16.0–32.0	13.0–26.0

* Calcium enrichment is also required for self-rising flour.
† A maximum level of iron enrichment for farina has not been established.
‡ Levels of enrichment allow for 30–50 per cent losses in preparation.
§ Because of technical difficulties in the application of riboflavin, the enrichment levels for this vitamin in rice are optional pending further study and hearings.

Food and Drug Administration so that the consumer will not become too confused by advertising claims. Federal and state laws require labeling statements concerning enrichment, a typical label reading as follows:

One-half pound of this bread supplies you with at least the following percentages of your Minimum Daily Requirements for these essential food substances: Thiamine (Vitamin B_1) 55%, Riboflavin (Vitamin B_2) 30%, Niacin (another "B" vitamin) 50%, Iron 40%.

The Minimum Daily Requirements (MDR) are levels established by the Food and Drug Administration for labeling purposes (see p. 316) and should not be confused with the Recommended Dietary Allowances. For instance, the MDR for thiamine is 1 mg; the one-half pound of bread cited in the sample labeling above would thus contain 0.55 mg of thiamine.

Vitamin A. The standard of fortification of margarine has been established at 15,000 I.U. per pound, a level similar to the average vitamin-A content of butter. The fortification of margarine is on a voluntary basis.

Vitamin D. Evaporated milk, almost all homogenized milk, and substantial proportions of plain pasteurized milk are now fortified on a voluntary basis with 400 I.U. vitamin D per quart, the established standard, and also the daily recommended allowance for the infant and child.

Iodine. The addition of small amounts of iodine to salt (1 part sodium or potassium iodide to 5000 parts salt) represents one of the earliest efforts to improve a staple food. Approximately one-half of the table salt in this country is now iodized.

Other nutrients. Ascorbic acid is now being added to some fruits and fruit juices, and lysine to certain breads, although no regulations have yet been established for these additions.

EMERGENCY FEEDING

Following a natural or man-made disaster, the goals of emergency feeding are: "to keep people alive, to restore and maintain morale, and to provide adequate and familiar food that will keep people at work or enable them to return to work." * The American Red Cross assumes responsibility for emergency feeding in a natural disaster such as a flood, while the civil defense and welfare services carry out feeding during disaster from war.

Problems associated with emergency feeding. Because of a lack of interest on the part of the public in planning and preparing for emergency, additional hundreds or thousands of people may become dependent upon mass feeding. The nurse, dietitian, and other professional workers can play a valuable role in educating the public to the importance of maintaining their own emergency supplies of food.

Disruption of one or more utilities may make it impossible to cook foods or to use water. Stock piles must be so planned that some foods not requiring heating are available. The lack of water limits the kinds of foods which can be cooked, and seriously interferes with cleaning and waste disposal.

The dietary needs of special groups require preplanning. Infants and young children are especially vulnerable to the lack of food, and parents are likely to become panic stricken if their children are not cared for. Dry and evaporated milk supplies are vital for infants and children. When no water is available for formula preparation, Bovee has suggested that canned fruit juices and even carbonated beverages might be used. The ill and the aged should also be considered. Most patients on modified diets can survive a short period when some foods needed by them are not available. For example, patients with peptic ulcer may get along quite satisfactorily if it is at all possible to eat a food such as bread at more frequent intervals. Every diabetic should be fully instructed on what to do when he is unable to get his food or his insulin.

The worker in a disaster—fire fighter, rescue worker, or the person restoring facilities—must receive sufficient food allowances so that he can keep his work at a maximum output; this may require 3000 to 3500 calories daily.

* Bovee, D. L.: "Emergency Feeding in Disaster," *Am. J. Clin. Nutrition,* **6:**77, 1958.

A disaster is no time to give unfamiliar foods, since the stress of the emergency will usually lead to refusal. Therefore, local foods which are familiar and well liked should be used.

During the first few days following a disaster, food to allay hunger and to sustain morale takes precedence over meeting nutritional needs. A cup of hot coffee to the adult and milk to the child given as soon as possible are tangible evidence that someone is caring for them and that some community facilities are functioning. When an emergency is of more than a few days duration, nutrient needs must be considered. The recommended allowances, however, are likely to provide unrealistic goals when there are food shortages; rationing priorities must be defined.

Safety of food supplies. Following a nuclear attack, the hazards of radioactive contamination of food and water must be appreciated. Foods which are in sealed, unbroken packages or in cans are safe for use, as are those in a refrigerator or freezer which has remained closed. However, the outside of the food container or utensil for cooking and eating must first be washed in detergent solution to remove the radioactive substances. Wash water and cloths used for cleaning must be buried.

If no refrigeration facilities are available, food spoilage occurs rapidly and food poisoning may affect large numbers of people. Cream fillings, milk, ground meat, sandwich fillings, and salads mixed with mayonnaise are especially likely to spoil. Infant formulas may be prepared from dry milk just before use if they cannot be refrigerated.

GUIDE FOR AN EMERGENCY SHELF FOR THE FAMILY *

General considerations

1. Allow about 2 quarts liquid per person per day—fruit and vegetable juices, bottled water, soft drinks.

2. Plan menus in advance using foods the family likes, and keeping these situations in mind: (1) no fuel available and water is limited; (2) no fuel available but there is sufficient water; (3) cooking facilities but little water; (4) cooking facilities and ample water.

3. Stock foods on the basis of menus planned. Avoid those foods which increase thirst. A 2-week supply of foods is recommended.

4. Rotate food supplies at least every 6 months so that the stock is always fresh.

5. Use only air-tight containers—metal, plastic, or heavily waxed cardboard. Glass is not satisfactory since it may shatter.

6. Consider emergency cooking facilities.

* Adapted from "Confidentially Speaking—A Report on Emergency Feeding," Nutrition Section, Louisiana State Department of Health, August, 1957.

Suitable foods from which to select (all in air-tight containers)

Liquids: fruit juices including citrus juices; vegetable juices; carbonated beverages; water

Milk: nonfat dry and evaporated

Canned foods: fruits; vegetables; soups; stews; baked beans; spaghetti and other pastes with sauces; chicken, meat balls, sea food, pressed pork; peanut butter; cheese; oils; shortening; jelly, jam, preserves

Dried foods: dried fruits; legumes

Cereals and breads: dry cereals; ready-to-eat cereals; spaghetti, macaroni, rice, noodles; flour; canned or frozen breads; cookies

Infant foods: dry milk, cereals, fruits, vegetables, strained meats

Miscellaneous foods: instant coffee, tea, salt, pepper, sugar, candy, pickles

Supplies: cooking and eating utensils, paper dishes, matches, candles, bottle and can openers, covered cans for waste disposal, water containers, paper towels and napkins, detergent powder

INTERNATIONAL PROGRAMS IN NUTRITION

Food and Agriculture Organization. Of all international agencies, the Food and Agriculture Organization of the United Nations (FAO) is most directly concerned with food. It was founded in Quebec, Canada, in October, 1945, the aims being:

to help the nations raise the standard of living;
to improve the nutrition of the people of all countries;
to increase the efficiency of farming, forestry, and fisheries;
to better the condition of rural people;
and, through these means, to widen the opportunity of all people for productive work.*

The headquarters office of FAO is in Rome where the work of the organization is supervised by the Director-General. A conference in which each member nation (76 countries in 1959) has one vote meets every 2 years to develop the program of work. A smaller group, the Council, with representatives from 24 member nations, meets every spring and fall and acts as the interim governing body. Regional offices are located in various parts of the world, the one in the United States being situated in Washington.

FAO provides assistance to its member states by maintaining an intelligence service which gathers, analyzes, and distributes information on which action can be based, and by developing programs of action in cooperation with the governments of a given country. An informational and educational

* *Food and Agriculture Organization—What It Is—What It Does—How It Works,* Leaflet, Food and Agriculture Organization of the United Nations, Rome, 1956.

division is responsible for library services and publications and for the dissemination of information to the public.

Technical assistance is provided through five divisions—agriculture, economics, fisheries, forestry, and nutrition. All of the participating countries supply technical experts so that the team going to any given locality truly gives an international approach. A technical team is not sent to a country until the local government makes a request for assistance and gives evidence that it will continue the program after the experts have completed the assignment. The local government shares in the cost of the project and of facilities for work, while FAO covers travel expenses and salaries of the experts and provides a minimum of demonstration equipment. Of the hundreds of projects completed since the inception of FAO, the following are examples:

Education

　　Establishment of home economics department: Queen Aliya College, Iraq
　　School feeding programs: Costa Rica, Colombia, Iraq
　　Nutrition training programs for teachers: Ecuador

Agriculture

　　Weed elimination: Chile
　　Development of rust-resistant wheat: Near East
　　Inland fish culture in ponds, rice fields: Haiti, Thailand, Israel
　　Control of locusts and other plant perils: Near East, Central America, Yugo-
　　　slavia, Syria, Iraq
　　Control of animal diseases: Far East, Near East, Central America

Technology

　　Improved bread-baking techniques: Chile
　　Pilot plant production of saridele (liquid soybean "milk"): Indonesia
　　Large-scale canning: India

Engineering

　　Irrigation, drainage, land reclamation: Pakistan, Ceylon
　　Machine shops and tractor stations: India, Ceylon

World Health Organization. The World Health Organization (WHO) was created in 1948 and now includes 88 member countries. Its work is directed by a Director-General with headquarters in Geneva, Switzerland, and with six regional offices, one of which is in Washington, D.C.

WHO is "the directing and coordinating authority for international health work." It is governed by two principles defined in its constitution:

Universality: The health of all peoples is fundamental to the achievement of peace and security. The enjoyment of the highest attainable standard of health is one of the fundamental rights of every human being without distinction of race, religion, political belief, economic or social condition.

Concept of health: Health is a state of complete physical, mental and social well-being and not merely the absence of disease or infirmity.*

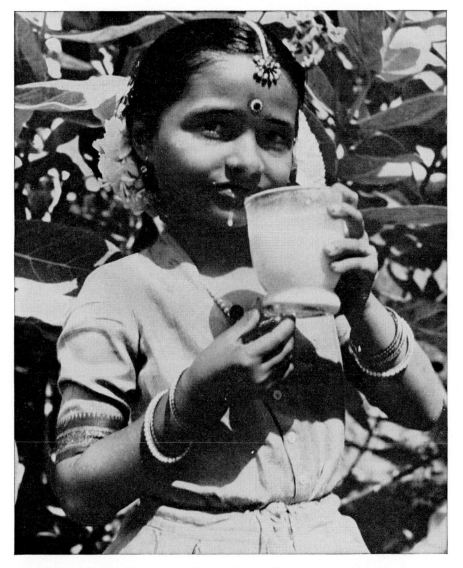

Fig. 22-3. The distribution of milk to children all over the world has been an important work of UNICEF. (*Courtesy, United Nations Children's Fund.*)

* *World Health Organization—What It Is—What It Does—How It Works,* Leaflet, World Health Organization, Geneva, 1956.

The assistance which WHO renders to governments includes:

. . . strengthening national health services; establishing and maintaining epidemiological and statistical services; controlling epidemic and endemic diseases; maternal and child health; promotion of mental health to foster harmonious human relations; improvement of sanitation and of preventive and curative medical services.*

Major efforts of WHO have been directed to the eradication of malaria, tuberculosis, venereal diseases, and yaws. These crippling diseases yearly reduce by thousands the number of workers available to produce food; the return of these people to productivity has incalculable effects on improving the food supply. The improvement of the sanitary standards—pure water supplies, pure milk and other food, insect control, housing, waste disposal— is likewise concerned with the improvement of nutrition.

United Nations Children's Fund. To children in different countries UNICEF means different things. It may mean an injection to cure them of yaws, a crippling disease, or vaccination to protect against tuberculosis; but to all children in these countries UNICEF has come to mean milk (see Fig. 22-3).

Organized in 1947, UNICEF continued the emergency feeding in war-devastated countries of Europe, with emphasis on protein-rich foods, especially milk. Now, all over the world, children are benefited by milk distributions through emergency relief, school feeding, and maternal and child health centers. Nonfat dry milk has been donated from the surplus in the United States, while UNICEF has provided for its transportation and distribution.

While UNICEF continues to provide emergency relief, most of its funds are now diverted to long-range programs, for it is realized that countries must be able to solve their own nutritional programs. With UNICEF funds demonstration programs, such as acceptance tests of fish flour, have been initiated with the cooperation of FAO and WHO.

PROBLEM AND REVIEW

1. How could you determine what nutritional problems exist in your school? In your community?

2. List superstitions concerning food with which you are familiar. What facts can you give to establish that they are erroneous ideas?

3. What are the dangers of food faddism and quackery?

4. What are some of the criteria by which you could tell whether a person is a food quack?

5. List the public and voluntary agencies in your own community who work for better nutrition in one way or another. If possible, arrange for an interview to learn more of the activities of one of these.

* *World Health Organization—What It Is—What It Does—How It Works,* Leaflet, World Health Organization, Geneva, 1956.

6. Select one of the organizations listed in this chapter and prepare a report of its objectives and its activities.

7. *Problem.* Prepare a 1-day menu for each of the four limitations listed on page 318 with respect to emergency feeding.

8. Suggest ways by which nutrition education can be made more effective for teenagers. What methods might appeal to a group of people over 65 years?

9. Discuss the activities of FAO; WHO; UNICEF.

THERAPEUTIC NUTRITION /

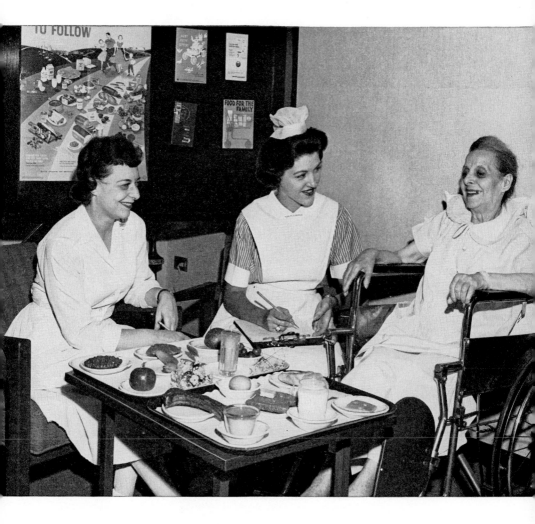

UNIT VI /
Introduction to the Study of Therapeutic Nutrition

CHAPTER 23 /

Therapeutic Nutrition: Factors in Patient Care and Rehabilitation

"The best doctors in the world are Doctor Diet, Doctor Quiet, and Doctor Merryman."—Jonathan Swift.

Good nutrition is a prerequisite to health. Man has probably always associated food, in one way or another, with health or illness. In fact, many of the ideas held by people for preventing or curing disease are based on folklore. The attributes of good nutrition and the principles and practices for achieving them have been discussed for all age categories in Units I–IV of this text. The failure to ingest an adequate supply of the proper nutrients, or inability to digest, absorb, or metabolize foodstuffs, invariably leads to deficiency diseases (see Chap. 26). These, in turn, may initiate or aggravate diseases of non-nutritional origin because of the body's lowered resistance.

Many illnesses such as infections, injuries, and metabolic disturbances lead to deficiencies even in persons normally possessing good nutritional status, because the individual is unable to ingest sufficient food or because the disease process imposes greatly increased demands for most, if not all, of the nutrients. Thus, a vicious cycle of disease, malnutrition, and prolonged convalescence is created. It should be apparent that proper attention to nutrition not only can prevent illness but also can remarkably alter the course of illness when it does occur.

Therapeutic nutrition. Diet therapy is concerned with the use of food as an agent in effecting recovery from illness. In most instances the patient's diet supplements the medical or surgical treatment; that is, the rate of recovery —or failure to recover—may be determined, at least in part, by the patient's acceptance or rejection of food. In some situations such as diabetes mellitus, for example, a modified diet rather than medical or surgical therapy is the most important aspect of the patient's treatment.

The purposes of diet therapy may be stated thus: (1) to maintain good nutritional status; (2) to correct deficiencies which may have occurred; (3) to afford rest to the whole body or to certain organs which may be affected; (4) to adjust the food intake to the body's ability to metabolize the nutrients; and (5) to bring about changes in body weight whenever necessary.

328

Diet is an integral part of total patient care. In her care of the patient, the nurse accepts certain responsibilities related to ensuring comfort and providing therapy according to the physician's orders. Included in these aspects of the patient's care are the daily meals and plans for dietary instruction.

The feeding of the patient involves the coordinated activities of the nursing, medical, and dietary staff, but the nurse is a central figure in a number of ways since she has the closest and the most constant association with the patient.

1. She assists the patient at mealtimes as the situation may require.

2. She serves as a liaison between the physician and patient or the dietitian and patient by:

   a. Helping the patient to select his menu when a selective menu is available;

   b. Interpreting the patient's attitudes and problems to the nursing, medical, and dietary staff;

   c. Observing the patient's acceptance or rejection of food, noting the response on the patient's record, and assuming responsibility for calling problems to the attention of the physician, dietitian, or both, as may be needed;

   d. Interpreting the prescribed diet to the patient, and developing his understanding and acceptance.

3. She assists in or assumes sole responsibility for dietary instruction of the patient.

Factors to consider in the study of diet therapy. If the nurse is to assume the role described above in patient care, it will be seen that certain understandings and abilities must be developed. An appreciation and knowledge are required of (1) the underlying disease conditions which require a change in diet, (2) the possible duration of the disease, (3) the factors in the dietary which must be altered to overcome these conditions, and (4) the patient's tolerance for food by mouth.

The planning of a therapeutic diet implies the ability to adapt the principles of normal nutrition to the various regimens for adequacy, accuracy, economy, and palatability. This may necessitate the calculation of one or more nutrients. Also essential is a recognition of the need for dietary supplements such as vitamin and mineral concentrates when the nature of the diet imposes severe restrictions, the patient's appetite is poor, or absorption and utilization are impaired.

A correctly planned diet is successful only if it is eaten. The dietitian or nurse must be able to apply the principles pertaining to the preparation and service of appealing, palatable, and nutritious food. She must have the necessary understanding of the psychologic and emotional factors influencing food acceptance.

Patient care includes planning for his full rehabilitation. For some patients a modified diet may be required for weeks, months, or even a lifetime; for others, guidance may be desirable in the improvement of a normal diet. Such planning necessitates consideration of social, religious, and cultural patterns, availability of foods, cost of food, suitable methods of food preparation, and so on.

EFFECT OF ILLNESS ON FOOD ACCEPTANCE

The physiologic, psychologic, and emotional factors governing food acceptance have been discussed in Chapter 15. Likewise, a number of cultural food patterns have been presented in Chapter 16. Illness may modify or accentuate the influence of any of these factors.

Illness modifies food acceptance. The disease process itself may have a profound effect on food acceptance. Some foods may produce marked anorexia, others may be distending, while still others may be irritants to the gastrointestinal tract. According to Moore [116] and others, the illness may turn the preferences back to those of earlier years. These may be the bland foods of childhood, but they might be the special dishes associated with one's ethnic origin.

The sick person has many fears: those relating to the outcome of the illness itself; economic concerns for himself and his family; emotional adjustments to having to depend on others during the illness; anxiety about loss of love and self-esteem.

When illness takes the individual from the home to the hospital, food acceptance becomes much more difficult. When the patient most needs the comfort and companionship of family and friends, he is relegated to eating alone. Perhaps the meal hours are different than those to which he is accustomed; the foods appearing on his tray may be unlike those he usually eats with respect to choice, or flavoring, or size of portion; a single food to which he has a strong aversion may so upset him that he is unable to eat anything served with it; managing a tray and the utensils for eating may be awkward when one is in bed; his expressed needs are often minimized or brushed aside.

Modified diets impose additional problems. When a patient is confronted with the need for a therapeutic diet, he may respond with comments such as these: "I just can't get it down." "This food is tasteless." "I can't afford such food when I go home." "Who is going to prepare my food at home?" "I can't buy these foods at work." These reactions and many others must be met by the nurse or dietitian during instruction by providing help in budgeting, arrangements for preparation, suggestions for palatability, etc.

Babcock [117] has pointed out that remarks such as the above also imply many responses to the diet: unwillingness to accept change; anger at those associated with the diet—nurse, dietitian, physician, or even mother or wife who have nagged about the food habits at home; fear of having to eat disliked foods or those foods to which he has a strong aversion; sense of deprivation with respect to choice of foods; fear of loss of social status and self-esteem; and the feeling that diet is, in some way, a punishment of him.

Young [118] states that the patient may express fear by being angry, self-conscious, talkative or reticent, uneasy, depressed, indifferent, impatient, hostile, apologetic for his failure, or resentful. Some patients may use diet as a means of gaining the attention from hospital personnel and later from the family who must provide this food. They may insist upon meticulous attention to the minutest of details, in order to gain this attention. They may actually enjoy the trouble this may be to others, and the release of responsibility for their welfare to others. Occasionally, one may actually prefer not to get well!

INTERPERSONAL RELATIONSHIP WITH THE PATIENT

The nurse, dietitian, or homemaker by her warmth and sincere interest in the welfare of the patient can do much to allay the anxieties of the ill person. Her work is often more successful if she can place herself in the patient's role, although she must guard against overidentification; if she does the latter, she may accept the patient's reactions as being always so reasonable that she is unable to do anything about changing them.

Listening. She who cares for the patient must learn to listen carefully—not only to the words themselves but also to their tone and inflection. By taking time to listen, she may be made aware of a legitimate complaint about something wrong with the trays a patient receives—for example, cold coffee, an egg not cooked to his liking, or a vegetable which he thoroughly dislikes. Such details are relatively easy to correct, and the patient is thereby made quite comfortable and satisfied. The seemingly casual conversation with the patient may bring to light that the past diet has been inadequate for a long period of time because of lack of teeth, poor health, inadequate income, inability to prepare food. Permitting the patient to talk about other things as well as the diet will often reveal that the problems encountered in food acceptance are actually a by-product of the deep anxieties caused by other problems; through understanding, the patient can often be helped.

Recognition of attitudes. How does the nurse or dietitian feel about the patient who doesn't eat his food, who eats too much, or who complains about his food a great deal? When the patient expresses resentment or hostility toward her, does she realize that this may be against the restrictions the diet puts upon him and not against her as an individual? It is important that she recognize her own attitudes toward the patient, lest she show him that she is pitying, superior, intolerant, resentful, or critical of him. Moreover, she must avoid an expression of any negative attitudes she may have toward food.

Encouragement to the patient. When adjustments are made with difficulty, praise for even a little progress and encouragement to keep on trying will usually accomplish more than a critical, scolding approach. Regard for the patient as a mature individual, and allowing him to protect his self-esteem will help to gain his confidence. Reassurance with respect to the diet is essential, but it must be realistic in terms of the difficulties of adjustment to it and its legitimate role in the total therapeutic program. To illustrate, appropriate diets for obesity and diabetes are basic to treatment, but some patients may find the adjustment to the restrictions extremely difficult; to minimize the problems involved is to invite failure. A low-fat diet may be helpful to the patient with gallstones, but it should never be held as a guarantee that surgery would not be required at a later time. Likewise, benefit may accrue to a patient with cardiovascular disease who is placed on a diet with modification of the amount and nature of the fat, but success is so variable that promises of marked improvement would be ill-advised and rash.

FEEDING THE PATIENT

Environment for meals. Time and effort directed toward creating an atmosphere conducive to the enjoyment of food is well spent. Such an environment implies that the surrounding areas are orderly and clean; that ventilation is good; and that distracting activities such as treatment of patients, doctors' rounds, etc., are not occurring at mealtime except as emergencies may arise.

Patients who are ambulatory enjoy eating with others. In some hospitals a dining room is provided for patients, while in others food service may be easily arranged at small tables set up in the patients' lounge.

The appearance of the tray itself is of major importance. The essentials of good tray and meal service are fully described in Chapter 42.

Readiness of the patient. The patient should be ready for his meal whether he is in bed or ambulatory. This may entail mouth care, the washing of the hands, and the positioning of the patient so that he can eat with comfort. If tests or treatment unavoidably delay a meal, arrangements must be made to hold trays so that the food can be fresh and appetizing when the patient is ready to eat.

Assistance in feeding. Some patients may require assistance in the cutting of meat or other foods, the pouring of a beverage, or the buttering of a piece of toast. Very ill or infirm patients must be fed. It is well for the nurse to sit down while she feeds the patient so that she can be at ease and avoid undue haste. Food will be enjoyed more if it can be eaten with reasonable leisure and if there is some conversation. Obviously, if the nurse is responsible for feeding several patients, she will make arrangements to delay tray service or to keep foods hot for those who must await their turn.

DIETARY INSTRUCTION

The plan for rehabilitation of many patients includes instruction regarding the improvement of a normal diet, or adjustment to a modified diet. The satisfactory relationship of the dietitian or nurse with the patient, as discussed earlier in this chapter, is fundamental to a successful outcome. References in the Appendix pertaining to techniques for successful dietary instruction are especially helpful to the student.

Instruction begins early. For the in-patient, dietary instruction should be planned well in advance, for little can be accomplished when a so-called "discharge" diet is given just as the patient is ready to leave the hospital and is concerned about his trip home, the medicines he is to take, and the readjustment to normal activities. The process of instruction, in fact, is part of the daily care of the patient. For example, the diabetic tray becomes, at each meal, a lesson in the use of the meal exchange lists; a complaint about unsalted food may provide opportunity to tell about the use of other flavoring aids. Such informal instruction provided day by day gives the patient opportunity to get used to the idea of the diet, to reflect on it, and to ask questions when they occur to him.

Establishing rapport. The nurse and dietitian have ample opportunity for establishing good rapport with the patient in the hospital, but in the clinic the patient may be seen for only a short time. The interviewer, then, must make every effort to make the patient feel comfortable and at ease before proceeding with the instruction. She must be cheerful, genuinely interested, and inspire confidence.

A quiet, pleasant room where privacy can be assured is essential. The patient and interviewer should be comfortably seated, preferably at a table or desk.

In establishing rapport, the interviewer gradually encourages the patient to talk about himself.[119] Initial questions may well be of a general nature such as: the patient's address; occupation; height; weight; age. The conversation is then directed to the food habits and should bring out the home situation and possibly give some clues to the patient's emotional state.

Timing is important. According to Hildreth,[120] choosing the right time of day for instruction is important. Just before or during meals, the patient is directed to familiar foods which have satisfied his hunger in the past, and he will resist efforts to divert him from them. Immediately following the satisfaction of hunger, he will have little interest in, and may even be nauseated by, the further mention of food. Therefore, some time should elapse after the meal when food can be discussed objectively. Instruction should come at a time when the patient need not be interrupted for routine care, treatments, etc. The instructor must have sufficient time for calm, unhurried teaching.

The dietary history. The individualization of the therapeutic diet necessitates information concerning the patient's practices: Where does he eat meals? When? With whom? Who prepares the food? What are the shopping, storage, and preparation facilities? How much money can be spent for food? What are some typical meal patterns at home? What amounts of food are eaten? Is food eaten between meals? If so, when? What foods? What are some favorite foods? Which foods are disliked? Has he ever been on a diet before? If so, how long? What was the outcome?

On the basis of the dietary history an evaluation may be made of the approximate adequacy of previous diets, and suggestions may be made for improvement. The prescribed diet may be adjusted realistically to the patient's home situation.

Dietary instruction based on patient needs. A fundamental tenet is to begin where the patient finds himself. Something good can be found in every diet, and every effort should be made to impose as few changes as necessary—not a complete discarding of the old pattern. The instruction should be in simple terms readily understood by the layman. Some judgment concerning the amount of detail which may be included is essential, for a weary patient may remember little when he gets home.

The patient will require guidance with respect to choice of foods, methods of preparation, kinds of seasonings which may be used, amounts of food allowed, the number of meals, and time for meals. A written meal pattern which has been developed with the patient is essential. Printed menus which have little or no regard for individual preferences are of doubtful value.

While the emphasis should always be directed to the foods which the patient may have, in some instances, such as the sodium-restricted diets, it may be desirable also to provide a list of foods which are contraindicated. Printed aids such as the meal exchange lists are useful and time saving, but they should always be accompanied with appropriate explanation. Illustrations, posters, and food models are helpful in clarifying instruction; even films may be used where group instruction is used as for pregnant women, the obese, diabetics, and others.

Other members of the family must often be included in the instruction. The wife or mother of the patient may not understand the reasons for the diet, may feel that the diet is an imposition upon her, and may not understand the methods for preparing the necessary foods unless she is present at the time of instruction. For some patients it is necessary to plan a food budget, to make arrangements for meals carried to work, or to make suggestions for a conference with the employer.

Follow-up visits. Dietary instruction is time consuming. The effort is often wasted when no opportunity is given for follow-up visits. The interval for such visits depends upon the patient's ability to understand the instruction, the nature of the diet, its duration, and how well the patient can adhere to his diet. These visits serve to extend and clarify the instruction itself, to provide reassurance, to check progress, and to recognize any tensions which are building up in the patient.

Group instruction. In a food clinic or health center, classes may be held for groups with similar diet problems: pregnant women, mothers with preschool children, diabetic patients, those requiring sodium restriction, and so on. Economy of time for the professional worker is an apparent advantage of using group instruction. Many patients are helped by this approach inasmuch as they learn to appreciate that others have similar problems and that they can share experiences with one another. The person who is given to much self-pity may receive encouragement toward a more positive outlook on his problems if proper guidance is provided in the group setting. Group instruction may be supplemented by individual teaching, particularly with respect to problems of finance and emotional reactions to the diet.

Group instruction must be a democratic process in which everyone feels free to participate. The nurse or dietitian cannot be authoritarian, the talkative patient should not monopolize all of the time, and the self-conscious, shy patient should not be made uncomfortable by having to respond when he is not ready. Verbal instruction should be coordinated with visual aids, including dietary lists, leaflets, posters, food models, and films as the occasion may warrant. The leader of the group cannot change the individual or the group; she can only help them to recognize their own goals and to make their own decisions for change.

PROBLEM AND REVIEW

1. What purposes are served by diet therapy?

2. Discuss the role of diet in total patient care.

3. How can you be sure that the diet prescribed for your patient is meeting his needs?

4. *Problem.* Keep a record of comments that your patients make about their meals. On the basis of these comments what can you do to ensure that your patients enjoy maximum comfort and optimum therapy insofar as their diets are concerned?

5. Discuss reasons why a patient's nutritional status may be unsatisfactory when he comes to the hospital.

6. A patient complains to you that his food is always cold. What steps can you take to correct this?

7. If a patient is having laboratory studies which will extend beyond the lunch hour, what arrangements will you make for the service of his meal?

CHAPTER 24 /

Therapeutic Adaptations of the Normal Diet

Normal, Soft, and Fluid Diets

Therapeutic nutrition begins with the normal diet. No diet is more important in the care of the sick than is the normal diet. In the first place, the majority of ill persons require no modification of the normal diet, but recovery may be hastened when particular attention is given to supplying the needs of normal nutrition. Secondly, therapeutic diets are adaptations of the normal diet and should be so planned that they maintain, or restore, good nutrition in any given situation.

The nutritive value of a basic diet composed of minimum amounts from each of the Four Food Groups is shown on page 327. One of the many ways in which such a foundation diet may be amplified to meet fully the Recommended Dietary Allowances is shown in the calculation on page 341. It will be readily seen that this plan provides for meal patterns which are typical of those used in many hospitals. The additional cup of milk is desirable because it provides so many nutrients required in greater than normal amounts by most individuals recovering from an illness and because milk, contrary to popular opinion, is one of the best-accepted foods in the hospital dietary.

For the sake of convenience in comparing one diet with another, this plan will be used as the basis for dietary evaluation throughout this unit of diet therapy. However, it is emphasized that other equally desirable plans could be used; for example, 2 cups of milk instead of 3 cups; a more generous allowance of meat; more or less fruit, vegetables, cereals, and so on. It must also be remembered that the normal diet does not necessarily represent ideal allowances in illness since past state of nutrition, modification of activity, increased or decreased metabolic demands brought about by the illness, changes in absorption, etc., may increase or decrease the needs for one or more nutrients.

When the normal diet is used as the basis for planning therapeutic diets, it is easy to see what the effects of omissions or additions of specific foods may have on the nutritive value by consulting the calculation for the normal

336

NUTRITIVE VALUE OF THE NORMAL DIET PATTERN AS A BASIS FOR THERAPEUTIC DIETS *

FOOD	MEASURE	WEIGHT gm	ENERGY calories	PROTEIN gm	FAT gm	CARBOHYDRATE gm	MINERALS Ca mg	Fe mg	A I.U.	Thiamine mg	Riboflavin mg	Niacin mg	Ascorbic Acid mg
Milk	3 cups	732	495	27	30	36	855	0.3	1170	0.24	1.26	0.6	6
Meat group													
Egg	1	50	80	6	6	tr	27	1.1	590	0.05	0.15	tr	0
Meat, fish, poultry (lean)	4 ounces	120	300	33	16	tr	16	4.0	2220 †	0.39	0.43	8.7	tr
Vegetables													
Potato	1 medium	122	90	3	tr	21	9	0.7	tr	0.11	0.04	1.4	20
Leafy green or deep yellow	½–⅔ cup	100	30	2	tr	6	70	1.2	9280	0.06	0.12	0.6	30
Other vegetable	½–⅔ cup	100	40	2	tr	8	20	0.6	660	0.06	0.06	0.6	16
Fruits													
Citrus fruit ‡	1 serving	100	45	1	tr	12	27	0.4	120	0.07	0.03	0.2	47
Other fruit	2 servings	200	120	2	tr	32	24	1.0	1200	0.08	0.08	0.8	18
Bread-cereal													
Cereal, enriched, or whole-grain	½ cup	20 (dry)	75	2	tr	16	8	0.6	0	0.11	0.03	0.7	0
Bread, enriched, or whole-grain	3 slices	69	180	6	3	36	57	1.8	tr	0.18	0.15	1.8	0
Butter or margarine	2 tablespoons	28	200	tr	22	tr	6	tr	920	—	—	—	—
TOTAL OF LISTED FOODS (page 338)			1655	84	77	167	1119	11.7	16,160	1.35	2.35	15.4 §	137
Additional foods													
Sugars, sweets	3 tablespoons	36	150	0	0	36	0	0	0	0	0	0	0
Dessert **	1 serving	varies	190	4	6	30	70	0.3	190	0.03	0.10	0.1	tr
Bread	3 slices	69	180	6	3	36	57	1.8	tr	0.18	0.15	1.8	0
			2175	94	86	269	1246	13.8	16,350	1.56	2.60	17.3	137

* The nutritive values of the foods listed for the normal diet, page 338, have been calculated using Table 1 in the Appendix. The additional foods listed at the bottom of the table suggest one of many ways to complete the diet.

† The vitamin-A value is reduced to a trace if an average of 1 ounce liver is not consumed weekly.

‡ Other ascorbic acid-rich foods such as cantaloupe, strawberries, etc., are also included.

§ The tryptophan content of this diet is about 840 mg, equivalent to about 14 mg niacin, thus providing a niacin equivalent of 29.4 mg.

** Desserts include plain gelatin, pie, cake with icing, custard, ice cream, cookies, and plain pudding.

337

pattern on page 337. For example, if an individual is allergic to milk, it becomes immediately apparent that some other means must be sought to provide especially for the calcium, riboflavin, and protein. If vegetables were contra-indicated, as in some very low-residue diets, it is obvious that there will be a deficiency in vitamin A and in ascorbic acid.

The use of the normal diet as a basis for planning therapeutic diets is psychologically advantageous. When as much of the normal diet is retained as possible, the patient is not set apart from his family and friends. Moreover, many foods can usually be used by all persons in the group so that food preparation procedures can be simplified in the home.

The normal diet in the hospital is variously described as regular, general, house, or full diet. It may consist of any and all foods eaten by the person in health. Fried foods, pastries, strongly flavored vegetables, and spices or relishes are not taboo, but good menu planning means that these foods are used judiciously.

REGULAR OR NORMAL DIET

Include these foods, or their nutritive equivalents, daily:

3 cups milk
5 ounces (4 ounces cooked weight) meat, fish, or poultry; cheese, additional
    egg or milk, or legumes may substitute in part
1 egg
4 servings vegetables including:
    1 medium potato
    1 serving dark green leafy or yellow vegetable
    1–2 servings other vegetable
    One of the above vegetables to be served raw
3 servings fruit including:
    1 serving citrus fruit, or other good source of ascorbic acid
    2 servings other fruit
1 serving enriched or whole-grain cereal
3 slices enriched or whole-grain bread
2 tablespoons (1 ounce) butter or fortified margarine

Additional foods such as soups, desserts, sweets, salad dressings, or increased
    amounts of foods listed above will provide adequate calories. See calculation
    on page 337.

MEAL PATTERN   SAMPLE MENU

Breakfast

Fruit   Sliced banana in orange juice
Cereal, enriched or whole-grain   Oatmeal

Milk and sugar for cereal	Milk and sugar
Egg	Soft-cooked egg
Whole-grain or enriched roll or toast	Whole-wheat toast with butter
Butter or margarine	
Hot beverage with cream and sugar	Coffee with cream and sugar

Luncheon or supper

Soup, if desired	
Egg or a substitute of cheese, meat, or fish	Cheese soufflé
Potato, rice, noodles, macaroni, spaghetti, or vegetable	Buttered peas
Salad	Lettuce and tomato salad
	Russian dressing
Enriched or whole-grain bread	Hard roll with butter
Butter or margarine	
Fruit	Royal Anne cherries
Milk	Milk

Dinner

Meat, fish, or poultry	Meat loaf with gravy
Potato	Mashed potato
Vegetable	Buttered carrots
Enriched or whole-grain bread	Enriched white, rye, or whole-wheat bread with butter
Butter or margarine	
Dessert	Apple Betty
Milk	Milk
Coffee or tea, if desired	

Therapeutic modifications of the normal diet. The normal diet may be modified (1) to provide change in consistency as in fluid and soft diets to be described below; (2) to increase or decrease the energy values; (3) to include greater or lesser amounts of one or more nutrients, for example, high protein, low sodium, etc.; (4) to increase or decrease bulk—high- and low-fiber diets; (5) to provide foods bland in flavor; (6) to include or exclude specific foods, as in allergic conditions; and (7) to modify the intervals of feeding.

The use of diet patterns. Throughout this text diets in use at various hospitals have been adapted insofar as practical to a standard style of presentation. The list of foods to include, detailed lists of foods permitted and contraindicated, a typical meal pattern, and sample menu are intended to be used as a guide. Such a presentation is intended to aid the student in rapidly comparing a given regimen with the normal diet, but it is of the utmost importance that this, or any other pattern, not be accepted as a final system which cannot be changed. In a given hospital the dietary patterns in general use will be governed by many factors—ethnic groups served, kind of hospital, economic factors, service facilities, etc. Moreover, the established pattern itself will need to be modified so that the patient's dietary needs can be satisfied even though problems of race, religion, economy, occupation, and idiosyncrasies enter in. Let the diet patterns, then, be a guide—not an inflexible rule!

The modified diets discussed in succeeding chapters of this text are summarized in the tables on pages 348–59.

Nomenclature of diets. Several practices have been, and still are, common in the naming of diets. The literature is replete with illustrations of diets named for their originators. The Sippy diet is a classic example, but there have been many others from time to time. Unfortunately, such nomenclature tells nothing about the nature of the diet, and it would seem to be wise to discourage this practice just as it is generally wise to discourage naming a disease for the doctor who first describes it.

Others have used the name of a disease condition to specify a given diet; thus we have ulcer, nephritic, cardiac diets, etc. Psychologically, this is not good, for the patient should not need to be reminded of his disease every time he looks at his diet list, or every time he notes his tray card in the hospital. Moreover, many of the diets used for some of these conditions are suitable for other purposes as well, and the uninitiated may overlook the full usefulness of a given dietary regimen by such limited terminology.

It will be the practice in this text, insofar as possible, to use a nomenclature which describes the modification in consistency, in nutrients, or in flavor which has been made in the diet. Thus, "bland diet" will replace "ambulatory ulcer diet," "sodium-restricted diet" will replace "cardiac diet," and "moderate-fat-diet" will replace "gallbladder diet," etc.

When the quantity of one or more nutrients is important to the success of the diet, it is essential that these quantities be specified in the diet prescription. Thus, the term "diabetic diet" has little meaning, while a prescription such as: protein, 80 gm; fat, 90 gm; carbohydrate, 200 gm, can be accurately interpreted. Likewise, a "sodium-restricted diet" gives no indication of the exact level of restriction required, while the designation "500 mg sodium diet" leaves no room for misinterpretation.

Mechanical soft diet. Many persons require a soft diet simply because they have no teeth. The objective of dietary planning for such individuals is to modify the normal diet so that foods require little chewing. It is neither desirable nor essential to restrict the patient to the selection allowed on the customary Soft Diet (p. 341) employed for a postoperative patient or for a patient with a gastrointestinal disturbance. For example, stewed onions, baked beans, and apple pie are foods considered to be quite unsuitable for the latter patients but which may be enjoyed by those who simply require foods that are soft in texture. The terms "mechanical soft" and "dental soft" are used in some diet manuals to describe such a dietary modification. The following changes in the normal diet will usually suffice for individuals without teeth:

Meats should be finely minced or ground.

Soft breads are substituted for crusty breads.

Cooked vegetables may be used without restriction, but dicing or chopping may be desirable for some; for example, diced beets, chopped spinach, corn cut from cob.

Most raw vegetables are omitted; raw tomatoes, cut finely, may usually be used. Sometimes finely chopped lettuce in a sandwich may be accepted.

Many raw fruits may be used: banana, orange, grapefruit, soft berries, soft pear, apricots, peaches, grapes with tender skins.

Hard raw fruits such as pineapple and apple are usually avoided; but finely diced apple in fruit cup may be used.

Tough skins should be removed from fruits: raw, soft pear, or baked apple, etc.

Nuts and dried fruits, when used in desserts or other foods, are acceptable if finely chopped.

Soft diet. This diet represents the usual dietary step between the full fluid and normal diet. It may be used in acute infections, some gastrointestinal disturbances, and following surgery. The diet is soft in consistency, easy to chew, made up of simple, easily digested food, and contains no harsh fiber, no rich or highly flavored food. It is nutritionally adequate when planned on the basis of the normal diet.

SOFT DIET

Include these foods, or their nutritive equivalents, daily:

3 cups milk

5 ounces (4 ounces cooked weight) very tender or ground meat, fish, or poultry; soft cheese, or additional eggs or milk may substitute in part

1 egg

4 servings vegetable including:
    1 medium potato
    1 serving dark green or yellow vegetable—tender chopped or strained
    2 servings other vegetable—tender chopped or strained

3 servings fruit including:
    2 servings citrus fruit or juice
    1 serving banana, cooked fruit without skin or seeds, or strained cooked fruit

1 serving enriched or strained whole-grain cereal

3 slices enriched or fine whole-grain bread

2 tablespoons butter or fortified margarine

Additional foods such as soups, desserts, sweets, or increased amounts of the above will provide adequate calories.

Nutritive value: See calculation for the normal diet on page 337.

Foods allowed:	**Foods to avoid:**
All beverages	
Bread—white, fine whole-wheat, rye without seeds; white crackers	*Bread*—coarse dark; whole-grain crackers; hot breads; pancakes; waffles
Cereal foods—dry, such as cornflakes, Puffed Rice, rice flakes; fine cooked, such as corn meal, farina, hominy grits, macaroni, noodles, rice, spaghetti; strained coarse, such as oatmeal, Pettijohn's, whole-wheat	*Cereals*—bran; coarse unless strained
Cheese—mild, soft, such as cottage and cream; Cheddar; Swiss	*Cheese*—sharp, such as Roquefort, Camembert, Limburger
Desserts—plain cake, cookies; custards; plain gelatin or with allowed fruit; Junket; plain ice cream, ices, sherbets; plain puddings, such as bread, cornstarch, rice, tapioca	*Desserts*—any made with dried fruit or nuts; pastries; rich puddings or cake
Eggs—all except fried	*Eggs*—fried
Fats—butter, cream, margarine, vegetable oils and fats in cooking	*Fats*—fried foods
Fruits—raw: ripe avocado, banana, grapefruit or orange sections without membrane; canned or cooked: apples, apricots, fruit cocktail, peaches, pears, plums—all without skins; Royal Anne cherries; strained prunes and other fruits with skins; all juices	*Fruits*—raw except as listed; stewed or canned berries; pineapple; with tough skins
Meat—very tender, minced, or ground; baked, broiled, creamed, roast, or stewed: beef, lamb, veal, poultry, fish, bacon, liver, sweetbreads	*Meat*—tough with gristle or fat; salted and smoked meat or fish, such as corned beef, smoked herring; cold cuts; frankfurter; pork
Milk—in any form	
Soups—broth, strained cream or vegetable	*Soups*—fatty or highly seasoned
Sweets—all sugars, sirup, jelly, honey, plain sugar candy without fruit or nuts, molasses Use in moderation.	*Sweets*—jam, marmalade, rich candies with chocolate
Vegetables—white or sweet potato without skin, any way except fried; young and tender asparagus, beets, carrots, peas, pumpkin, squash without seeds; tender chopped greens; strained cooked vegetables if not tender; tomato juice	*Vegetables*—raw; strongly flavored, such as broccoli, Brussels sprouts, cabbage, cauliflower, cucumber, onion, radish, sauerkraut, turnip; corn; dried beans and peas; potato chips

Foods allowed (*continued*)

Miscellaneous—salt, seasonings and spices in moderation, gravy, cream sauces

Foods to avoid (*continued*)

Miscellaneous—pepper and other hot spices; fried foods; nuts; olives; pickles; relishes

MEAL PATTERN

Breakfast

Fruit or fruit juice
Cereal—strained, if coarse
Milk and sugar for cereal
Egg
Soft roll or toast
Butter or fortified margarine
Hot beverage with cream and sugar

SAMPLE MENU

Orange sections and banana slices
Oatmeal
Milk and sugar for cereal
Soft-cooked egg
Buttered toast

Coffee

Luncheon or supper

Strained soup, if desired
Egg or substitute of mild cheese, tender or ground meat, fish, or poultry
Potato without skin, rice, noodles, macaroni, or spaghetti; or
Cooked vegetable
Enriched bread
Butter or fortified margarine
Fruit
Milk
Coffee or tea, if desired

Cream of tomato soup
Cheese soufflé

Tender peas
Soft roll
Butter
Royal Anne cherries
Milk
Coffee or tea, if desired

Dinner

Orange, grapefruit, or tomato juice
Tender or ground meat, fish, or poultry

Potato, any way except fried
Cooked vegetable
Enriched bread
Butter or fortified margarine
Dessert
Milk
Hot beverage with cream and sugar, if desired

Grapefruit juice
Meat loaf (no onion or pepper) with gravy
Mashed potato
Buttered carrots
Rye bread without seeds
Butter
Baked apple without skin; cream
Milk
Tea with sugar and lemon

Liquid diets. Fluid diets are used in febrile states, postoperatively, or whenever the patient is unable to tolerate solid foods. The degree to which these diets are adequate will depend upon the type of liquids permitted.

Clear-fluid diets. Whenever an acute illness or surgery produces a marked intolerance for food as may be evident by nausea, vomiting, anorexia, distention, and diarrhea, it is advisable to restrict the intake of nutrients. A clear-fluid diet is usually used for 1 to 2 days, at the end of which time the patient is commonly able to retain and utilize a more liberal liquid diet.

Tea with lemon and sugar, coffee, fat-free broth, carbonated beverages, and cereal waters are the usual liquids permitted. In addition, strained fruit juices, fruit ices, and plain gelatin are often included. A more liberal clear-fluid diet permits the addition of egg white, whole egg, and gelatin to strained fruit juices and other beverages. The recipes for beverages (p. 669) will prove to be of value in the planning and preparation of this diet.

The amount of fluid in a given feeding on the clear-fluid diet is usually restricted to 30 to 60 ml per hour at first, with gradually increasing amounts being given as the patient's tolerance improves. Obviously, such a diet can accomplish little beyond the replacement of fluids.

Full-fluid diet. This diet is indicated whenever a patient is acutely ill or is unable to chew or swallow solid food. It includes all foods liquid at room temperature and at body temperature. It is free from cellulose and irritating condiments.

When properly planned, this diet can be used for relatively long periods of time. From the stated nutritive values on page 345 it appears that iron, thiamine, and niacin are provided at inadequate levels. The excellent quality of protein in this diet may be counted upon to supply tryptophan amounting to about 850 mg daily, or niacin equivalent to 14 mg, thus bringing the total niacin to 19 mg. Two additional eggs would improve the iron and thiamine levels; brewers' yeast might also be used; or a supplement might be prescribed.

FULL-FLUID DIET

General rules:

Give six or more feedings daily.

The protein content of the diet can be increased by incorporating whole egg, egg white, nonfat dry milk in beverages and soups. Strained canned meats (used for infant feeding) may be added to broths.

The caloric value of the diet may be increased by: (1) substituting 10 per cent cream for part of the usual milk allowance; (2) adding butter to cereal gruels and soups; (3) including glucose in beverages; (4) using ice cream as dessert or in beverages.

If a decreased volume of fluid is desired, nonfat dry milk may be substituted for part of the fluid milk.

Include these foods, or their nutritive equivalents, daily:

6 cups milk
2 eggs
1–2 ounces strained meat
½ cup strained cooked cereal for gruel
¼ cup vegetable purée for cream soup
1 cup citrus fruit juice
½ cup tomato or vegetable juice
1 tablespoon cocoa
3 tablespoons sugar
1 tablespoon butter
2 servings plain gelatin dessert, Junket, custard, ices, or plain ice cream
Broth or bouillon

Nutritive values of foods specified above: Calories, 1950; protein, 85 gm; calcium, 2.1 gm; iron, 7.7 mg; vitamin A, 7150 I.U.; thiamine, 1.1 mg; riboflavin, 3.2 mg; niacin, 5.0 mg; ascorbic acid, 160 mg.

Foods allowed: *Avoid all foods not specifically listed below*

Beverages—carbonated, cocoa, coffee or substitute, tea
Cereal—fine or strained whole-grain: in gruels only
Dessert—soft or baked custard, gelatin without fruit or nuts, plain ice cream, ice, sherbet, Junket, plain cornstarch puddings
Eggs—raw in broth, with fruit juice, or in milk; soft-cooked
Fruit—all strained juices
Meat—strained in soups
Soup—strained cream, meat, or vegetable; no pepper or onion
Vegetables—purée for soups; juices
Miscellaneous—butter, cocoa, flavoring extracts, sugar, salt

MEAL PATTERN	SAMPLE MENU
Breakfast	
Citrus juice	Orange juice
Cereal gruel with butter, sugar	Cream of wheat with milk, butter, and
Milk	sugar
Beverage with cream, sugar	Coffee with cream and sugar
Midmorning	
Fruit juice with egg	Lemonade with egg white
or	
Milk, plain, malted, chocolate,	
or eggnog	

MEAL PATTERN	SAMPLE MENU

Luncheon or supper

Strained soup	Beef broth with strained meat
Tomato juice	Tomato juice
Custard, Junket, ice cream, sherbet, ice, gelatin dessert or plain pudding	Maple Junket
Eggnog, milk, or cocoa	Milk
Tea with sugar, if desired	Tea with sugar and cream

Midafternoon

Same as at midmorning	Pineapple eggnog

Dinner

Strained cream soup	Cream of carrot soup
Citrus juice	Grapefruit juice
Custard, Junket, ice cream, ice, sherbet, or gelatin dessert	Vanilla ice cream
Milk or cocoa	Cocoa
Tea, if desired	Tea with sugar and lemon

Evening nourishment

Same as at midmorning	Hot malted milk

Other methods of feeding. Food by mouth is the method of choice when the patient can eat, digest, and absorb sufficient food to meet his nutritive requirements. In illness, however, it may be occasionally necessary to augment the oral intake by giving parenteral feedings of one type or another.

When the patient is unable to chew or swallow because of deformity or inflammation of the mouth or throat, corrosive poisoning, unconsciousness, paralysis of the throat muscles, etc., tube feeding is used (see p. 401).

Intravenous feeding is used when it is necessary to rest the patient's stomach completely. Fluids given by such means include solutions of glucose, amino acids, salts, and vitamins. Fat emulsions have been employed successfully by a few, thus making it possible to provide sufficient calories as well as protein, minerals, and vitamins. Transfusions of whole blood or of plasma are commonly used.

PROBLEMS AND REVIEW

1. Why is the normal diet used as a basis for planning therapeutic diets?
2. What is meant by routine house diets?
3. What are the advantages of developing dietary patterns for a given individual, or institution? What are the limitations?

4. What objections can you see to the following examples of dietary nomenclature: nephritic diet; low-protein diet; Kempner diet; ulcer discharge diet? Examine the nomenclature used in your hospital and suggest ways in which it might be improved.

5. *Problem.* Write a menu for 1 day for a patient who is to receive a regular diet. Indicate the changes you would make in this menu to make it suitable for another patient requiring a soft diet.

6. *Problem.* Plan a full-fluid diet for 1 day which will provide 2500 calories. Calculate the protein, calories, iron, and ascorbic acid. Compare with the recommended allowances for a 45-year-old man.

7. What foods are usually allowed on a clear-fluid diet? What nutrients are lacking in this diet?

8. From your work with patients up to this time, what modifications of the normal diet have you observed so far?

SUMMARY OF ROUTINE AND THERAPEUTIC DIETS

TYPE OF DIET	INDICATIONS FOR USE OF DIET	CHARACTERISTICS OF THE DIET	FOOD SELECTION
Regular or Normal Diet (Chap. 24)	Most frequently used of all diets; used for all ambulatory and bed patients whose condition does not necessitate a modified diet. Many modified diets progress ultimately to the regular diet All therapeutic diets are based upon the normal diet	This diet provides recommended allowances of all nutrients, permits the use of all foods, and follows the principles of good meal planning and preparation for any normal diet	*Basic foods included:* 2–3 cups milk 1 egg 4 ounces meat, poultry, fish 1 medium potato 1 serving green leafy or deep yellow vegetable 1 serving other vegetable 2 servings fruit including 1 citrus 1 serving enriched or whole-grain cereal 3 slices bread Others as desired for sufficient calories
Soft Diet (Chap. 24)	One of the most frequently used routine diets; many patients are placed on this until diagnosis is made. It bridges the gap between acute illness and convalescence	This diet is nutritionally adequate; it is soft in texture and bland in flavor A mechanical soft diet is a regular diet modified in texture for a person who cannot chew satisfactorily	*Foods included:* Milk, cream, mild cheese; eggs, except fried; tender, minced, or ground meat, poultry, fish; cooked, mild-flavored, low-fiber vegetables; cooked fruits without seeds or skin, citrus juices and sections, ripe banana; white or fine-grained breads and cereals; plain cakes, cookies, puddings; fats; sweets *Foods to avoid:* Those with skin, seeds, coarse fiber; raw fruit, except citrus and banana; raw and strongly flavored vegetables; coarse cereals and breads; rich pastries; fried foods; tough meats; highly seasoned food *Intervals of feeding:* Usually three meals; intermediate feedings if needed

Diet	Description	Used in / Indications	Foods included
Clear-fluid Diet (Chap. 24)	The diet is made up of clear liquids that leave no residue; it is nondistending, nonirritating, and nonstimulating to peristaltic action. This diet is entirely inadequate from a nutritional standpoint; its use is usually limited to 24 to 48 hours	In acute infections before diagnosis; in acute inflammatory conditions of the intestinal tract; in acute diarrhea; following operations on the colon or rectum when it is necessary to prevent evacuation for several days. To relieve thirst, to supply water to the tissues	*Foods included:* Tea, coffee, and coffee substitutes; fat-free broths; carbonated beverages; cane sugar or glucose in moderation. *Occasionally permitted:* Fruit juices, egg white, whole egg, gelatin, thin water gruels. *Intervals of feeding:* Small amounts every 1 to 2 hours
Full-fluid Diet (Chap. 24)	The normal diet is restricted to those foods which are liquid or which become liquid on reaching the stomach. This diet may be made adequate with careful planning and may be used for an extended period of time	This diet bridges the gap between the clear-fluid and soft diet. It is used in acute infections, gastritis, diarrhea when milk is permitted, following surgery, and for patients too ill to eat solid or semisolid foods	*Foods included:* All liquids included on the clear-fluid diet plus milk in all forms including malted milk, milk shakes, chocolate milk or cocoa, eggnogs; soups; soft custard; plain ice cream; Junket; tomato juice and fruit juices; plain gelatin. *Intervals of feeding:* Usually 2- to 4-hour intervals
Tube Feeding (Chap. 29)	A liquid diet providing normal nutritional requirements. May be modified for one or more nutrients such as protein, fat, carbohydrate, sodium, etc. Fiber is carefully removed. May be prepared from calculated formula of selected foods; or may be prepared by liquefying foods of a normal diet in a blender and storing	Inability to chew or to swallow; obstruction of esophagus; anorexia nervosa; severe burns; gastric surgery	*Foods included:* All foods of a normal diet which are liquid or which can be liquefied in a blender. *Intervals of feeding:* Hourly at first with small feedings; then every 3 to 4 hours
Very Low-residue Diet (Chap. 31)	This diet is made up of foods which can be completely absorbed, thereby leaving little or no residue for formation of feces. Insufficient minerals and vitamins are provided; if used for more than a few days it must be supplemented	Severe diarrhea to afford rest to the gastrointestinal tract. Ulcerative colitis in initial stages. Preceding and following operations on the colon or rectum when no movement is desired for several days. Partial intestinal obstruction	*Foods included:* Eggs; tender meat, fish, or poultry; fruit juices; refined cereals and breads; butter or margarine; sugar; fat-free clear soups; plain gelatin desserts; coffee, tea

349

(continued)

SUMMARY OF THERAPEUTIC DIETS (continued)

TYPE OF DIET	INDICATIONS FOR USE OF DIET	CHARACTERISTICS OF THE DIET	FOOD SELECTION
Very Low-residue Diet (cont.)		Usually progresses to Bland Diet, IV and V	*Foods to avoid:* Milk; cheese; vegetables; fruits (except juices); coarse breads and cereals; tough meats; rich desserts; fried foods or excessive fat; condiments; relishes; excessive sweets. *Intervals of feeding:* Usually three meals; intermediate feedings if necessary
Bland Diet Stages IV and V (Chap. 30)	This diet is used to neutralize acid, to reduce gastric secretion and motility, and to avoid gastrointestinal irritation 1. Gastric and duodenal ulcers 2. Gastritis 3. Diarrhea 4. Ulcerative colitis (see High-protein Diet)	Five stages of this diet are described in the text. Stages IV and V are nutritionally adequate. This diet is mechanically, chemically, and thermally nonirritating. When used for the treatment of ulcers, small frequent feedings are necessary. Rest, relaxation, and a happy environment are essential to success of dietary treatment	*Foods included* (stages IV and V): Milk, cream, butter, mild cheeses; eggs; tender meat, fish, poultry; cooked fruits and vegetables; citrus fruits, fruits, banana; enriched bread; refined cereals; white potato, macaroni, rice, etc.; plain desserts. *Foods to avoid:* Foods with seeds, skin, coarse fiber; strongly flavored vegetables most raw fruits and vegetables, berries, pineapple; meat extractives and sauces; spices, and seasonings in excess; relishes, pickles; caffeine-containing beverages; alcohol. *Intervals of feeding:* Three meals with three intermediate feedings

High-fiber Diet (Chap. 31)	When there is marked stasis in the colon resulting from impairment in the tone of the muscles lining the tract—atonic constipation	Normal diet with fiber increased to 10 to 11 gm daily Fluid intake increased to 2000 ml or more daily; 1 to 2 glasses water before breakfast Concentrated foods replaced by those of greater bulk	*Foods included:* All foods of the normal diet with emphasis on long-fibered vegetables such as greens, kale, cabbage, celery; raw vegetable salads; raw and cooked fruits; whole-grain cereals and breads *Foods to restrict:* Highly refined and concentrated foods; excessive amounts of rough bran; excessive seasonings *Intervals of feeding:* Three meals daily
High-calorie Diet (Chap. 27)	This diet is used especially in fevers, in diseases with high metabolic rate such as hyperthyroidism, following prolonged or severe illness which has resulted in loss of weight and undernutrition	This is a normal diet with an increase in the caloric level to 3000 to 5000 daily Reinforcements such as sugars and fats are used. If appetite is poor, small servings of highly reinforced foods are given The diet may be modified in consistency and flavor according to specific needs	*Foods included:* All foods of the normal diet with added glucose and other sugars and sweets; increased amounts of cereals, breads, potatoes, etc.; butter, cream, and other fats *Foods to avoid:* Excessive amounts of bulky, low-calorie foods; fried foods or others which may interfere with appetite *Intervals of feeding:* Four to six meals daily
Low-calorie Diet (Chap. 27)	Treatment of obesity, especially important in: 1. Diabetes mellitus 2. Cardiovascular and renal diseases 3. Hypertension 4. Gout 5. Gallbladder disease 6. Preceding surgery	Normal diet with energy value reduced to 1500, 1200, or 1000 calories Protein levels at 65 to 100 gm Fats and carbohydrate restricted to caloric limit of the diet Low-carbohydrate fruits and vegetables are used, with restriction of concentrated sugars, fats	*Foods included:* (1200 calorie diet) 3 cups milk 2 group A vegetables (Appendix, Table 4) 1 group B vegetable 3 fruit exchanges 2 bread exchanges 5 meat exchanges 1 fat exchange

(continued)

SUMMARY OF THERAPEUTIC DIETS (*continued*)

TYPE OF DIET	INDICATIONS FOR USE OF DIET	CHARACTERISTICS OF THE DIET	FOOD SELECTION
Low-calorie Diet (*cont.*)		Concentrates of vitamin A and thiamine usually required for diets below 1000 calories	*Foods to avoid:* All except those allowed in the exchange lists *Intervals of feeding:* Three meals daily; may use six smaller meals, if desired
High-protein Diet (Chap. 26)	Protein deficiency following inadequate intake, before and after surgery, injury, burns, high fevers, increased metabolic rate (see High-calorie Diet)	This is a regular diet with protein increased to 100–150 gm or more daily It may be planned as a soft or fluid diet when necessary Each meal should contain complete protein for optimum utilization Carbohydrate and fat must be liberal to cover energy needs	*Foods included:* All foods on regular diet with emphasis on dry and liquid milk; eggs; cheese; lean meat, fish, poultry *Intervals of feeding:* Three meals with evening feeding. Midmorning and midafternoon feedings of high-protein beverages may also be used
(Chap. 40)	Nephrosis, chiefly in children	Protein allowance of 3 to 4 gm per kg Sodium restriction when marked edema is present	Low-sodium milk may replace regular milk if sodium is restricted; foods cooked without salt
(Chap. 37)	Chronic nephritis to cover protein losses in the urine Not indicated when there is marked nitrogen retention	Protein for a normal diet plus allowance to cover loss in the urine; usually 80 to 100 gm daily Ample calories essential to reduce tissue catabolism Mild to moderate sodium restriction often needed	
(Chap. 38)	Pernicious anemia (see also Bland Diet)	About 100–150 gm protein daily Fat is often poorly tolerated A soft diet may be needed	*Foods to avoid:* Fatty meats; fried foods; salad dressings; gravies and sauces; rich cakes, cookies, desserts; high-fiber fruits, vegetables, cereals; excessive seasonings

(Chap. 31)	Ulcerative colitis (see also Bland Diet)	100–150 gm protein daily 3500–4000 calories Bland, low-fiber foods	Food selection as for the Bland Diet, usually Stages IV and V. Milk often poorly tolerated; may be evaporated, homogenized, boiled. If omitted, must provide liberal lean meat and eggs
(Chap. 32)	Hepatitis Cirrhosis of the liver without hepatic coma	100–150 gm protein 100–150 gm fat 300–400 gm carbohydrate Sodium restricted to 250 mg daily if ascites present Soft diet without coarse fiber when esophageal varices are present	All foods on regular diet with emphasis on milk, eggs, lean meat, fish, poultry *Foods to avoid:* If sodium is restricted, regular milk, salted foods in cooking or at table (see Sodium-restricted Diet)
(Chap. 34)	Hyperinsulinism (see Low-carbohydrate Diet)		
(Chap. 29)	Dumping syndrome (see Low-carbohydrate Diet)		
(Chap. 40)	Celiac disease Cystic fibrosis	6 to 8 gm protein per kg; gradual return to normal in celiac disease Fat is markedly restricted; some unsaturated fats tolerated in mild celiac syndrome Carbohydrate restricted to formula at first; then simple sugars in small amounts; starch only after 6 to 12 months without severe diarrhea Puréed foods with gradual return to normal foods by 3 to 4 years of age Vitamin supplements always used Pancreatin for patients with cystic fibrosis	*Food selection:* High-protein formula with glucose or banana powder Gradual additions of ripe banana, applesauce; strained meat, low-fat cottage cheese; puréed carrots, green beans; egg yolk; gelatin; citrus juices Diet is gradually liberalized according to individual progress (see schedules in Chap. 40)

(continued)

TYPE OF DIET	INDICATIONS FOR USE OF DIET	CHARACTERISTICS OF THE DIET	FOOD SELECTION
Protein-restricted Diet (Chap. 37)	Hepatic coma Chronic uremia Acute glomerulonephritis	Protein is restricted to 20 to 60 gm daily Carbohydrate is liberal Adequate calories for maintenance should be derived from carbohydrate and fat to avoid burning of body tissue Sodium may be restricted to 500 mg or less This diet may be of soft, liquid, or regular consistency	*Foods included* (40 gm protein) ½ cup milk ½ cup cream, light 1 egg 1 ounce meat 2 potatoes 2–3 servings vegetables 3 servings fruit 1 cup fruit juice 1 serving cereal 4 slices bread 3 tablespoons butter *Foods to avoid:* In excess of amounts stated above: meat; eggs; milk; bread; cereal Avoid entirely: legumes; nuts; gelatin At 20 gm protein level omit all milk, meat, egg
Protein-free Diet (Chap. 37)	Hepatic coma Acute anuria	This diet provides carbohydrate and fat for about 1500 to 2000 calories daily The diet is used only as an emergency measure, and is then progressed to 20 gm, 40 gm, and 60 gm protein	*Foods included:* Fruit juices with glucose if potassium is not restricted Butter-sugar mixture Sugar-fat emulsions
High-carbohydrate Diet (Chaps. 17, 32, 37)	Toxemias of pregnancy Liver disturbances (see High-protein diets) Acute glomerulonephritis Uremia Addison's disease Preparation for surgery	To ensure sufficient calories to meet energy needs, minimizing tissue catabolism Other modifications depend upon condition for which diet is used; for example, low-protein in hepatic coma, or high-protein in hepatitis without coma	*Foods included:* High-carbohydrate foods: glucose; sucrose, sirups, jellies; fine cereals and breads; simple starchy puddings; fruits and vegetables high in carbohydrate Milk, eggs, lean meat, fish, poultry, fats according to diet prescribed *Intervals of feeding:* Three meals with interval feedings

Carbohydrate-restricted Diet (Chap. 33)	Diabetes mellitus	Most diabetic diets are now only moderately restricted in carbohydrate; nutrients are provided at levels for normal nutrition Each diet is individually prescribed for protein, fat, and carbohydrate	The diet is calculated using the exchange lists; daily meals are selected from these lists (see Table 4, Appendix)
(Chap. 34)	Hyperinsulinism	The carbohydrate level is drastically reduced to minimize the production of insulin Protein, fat, and small amounts of carbohydrate are evenly divided in three meals for uniform, gradual rate of absorption, and reduced stimulation to insulin production 120–140 gm protein 75–125 gm carbohydrate Fat to complete the caloric requirement	The diet is calculated using meal exchange lists (Table 4, Appendix). *Intervals of feeding:* Three meals with equal distribution of protein, fat, and carbohydrate at each meal
(Chap. 27)	Obesity (see Low-calorie Diet)		
(Chap. 35)	Epilepsy (see High-fat Diet)	Carbohydrate drastically reduced to 10–30 gm daily	
(Chap. 40)	Celiac disease (see High-protein Diet)		
(Chap. 29)	Dumping syndrome	Three routines are described in the text. The first is carbohydrate free, with gradual progression in routines II and III Six small meals high in protein and fat, and low in carbohydrate Carbohydrate foods are measured carefully Liquids are given only between meals Vitamin and iron supplementation is essential	*Foods included liberally:* Meat, poultry, fish, eggs, peanut butter Butter, margarine, bacon *Foods restricted:* Breads, cereals, pastes, vegetables, fruits *Foods omitted:* Sugar, candy, sirup, milk, ice cream, chocolate, gravies, rich sauces

(continued)

TYPE OF DIET	INDICATIONS FOR USE OF DIET	CHARACTERISTICS OF THE DIET	FOOD SELECTION
High-fat Diet (ketogenic) (Chap. 35)	To produce an acidosis: 1. Epilepsy for alleviation of seizures	Protein is limited to ⅔–1 gm per kg of body weight; carbohydrates are restricted to less than 30 gm per day, but not less than 10 gm; sufficient fat is provided for adequate energy, and to effect a state of ketosis. The diet must be calculated for each patient, and the daily food allowances must be weighed. Calcium, iron, and the water-soluble vitamins should be supplied in the form of concentrates. Fluids are usually restricted	*Foods included:* Cream (40 per cent); butter; bacon; salad oils and salad dressings; meat, eggs, cheese; small amounts of low-carbohydrate fruits and vegetables. Cellu bran wafers may be used for bulk. *Foods to avoid:* Breads and cereals; desserts; sugar, candy, sirups and all sweets; cakes, cookies, pastries; fruits and vegetables high in carbohydrate. *Intervals of feeding:* Three meals of equal carbohydrate, fat, and protein content
Moderate- to Low-fat Diet (Chaps. 27, 32, 40)	Gallbladder disturbances. Obesity (see Low-calorie Diet). Celiac disease, sprue, and pancreatic disease (see High-protein Diet). Intestinal disturbances when membranes show a sensitivity to fatty acids (see also Bland Diet)	For gallbladder disease, fats are moderately restricted, using those easily digested in amounts to ensure palatability. In obesity fats are restricted to ensure low caloric level. Fats are poorly tolerated in celiac disease and are severely restricted. When butter and whole milk are omitted, it is necessary to supply fat-soluble vitamin supplements, if there is inability to convert carotene to vitamin A	*Foods included:* Milk, whole or skim; egg; lean meat; cottage cheese; egg white; bread and cereals; fruits; vegetables. *Foods to avoid:* Fatty meat; gravies; salad dressings; rich desserts; pastries; fried foods. Strongly flavored vegetables, legumes, melons often poorly tolerated

Diet	Indications	Description	Foods
Modified-fat Diet (Chap. 36)	Atherosclerosis	A diet is planned to provide nutritional requirements with no more than 25–30 gm fat. The intake of polyunsaturated fatty acids is increased by adding 30 to 90 ml corn, cottonseed, soybean, or other oil rich in linoleic acid	*Foods included:* Skim milk; lean meat, fish, and poultry in measured amounts; fruits; vegetables; breads; cereals; sugars and sweets; Soybean, cottonseed, corn oil may be stressed for their linoleic acid content. *Foods to avoid:* Those rich in saturated fats: fat of meats, butter, hydrogenated fats; whole milk, etc.
Sodium-restricted Diet (Chap. 36)	To prevent edema in: 1. Nephritis 2. Nephrosis 3. Cardiac disease 4. Cirrhosis of the liver 5. Toxemia of pregnancy 6. ACTH therapy Hypertension	The basic diet for the adult using selected unsalted foods contains 500 mg sodium. When sodium is reduced to 200 mg, low-sodium milk is necessary. Protein should be sufficient for maintenance and repair. Bland, easily digested foods in small feedings are essential for critical illness	*Foods in specified amounts:* Milk, meat, eggs, fish, or poultry. *Unrestricted foods:* Unsalted cereals or breads; fruits; vegetables; unsalted fats; sugars. *Foods to avoid:* All salted foods: canned fish, meat, vegetables; pickles, relishes, meat sauces; salted butter, bread, nuts. Foods containing regular baking powder or soda: cakes, cookies, prepared mixes, quick breads. Spinach, beets, beet greens, kale, celery, chard, dandelion, carrots, sauerkraut
Acid-ash Diet (Chap. 37)	To aid in adjusting the reaction of the urine so that salts are held in solution: kidney stones—calcium and magnesium phosphates, carbonates, and oxalates	This diet, when carefully planned, meets the requirements for normal nutrition. Acid-ash foods are emphasized—flesh foods, eggs, cereals. Fruits and vegetables of low alkaline ash are chosen. Neutral foods may be used as desired	*Foods included:* Large servings of meat, fish, poultry, eggs, whole-grain cereals, soda crackers, bread, cake, rice, macaroni, noodles, corn, plums, prunes, cranberries. Limit: Milk, fruits, vegetables. Neutral foods as desired: butter, sugar, plain candies, tapioca, oils and fat, coffee, tea

(continued)

357

SUMMARY OF THERAPEUTIC DIETS (continued)

TYPE OF DIET	INDICATIONS FOR USE OF DIET	CHARACTERISTICS OF THE DIET	FOOD SELECTION
Acid-ash Diet (cont.)		Sodium is carefully calculated when used for cardiac edema. No salt is then used in food preparation	*Foods to avoid:* Legumes, spinach, greens, dried fruits, molasses, olives, parsnips, salty foods such as canned fish and canned vegetables, salted nuts, catsup, relishes
Alkaline-ash Diet (Chap. 37)	To aid in adjusting the reaction of the urine so that salts are held in solution: kidney stones—uric acid and cystine calculi	This diet meets the requirements of normal nutrition Alkaline-ash foods such as fruits, vegetables, and milk are emphasized Acid-ash foods are limited to those necessary for good nutrition Neutral foods may be used as desired	*Foods included:* Large amounts of fruits, vegetables, milk Limited amounts: 2 ounces meat 1 egg 1 serving cereal 1–2 slices bread As desired: butter, sugar, oils and fats *Foods to limit or avoid:* Meat, fish, fowl; eggs; cheese; prunes, plums, cranberries, corn; breakfast cereals, macaroni, rice; cakes, cookies, crackers
Calcium- and Phosphorus-restricted Diet (Chap. 37)	To reduce the absorption of calcium and phosphorus, and thus to minimize the tendency to form urinary calculi	This diet provides maintenance levels of calcium and phosphorus, and is otherwise adequate	*Foods included:* 1½ cups milk 1 egg 6 ounces meat 3 servings vegetables 3 servings fruit 2 servings cereals 6 slices bread 2 tablespoons fat

Diet	Disease	Description	Foods
			Foods to avoid: Those made with milk, cheese; whole-grain breads, cereals, flours; legumes; nuts; milk; eggs and meat in excess of allowance; collards, kale, turnip greens, oysters, clams, and other high-calcium or high-phosphorus foods
Low-purine Diet (Chap. 34)	Gout	This is usually a normal diet with restriction of foods containing purine. The amount of fat may be limited because fats interfere with the excretion of urates. Whenever obesity is present, a low-calorie diet is necessary (see Low-calorie diet)	*Foods included:* Milk, eggs, cereals and bread, potato, vegetables (note exceptions), fruits, butter in moderation. *Foods to avoid:* Meat extracts, bouillon, gravies; meats, especially organ meats; fish; anchovies; sardines; alcoholic beverages
Wheat-, Oat-, Rye-free Diet (Chap. 31)	Celiac disease Nontropical sprue	A nutritionally adequate diet from which all foods containing gluten and gliadin have been eliminated. Mineral and vitamin supplementation is often indicated in severe steatorrhea	*Foods included:* Milk, meat, fish, poultry, eggs, fruits, vegetables, fats, sweets, rice, corn, soybean breads and cereals. *Foods to avoid:* All wheat, oat, rye, or barley breads, cereals, and flours or foods containing them
Galactose-free Diet (Chap. 40)	Galactosemia	An infant formula using no milk is needed. Soybean preparations, synthetic formulas, and meat-base formulas may be used	*Foods included:* All foods suitable for infant feeding except milk and milk-containing foods
Low-phenyl-alanine Diet (Chap. 40)	Phenylketonuria	Protein foods contain about 5 per cent phenylalanine. Therefore, all protein foods are severely restricted to permit 15 to 40 mg phenylalanine per kg daily	*Foods included:* A proprietary formula low in phenylalanine is used. With increasing age of the child, small amounts of low-protein fruits and vegetables are gradually added

CHAPTER 25

Short Methods of Dietary Calculation Including Use of the Meal Exchange Lists

Need for quick methods of dietary calculation. Some therapeutic diets must be planned within a stated maximum of one or more nutrients, for example, the low-fat diet. For other diets, such as the diabetic diet, protein, fat, and carbohydrate levels must be kept within relatively narrow allowances of the prescription. Physicians sometimes request that the intake of one or several of the nutrients be charted from day to day for certain patients. Thus, the nurse and dietitian in their daily care of the nutritional needs of the patient are frequently expected to make quick, yet reasonably accurate, estimations of nutritive value.

The uses of Table 1 in the Appendix, page 720, were described in Chapter 3, and the student undoubtedly has had some experiences with dietary calculation on the basis of this table. Unquestionably of value for many purposes, it soon becomes evident that day-to-day calculations of all the listed nutrients—or for selected nutrients—are much too time consuming for the nurse or dietitian with many responsibilities. Such detailed calculations are not justified unless great care is also taken in carefully controlling the preparation procedures, and accurately measuring or weighing all food served to the patient and likewise all food which is returned on the tray. Moreover, the body itself varies from day to day in its net utilization of food, depending upon activity, endocrine balance, and the proportions of nutrients presented to it. Thus, it is evident that dietary calculation should be directed to reasonable assurances of control without time-wasting paper work. To this end, two short methods of dietary calculation will be discussed here.

Food composition table for short method. A number of short tables of food composition have been developed for determining nutritive values of diets used in group feeding situations. One of these is presented in Table 2 of the

Appendix, page 764. It will be noted that foods having similar nutritive values have been grouped together, thus assigning average energy, protein, mineral, and vitamin values to all foods within the group. For example, under *Cereals,* bread, crackers, breakfast cereals, and pastes such as macaroni have been grouped. Thus, one may count the total number of servings of cereal foods fed during the day, keeping refined and whole-grain or enriched cereals in separate categories. Suppose that the following cereal foods were eaten on a given day: ½ cup oatmeal, ½ slice whole-wheat bread, 1 soft enriched roll, 2 slices enriched toast, and macaroni and cheese (½ cup unenriched macaroni). The calculations would then be based on 1 serving unenriched cereal and 4½ servings whole-grain and enriched cereal, thereby avoiding the necessity of looking up five different items.

Uses for the short method. Once the student has become familiar with the arrangement of items in the table and learns to translate the amount of food actually served to the size of servings described in the table she will find that much valuable time is saved when the adequacy of a diet is to be determined. This table is especially useful in the periodic check that a dietitian gives to her menus served in the hospital, institution, school dormitory, or school lunchroom.

If a single diet is calculated by using the data of Table 1 and again with the short method of Table 2, some variations will be noted. However, these variations tend to cancel out when Table 2 is used for calculations of many menus. The differences are not significant for the purposes for which the short method is intended.

Procedure for calculation. The following steps are followed in using Table 2:

1. Record the amount of food served at each meal. If any food is refused, subtract it from the amount served.

2. Group the foods eaten according to the groupings of Table 2.

3. Total the number of servings for each food group.

4. Enter the total number of servings of each group on a calculation form, and multiply the values of the food groups in Table 2 by the number of servings.

5. Total the values for each column, and compare with the recommended allowances which apply to the particular individual.

Some mixtures of foods are not included in Table 2. A typical recipe may be consulted, grouping the ingredients in the corresponding classes of Table 2, taking care that the amount so recorded is representative of that eaten. Or, if nutritive values are given for such a mixture in Table 1, it may be simpler to use this source for the mixed dish.

As an example of the short method of calculation, the menu for the normal diet on page 363 has been selected. The foods of this menu were grouped as follows:

	Number of Servings		Number of Servings
Cereal products	5	*Fruit*	
oatmeal	1	banana	1
bread, rolls	3	citrus ($\frac{1}{4}$ cup)	$\frac{1}{2}$
toast (Apple Betty)	1	other	2
		apple (Betty)	
Dairy products		cherries	
butter	9		
2 teaspoons per meal		*Gravy,* white sauce	2
3 teaspoons for Apple		*Meat* loaf	$1\frac{1}{2}$
Betty and vegetables			
cheese (for soufflé)	1	*Sweets*	$4\frac{1}{2}$
cream (coffee)	$\frac{1}{2}$	in beverages	1
egg (breakfast and soufflé)	$1\frac{1}{2}$	Apple Betty	3
milk	$2\frac{1}{2}$	in cherries	$\frac{1}{2}$
cereal	$\frac{1}{2}$	*Vegetables*	
to drink	2	carrots	1
Fat (salad dressing)	1	peas	1
		potato, small	1
		tomato	1
		lettuce, 1 leaf	$\frac{1}{4}$

The nutritive values of this menu are calculated in the table on page 363.

MEAL EXCHANGE LISTS

Evolution of the meal exchange lists. Probably the classic example requiring rapid dietary calculations is afforded by the diabetic diet. At one time these calculations were time consuming. Far too much faith was placed on decimal point calculations, with too little understanding of the variability of food composition and of body utilization. A number of tables of food composition were developed for calculation of the diabetic diet, but to the patient the several approaches were confusing to say the least. Incorporating the best features of several methods in use, the meal exchange lists (Table 4, Appendix, p. 768) were evolved and published in 1950 by a joint committee of the American Dietetic Association, the American Diabetes Association, and the United States Public Health Service.[121] These lists are now the most widely used of any for diabetic calculations. They are equally applicable to the calculation of any diet for which protein, fat, and/or carbohydrate must be controlled; for example, the low-calorie diet. In Chapter 36 it will be noted that the sodium-restricted diet is also oriented about this method of dietary calculation. Because of their broad application, the meal exchanges

NUTRITIVE VALUE OF NORMAL DIET (Sample Menu, p. 362) CALCULATED BY SHORT METHOD *

FOOD	MEASURE †	ENERGY Calories	PROTEIN gm	FAT gm	CARBO-HYDRATE gm	MINERALS Ca gm	Fe mg	VITAMINS A I.U.	Ascorbic Acid mg	Thiamine mg	Riboflavin mg	Niacin mg
Cereal products	5	400	13	5	75	0.10	3.0	—	—	0.35	0.20	3.0
Butter	9	315		36				1485	—			
Cheese	1	125	8	10	1	.22	.3	420	—	.01	.13	—
Cream, light	½	30	1	3	1	.02	—	125	—	.01	.02	—
Egg	1½	120	10	9	—	.05	2.1	855	—	.08	.21	.2
Milk	2½	410	21	23	30	.70	.5	960	5	.25	1.02	.5
Fat	1	105	1	11	—	—	.2	15	—	.03	.02	.4
Banana	1	90	1	—	22	.01	.6	430	10	.04	.05	.7
Citrus fruit	½	20	—	—	5	.02	.2	60	22	.03	.01	.1
Other fruit	2	110	1	—	26	.02	.8	190	8	.08	.06	.4
Gravy	2	210	5	16	12	.14	.4	450	—	.08	.22	.4
Meat	1½	360	29	27	—	.02	3.5	—	—	.10	.25	5.5
Sweets	4½	250	—	—	63	—	—	—	—	—	—	—
Carrots	1	30	1	—	7	.03	.6	12,500	4	.05	.05	.4
Peas	1	70	4	—	13	.02	1.8	630	15	.25	.14	2.3
Potato	1	85	2	—	19	.01	.7	20	14	.09	.03	1.0
Tomato	1	20	1	—	4	.01	.5	1035	18	.05	.03	.8
Raw vegetable	¼	tr	tr	—	1	.01	.1	25	1	.01	.01	.1
		2750	98	140	279	1.38	15.3	19,200	97	1.51	2.45	15.8
Recommended Dietary Allowances:												
Man, 25 years		3200	70			0.8	10	5000	75	1.6	1.8	21
Woman, 25 years		2300	58			0.8	12	5000	70	1.2	1.5	17

* Calculations based on Table 2, Appendix, page 764.
† Measure is expressed as multiples of the amounts of food in each group, Table 2.

are discussed at this point; further detail on the method of calculation of diabetic diets is given in Chapter 33.

What is an exchange list? A grouping of foods which, for practical purposes, is approximately equal in carbohydrate, protein, and fat values is an *exchange* list. For example, in list 3, 1 small apple, or 2 prunes, or ½ small banana might be exchanged for ½ cup orange juice; that is, any of the fruits in the list, *in the amounts stated,* would provide 10 gm carbohydrate, and negligible protein and fat. To illustrate further, a patient allowed 5 bread exchanges a day might select as follows: ¾ cup dry cereal, 1 slice toast, 2 graham crackers, 1 small potato, and ½ cup cooked rice.

The sample menu for the normal diet on page 338 has been calculated according to the meal exchange lists as follows:

FOOD LIST		NUMBER OF EXCHANGES	CARBO-HYDRATE gm	PROTEIN gm	FAT gm
Milk		2½	30	20	25
Vegetable A					
lettuce, tomato		1	—	—	—
Vegetable B					
carrots, peas		2	14	4	—
Fruit		4½	45	—	—
banana	2				
citrus	½				
other	2				
Bread		6	90	12	—
bread, rolls	4				
oatmeal	1				
potato	1				
Meat		6½	—	46	33
meat loaf	4				
cheese	1				
egg	1½				
Fat		12½	—	—	62
butter	9				
salad dressing	3				
light cream	½				
			179	82	120
Sweets (Table 2)		4½ tbsp.	63		
Gravy, white sauce (Table 2)		2 servings	12	5	16
			254 × 4	87 × 4	136 × 9
TOTAL CALORIES		2588	1016	348	1224

Using the exchange lists. The procedure for quickly estimating the carbohydrate, protein, and fat content of the diet follows the same steps as outlined for the short method of dietary calculation, noting, however, that the food groups of Table 2 and of the exchange lists are not identical. It is important that the student learn early that the words *exchange* and *serving* are not synonymous. For example, 1 small banana, 6 prunes, and ½ grapefruit would generally be considered to be 3 servings of fruit, but they are equal to 6 exchanges of fruit. Again, 6 exchanges of meat might be distributed as 1 egg for breakfast, 2 ounces of chicken in a luncheon sandwich, and 3 ounces of roast beef at dinner.

The exchange lists do not include sweets or mixtures, but these values may be obtained from Tables 1 or 2, as indicated in the above calculation.

Assuring mineral and vitamin adequacy. Since the exchange lists do not provide information on mineral and vitamin values it becomes evident that some degree of discretion must be used in establishing the meal pattern and in selecting specific menus. For example, less than 2 milk exchanges daily will compromise the calcium and riboflavin levels of the diet, unless the daily selection from the meat list includes hard cheese. Likewise, the ascorbic acid intake might be too low if citrus fruits were never selected from the fruit exchanges. To be sure, cantaloupe, strawberries, and a few other fruits from this list are also good sources of vitamin C. A far too common error is that of omitting the vegetables of the A group, simply because their carbohydrate, protein, and fat values are negligible. To do so is to reduce the dietary intake of a number of valuable nutrients, especially vitamin A, ascorbic acid, and iron.

PROBLEMS AND REVIEW

1. How can you explain the fact that Cheddar and cottage cheese are listed as meat exchanges, but that they are both included in the milk group of the Four Food Groups (p. 29)?

2. Which vegetables in the A group are especially rich in vitamin A? In iron? In ascorbic acid?

3. Explain the placement of potatoes, corn, Lima beans, baked beans in the bread exchange list. Note also the group C vegetables in the Unit Lists of the sodium-restricted diet (p. 512).

4. *Problem.* Plan a menu for a lunch which permits the following exchanges: 1 milk; 2 A vegetable; 1 fruit; 3 bread; 2 meat; 3 fat.

5. *Problem.* Write three breakfast menus based on the following exchanges: 1 milk, 1 fruit, 2 bread, 2 meat, and 3 fat.

6. *Problem.* Keep a record of your food intake for 1 day, and calculate the nutritive values using Table 2.

7. *Problem.* Using the diet record of Problem 6, calculate the carbohydrate, protein, fat, and caloric value with the exchange lists. Compare these values with those obtained in Problem 6.

8. *Problem.* Refer to the calculation of the sample menu on page 363. If the calories and thiamine were to be increased to meet the recommended allowances for the man of 25 years, what foods could you add at least cost? Would the calculated thiamine level of this diet be adequate for a sedentary man, or one who is sick in bed? Explain.

9. *Problem.* Calculate the total niacin equivalent of the diet on page 363.

10. *Problem.* Examine the protein, fat, and carbohydrate values as calculated by Table 2 and by the exchange lists (see pp. 363 and 364). See if you can determine why these differences exist. Are they significant? Explain.

UNIT VII /
Modification of the Normal Diet for Energy, Protein, and Texture

CHAPTER 26 /

Nutritional Deficiencies and Their Correction

High-protein Diets

Nutritional diseases as problems of the national and international community have been discussed in Chapters 1 and 22, while the effects of deficiencies of the various nutrients have been described in the several chapters of Unit II pertaining to each of the specific nutrients. The purposes of this chapter are: (1) to discuss further the broad causes of nutritional deficiency; (2) to list signs which are suggestive of the existence of deficiency; and (3) to study the high-protein diet as an effective regimen for the correction of nutritional deficiency.

Some causes for nutritional deficiencies. Representative and important causes of nutritional diseases are listed here, and others will no doubt suggest themselves.

Inadequate intake of essential nutrients constitutes a major cause of all deficiency diseases. The intake may be inadequate for one or more of the following reasons.

1. Bad food habits are the result primarily of ignorance of the proper choice of foods. Too much of one type or too little of another type of food will lead to an unbalanced diet so that the required nutrients are not obtained in sufficient quantity. Energy-rich foods with little protein, minerals, or vitamins too often predominate in the dietary pattern.

2. Processing, marketing, and storage of foods may be such that important nutrients are lost. The restoration and enrichment of cereals have been of great significance in correcting deficiencies in thiamine, niacin, and iron. Generally speaking, the food supply in America today is of higher nutritive value than ever before.

3. Increased activity or body metabolism occurs without increase in intake. In pregnancy, lactation, and during childhood almost all nutrients are required in greatly augmented amounts. In fevers, hyperthyroidism, and under stress of surgery or injury the need for most nutrients is greatly increased.

368

4. Many diseases with accompanying poor appetite are responsible for grossly inadequate food intake. Some neuropsychiatric disturbances, pronounced food allergies, and the nausea of pregnancy are commonly accompanied by poor intake of food.

5. Faulty therapeutic diets, characterized by overzealousness of treatment for the disease condition rather than consideration of the patient as an individual, have led to omission of essential nutrients. For example, some regimens for treatment of ulcers have been low in protein, the B complex, and ascorbic acid; reduction diets have been low in protein, calcium, iron, and vitamins; and sodium-restricted diets have sometimes been grossly inadequate in protein, calcium, and riboflavin.

6. Chronic alcoholism is responsible for decreased intake of essential nutrients and is also known to impair various organs of the body so that utilization of the nutrients is interfered with.

Faulty utilization frequently produces deficiency even though the diet itself may have been adequate under normal conditions. Representative examples of factors which bring about poor absorption and metabolism are here given.

1. Achlorhydria may impair the absorption of iron, thiamine, and other factors.

2. Chronic gastrointestinal disorders such as sprue and colitis decrease the absorption of all nutrients to the point where the body's energy needs are not met, protein is inadequate for tissue repair, and mineral and vitamin deficiencies occur.

3. Pancreatic and hepatic disorders restrict fat digestion and absorption so that insufficient energy is available and the fat-soluble vitamins are absorbed poorly.

4. In some instances, such as diabetes mellitus, the liver is apparently unable to convert carotene to vitamin A. In uncontrolled diabetes, carbohydrate, protein, and fat metabolism is disrupted.

5. Excessive use of mineral oil may interfere with the absorption of carotene and other fat-soluble vitamins.

6. Extensive oral therapy with antibiotics or other drugs may modify or destroy the microorganisms of the intestinal tract so that certain vitamins are not synthesized.

Some signs of nutritional deficiencies. Positive diagnosis of most nutritional deficiencies is difficult in the early stages because the onset is often slow, insidious, and vague as to symptoms. The following may suggest deficiency, but most of them are not specific for nutritional diseases alone.

1. Loss of interest and desire for food, causing loss of weight

2. Difficulty in concentration and a progressive loss of interest in affairs formerly considered important

3. Insomnia

4. Nervousness and irritability

5. Frequent respiratory infections

6. Sore mouth and tongue, dermatitis, and other skin disturbances

7. Glossitis, gastrointestinal disturbances, including anorexia, diarrhea, or constipation

8. Sore, painful muscles and joints, muscular weakness, and inability to coordinate

9. Cheilosis—lesions at angles of the mouth and extending into the face with frequent eruptions occurring about the nose and ears

10. Poor wound healing; proneness to bed sores

11. Simple goiter

12. Dental caries

13. Bone deformities, especially of the long bones, the bones of the chest, spine, and pelvis; multiple fractures caused by fragility of the bones

14. Difficulty in seeing in a dim light, especially after leaving a brightly lighted room

15. Swollen congested eyelids, dry surface of the eye itself resulting from impairment of the lacrymal glands and the secretions therefrom and leading to infections of the eye and itching and burning sensations of the eye

A carefully taken dietary history is one of the most valuable aids in making a diagnosis of nutritional deficiency. There are many reliable laboratory tests which can be used in determining the existence of deficiencies in human subjects. Determination of protein, mineral, and vitamin levels of the blood may be made. The urinary excretion of certain minerals and vitamins may be studied with respect to intake or to certain test doses. X-ray studies indicate bone changes as in rickets or in scurvy. Special types of apparatus, such as the biophotometer which measures dark adaptation, may be used. These tests are primarily medical procedures and will not be discussed further here.

Treatment of deficiency diseases. Specific vitamin deficiencies are now treated with therapeutic doses of vitamin preparations.[53] The latter effect a cure much more rapidly than is possible with diet alone; they are less expensive than dietary sources of the vitamins; the concentrates are usable at a stage of illness when the patient may be able to take little if any food by mouth; and the amount which is given is precisely known. The student must bear in mind that vitamin concentrates are never a substitution therapy for a good normal diet but should be used in conjunction with the diet insofar as the patient is able to consume food. The ultimate aim is to restore the normal diet so that it can serve effectively in preventing future deficiencies.

Most patients exhibiting vitamin deficiencies also show signs of calorie or protein lack or both. The caloric modification of the diet will be discussed in Chapter 27 while the protein modification is discussed below.

PROTEIN DEFICIENCY

Disease factors leading to protein depletion. The effect of inadequate intake of proteins supplying the essential amino acids has been discussed in Chapter 4. However, a mild deficiency may be aggravated by a disease process, or conditioning factors may initiate a deficiency when none existed before.

Even though the diet may normally be adequate, *poor digestion and absorption,* as in chronic diarrheas of any origin, may provoke deficiency symptoms. Edema of the intestinal tract caused by inadequate protein leads to continued poor absorption, and thus a vicious cycle is maintained. There may be *excessive metabolism of protein* as in fevers, following surgery or wound healing of any type, following burns, in diabetic acidosis, and thyrotoxicosis. *Excessive loss of protein* from the body occurs in nephrosis, hemorrhage, burns, and in wound exudates. Then, finally, there may be a *failure to synthesize proteins* in a normal manner because of liver injury.

Detection of protein deficiency. The classic examples of protein deficiency are kwashiorkor (see Chap. 4) and marasmus, both of which are seen especially in children in underdeveloped countries of the world. Marasmus occurs when both protein and calories are severely lacking; it presents the signs described earlier for kwashiorkor, but there is also extensive wasting of the tissues.

Loss of weight to the point of emaciation also occurs in adults subjected to severe protein and calorie deprivation. Edema frequently but not always accompanies starvation and is also known as "hunger edema," "war edema," or "famine edema" because of the conditions under which it most frequently occurs.

Blood proteins may give a clue to the state of protein nutrition. In deficiency the total blood protein is reduced, the albumin fraction being especially affected. It is important to realize that these blood proteins are not decreased until the tissue stores have become so depleted that they can no longer supply protein for the important functions of the serum proteins; thus, a deficiency of plasma proteins reflects a much larger and more long-standing tissue protein depletion. Elman [122] has estimated that approximately 30 gm of tissue protein are lost for every gram of serum protein which is lost. To illustrate: If the total serum protein level has decreased from 7 to 6 gm per 100 ml, and the total circulating plasma volume is 2700 ml, this represents a loss of 27 gm of serum protein; it would represent, in addition, a loss of 30×27 gm or 810 gm of protein from the tissues.

The presence of edema cannot be explained entirely by changes in the hydrostatic and colloid osmotic pressure, and Keys [123] concludes that the condition is simply related to a low caloric intake. Keys and his associates believe further that the recovery from starvation is first of all a matter of supplying adequate calories. On the other hand, Benditt et al.[124] believe that the level of protein and the quality of protein are limiting factors in recovery from starvation, provided calories are also adequate. Their studies show that a certain minimum level of calories is necessary to ensure maximum tissue building. Beyond this minimum caloric level, there is no advantage in further increasing the intake of calories. For all practical purposes the High-protein Diet (p. 373), either in liquid, soft, or regular form, is suitable as a basis of therapy for starved individuals.

Modification of the diet. Few diets have greater usefulness in a wide variety of conditions than the high-protein diet, and the student will be well repaid for making a thorough study of the many variations which are possible and in acquiring skill in the planning of diets which will satisfy the most capricious of appetites. Food by mouth is the most effective method for the administration of protein when the patient is able to eat.

Protein. A diet which contains 100–125 gm of protein or more daily is generally considered to be high in protein. However, no arbitrary level can be established which will satisfy all circumstances. An amount of protein sufficient to maintain positive nitrogen balance is essential if satisfactory progress is to be made. The rate of synthesis of tissue protein is roughly proportional to the protein intake, providing the caloric level is adequate.[124] From 1.5 to 3 or even 4 gm of protein per kg of body weight are prescribed, depending upon the condition.

Not only must the level of protein be high, but the quality must be of the best. It is a good rule to select about two-thirds of the daily protein desired from complete protein foods. Moreover, all of the essential amino acids must be continuously available if maximum synthesis is to take place in the body. Thus, each meal should contain complete protein foods to supplement the incomplete protein foods.

Calories. Maximum protein utilization can occur only when the diet contains sufficient calories to provide energy for the needs of activity, basal metabolism, tissue synthesis, and waste. Benditt et al. have estimated that 1500 nonprotein calories per square meter of body surface are necessary for an afebrile individual at bed rest, or approximately 2600 calories for the average-size man. The calories commonly calculated for the protein portion of the diet are not included in this figure, since protein used for tissue synthesis will not at the same time yield energy.

Other nutrients. Protein foods, as a rule, are excellent sources of B-complex vitamins and iron, and hence the high-protein diet will contain liberal quantities of these nutrients. Normal amounts of vegetables and fruits together with milk will ensure sufficient ascorbic acid and calcium respectively.

Consistency and volume. A fluid, soft, or regular diet may be ordered, depending upon the condition of the patient. The starved individual such as was seen in many prisoner-of-war camps can tolerate neither the volume nor the texture of a regular diet. For these emaciated patients a liquid diet in which the beverages have been highly reinforced with concentrated protein so as to keep the volume at a minimum is prescribed until the gastrointestinal tract again becomes accustomed to handling more food, and until the heart and circulatory system can cope with the additional demands made on it.

Management of the diet. Patients with a good appetite can eat a diet containing 100 to 150 gm of protein, as it occurs naturally in foods, without difficulty. Continuous and determined effort on the part of the nurse can be very helpful in achieving the desired protein intake even by many patients with an impaired appetite. The amounts of food must often be increased gradually. The severely depleted individual often finds it impossible to consume large amounts of food at one time. For some, small meals with between-meal feedings may be most suitable. Others may achieve a greater intake by eating three meals and an evening feeding. High-protein beverages (see beverage recipes, p. 672) are effective in achieving maximum protein intake with a minimum of volume. The patient must be watched carefully lest he become anorexic.

HIGH-PROTEIN DIET

Characteristics and general rules:

Complete protein foods should be emphasized in this diet. Those of best quality include milk, cheese, eggs, and meat products.

Nonfat dry milk and egg white are effective reinforcing agents whenever it is difficult for the patient to eat the amounts of protein foods listed below. See recipes for high-protein beverages, pages 671–72.

Include these foods, or their nutritive equivalents, daily:

4 cups (1 quart) milk
6 ounces (cooked weight) meat, fish, or poultry
3 eggs
1 ounce cheese
4 servings vegetables including:
    1 serving green or yellow vegetable
    1 to 2 servings potato
    1 to 2 servings other vegetable
    One vegetable to be eaten raw daily
2 servings fruit including:
    1 serving citrus fruit—or other good source of ascorbic acid
    1 serving other fruit
1 serving whole-grain or enriched cereal
5 slices whole-grain or enriched bread
2 tablespoons (1 ounce) butter or fortified margarine
Additional foods as required to meet caloric need may be selected from the above list of foods, or as desired from other foods.

Nutritive value: On the basis of specified amounts of foods above: protein, 125 gm; calories, 2500. All vitamins and minerals in excess of normal diet—see page 337.

MEAL PATTERN	SAMPLE MENU
Breakfast	
Fruit	Half grapefruit
Cereal	Oatmeal
Eggs—2	Fried eggs
Bread, whole-grain or enriched	Whole-wheat toast
Butter or margarine	Butter
Milk to drink and for cereal	Milk
Beverage	Coffee
Luncheon or supper	
Meat or substitute of egg, cheese, fish, or poultry—large serving	Chicken soufflé
	Mushroom sauce
Potato, macaroni, spaghetti, noodles, or vegetable	Buttered green beans
Salad with dressing	Shredded carrot and raisin salad
Bread with butter or margarine	Whole-wheat roll and butter
Fruit	Fresh peaches
Milk—1 glass	Milk
Dinner	
Meat, fish, or poultry—large serving	Broiled trout with parsley garnish
Potato	Creamed potato
Vegetable	Buttered spinach
Bread with butter or margarine	Rye bread with butter
Dessert	Lemon-flake ice cream
	Brownies
Milk	Milk
Beverage	Tea with lemon
Evening nourishment	
Eggnog—1 glass	Chocolate eggnog
Sandwich with cheese or equivalent	American cheese and tomato sandwich

HIGH-PROTEIN SOFT DIET

General rules:

Include foods in the amounts listed under High-protein Diet, page 373.

Select foods from those allowed for Soft Diet, page 341, or Bland Diet, page 420.

MEAL PATTERN	SAMPLE MENU

Breakfast

Cooked fruit, banana, or fruit juice	Grapefruit sections without membrane
Cereal—strained, if coarse	Strained oatmeal
Milk	Milk
Eggs—2	Scrambled eggs
Soft roll or enriched white toast	Toast
Butter	Butter
Sugar	
Beverage	Coffee

Luncheon or supper

Cream soup	Cream of asparagus soup
Ground meat or substitute of egg, cheese, poultry, or fish—large serving	Chicken soufflé
Potato, macaroni, spaghetti, noodles, rice or tender chopped vegetable	Buttered green beans
Enriched bread with butter or margarine	Enriched bread with butter
Cooked fruit	Stewed peaches
Milk—1 glass	Milk

Dinner

Orange, grapefruit, or tomato juice	Orange juice
Ground or flaked meat, fish, or poultry —large serving	Broiled trout
Potato	Creamed potato
Cooked vegetable—tender chopped or strained	Buttered chopped spinach
Enriched bread with butter or margarine	Rye bread without seeds; butter
Dessert	Lemon-flake ice cream
	Plain sugar cookie
Milk	Milk
Beverage, if desired	Tea with lemon

Evening nourishment

Milk—1 glass	Milk
Sandwich with tender or ground meat or cheese	Sandwich with flaked salmon and chopped egg

HIGH-PROTEIN FLUID DIET

Include these foods, or their nutritive equivalents, daily:

   3 cups milk
   3 cups high-protein milk or eggnog (see recipes, p. 672)

4 eggs
1–2 ounces strained meat
½ cup strained cereal—for use in gruel
1 cup citrus fruit juice
½ cup tomato juice
¼ cup vegetable purée for cream soup
2 or more servings plain dessert—gelatin, Junket, ice cream, custard
3 tablespoons sugar
1 tablespoon cocoa

Nutritive value: On the basis of specified amounts of foods above: protein, 110 gm; calories, 2100.

MEAL PATTERN	SAMPLE MENU
Breakfast	
Strained fruit juice	Grapefruit juice
Cereal gruel with milk and sugar	Strained oatmeal with milk and sugar
Hot beverage with cream and sugar	Cocoa
Midmorning	
Strained citrus juice with whole egg	Orange juice with whole egg
Luncheon or supper	
Cream soup	Cream of asparagus soup
Tomato juice	Tomato juice
High-protein milk, plain or flavored	High-protein milk with pineapple flavor
Fruit-juice gelatin, custard, Junket, or ice cream	Soft custard
Midafternoon	
Malted milk or eggnog	Chocolate eggnog
Dinner	
Broth with whole egg	Chicken broth with whole egg
Strained fruit juice	Apricot juice
High-protein milk or eggnog	High-protein milk
Ice cream, custard, Junket, or fruit-juice gelatin	Raspberry ice
Evening nourishment	
High-protein eggnog—plain or flavored	High-protein eggnog with nutmeg

Protein hydrolysates in therapy. Whole protein food by mouth is in every respect preferable, provided the patient is able to ingest sufficient food and can digest and absorb such food. However, when this ability is partly or completely broken down, hydrolysates of protein are useful as substitution therapy or as a supplement to the diet. The hydrolysate must be a mixture which contains all the essential amino acids in their correct proportions for tissue synthesis.

The oral hydrolysates are of especial value in infant allergies to milk, in ulcerative colitis, and chronic pancreatitis, and in supplementing the diet in conditions where it is impossible to accomplish a sufficiently high protein intake by the use of ordinary foods, as in surgery. Oral hydrolysates present certain practical difficulties: (1) they are usually more expensive than food proteins from the same source; (2) they are less palatable than natural food proteins, and it is often difficult to get the patient to take the necessary amounts for a prolonged period of time.

PROBLEM AND REVIEW

1. What are some symptoms which may suggest nutritional deficiency of one type or another?

2. A careful dietary history may be of diagnostic importance in detecting deficiency disease. Illustrate.

3. What are outstanding nutritional deficiencies in the United States today? What nutrients are most likely to be received in less than optimum amounts?

4. Feeding programs for starving populations have placed special emphasis on providing cereal grains. Why is this class of foods so important? What limitations may such a program have?

5. What is marasmus?

6. Deficiency diseases are usually treated by adjustment of the diet so that it is once again adequate and by using vitamin concentrates. Why are concentrates more satisfactory than a "high-vitamin" diet? What nutrients may be especially emphasized in the diet of such patients?

7. *Problem.* Jack, a 17-year-old boy, is recovering from a long illness. The doctor has prescribed a diet containing 150 gm of protein and 4000 calories. Jack is allergic to eggs. Using the High-protein Diet as a basis (p. 373), plan a diet which would be suitable for him.

8. What adverse effects is a protein deficiency likely to have upon recovery from illness?

CHAPTER 27

Overweight and Underweight

Low-calorie and High-calorie Diets

Importance of weight control. The greatest problem of preventive medicine today is obesity. Excessive weight is closely associated with cardiovascular and renal diseases, diabetes, degenerative arthritis, gout, and gallbladder disease. It constitutes a risk for the patient who needs surgical treatment. The complications of pregnancy and the hazards during childbirth are multiplied. The popular saying "The longer the belt, the shorter the life" is far too true.

Overweight is a physical handicap as well as a primary health hazard. Obese people are more uncomfortable during warm weather because the thick layers of fat serve as an insulator. More effort must be expended to do a given amount of work because of the increase in body mass. Because of their lessened ability, obese people are more susceptible to accidents. Fatigue, backache, and foot troubles are common complaints of the obese.

Obesity is no longer fashionable, although in times past moderate overweight was considered a sign of health and beauty. Emotional and psychologic problems stem from obesity, just as these problems may indeed be the cause of obesity. The obese individual may be the butt of jokes, is sometimes looked upon as one who is greedy or who has no will power, or may experience social humiliation and inability to get a job. He may lose his self-esteem and may withdraw from others in order to avoid embarrassment. Such attitudes may serve to reinforce the conditions that led to the obesity.

The national preoccupation with slimness is in itself—surprising as it may seem—a major problem. Too many people resort to fad diets, pills, and gadgets which result in nutritive inadequacy, economic loss, and sometimes serious effects on health. Medical supervision is not always sought and weight reduction may be ill advised for some. Many people resort to one merry-go-round after another of reducing diets, losing a little only to gain it again, thus submitting themselves to the repeated body stresses which accompany weight loss.

Underweight. Much less attention is directed to the problems of underweight, although many people in all age categories are not enjoying optimum health because of the undernutrition usually associated with extreme underweight. Fatigue and lowered resistance to infection are corollaries of underweight. Tuberculosis, especially, is found more frequently among young people whose weight is considerably below normal. Underweight at the beginning of pregnancy and failure to gain at a sufficient rate during pregnancy were found by Tompkins [78] to be even greater hazards than overweight.

Desirable weight. The best weight for a given individual's height, age, bone structure, and muscular development is not exactly known. Height-weight tables (see p. 785) currently classify people as having a large, average, or small frame. The person who is stocky may be 5 to 10 per cent above the weight for average build without being considered overweight, while the individual who has a small frame should weigh 5 to 10 per cent less than the desirable weight for average build.

A large proportion of people continue to gain weight until late middle life, but this is not physiologically necessary, nor need it be inevitable. On the basis of life insurance statistics the most nearly ideal weight to maintain throughout life is that which is proper at age 25 for one's height and body build. Therefore, height-weight tables no longer indicate figures beyond the ages of 25 to 30 years. Generally speaking, the best weight is likely to be that at which one both looks and feels his best.

Obesity, overweight, and underweight are somewhat arbitrary terms. A deviation of not more than 10 per cent above or below the desirable weight for a given individual is not considered significant. The term *overweight* is applied to individuals who are 10 to 20 per cent above desirable weight. This group is estimated to be roughly one-fifth of the population over 30 years in the United States. *Obesity* is applied to persons 20 per cent or more overweight, probably about 10 per cent of the population over 30 years. *Underweight* denotes those individuals who are more than 10 per cent below the established standards; those more than 20 per cent below these standards are considered to be seriously underweight.

It is probably not difficult to identify obesity which is marked, but height-weight tables provide only approximations on the degree of fatness. For example, a football player may be overweight by such standards but has a well-developed musculature and does not have excessive fat deposits. Research studies have employed techniques which measure body density by weighing in water and in air, but they are not applicable to routine measurements. The thickness of subcutaneous layers of fat may be measured by means of calipers. As data are accumulated from such studies they may be more applicable than height-weight tables in determining the degree of obesity.

Estimation of weight gain or loss. Each gram of body fat represents the storage of approximately 9 calories. Thus, if an individual consumes an amount of food which provides 100 calories in excess of his energy requirement, there will be deposited 78 gm (700 ÷ 9) of fat each week, or approximately 9 pounds (4056 ÷ 454) in a year. If one were to overeat consistently by this amount for 5 or 10 years, it is obvious that obesity would be the result even though the person maintained he "didn't eat such large amounts of food"! It would take only 3 teaspoons butter, or two 1-inch squares of fudge, or an oatmeal cookie to supply this additional 100 calories each day.

Conversely, the removal of 1 gm body fat requires the expenditure of 9 calories not provided by the diet. If the diet each day provides 1000 calories less than the daily energy requirement, the weekly weight loss is roughly 780 gm (7000 ÷ 9) or 1¾ pounds (780 ÷ 454). In practice weight loss does not follow a predicted straight line because of day-to-day variations in water balance and activity.

OBESITY

Cause. Obesity is invariably caused by an intake of calories beyond the body's need for energy. Such a statement, however, tends to oversimplify the problem of obesity, for one might infer that its correction might be easily achieved by bringing the energy intake and expenditure into balance. The reasons for an existing imbalance are many and complex, and some understanding of the problems of the individual must be gained before therapy can be effectively instituted. A thorough physical examination, a dietary history, and an investigation of habits relating to activity, rest, and family and social relationships are indicated.

Mayer [125] has studied the effect of genetic, traumatic, and environmental factors in causing obesity in experimental animals. While his studies on genetic and traumatic elements cannot be directly related to man at the present time, they cannot be wholly discounted. Many environmental factors help to explain the incidence of obesity.

Eating too much becomes a habit for some people. It may result from family customs in using concentrated high-calorie foods, or having to maintain social relationships including rich party foods in addition to usual mealtime eating, or eating excessive amounts of carbohydrate foods because they are cheaper, or maintaining irregular habits of eating, including snacks all day long.

Numerous persons continue to gain weight throughout life because they fail to adjust their appetites to reduced energy requirements. The many labor-saving devices in the homes and in industry reduce the energy requirement. Most people enjoy sports as spectators rather than as participants. Riding rather than walking to school or work is common practice even for short distances. Other circumstances may further reduce the energy needs: (1) basal metabolism is gradually decreased from year to year (see p. 87); (2) changes in occupation may result in reduced activity; (3) the middle years of life sometimes bring about a repose and consequent reduction of muscle tension; (4) periods of quiet relaxation and sleep may be increased; and (5) disabling illness such as arthritis or cardiac disease may reduce markedly the need for calories.

Recent years have brought an increasing awareness of the psychologic aspects of obesity. Numerous articles in current journals emphasize that eating is a solace and a pleasure to the individual who is bored, feels lonely or unloved, has become discontented with his family, social, or financial standing, has experienced deep sorrow, or needs an excuse to avoid the realities of life.

Obesity resulting from disturbances of the glands, such as the thyroid or pituitary, accounts for less than 5 per cent of the total incidence. The basal metabolism is lowered in this group of persons so that weight gain results unless the diet provides fewer calories than is usually considered normal.

Treatment. Ultimately, the correction of obesity is dependent upon the reduction of energy intake below the energy requirements of the body. Weight reduction is difficult to achieve and maintain, and may be fraught with danger if the medical, psychologic, and dietary aspects of the program are not properly integrated.

Weight reduction should be guided by a physician since the physiologic and psychologic stress are not equally borne by all. Some persons, according to Young,[126] will lose weight satisfactorily when shown how to keep the caloric intake within the prescribed limits; others need help in relieving their tensions before a dietary regimen will be effective; still others have such deep emotional problems that weight loss should not be attempted until these problems have been corrected by psychiatric help.

A diet prescription will prove worthless unless the patient has some motivation for losing weight, such as the maintenance or recovery of health, the ability to win friendship, admiration, and affection, the importance of normal weight in being able to earn one's livelihood or in being considered for occupational advancement, as the case may be. The patient must have the capacity for self-discipline, patience, and perseverance. The physician, nurse, and dietitian, however, can be of immeasurable help by providing encouragement and guidance at frequent follow-up visits. Helping the patient to maintain self-esteem and treating him with dignity can scarcely be overemphasized. Chiding him, on the other hand, for his failure rarely accomplishes anything.

Keeping a weight chart with a record of progress from week to week is most helpful. It must be explained to the patient that weight losses may be irregular even though the diet is carefully kept, inasmuch as variations in water balance occur. The temporary retention of water for 2 or 3 weeks at the beginning of a reduction program may lead the patient to abandon the program if he is not aware of these irregularities.

Exercise. Moderate exercise taken consistently and often can be an important aid in losing weight, providing that there are no contraindications to it such as cardiovascular disease. It can result in better muscular tone and a sense of well-being. Exercise is not necessarily accompanied by an increase in appetite, nor does a diminution of activity always lead to a decreased appetite.[127] It has been said by some that the best exercise is the exercise of the will power; that is, in pushing away from the table before the appetite is completely satisfied!

Hormones and drugs. Most overweight persons have no deficiency of endocrine secretions and should not be led to believe that they have glandular disturbances; nor should they be exposed to the increased nervousness and irritability which results from such medication. The occasional patient with thyroid deficiency who requires thyroid extract should be treated only by a physician.

Amphetamine sulfate, sometimes prescribed by a physician because of its ability to dull the appetite, is also a stimulant. It may produce insomnia, excitability, gastrointestinal disturbances, and other toxic manifestations. Other drugs are also used to dull the appetite. Some preparations include methyl cellulose which has the ability to absorb water and to provide a feeling of satiety.

Many so-called reducing pills advertised in the press and on radio and television programs are preparations of glucose or other sugars, nonfat dry milk, and various combinations of vitamins. They have no effect whatsoever on the control of weight, but are usually sold at exorbitant prices. Some preparations contain laxative or diuretic drugs so that weight is lost, but at the expense of body water—not body fat.

Group therapy. Individual instruction of the obese is expensive and often ineffectual. Moderate success has been realized when groups of individuals met to discuss their common problem of obesity at weekly intervals during the weight-reducing program.[128,129] The group approach to weight reduction gives people an opportunity to share and discuss with one another their problems in losing weight. The members of the group provide understanding, a spirit of competition, encouragement, and support to the efforts of the individual.

Modification of the diet. The objectives of a reducing diet should be (1) to maintain, or restore, good nutrition; (2) to bring about gradual loss of weight; and (3) to correct faulty food habits. The low-calorie diet should permit the use of everyday foods in a reasonable variety and at moderate cost. It should promote a sense of well-being and be palatable, but it is not necessary to use unusual recipes which require much preparation time or additional expense.

Many persons who enter upon a reducing program have had prolonged deficiencies of several nutrients. Moreover, carefully controlled studies [130–133] on young women have shown that weight reduction in itself imposes considerable stress on the body. Even though the diets used in these investigations were planned to meet or exceed the Recommended Dietary Allowances, there were negative calcium, phosphorus, and nitrogen balances as weight loss progressed. It is obvious that there is no room for the numerous, nutritionally inadequate fad diets which make such extravagant claims. On the other hand, a good reducing diet is often better nutritionally than the diet on which the patient gained so much weight.

Energy. A gradual loss of 6 to 8 pounds monthly is desirable since the patient need not experience the severe hunger, nervous exhaustion, and weakness which often accompany drastic reduction regimens. Such a weight loss requires that the daily intake be reduced 800 to 1000 calories below the daily energy requirement; thus, an individual whose normal activity requires 2400 calories may use a 1400 to 1600 calorie diet. For moderately active individuals weight loss can be achieved at diet levels of 1200 to 1600 calories.

Diets supplying 1000 calories or less are rarely necessary except for individuals who are kept in bed. Such drastic restrictions, used far too often, are likely to be inadequate in several nutrients.

Protein. The allowance of protein should be at least 1 gm per kilogram of ideal body weight, but an allowance of $1\frac{1}{2}$ gm per kilogram improves the satiety value of the diet and minimizes tissue nitrogen loss. Most diets can be planned to include 70 to 100 gm protein.

Fat and carbohydrate. The conventional diets used for many years have sharply curtailed the intake of fat and restricted the carbohydrate to moderate levels, as shown in the 1000-calorie diet listed on page 384. Recent work [130,132,134] has indicated that the patient experiences a greater sense of satisfaction when a somewhat more liberal intake of fat and a greatly reduced carbohydrate level is employed. About half of the calories of such a diet are provided by fat.

Because some individuals may request the inclusion of alcoholic beverages, it should be remembered that each gram of alcohol yields 7 calories, and that allowance must therefore be made in the total calories permitted each day. The beverages are used only according to the physician's orders.

Minerals and vitamins. When diets containing 1000 calories or less are prescribed, supplements of iron salts, and possibly calcium, together with a multivitamin preparation are indicated. Low-calorie diets for obese children and for pregnant women must be planned with the increased mineral and vitamin requirements in mind. For that reason the diets used are usually somewhat less stringent.

Satiety value of the diet. The patient must have a sense of satisfaction and well-being, which can be effected by considering the satiety value of foods. Proteins and fats remain in the stomach longer and their use delays the return of hunger. The protein allowance should be divided approximately equally between the three meals. Thus, an egg and milk at breakfast, lean meat, cheese, or egg at lunch, and lean meat at dinner are desirable.

Some individuals prefer small meals and a between-meal snack to a three-meal schedule. There is no reason why this should not be permitted if the patient adheres to his food allowance. Part of the success of a reducing diet depends on learning to be content with smaller portions of food and less concentrated foods.

The intake of concentrated foods, especially quickly-metabolized carbohydrates, is reduced to a minimum. While bulky fruits and vegetables may give satisfaction to some degree, the use of fibrous foods should not be excessive. Tea, coffee, and fat-free broth are useful in maintaining satisfaction.

Rich sauces, cream, and fats are obviously contraindicated in food preparation. Nevertheless, foods may be prepared in a great variety of ways. Vegetables and meats may be seasoned with tomato sauces, broth, spices, and herbs. A list of such seasonings is given on page 516. Instead of sugar, artificial sweetening agents such as saccharin or Sucaryl may be used in beverages, with fruits and cereals, and in a variety of low-calorie desserts.

Planning the daily diet. The diets below are planned on the basis of the exchange lists (Table 4, p. 768). These lists permit a flexibility of choice according to individual desires. A comparison with the basic diet on page 337 shows that the mineral and vitamin values will equal or exceed recommended allowances. The low-calorie diets include an additional cup of milk, thus enhancing the calcium value.

LOW-CALORIE DIETS

FOOD FOR THE DAY	NORMAL PROTEIN, MODERATE CARBO-HYDRATE, LOW TO MODERATE FAT			HIGH PRO-TEIN, LOW CARBOHYDRATE, MODERATE FAT
	1000 calories	1200 calories	1500 calories	1500 calories
Milk, whole, cups	3 (skim)	3	3	3
Vegetable, Group A	1 cup	1 cup	1 cup	1 cup
Group B	1/2 cup	1/2 cup	1/2 cup	1/2 cup
Fruit, unsweetened, exchanges	4	3	4	2
Bread, exchanges	2	2	4	2
Meat, exchanges	5	5	5	9
Fat, exchanges	1	1	3	2
Nutritive Value				
Protein, gm	65	65	69	93
Fat, gm	30	60	70	85
Carbohydrate, gm	113	103	143	93
Calories	980	1210	1480	1510

Foods to restrict or avoid. The patient who learns to select his foods in appropriate amounts from the exchange lists does not require specific lists of foods to avoid. For some persons, however, it may help to create calorie consciousness if listings of concentrated foods are provided. Some of the foods listed below are permitted in specified amounts in the exchange lists, but others are best avoided altogether.

High-fat foods: butter, cheese, chocolate, cream, ice cream, fat meat, fatty fish, or fish canned in oil, fried foods of any kind such as doughnuts and potato chips, gravies, nuts, oil, pastries, and salad dressing

High-carbohydrate foods: breads of any kind, candy, cake, cookies, corn, cereal products such as macaroni, noodles, spaghetti, pancakes, waffles, sweetened or dried fruits, legumes such as Lima beans, navy beans, dried peas, potatoes, sweet potatoes, honey, molasses, sugar, sirup, rich puddings

Beverages: all fountain drinks, including malted milks and chocolate, carbonated beverages of all kinds, rich sundaes, alcoholic drinks

SAMPLE MEAL PATTERNS

Normal Protein, Moderate Carbohydrate, Moderate Fat
1500 Calories

High Protein, Low Carbohydrate, Moderate Fat
1500 Calories

Breakfast

Unsweetened citrus fruit—1 exchange
Egg—1
Bread—1 slice
Butter—1 teaspoon
Milk, whole—1 cup
Coffee or tea

Unsweetened citrus fruit—1 exchange
Eggs—2
Bread—1 slice
Butter—1 teaspoon
Milk, whole—1 cup
Coffee or tea

Lunch

Meat, poultry, or fish—2 ounces
Vegetable, raw or cooked,
  group A—1 serving
Milk, whole—1 cup
Bread—1 slice
Butter—1 teaspoon
Unsweetened fruit—1 exchange

Meat, poultry, or fish—4 ounces
Vegetable, raw or cooked,
  group A—1 serving
Milk, whole—1 cup

Dinner

Meat, poultry, or fish—2 ounces
Potato—1 small
Vegetable, group B—½ cup
          group A—1 serving
Milk, whole—1 cup
Bread—1 slice
Butter—1 teaspoon
Unsweetened fruit—2 exchanges
Coffee or tea, if desired

Meat, poultry, or fish—3 ounces
Potato—1 small
Vegetable, group B—½ cup
          group A—1 serving
Milk, whole—1 cup

Butter—1 teaspoon
Unsweetened fruit—1 exchange

Maintenance of weight. To lose weight is by no means easy; to maintain the desirable level of weight is even more difficult. The low-calorie diet which has been planned with regard for the patient's pattern of living also provides the basis upon which to build the diet for maintenance. The patient must learn that a change in food habits is essential not only for weight loss, but that such a change must also continue throughout life if desirable weight is to be maintained. Thus, additions of foods should be made judiciously until weight is being kept constant at the desired level. It is important for the patient to weigh himself at weekly intervals or so in order to be sure that the foods added are in appropriate amounts.

If foods added for maintenance are also selected from the Four Food Groups, the quality of the diet with respect to protein, minerals, and vitamins is thereby enhanced. On the other hand, the additions of concentrated high-calorie foods may be more difficult to control in amounts suitable for maintenance. For example, the sedentary person of middle age must continue to forego rich desserts and sweets except on rare occasions.

UNDERWEIGHT

Causes. Underweight results when the energy intake does not fully meet the energy requirements. Not infrequently this occurs in people who are very active, tense, nervous, and who obtain too little rest. Sometimes irregular habits of eating and poor selection of foods are responsible for an inadequate caloric intake.

Just as psychologic factors have been noted as contributing to overeating, so they may contribute to eating too little food. Some patients with mental illness reject food to such an extent that severe weight loss results; this condition is referred to as *anorexia nervosa*.

Underweight also occurs in many pathologic conditions such as fevers in which the appetite is poor but the energy requirements are increased; gastrointestinal disturbances characterized by nausea, vomiting, and diarrhea; and hyperthyroidism in which the metabolic rate is greatly accelerated.

Modifications of the diet. Before weight gain can be effected, the direct cause for the inadequate caloric intake must be sought. As in obesity, these causes in relation to the individual must be removed and a high-calorie diet provided.

Energy. Approximately 500 calories in excess of the daily needs will result in a weekly gain of about 1 pound. For moderately active individuals diets containing 3000 to 3500 calories will bring about effective weight gain. Somewhat higher levels are required when fever is high, or gastrointestinal disturbances are interfering with absorption, or metabolism is greatly increased.

Protein. A daily intake of 100 gm protein or more is usually desirable since body protein as well as body fat must be replaced.

Minerals and vitamins. If the quality of the diet resulting in weight loss was poor, considerable body deficits of minerals and vitamins may likewise have occurred. Usually the high-calorie diet will provide liberal levels of all of these nutrients. When supplements are prescribed, it is important that the patient understand that they are in no way a substitute for the calories and protein provided by food.

Planning the daily diet. A patient cannot always adjust immediately to a higher caloric intake. It is better to begin with the patient's present intake and to improve the diet both qualitatively and quantitatively day by day until the desired caloric level is reached. Nothing is more conducive to loss of appetite than the appearance of an overloaded tray of food.

The caloric intake may be increased by using additional amounts of foods from the Four Food Groups, thus increasing the intake of protein, minerals, and vitamins. For example, 500 calories might be added to the patient's present intake as follows:

1 glass milk, ½ cup ice cream, 1 small potato, 1 small banana; *or*
2 slices bread, 2 ounces meat, 1 ounce cheese, ½ cup Lima beans.

The judicious use of cream, butter, jelly or jam, and sugars will quickly increase the caloric level, but excessive use may provoke nausea and loss of appetite.

Some patients make better progress if given small, frequent feedings; but for many patients midmorning and midafternoon feedings have been found to interfere with the appetite for the following meal. Bedtime snacks, however, may be planned to provide 300 to 800 or so calories, thus making it possible to follow a normal pattern for the three meals.

The following list of foods illustrates one way in which the Four Food Groups may be adapted to a high-calorie level. The meal patterns outlined for the High-protein Diet (p. 373) suggest suitable arrangements of these foods.

3 to 4 cups milk
1 cup light cream
4 to 6 ounces meat, fish, or poultry
2 eggs
4 servings vegetables including:
    1 serving green or yellow vegetable
    2 servings white or sweet potato, corn, or beans
    1 serving other vegetable
2 to 3 servings fruit, including one citrus fruit
1 serving whole-grain or enriched cereal
3 to 6 slices whole-grain or enriched bread
4 tablespoons or more butter or fortified margarine

High-calorie foods to complete the caloric requirement: cereals such as macaroni, rice, noodles, spaghetti; honey, molasses, sirups; hard candies; glucose;
salad dressings; cakes; cookies, and pastry in moderation; ice cream, puddings,
sauces.

PROBLEMS AND REVIEW

1. Why is obesity such a serious handicap to health?

2. Eating in excess of one's caloric requirement is the cause of all obesity. List
eight situations in which overeating is especially apt to occur.

3. *Problem.* Walking at the rate of 3¾ miles per hour requires an energy expenditure of 285 calories for 1 hour by an individual who weighs 150 pounds.
How many miles would an individual have to walk in order to lose 1 pound of
body fat?

4. *Problem.* Jon requires 2600 calories daily but is now getting 1800 calories
a day. How much weight would you expect him to lose in a month?

5. Obesity can be overcome by strict adherence to a low-calorie diet. What
factors must be considered in order to obtain the patient's cooperation? What points
would you consider in planning a low-calorie diet?

6. *Problem.* Plan a low-calorie diet for a woman who is 5 feet 2 inches tall and
who weighs 165 pounds. Include 90 gm of protein and 1500 calories.

7. What is meant by the satiety value of foods? Which foods are high in satiety
value?

8. Miss R. has adhered carefully to a 1200-calorie diet for 3 weeks but has
lost no weight. What advice can you give her?

9. Mrs. A. has brought her weight within normal limits. What measures are
now necessary to maintain this normal weight?

10. What is the relative importance of exercise in a low-calorie regimen? Of
drugs? Of psychotherapy?

11. *Problem.* Jane, a 23-year-old girl who is 30 pounds underweight, needs
some help in planning a diet which will include 3000 calories and at least 90 gm of
protein. Her present daily intake averages 55 gm protein and 1800 calories. Show
how she can increase her intake with a minimum of bulk. What factors may help
to improve her appetite?

12. What are some of the factors which may contribute to loss of weight?

13. *Problem.* Using the meal exchange lists, calculate the protein, fat, and carbohydrate value of the list of foods suggested for weight gain on page 387. How
many calories are provided?

14. *Problem.* Plan three bedtime snacks which will each provide about 500
calories.

CHAPTER 28 /

Diet in Fevers and Infections

Classification of fevers. Fever is an elevation of temperature above the normal and results from an imbalance between the heat produced in the body and the heat eliminated from the body. Fevers may be (1) acute, or of relatively short duration, such as colds, tonsillitis, influenza, pneumonia, chicken pox, scarlet fever, and typhoid fever, or (2) chronic, such as tuberculosis, lasting for years. The acute phases of rheumatic fever and poliomyelitis are of short duration, but the nutritional problems may be prolonged. Some fevers are accompanied with such a high temperature that they are extremely debilitating, typhoid fever and malaria being examples.

Metabolism in fevers. The more important changes in fevers which may affect nutrition are:

1. Increased metabolic rate amounting to 7 per cent for every degree Fahrenheit rise in body temperature;

2. Decreased glycogen stores;

3. Increased protein metabolism, which is especially excessive in typhoid fever, malaria, typhus fever, and others—the additional end products of protein metabolism, excreted as urea, place a heavy burden upon the kidneys;

4. Accelerated loss of body water owing to the increased perspiration and the excretion of body wastes;

5. Increased excretion of sodium chloride and of potassium;

6. Decreased motility and reduced absorption of nutrients.

General dietary considerations. The diet in fevers depends upon the nature and severity of the existing pathologic conditions and upon the length of convalescence. In general it should meet the following requirements:

Energy. The caloric requirement may be increased as much as 50 per cent or even more, depending upon the temperature, the degree of destruction of tissues, and the amount of restlessness. The body's need for calories will probably not be met during the height of the fever, but a high-calorie diet with intermediate feedings should be used as soon as possible.

Protein. It is usually desirable to give 100 to 150 gm protein per day. The most easily digested and most efficiently used protein foods such as milk and eggs should be utilized liberally in order to minimize tissue losses. High-protein beverages (recipes, p. 672) are desirable.

Carbohydrates. Glycogen stores are most efficiently replenished by a liberal intake of carbohydrate. Any sugars such as glucose, corn sirup, cane sugar, and lactose may be used to increase the carbohydrate intake. However, glucose is less sweet than some other sugars and more of it can consequently be used. Furthermore, it is a simple sugar which is absorbed into the blood stream without the necessity for enzyme action. Lactose is sometimes used, but it is relatively expensive, dissolves poorly in cold solutions, and when used in large amounts may increase fermentation in the intestine resulting in diarrhea.

Fats. The emulsified fats of cream, butter, whole milk, and egg yolk are easily digested and provide energy in concentrated form. Occasionally, nausea makes it inadvisable to use much fat, in which case carbohydrate must be relied upon to provide most of the calories. Skim milk may then be used in preference to whole milk.

Vitamins. Increased intake of vitamin A, ascorbic acid, and the B complex is advisable during fevers owing to the accelerated metabolism.

Salt. A sufficient intake of sodium chloride is accomplished by the use of salty broth and soups and by liberal sprinklings of salt on other food. Generally speaking, foods are a good source of potassium, but a limited food intake might result in potassium depletion whenever fever is high and prolonged. Fruit juices and milk are relatively good sources of this element.

Fluid. Approximately 2500 to 5000 ml fluid per day are necessary, including beverages, fruit juices, soups, and water.

Ease of digestion. Bland, readily digested foods should be used to afford maximum rest to the body, to facilitate ready digestion and rapid absorption, and to ensure adequate fluid intake. Usually a full fluid diet is used initially with progression to a soft diet and then a regular diet as the appetite improves.

Several points are of importance in deciding whether to use a liquid diet initially: (1) most liquid diets occupy bulk out of all proportion to their caloric and nutrient values, so that reinforcement of liquids is essential; (2) a liquid diet may sometimes increase abdominal distention to the point of acute discomfort, whereas solid foods may be better tolerated; (3) many patients experience less anorexia, nausea, and vomiting when they are taking solid foods.

Intervals of feeding. Small quantities of food at intervals of 2 to 3 hours will permit adequate nutrition without overtaxing the digestive system at any one time. With improvement, many patients consume more food if given three meals and a bedtime feeding.

Diet in fevers of short duration. A high-calorie high-protein fluid diet given in small, frequent feedings is suitable during the acute stage of illness. Initially, the patient may not be able to ingest enough food to meet his full nutrient needs, but emphasis should be placed upon adequate fluid intake. The pattern for the High-protein Fluid Diet on page 375 is suitable, using cream, additional butter, and sugar for increase in the calories. When the patient's condition improves, the High-protein Soft Diet, page 374, may be used with similar supplements of sugars and fats for additional calories.

Diet in typhoid fever. Improved sanitation has greatly reduced the incidence of typhoid fever, while antibiotic therapy has shortened the acute stage of the disease. Nevertheless, short and uneventful convalescence is determined to an important degree by adequate nutrition.

The febrile period may cause loss of tissue protein amounting to as much as ½ to ¾ pound of muscle a day. The body store of glycogen is quickly depleted, and a probable upset in water balance occurs.

The intestinal tract becomes highly inflamed and irritable, and diarrhea which is a frequent complication interferes with the absorption of nutrients. The ulceration may be so severe that hemorrhage and even perforation of the intestines may occur.

The dietary considerations outlined on page 389 apply as in other fevers. Special emphasis must be placed upon a caloric intake of 3500 or more, and a protein intake in excess of 100 gm. Because of the intestinal inflammation, great care must be exercised to eliminate all irritating fibers. The high-protein fluid diet may be used as a basis in dietary planning. In addition, low-fiber foods including white breads and crackers, refined cooked and dry cereals, eggs, cheese, tender meat, fish, and poultry, potato, and plain desserts may be used. The foods permitted for Bland Diet III, page 418, with the exception of fruits are suitable for the patient with typhoid fever. In addition, broths are useful for their salt content. A representative meal pattern is as follows:

HIGH-PROTEIN HIGH-CALORIE LOW-FIBER DIET

MEAL PATTERN	SAMPLE MENU
Breakfast	
Citrus juice with glucose—1 glass	Orange juice with glucose
Cereal with cream and sugar	Cream of Wheat with cream and sugar
Egg, soft-cooked or poached	Poached egg on
White toast with butter	Buttered white toast
Beverage	Cocoa
Midmorning	
Eggnog	Eggnog made with cream
Luncheon or supper	
Broth or strained cream soup	Cream of tomato soup
Potato with butter	Baked potato (no skin) with butter

MEAL PATTERN   SAMPLE MENU

Luncheon or supper (continued)

White bread with butter	Buttered white toast
Dessert	Vanilla ice cream
High-protein beverage	High-protein milk

Midafternoon

Citrus juice	Orange juice with egg
Saltines	Saltines

Dinner

Cream soup or broth	Consommé with gelatin
Egg or cheese	Soft-cooked egg
Potato or cereal	Boiled rice with sugar and cream
White bread with butter	Buttered white toast
Dessert	Tapioca cream
Milk	Milk

Bedtime

High-protein beverage	Chocolate malted milk
Plain pudding, bread, or crackers	Cream-cheese sandwich on white bread

Diet in rheumatic fever. This is one of the leading causes of chronic illness in children. It will permanently damage the heart if it is not recognized early and treated promptly. Rheumatic fever follows streptococcus infections and is more common among poorer classes of people. However, all attempts to correlate the incidence of the disease with specific nutrient deficiencies have so far failed.

The soft and liquid diets described in Chapter 24 are suitable during the acute phase of rheumatic fever. When cortisone or ACTH therapy is used, the diet must be restricted in sodium to approximately 1000 mg or less to avoid sodium retention and edema formation (see Chap. 36).

The acute stage may last only a few weeks, but absolute bed rest is essential for many weeks or months. The chief problem in nutrition is that of maintaining an adequate intake of nutrients during the prolonged period of bed rest. Because the appetite may be poor, it has been suggested [135] that cereal foods and sweets be restricted as a means of ensuring adequate intake of milk, eggs, citrus fruits, and other essential foods. The diet is planned according to the principles of the normal diet described in Chapter 19.

Diet in poliomyelitis. Spinal poliomyelitis requires essentially the same dietary attention during the acute phase as that for other acute fevers. However, convalescence is prolonged, and tissue destruction occurs. Immobilization leads to excessive excretion of calcium and the frequent incidence of urinary calculi (see Chap. 37).

Physical handicaps may interfere seriously with the ability to manage the foods served and may lead to discouragement and poor food intake. The nurse must assume responsibility not only for helping the patient through giving him foods he can manage or in feeding him, if required, but she must also give the necessary encouragement and psychologic support which brings the patient to make every effort to help himself, difficult though it may be.

The chief dietary problem in bulbar poliomyelitis is the difficulty or failure in swallowing food and the possibility of choking or aspiration. After the initial feedings by the parenteral route, a four-stage feeding program has been described by Seifert: *

Stage I. Tube feedings of 30–50 ml up to 150–200 ml are alternated every 2 hours with water. The tube feedings consist of skim milk-egg-sugar formulas or milk-cream-orange juice-sugar mixtures with or without added protein foods and oral fat emulsions.

Stage II. Tube feedings are continued. Ability to swallow is cautiously tested by giving 1 to 2 teaspoons of grape juice and noting whether the juice is seen in the tracheotomy opening. If swallowing is successful, broth, tea with sugar, apple juice, flavored gelatin, and diluted, strained juices are cautiously tried.

Stage III. A soft, low-fiber diet of easily digested foods is started. Tube feeding is continued until sufficient amounts of food can be swallowed. Sticky foods especially must be avoided. The foods which may be permitted include:

All foods from tube feedings in stages I and II
Beverages: tea with sugar, water, or coffee
Cereals: Cream of Wheat or farina with large amounts of sugar and a little milk
Desserts: custard, flavored gelatin, sherbet
Eggs: soft-cooked or poached
Fats: butter
Fruits: puréed, cooked, or canned (without seeds, skin or fiber) strained fruit
   juices
Meats: strained
Soups: bouillon or strained meat soup
Vegetables: well-cooked or puréed

Foods to avoid are:

Fish
Fried foods
Milk

* Adapted from Seifert, M. H.: "Poliomyelitis and the Relation of Diet to Its Treatment," *J. Am. Dietet. A.,* **30:**671, 1954.

Pastries
Potatoes
Raw fruits and vegetables
Seeds as in berries, tomatoes
Spicy or highly seasoned foods
Starchy products: macaroni, rice, spaghetti
Sticky foods: cheese dishes, ice cream, oatmeal
Strongly flavored vegetables

Stage IV. More solid foods, including ground meat, bread, and milk products, are introduced when the patient can take stage III without mishap. In addition to stage III, the following foods are permitted:

Breads: soda crackers, white bread, or toast with butter
Desserts: plain cornstarch puddings and ice cream
Fruits: cooked or canned applesauce, apricots, peaches, or pears
Meats: ground beef, chicken, lamb, or turkey with light gravies or mayonnaise
Milk alone or with protein supplements
Vegetables: well-cooked but not puréed asparagus, French-cut green beans, carrots, canned peas, squash, or chopped spinach

Foods to avoid are:

Fish
Potatoes
Starchy products
Sticky foods—casserole dishes

Diet in tuberculosis. Pulmonary tuberculosis is an inflammatory disease of the lungs accompanied by a wasting of the tissues, exhaustion, cough, expectoration, and fever. In its acute form it resembles pneumonia, because the temperature is high and circulation and respiration are increased. The metabolic rate in tuberculosis is not as high as in other fevers except when the fever is high, but wasting may be considerable because of the length of the illness. A tendency to develop gastrointestinal disturbances is characteristic of the disease. The normal diet is modified as follows:

Energy. Since the metabolic rate is not as high as in other fevers, satisfactory weight can be maintained, as a rule, at 2500 to 3000 calories. It is not desirable to gain more than 10 per cent above the ideal weight for the body frame.

Protein. A protein intake somewhat in excess of normal requirements is necessary in tuberculosis, since the serum albumin value, especially in advanced tuberculosis and in cases of long standing, may be low.[136] The daily level may range from 80 to 120 gm.

Minerals. Calcium, especially, should be provided liberally since it is essential for the healing of tuberculous lesions. At least 1 quart of milk should be taken daily.[137] The iron needs may also be increased if there has been hemorrhage.

Vitamins. The metabolism of vitamin A is adversely affected in tuberculosis. Carotene appears to be poorly converted to vitamin A so that the diet should be planned to provide vitamin A as such.[136] The weekly inclusion of liver and dietary supplementation with vitamin A are essential.

Ascorbic acid deficiency is present even in patients with slight tuberculous involvement and becomes more marked with the progression of the disease. Increased amounts of orange juice may be given, but ascorbic acid is frequently also prescribed. Isoniazid has been found to be an effective drug in the treatment of tuberculosis, but it is also an antagonist of vitamin B_6, thereby increasing the requirement. When this therapy is used, vitamin B_6 supplementation is essential.

Selection of foods. During the acute stage of the illness, a high-protein high-calorie fluid diet may be given as in other acute fevers, progressing to the soft and regular diets when improvement occurs. Most patients have very poor appetites. For some a six-meal routine is best, while others eat better if they receive three meals and a bedtime feeding. The individuals responsible for planning meals should respect the patient's food idiosyncrasies. To this

HIGH-PROTEIN, HIGH-CALORIE DIET *

Breakfast	*Luncheon or supper*	*Dinner*
Citrus fruit or juice	Cream soup	Clear soup or fruit juice
Cereal—⅔ cup	Meat, fish, poultry, eggs, or cheese—2 ounces	Meat, poultry, or fish—3 ounces
Cream, light—½ cup	Potato or substitute	Potato
Egg—2	Green leafy or yellow vegetable	Cooked vegetable
Toast or roll—1 to 2 slices	Salad	Bread or roll—1 to 2 slices
Butter or fortified margarine—2 teaspoons	Salad dressing	Butter or fortified margarine—2 teaspoons
Jelly—1 tablespoon	Bread or roll—1 to 2 slices	Dessert
Milk—1 cup	Butter or fortified margarine—2 teaspoons	Milk beverage
Sugar—3 teaspoons	Milk—1 cup	
Hot beverage	Fruit	
Midmorning	*Midafternoon*	*Evening*
Milk beverage	Citrus fruit juice	Milk beverage
	Crackers or plain cookies	Sandwiches, plain dessert, cookies, or crackers

* Approximately 130 gm protein, 3500 calories.

end, a selective menu from which the patient chooses his foods each day is helpful. Other patients may eat better when they are not consulted in advance about their diets, thus introducing an element of surprise. Needless to say, every attention must be given to making meals as appetizing in appearance and taste as possible. A pattern for a high-protein high-calorie diet is given on page 395.

Instruction of the patient. Time and again throughout this text the value of instruction has been pointed out. In no situation is this of greater value than for the patient who has recovered from tuberculosis. Wilson and her associates [138] have pointed out that failure of the patient to secure the essentials of a good diet leads to a great increase in recurrence and repeated hospitalization. The characteristics of a normal diet, with special emphasis on a liberal milk intake, protein-rich foods, fruits and vegetables must be pointed out. When there is financial need it is not enough to secure additional allowances to purchase the required foods, but practical measures for budgeting the food allowance must be recommended.

PROBLEMS AND REVIEW

1. How great is the increase in energy metabolism brought about by fever? What other changes in metabolism of nutrients take place during fever? In view of these changes criticize the commonly held belief "Starve a fever."

2. Give examples of reinforcing agents used for increasing the protein of the diet, the carbohydrate, and the fat.

3. *Problem.* Plan a diet for a patient with pneumonia which contains 80 gm protein and 2500 calories. What principles are observed in planning a diet for such a patient?

4. What are the principles of dietary management in poliomyelitis?

5. Satisfactory dietary treatment in tuberculosis must consider very carefully the patient's attitude to his diet, since appetite is often very poor. What are the advantages and disadvantages of using a selective menu for such patients?

6. *Problem.* Plan a diet for a patient with tuberculosis which contains 100 gm protein and 3000 calories. List a number of ways in which you would try to bring about this intake of food.

7. What is the basis for recommending sodium restriction for some patients with rheumatic fever?

CHAPTER 29

Nutrition in Surgical Conditions

Tube Feedings; High-protein, High-fat, Low-carbohydrate Diet (for Dumping Syndrome)

Good nutrition prior to and following surgery assures fewer postoperative complications, better wound healing, shorter convalescence, and lower mortality.

Effects of surgery on the nutritive requirements. Surgery or injury brings about a greatly increased need for nutrients as a result of loss of blood, plasma, or pus from the wound surface; hemorrhage from the gastrointestinal or pulmonary tract; vomiting; and fever. During immobilization, the loss of some nutrients such as protein is accelerated.

A fairly simple operation often involves moderate or marked deficiency in food intake for 3 to 8 days following operation. Even though some nutrients may be supplied by parenteral fluids, the full needs of the body usually cannot be met by that means alone. Moreover, when foods are permitted following surgery, the choice and amount are sometimes too limited to permit nutritive balance.

Far more serious is the problem of the patient whose poor nutritional state prior to surgery imposes a severe additional strain. Chronic infection as in bronchiectasis or heightened metabolism as in hyperthyroidism may lead to increased requirements. Poor appetite and inadequate intake of nutrients are the rule in many diseases. Especially in liver diseases and in sprue absorptive failure may be serious. Extensive losses of nutrients and fluids may have occurred through hemorrhage, vomiting, or diarrhea. The extent of the deficiency is manifested by weight loss, poor wound healing, decreased intestinal motility, anemia, edema or dehydration, and the presence of decubitus ulcers. The circulating blood volume and the concentration of the serum proteins, hemoglobin, and electrolytes may be reduced.

Nutritional considerations. The objectives in the dietary management of surgical conditions are (1) to improve the preoperative nutrition whenever the operation is not of an emergency nature, (2) to maintain correct nutrition after operation or injury insofar as possible, and (3) to avoid harm from the injudicious choice of foods.

Protein. A satisfactory state of protein nutrition ensures rapid wound healing by providing the correct assortment and quantity of essential amino acids, increases the resistance to infection, exerts a protective action upon the liver against the toxic effects of anesthesia, and reduces the possibility of edema at the site of the wound. The presence of edema is a hindrance to wound healing and, in operations on the gastrointestinal tract, may reduce motility thus leading to distention.

Crandon [139] suggests that it is not always realistic to fully replace protein losses prior to surgery because the disease process itself may be such as to preclude a satisfactory intake of food. He believes that improved surgical results of recent years have come about through adequate replacement of blood volume and better operative techniques rather than preoperative protein replacement. The extent to which surgery should be delayed in order to improve the nutritional state is obviously a highly individual matter.

Immediately following surgery or injury and for several days thereafter, protein catabolism is increased and patients are characteristically in negative nitrogen balance even though the protein intake might be appreciable. Such losses, paradoxically, are greatest in patients who have been well nourished and are least in those who are poorly nourished.[139]

The level of protein to be used in preoperative and postoperative diets depends upon the previous state of nutrition, the nature of the operation, and the extent of the postoperative losses. Intakes of 100 gm protein, and frequently much more, are necessary as a rule.

Energy. The weight status is an important pre- and postoperative consideration, for it serves as a guide to the caloric level to be recommended. Without sufficient caloric intake, tissue proteins cannot be synthesized. Excessive metabolism of body fat may lead to acidosis, while depletion of the liver glycogen may increase the likelihood of damage to the liver.

When hyperthyroidism or a fever is present, as much as 4000 calories daily may be essential to bring about weight gain. Other patients will make satisfactory progress at 2500 to 3000 calories.

Obesity constitutes a hazard in surgery. Whenever possible, it should be corrected, at least in part, by using one of the low-calorie diets (see p. 384).

Minerals. Phosphorus and potassium are lost in proportion to the breakdown of body tissue. In addition, derangements of sodium and chloride metabolism may occur from vomiting, diarrhea, perspiration, drainage, anorexia, and diuresis or renal failure. The detection of electrolyte imbalance and appropriate parenteral fluid therapy requires careful study of clinical signs and biochemical evaluation.

If absorption has been faulty or if blood losses have been high, iron-deficiency anemia may occur. Diet alone is ineffective in its correction, but iron salts may be administered together with a liberal dietary intake of protein and ascorbic acid. Such therapy is of value in convalescence, but transfusions are usually required for severe reduction in hemoglobin level.

Fluids. A review of the maintenance of water balance (see p. 162) will bring to the attention of the student the large amounts of fluid lost daily by the normal individual and the several sources of water to the body. The fluid balance may be upset prior to and following surgery owing to failure to ingest normal quantities of fluids and to increased losses from vomiting, exudates, hemorrhage, diuresis, and fever. A patient should not go to operation in a state of dehydration since the subsequent dangers of acidosis are great. When dehydration exists prior to operation parenteral fluids are administered if the patient is unable to ingest sufficient liquid by mouth. Following major surgery the fluid balance is maintained by parenteral fluids until satisfactory oral intake can be established.

Vitamins. Ascorbic acid is especially important for wound healing and should be provided in increased amounts prior to and following surgery. Vitamin K is of concern to the surgeon since the failure to synthesize vitamin K in the small intestine, the inability to absorb it, or the defect in conversion to prothrombin is likely to result in bleeding. Hemorrhage is especially likely to occur in patients who have diseases of the liver.

Planning the preoperative diet. Patients who have lost much weight prior to surgery may benefit considerably by ingesting a high-protein high-calorie diet (see p. 373) for even a week or two prior to surgery. The diet may be of liquid, soft, or regular consistency depending upon the nature of the pathologic condition. In addition, the maintenance of metabolic equilibrium as in diabetes or other diseases must not be overlooked.

When surgery is delayed in order to improve the nutritional status, each day's intake should represent such improvement in nutrition that the delay is justified. This necessitates constant encouragement by the nurse and dietitian; it likewise requires imagination in varying the foods offered to the patient and ingenuity in getting the patient to eat. Foods which provide a maximum amount of nutrients in a minimum volume are essential. Small feedings at frequent intervals are likely to be more effective than large meals which cannot be fully consumed.

For additional protein, milk beverages may be fortified with nonfat dry milk, whole egg, and egg whites. Strained meat in broth may be used when patients are unable to eat other meats. Fruit juices fortified with glucose, high-carbohydrate lemonade (p. 673), jelly with crackers and bread, and hard candy may be used to increase the carbohydrate intake and to facilitate storage of glycogen. Butter incorporated into foods and light cream mixed with equal amounts of milk are also useful for increasing the caloric intake. The excessive use of sugars and fats may provoke nausea, however.

Food and fluid are generally allowed until midnight just preceding the day of operation, although a light breakfast may be given when the operation is scheduled for afternoon and local anesthesia is to be used. It is essential that the stomach be empty prior to administering the anesthesia so as to reduce the incidence of vomiting and the subsequent danger of aspiration of vomitus. When an operation is to be performed on the gastrointestinal tract, a diet very low in residue (p. 429) may be ordered for 2 or 3 days prior to operation. In acute abdominal conditions such as appendicitis and cholecystitis, no food is allowed by mouth until nausea, vomiting, pain, and distention have passed in order to prevent the danger of peritonitis.

Planning the postoperative diet. During the first 24 to 48 hours postoperatively gastrointestinal secretions and peristalsis are inhibited, and feeding may lead to vomiting and adynamic ileus. At this time the fluid and electrolyte balances are maintained by means of parenteral fluids if necessary. Glucose, amino acids, vitamins, and sometimes fat emulsions are given intravenously to support the nutritive needs if oral feeding is unduly delayed. Usually, the complete nutritive requirements cannot be met until oral feeding is resumed.

Postoperative feeding can be initiated as soon as there is evidence of peristaltic sounds of normal quality, the movement of material along the gastrointestinal tract, and evacuation of the colon. Early ambulation of the patient contributes to a more rapid return of gastrointestinal activity. As soon as gastrointestinal function returns, the digestive fluids which amount to several liters daily place a burden on the gastrointestinal tract. The ingestion of food at this time serves to move the gastrointestinal contents along and to prevent gastric retention.[140] The nature of the operation determines the rapidity of the dietary progression and will be presented in more detail in the discussion of specific surgical conditions below. A low-residue, soft, or normal diet is often ordered as early as the second day with the patient eating from such diets as he is able. It is believed by many that liquid diets retard emptying of the gastrointestinal tract and thus contribute to distention.

TUBE FEEDING

Tube feeding is required in a variety of circumstances: surgery of the mouth; gastrointestinal surgery; obstruction of the esophagus; in severe burns; in anorexia nervosa; and in the comatose patient. A satisfactory tube feeding must be: (1) nutritionally adequate; (2) well tolerated by the patient so that vomiting is not induced; (3) easily digested with no unfavorable reactions such as distention, diarrhea, or constipation; (4) easily prepared; and (5) inexpensive.

Numerous formulas have been developed for tube feeding, one of which is presented in the table on page 401. This formula provides approximately 1 calorie per ml. The usual daily intake of this formula would be about 2000 ml, thus providing a liberal protein intake. The formula may be modified in

TUBE FEEDING

FOOD	MEASURE	WEIGHT gm	ENERGY calories	PROTEIN gm	FAT gm	CARBO-HYDRATE gm	MINERALS			A I.U.	VITAMINS			
							Ca mg	Fe mg	Na mg		Thia-mine mg	Ribo-flavin mg	Niacin mg	Ascorbic Acid mg
Nonfat dry milk	1½ cups *	150	544	54	2	78	1950	1.0	788	60	0.54	2.94	1.8	10
Eggs	2	100	154	13	12	tr	54	2.7	130	1140	0.10	0.29	0.1	0
Sugar	¼ cup	60	240	0	0	60	0	0	0	0	0	0	0	0
Molasses, medium	¼ cup	60	139	0	0	39	174	3.6	0	0	0	0.07	0.7	0
Brewers' yeast	5 teaspoons	13	35	5	tr	5	13	2.4	20	0	1.27	0.72	4.7	0
Water	3 cups	720												
TOTAL (approximately 1000 ml)			1112	72	14	182	2191	9.7	938	1200	1.91	4.02	7.3	10

* The measure of dry milk varies, depending upon brand.

To Prepare. Put water in bowl, and add dry milk powder. Mix well with rotary beater. Beat eggs, add sugar, molasses, and yeast. Add gradually to milk and beat until smooth. Strain through fine mesh. Store in covered bottles in the refrigerator. Use within 24 hours.

To Feed. Heat enough formula for one feeding over hot water to 100° F (lukewarm). Overheating leads to curdling.

Supplements. Give 6 to 8 ounces orange juice daily as a separate feeding. Add cod-liver oil or vitamin-A concentrate to one of the feedings each day. Salt may be added to the formula if there appears to be increased need.

Variations. Reduce the concentration of the formula by using 100 gm nonfat dry milk instead of 150 gm. Increase the calories of the formula by substituting light cream for part of the water.

Sodium deficient dry milk may be substituted for nonfat dry milk if a low-sodium intake is required.

If diarrhea occurs, 1 tablespoon fruit pectin or 2 tablespoons applesauce or apple powder may be added to each liter of formula.

a number of ways for protein and caloric content, and for reduction in sodium.

Tube feedings may also be prepared by blending strained baby meats and vegetables with milk, eggs, and fruit juices. A simple feeding consisting of canned soybean milk (Mull-Soy) diluted with an equal volume of water and supplemented with a vitamin concentrate was found to be satisfactory by Krehl.[141]

Blenderized feedings. Natural whole foods commonly appearing on a regular diet may be liquefied in a mechanical blender for use as a tube feeding. Such feedings more nearly approach the customary food intake of the patient, are well tolerated, and are believed to result in lesser incidence of diarrhea. To prepare such feedings the following procedures are followed: [142]

1. Food is mixed with sufficient liquid in the blender to facilitate homogenization and liquefaction.

2. Homogenized milk should be used in the blender since plain milk will form butter.

3. About 4 to 5 minutes is usually required for homogenization.

4. The homogenate must be strained several times through a fine mesh wire sieve to remove all fibrous material which might clog the tube.

Administration of tube feedings. Depending upon its nature, the feeding may be heated over hot water to body temperature, taking care that curdling does not occur with certain mixtures. Initially, small amounts of a dilute formula (50 ml) are given at hourly intervals. It is important that the feeding be given at a slow constant rate. Barron [142] recommends the use of a food pump with blenderized feedings. In patients who do not have an adequate swallowing mechanism or who are comatose, special care must be taken to avoid vomiting and aspiration of the vomitus. The patient should be positioned to prevent aspiration, and suction should be readily available at the bedside if vomiting occurs.[141]

When the small feedings are satisfactorily tolerated, the concentration and amount of the formula is gradually increased, with feedings not exceeding 12 ounces per 3- to 4-hour interval.

DIET IN SPECIFIED SURGICAL CONDITIONS

Diet following operations on the mouth, throat, or esophagus. The extraction of teeth, the period of waiting for dentures, and the time required to become accustomed to new dentures could result in nutritive inadequacy if suggestions for adequate diet are not given to the patient. For 1 or 2 days following the extraction of teeth, it may be necessary to restrict the diet to liquids taken through a drinking tube. Thereafter, any soft foods which require little if any chewing may be used for 3 weeks or longer.

Radical surgery of the mouth necessitates the use of a full fluid diet, but immediately after surgery one of the regimens for tube feeding described in the previous section may be used. Tube feeding is likewise required for an operation on the esophagus, the tube being inserted directly into the stomach.

Following tonsillectomy the patient may be given cold fluids including milk, bland fruit juices, ginger ale, plain ice cream, and sherbets. Tart fruit juices and fibrous foods must be avoided. On the second day, soft foods such as custard, plain puddings, soft eggs, warm but not hot cereals, strained cream soups, mashed potatoes, and fruit and vegetable purées may be tolerated. As a rule, the regular diet is swallowed without difficulty within the week.

Diet following gastrectomy. A number of problems arise following gastrectomy and their treatment should be anticipated. More than half of all patients who have had gastric surgery fail to regain weight to desirable levels.[143] The loss of a reservoir for food means that small feedings given at frequent intervals must be used if sufficient nutrients are to be ingested. Moreover, the absence of pepsin and hydrochloric acid entails the entire digestion of protein by the enzymes of the small intestine. Fat utilization is often impaired because of inadequate biliary and pancreatic secretions or from defective mixing of food with the digestive juices. Intestinal motility is frequently increased.

Iron is less readily absorbed and hypochromic microcytic anemia is common. In the absence of gastric juice and its intrinsic factor vitamin B_{12} cannot be absorbed from the intestine, thereby leading to macrocytic anemia in 2 to 5 years after operation unless injections of vitamin B_{12} are given.

Dietary progression. The oral feeding of the patient varies widely from patient to patient, but the following illustrates a typical sequence.

Day 1. 60 to 90 ml water hourly as tolerated

   2. 60 to 90 ml clear fluids hourly as tolerated

   3. 60 to 90 ml full fluids hourly as tolerated (see p. 344)

   4. Six small meals of bland foods

14–28. Normal diet, using six small meals

Lewis and her associates [144] found that patients made more satisfactory progress beginning with the fourth postoperative day when the following dietary characteristics were in effect:

1. The diet progresses from day to day according to the patient's tolerance for food.

2. The protein and fat content of the foods is emphasized by including these nutrients in the smallest practical volume.

3. The carbohydrate is kept relatively low.

4. Five to six small meals are given daily consisting of soft, low-fiber foods. Eggs, custards, thickened soups, cereals, crackers, milk, and fruit purées are used on the fourth and fifth days. The next additions are tender chicken, cottage cheese, puréed vegetables. The selection of foods afforded by Bland Diet II (see p. 418) may be used initially with progression to Bland Diet III and Bland Diet IV.

Diet following intestinal surgery. When intestinal function is resumed, small feedings of very low-residue foods may be cautiously tried. Such foods include white bread, refined cereals, eggs, tender meat, rice, plain puddings, custards, and plain gelatin desserts. See page 429 for full description of such a diet.

Following operation on the rectum, bowel movement is avoided for 4 or 5 days by using a Very Low-residue Diet (p. 429). This is followed by a moderately low-fiber diet (see Bland Diet III and IV, pp. 418 and 420).

Diet following other abdominal operations. The principles outlined on page 397 pertain to the planning of diet following appendectomy, cholecystectomy, and other abdominal operations. Adynamic ileus is present longer following cholecystectomy and hysterectomy than after removal of the appendix. Patients who have had the gallbladder removed may require a low-fat diet for 3 months or longer, after which a regular diet is used.

Following peritonitis and intestinal obstruction, nothing whatever is given by mouth until gastrointestinal function has been resumed. Drainage of the stomach and upper intestine is essential until there is reduction of distention and passage of gas. This may require 4 to 6 days, during which time nutrition is maintained by complete intravenous therapy. When the patient shows tolerance for water, broth, and weak tea a very low-residue diet may be introduced cautiously.

Diet following burns. Tremendous losses of protein, salts, and fluid take place when large areas of the body have been burned. Greatly increased nutritive requirements exist for weeks or months following burns. Severe hypoproteinemia, edema at the site of injury, failure to obtain satisfactory skin growth, and gastric atony are among the nutritional problems encountered.

When vomiting and diarrhea are severe, reliance must be placed primarily on complete intravenous therapy. Tube feeding may precede oral feeding and is continued until the high nutritive requirements can be met by the usual feeding procedures. At least 150 gm protein, and often as much as 300 gm protein, is required daily together with 3500 to 5000 calories. High-protein meals supplemented with high-protein beverages are used. (See diet, p. 373, and high-protein recipes, p. 672.) Oral fat emulsions taken as a beverage or given by tube are useful in maintaining a high-caloric intake.[145] The need for as much as 1.0 gm ascorbic acid has been definitely established, while additional B-complex vitamins are also considered essential.

Diet following fractures. Following fractures there is a tremendous catabolism of protein, which may not be reversed for several weeks. Nitrogen loss is accompanied by loss of phosphorus, potassium, and sulfur. Fever and infection may further accentuate such losses.

Calcium loss is also great but is not corrected by the administration of calcium. In fact, calcium therapy may lead to the formation of renal calculi and should not be attempted until the cast is removed and some mobilization is possible.

The chief need is for a liberal protein intake—approximately 150 gm daily

—to permit restoration of the protein matrix of the bone so that calcium can be deposited.[146] In addition approximately 3000 nonprotein calories are recommended.

DUMPING SYNDROME

Nature of the dumping syndrome. Following convalescence from gastric surgery a relatively high proportion of patients experience distressing symptoms after eating. There is a sense of fullness in the epigastrium with weakness, nausea, sweating, and dizziness. Vomiting and occasionally diarrhea may be present. Failure to gain weight is commonly observed because the patient eats less food.

Since no reservoir exists for food when gastrectomy has been performed, the food is dumped into the small intestine. The exact mechanisms which cause the syndrome are not fully understood, but a high concentration of carbohydrate in the small intestine aggravates the condition. The rapidly digested carbohydrates produce a hyperosmolar mixture which is made isotonic in the small intestine by withdrawing water from the blood circulation. As a result the blood volume and blood pressure are markedly reduced and cardiac insufficiency results.

Modification of the diet. A number of dietary regimens developed in recent years to alleviate the symptoms of the dumping syndrome emphasize: (1) avoidance of sugar and concentrated forms of carbohydrate, (2) liberal protein, (3) small frequent feedings, and (4) dry meals with fluids taken only between meals. The regimen of Pittman and Robinson is described below:

HIGH-PROTEIN, HIGH-FAT, LOW-CARBOHYDRATE DIET *

Characteristics and general rules:

1. Three routines are employed, with progression from one to another as the patient's condition warrants. The composition of the three routines is approximately:

	Routine I	Routine II	Routine III
Carbohydrate, gm	0	100	100
Protein, gm	115	150	150
Fat, gm	170	225	225
Calories	2000	3000	3000
Calorie Ratio:			
Carbohydrate	0	1	1
Fat	5	5	5
Protein	1.5	1.5	1.5

* Pittman, A. C., and Robinson, F. W.: "Dumping Syndrome—Control by Diet," *J. Am. Dietet. A.,* **34:**596, 1958.

2. Multiple vitamin supplements are prescribed; iron may be necessary.

3. Six small dry meals are given daily; meals must be eaten regularly without omissions.

4. Liquids are taken 30 to 45 minutes after meals.

5. Carbohydrate foods are severely restricted. Those allowed must be measured accurately.

6. Liberal portions of meat are used; 1 pat margarine or butter should be eaten with each ounce of meat.

7. Foods to avoid include: milk, ice cream and other frozen desserts; sugars, sweets, candy, sirup, chocolate; gravies and rich sauces.

8. Rest before meals, eating slowly and chewing well, and relaxation are essential.

Foods Allowed for Patients with the Dumping Syndrome

ROUTINE I

Beverages: never at meals. 30 to 45 minutes *after* meals; small amounts of cool (not cold) water, or coffee, tea, limeade, or lemonade without sugar. Use artificial sweetener

Eggs: 2 to 3; poached, scrambled, coddled, shirred, hard-cooked

Fats: 1 pat margarine or butter per ounce meat; 2 to 3 strips crisp bacon

Lean meat: beef, lamb; fresh lean pork; yearling veal; birds (quail, dove, etc.); chicken; turkey; ham; rabbit; venison; fresh fish of all kinds; crabmeat; clams; oysters; shrimp; crayfish. Meats to be broiled, baked, poached, stewed, or grilled—not fried. *Limited amounts,* if tolerated: baked duck or goose; fresh brains

ROUTINE II

Use all foods in Routine I with the following additions:

Breads: made without sugar, if possible. Only 1 slice with each feeding; enriched day-old white toast, zwieback, soda crackers, Melba toast

Bread substitutes: for 1 slice bread, use one of these:

½ cup fresh Lima beans

⅓ cup sweet corn

½ cup cooked dried beans and peas, including Lima, navy, red, split peas, cowpeas

Crackers

    5 saltines (2 in.)

    2 soda (2½ in.)

    20 oysterettes

2½ tbsp flour

½ cup grits

½ cup noodles

½ cup macaroni

½ cup cooked rice

ROUTINE III

Use all foods in Routines I and II. Add the following:

Fruits: without sugar! Fresh, canned, frozen, stewed: all drained of liquid. Applesauce; baked apple; ripe or baked banana; peeled apricots; white cherries; canned pears, peaches; orange and grapefruit sections

Note: Fruit juices must be taken 30 to 40 minutes after meals

ROUTINE I

or sweetbreads; luncheon meats without added cereal; frankfurters; Spam; sardines; tuna; salmon

Miscellaneous: salt; lemon or lime juice on fish, oysters, etc.

ROUTINE II

$\frac{1}{2}$ cup spaghetti
$\frac{2}{3}$ cup parsnips
1 small boiled potato (2 in. diam.)
$\frac{1}{2}$ cup mashed potato
$\frac{1}{4}$ cup sweet potato
Note: no excess gravy or sauces with pastes

Cereals: cooked thick; only 1 serving: Cream of Wheat; farina; cornmeal mush; rice; grits; oatmeal, etc.

Fats: heavy (30–40 per cent) cream in small amounts; cream cheese

Nuts, when tolerated, plain or salted: pecans; almonds; cashews; peanuts; walnuts; peanut butter, etc. Chew thoroughly

Vegetables: not more than one average serving per meal. All kinds —fresh, frozen, or canned without sugar: potatoes, asparagus, beets, carrots, celery hearts, cauliflower, eggplant, greens of all kinds, green beans, lettuce, peas, okra, squash

Miscellaneous: olives; pimiento

Sample Menu Plans for Patients with Dumping Syndrome

ROUTINE I	ROUTINE II	ROUTINE III
Morning		
2 eggs with	2 scrambled eggs with	2 scrambled eggs with
2–3 pats margarine or butter (or more)	3 pats margarine or butter	3 pats margarine or butter
2 or more strips crisp bacon	2 slices crisp bacon	2 strips crisp bacon
	1 average slice bread	$\frac{1}{2}$ slice bread

Sample Menu Plans for Patients with Dumping Syndrome (*continued*)

ROUTINE I	ROUTINE II	ROUTINE III
Morning		
	1 pat margarine or butter	1 pat margarine or butter
		½ cup orange sections (no liquid)
Midmorning		
3 oz meat with	2 oz meat with	2 oz meat with
3 pats margarine or butter, if possible	1 pat margarine or butter	1 pat margarine or butter
	2 thin slices of bread for sandwich	2 thin slices bread for sandwich
Noon		
2 beef patties or hamburger, steak, chops, roast with	4 oz chicken with	4 oz chicken with
3 pats margarine or butter (or more)	2 pats margarine or butter	3 pats margarine or butter
	½ cup string beans with	½ cup string beans with
	1 pat margarine or butter	1 pat margarine or butter
	1 slice bread with	½ slice bread with
	2 pats margarine or butter	1 pat margarine or butter
		½ small banana
Midafternoon		
Meat or eggs with	2 oz meat or 4 tbsp peanut butter with	2 oz meat or 4 tbsp peanut butter
3 pats margarine or butter	1 pat margarine or butter	1 pat margarine or butter
	2 thin slices bread for sandwich	2 thin slices bread for sandwich
Evening		
Same as at noon	4 oz broiled fish with	4 oz broiled fish with
	2 pats margarine or butter	3 pats margarine or butter
	Asparagus tips with	Asparagus tips with
	1 pat margarine or butter	1 pat margarine or butter
	1 average slice bread	½ slice bread
	1 pat margarine or butter	½ cup applesauce
Bedtime		
Same as midafternoon	Same as midafternoon	Same as midafternoon

PROBLEMS AND REVIEW

1. List a number of symptoms and laboratory findings which may require attention in preoperative dietary treatment. What measures can be taken to treat these symptoms?

2. What are some reasons why such great emphasis must be placed on adequate protein therapy prior to and following surgery?

3. Give at least two reasons why an increased intake of carbohydrate prior to and following surgery is important.

4. Which vitamin is most directly related to wound healing?

5. Outline a specific plan for a high-carbohydrate intake prior to operation.

6. *Problem.* Prepare a chart showing ingredients and methods of preparation for six high-protein beverages. Calculate the protein content for 100 ml of each of these beverages.

7. *Problem.* Prepare a chart showing the customary preoperative and postoperative dietary progressions for each of the following operations: appendectomy, gastric resection, colostomy, tonsillectomy, cholecystectomy, and hemorrhoidectomy. Indicate in each instance (a) the approximate length of time each diet might be used, and (b) the factors which require particular emphasis.

8. *Problem.* Select any two patients who have just had a major operation and note the actual progression of diets in each instance for 7 to 10 days. Indicate the kinds and amounts of intravenous therapy used, if any. Note any vomiting or complaints of nausea and distention.

9. *Problem.* Prepare a list of parenteral feedings used in your hospital and enumerate the chief contributions made by each.

10. If a patient who requires a tube feeding is allergic to milk, in what way could nutrition be maintained?

11. What is meant by the dumping syndrome? What dietary modifications are required for patients with this condition?

UNIT VIII /
Diet in Disturbances of the Gastrointestinal Tract

CHAPTER 30

Diet in Diseases of the Stomach and Duodenum

Bland Diet (Five Stages)

The gastrointestinal tract, on which the entire body depends for adequate nourishment, assumes a most essential role in the maintenance of body health. The stomach is the first important organ of digestion, since the food stays too short a time in the mouth to accomplish much by way of adequate preparation. The work of the stomach is accomplished by chemical and physical means. A review of the subject of digestion in Chapter 13 will enable the student to understand more readily the rationale for diet therapy in gastrointestinal diseases.

Secretory and motor activity of the stomach. The gastric secretion consists of hydrochloric acid, the protein-splitting enzyme pepsin, intrinsic factor to facilitate the absorption of vitamin B_{12}, small amounts of lipase, and other substances. The contraction and relaxation of the muscular walls of the stomach and the peristaltic waves which assist in mixing the food mass with the gastric juices constitute the motor activity of the stomach. The rate of secretion of gastric juice as well as the motility and tone of the alimentary tract are affected by many physiologic and psychologic factors. Some of these are listed in the table on page 413. It will be noted that individuals may differ in their response to certain stimuli, increased activity being produced in some and decreased activity in others.

Disorders of the stomach and duodenum. Gastric and duodenal disturbances are functional or organic in character. Functional disturbances present no pathologic lesions and are frequently caused by errors in diet or neuroses. Pathologic lesions are present in the organic diseases such as peptic ulcer and carcinoma. Modifications in secretory and motor activity are characteristic of both types of gastrointestinal disorders.

Hyperchlorhydria means a secretion of acid in excess of normal and is often accompanied by epigastric distress. Of the total acid which is secreted by the stomach, some combines with protein, while that which remains un-

FACTORS WHICH MODIFY ACID SECRETION AND GASTROINTESTINAL MOTILITY AND TONE

INCREASED FLOW OF ACID AND ENZYME PRODUCTION	DECREASED FLOW OF ACID AND ENZYME PRODUCTION
1. Chemical stimulation—meat extractives, seasonings, spices, alcohol, acid foods 2. Attractive, appetizing, well-liked foods 3. State of happiness and contentment 4. Pleasant surroundings for meals	1. Large amounts of fat, especially as fried foods, pastries, nuts, etc. 2. Large meals 3. Poor mastication of food 4. Foods of poor appearance, flavor, or texture 5. Foods acutely disliked 6. Worry, anger, fear, pain *

INCREASED TONE AND MOTILITY	DECREASED TONE AND MOTILITY
1. Warm foods 2. Liquid and soft foods 3. Fibrous foods, as in certain fruits and vegetables 4. High-carbohydrate low-fat intake 5. Seasonings; concentrated sweets 6. Fear, anger, worry, nervous tension	1. Colds foods 2. Dry, solid foods 3. Low-fiber foods 4. High-fat intake, especially as fried foods, pastries, etc. 5. Vitamin-B-complex deficiency, especially thiamine 6. Sedentary habits 7. Fatigue 8. Worry, anger, fear, pain

* In certain individuals these emotional disturbances may stimulate the flow of gastric juice.

combined is known as "free" hydrochloric acid. There is a great variation in the amount of acid secreted under various conditions and in different people. Many people continually secrete more gastric juice than normal and never experience any discomfort. Hyperchlorhydria may be associated with emotional or nervous upsets, or it may accompany organic disease such as peptic ulcer or cholecystitis.

Hypochlorhydria denotes a diminished amount of free acid, while in achlorhydria there is no free acid present whatsoever, although there is some peptic activity. *Achylia gastrica* refers to the absence of both free and combined acid and of enzyme activity. Hypochlorhydria may be present indefinitely in perfectly healthy people. However, when a physician finds this condition he always tries to determine its cause, since it also accompanies diseases such as pernicious anemia and is a common finding in sprue, chronic gastritis, and pellagra. More occasionally, it also occurs in cancer, nephritis, cholecystitis, and diabetes.

Gastric atony is characterized by lack of normal tone of the muscles of the stomach. The contractions are not of sufficient strength to move the food mass out of the organ at a normal rate. Larger pieces or fragments of food are not adequately disintegrated and mixed with the stomach juices.

Hyperperistalsis refers to an increased action of the musculature of the stomach and intestines. This may be brought about by excessive amounts of fibrous foods, psychologic factors such as worry or fear, or nervous stimulation.

PEPTIC ULCER

Peptic ulcer is an important medical problem which occurs in one person of every ten on a lifetime basis.[147] It may be defined as an open lesion upon the mucous lining of the stomach or duodenum, with gradual disintegration and necrosis of the tissue. Gastric and duodenal ulcers provoke symptoms which are similar and respond to the same treatment; hence, for the purposes of diet therapy they may be considered together. A thorough understanding of dietary regimens in peptic ulcer will also provide a basis for consideration of other functional and organic gastrointestinal disorders to be discussed subsequently.

Etiology. The exact cause of peptic ulcer remains unknown. For some reason the mucosa of the stomach and duodenum becomes unable to resist the action of the digestive juices, part of the tissue is digested away, and an ulcer develops. In gastric ulcer the amount of acid is not increased, but resistance of the tissue appears to be reduced. In duodenal ulcer an excess production of acid and pepsin results in ulceration of tissue believed to be normal in its resistance.

Possibly trauma plays a role. Repeated irritation from frequent dietary indiscretion or alcoholism may result in a devitalized area which is more subject to the eroding effect of the gastric juice.

People who are highly nervous and emotional and who are given to worry, fear, and anxiety seem to be particularly susceptible. These emotional and nervous factors in turn may lead to hypersecretion and hypermotility of the stomach. Individuals of a nervous temperament not only develop ulcers in the first place but are likely to have flare-ups when undergoing strong emotional stress, even after the ulcer has healed. The fact that peptic ulcer has its greatest incidence between 20 and 40 years of age suggests an important link between the stresses of life and the occurrence of the ulcer.

The nervous control of the vascular system in the gastric or duodenal walls may be so disturbed that there is a diminution in the blood supply to the mucosa of the stomach and duodenum. The acid of the stomach brings about erosion and eventually ulceration.

Symptoms and clinical findings. The diagnosis of peptic ulcer is based upon the patient's symptoms, the results of gastric analysis (see pp. 577–79), gastroscopy, and x-rays. Most patients with ulcers present the following signs.

1. Gastric tone is increased, with deep hunger contractions occurring when the stomach is empty. Characteristic gnawing pains make their appearance

2 or 3 hours after meals or in the middle of the night. Relief is usually prompt when one takes food or alkalies.

2. The presence of unneutralized acid and hypermotility is believed to be responsible for the pain. The volume and concentration of hydrochloric acid are usually increased in duodenal ulcer, but may be normal in gastric ulcer.

3. Distention follows ingestion of quantities of fluid or solid food in the majority of patients. The gastric mucosa may be sensitive to hot spices, acids, and coarse fibers.

Various deficiency manifestations are often encountered. Gastrointestinal diseases are second only to a faulty food intake as a cause of protein deficiency.[148] The patient very often has a moderately low, and at times a very low, serum protein level. In addition to the usual implications of protein deficiency (see Chap. 26), such low levels of protein are incompatible with rapid healing of the ulcer. Even when healing does occur, the ulcer breaks open with the least irritation.

Loss of weight and iron-deficiency anemia are common. The intake of thiamine, niacin, and ascorbic acid tends to be low when vegetables have been restricted for a long time.

In some patients the first indication of an ulcer may be hemorrhage. In other patients the ulcer may erode through (perforate) the gastrointestinal wall, thus necessitating immediate surgery. The possibility that the lesion is malignant must always be kept in mind when the ulcer occurs in the stomach. X-ray and the rate of response to healing by conservative measures are important in differentiating between benign and malignant lesions.

Rationale for treatment. Treatment of the patient rather than the ulcer is the keystone to success. Especially important is consideration of good physical and mental hygiene. Improvement may be rapid if the patient can be relieved of worry, anxiety, or other factors which create nervous tension. On the other hand, the failure to help the patient in dealing constructively with his day-to-day problems may nullify the beneficial effects which might be expected from the dietary program. Many patients require complete bed rest for a time. Others can be satisfactorily treated while continuing light employment.

Antacids are prescribed to aid in neutralizing the gastric contents; *anticholinergic* drugs reduce the secretion of gastric juice; and *antispasmodics* reduce gastrointestinal activity.

Modification of the diet. In 1915 Sippy [149] first outlined his regimen of hourly 3-ounce milk and cream feedings. Bland, easily digested foods such as eggs and cereal were added on the second and third day, with other additions being made from time to time until a full bland diet was being taken. An important feature of the therapy was the continual neutralization of free hydrochloric acid by giving alkali (antacid) midway between each feeding.

Numerous modifications of the Sippy regimen have been developed since

Sippy's diet was described. The generally accepted aims in the dietary management have been and are: (1) to provide adequate nutrition; (2) to afford rest; (3) to maintain continuous neutralization of the gastric acid; (4) to inhibit acid production; and (5) to reduce mechanical, chemical, and thermal irritation.

Adequate nutrition. The caloric, protein, mineral, and vitamin needs of patients with peptic ulcer are similar to those of persons in health. Some patients who have limited their intake to a few foods because they have been afraid to eat a variety may require additional protein to restore depleted tissues, as well as supplementary minerals and vitamins.

The rapid healing of the ulcer depends especially upon the correct assortment of essential amino acids and sufficient ascorbic acid. Iron absorption is dependent upon an acid medium, and is facilitated by the presence of ascorbic acid; however, neutralization of stomach acid interferes with iron absorption. Yet, protein, ascorbic acid, and iron are the very nutrients provided in suboptimal amounts by the customary milk and cream feedings. Today, most clinicians favor a liberal selection of foods even from the first few days of treatment, thus ensuring a more nearly adequate nutrient intake.

Stages I and II to be described below, when used at all, should be limited to a few days. The protein intake may be increased by adding nonfat dry milk to the milk-cream mixture; iron and vitamin supplements should also be prescribed.

Amount of food. No single feeding should be so large that pressure on the stomach walls with subsequent distention and increased peristalsis results. Initially, feedings of 3 to 4 ounces may be used with gradually increasing amounts as the interval between feedings is lengthened. Even after the ulcer has healed the patient should remember to eat meals of moderate size.

Intervals of feeding. Constant dilution of the stomach contents and neutralization of acid are achieved by giving punctual feedings at frequent intervals. Initially, feedings may be given at 1- to 2-hour intervals with progression to six meals a day.

Neutralization of acid. Protein foods such as milk, eggs, and meat have a high acid-buffering capacity. Milk, soft cheeses, and eggs are permitted in early stages of treatment. Some stimulation may be expected from the extractives of meat, but that appears to be more than balanced by the effective neutralizing action of the meat proteins.

Inhibition of acid production. The presence of easily digested fat such as cream, butter, and egg yolk in the stomach inhibits gastric secretion and reduces motility.

Mechanically irritating foods are those which increase peristaltic action because of their coarse, fibrous nature. They include whole-grain breads and cereals, skins and seeds of fruits, and coarse vegetable fibers. The cooking of food softens these fibers and disintegrates them to some extent. By using only refined breads and cereals and by pressing cooked fruits and vegetables through a strainer, coarse fibers are removed. The omission of all fruits and vegetables, as in Stages I and II, results in an essentially fiber-free diet.

Chemically irritating foods are those that stimulate the flow of gastric juices and that may cause some pain to the patient. They include meat extractives, meat soups, gravies, certain spices, caffeine-containing beverages (coffee, tea, cola beverages), and alcohol.

Vegetables as a class are a frequent cause of indigestion, nausea, and epigastric pain. This is due to the inclusion of improperly cooked, strongly flavored vegetables in the diet. When properly cooked (see p. 634), even strongly flavored vegetables are tolerated by many people. Excessive amounts of concentrated sweets and of salt may also be irritating to the gastric mucosa, and increase the rate of secretion.

Thermal irritation refers to the effect of eating very hot or very cold foods. It may be avoided by reminding the patient to eat more slowly.

A four-stage diet. A flexible four-stage diet which embodies the principles discussed above is given here. Generally, the first three stages are used during the time the patient is at bed rest; the fourth stage may be prescribed for the ambulatory patient and may be used for an indefinite period of time. A more liberal diet is described on page 423; it may be used following the fourth stage, or it may be used early in therapy according to the individual patient's response to diet.

FOUR-STAGE BLAND DIET

Characteristics and general rules:

This four-stage diet provides for gradual increases in kinds and amounts of food:

Diet I: milk and cream at hourly intervals

Diet II: seven to eight feedings, 6 ounces each; with additions of breads, cereals, eggs, desserts, cream soups

Diet III: six to seven feedings, 10 to 12 ounces each; additions of strained fruit

Diet IV: three small meals and three intermediate feedings; additions of meat and more liberal selection of foods

The foods used are restricted to those known to be mechanically and chemically nonirritating.

Patients should progress as rapidly as possible. Many patients can be started on stage III or even stage IV.

The protein level can be increased by substituting high-protein beverages for part or all the milk and cream feedings. Recipes for such beverages are found on page 672.

Stages I, II, and III should be supplemented with B-complex vitamins, ascorbic acid, and iron. Stage IV is nutritionally adequate.

DIET I

Give 3 ounces of milk and cream mixture or high-protein beverage every hour from 6 or 7 A.M. to 9 or 10 P.M. and during the night if the patient awakens.
Milk-cream mixture: Mix equal parts of milk and light cream.
High-protein mixture: Mix 3 parts high-protein milk (recipe, p. 672) with 1 part light cream.

Nutritive value: With milk-cream mixture, 15 hourly feedings, 3 ounces each: protein, 43 gm; calories, 1860. With high-protein mixture, 15 hourly feedings: protein, 81 gm; calories, 1700.

SELECTION OF FOODS FOR BLAND DIETS II AND III

BLAND DIET II	BLAND DIET III
Breads—enriched toast; milk toast; saltines; soda crackers	*Breads*—enriched toast; milk toast; saltines; soda crackers
Cereals—corn meal; farina; rice; strained oatmeal	*Cereals*—corn meal; farina; rice; strained oatmeal; corn flakes; rice flakes; macaroni, noodles, spaghetti
Cheese—none	*Cheese*—mild American in sauces; cottage, cream
Desserts—custard; fruit whip; gelatin; Junket; bread, cornstarch, rice, or tapioca pudding without raisins or nuts	*Desserts*—custard; fruit whip; gelatin; Junket; bread, cornstarch, rice, or tapioca pudding without raisins or nuts
Eggs—poached or soft-cooked	*Eggs*—any way except fried
Fats—butter, cream, margarine	*Fats*—butter, cream, margarine
Fruits—none	*Fruits*—strained cooked apples, apricots, peaches, pears, plums, prunes
Milk—plain; with cream; eggnog	*Milk*—plain; with cream; eggnog; weak cocoa
Seasonings—salt	*Seasonings*—salt
Soups—strained cream without any meat or chicken stock	*Soups*—strained cream without any meat or chicken stock
Sweets—sugar in moderation	*Sweets*—sugar and jelly in moderation
Vegetable—white potato without skin	*Vegetable*—white potato without skin

MEAL PATTERNS FOR BLAND DIETS II AND III

	BLAND DIET II (6 oz feedings)	BLAND DIET III (10–12 oz feedings)
On awaking	Milk and cream—6 oz	Milk—8 oz
Breakfast (8 A.M.)	Refined or strained cereal—4 oz	Refined or strained cereal—4 oz

	BLAND DIET II (6 oz feedings)	BLAND DIET III (10–12 oz feedings)
	Milk or cream—2 oz Sugar	Milk—4 oz Sugar Egg—1 White toast—1 slice Butter
Midmorning (10 A.M.)	Milk and cream—6 oz	Milk, milk and cream, eggnog, or weak cocoa—8 oz Crackers, custard, gelatin, Junket, or plain pudding—3 oz
Luncheon	Cream soup—4 oz Crackers—2 Butter Dessert—2 oz	Cream soup—4 oz Crackers—2 Butter Dessert—3 to 4 oz Egg—1; or soft cheese—1 oz White toast—1 slice Butter Orange juice—3 oz
Afternoon (2 P.M.) (3 P.M.) (4 P.M.)	Milk and cream—6 oz Milk and cream—6 oz	 Milk or milk beverage—8 oz Crackers or dessert—3 oz
Dinner (6 P.M.)	Egg—1; or soft cheese—1 oz White potato with butter—3 oz Toast—1 slice Butter	Egg—1; or soft cheese—1 oz White potato with butter—3 oz Toast—1 slice Butter Strained fruit—3 oz Milk or cream soup—4 oz
Evening (8 P.M.) (10 P.M. if awake)	Milk and cream—6 oz Milk and cream—6 oz	Milk beverage—8 oz Crackers or dessert—3 oz
PROTEIN, gm	60	85
CALORIES	1600	2100

BLAND DIET IV

Include these foods, or their nutritive equivalents, daily:

4 cups milk
4 ounces tender meat, fish, or poultry
2 eggs; or 1 egg plus additional meat, cheese, or milk
3 servings vegetables including:
    1 serving cooked leafy green or deep yellow
    1 serving potato
    1 serving other vegetable
3 servings fruit including:
    1 cup (8 ounces) citrus or tomato juice
    1–2 servings cooked fruit without seeds or skin
1 serving enriched cereal
3 slices enriched bread
2 tablespoons butter or margarine
Additional foods as required to meet caloric needs may be selected from the
    list of foods allowed.

Nutritive value: On the basis of specified amounts of foods above: calories, 1945; protein, 100 gm; calcium, 1.45 gm; iron, 13.3 mg; vitamin A, 17,250 I.U.; thiamine, 1.6 mg; riboflavin, 2.9 mg; preformed niacin, 15.8 mg; niacin equivalent, 32.5 mg; ascorbic acid, 186 mg.

Foods allowed:

Beverages—all milk beverages; fruit juices; coffee or tea with half milk— 1 cup daily

Breads—bread, plain rolls, toast made from enriched, rye, or fine whole-wheat flour; saltines; soda crackers; zwieback

Cereals—corn flakes, corn meal, farina, hominy grits, infant cereals, macaroni, noodles, Puffed Rice, rice, rice flakes, spaghetti, strained oatmeal or whole-wheat cereal

Cheese—mild American; cottage; cream

Desserts—plain cake and cookies; custard; fruit whip; gelatin; plain ice cream; Junket; bread, cornstarch, rice, or tapioca pudding

Eggs—any way except fried

Fats—butter, cooking fat, cream, margarine, peanut butter if smooth, vegetable oils

Foods to avoid:

Beverages—alcohol; carbonated and cola beverages

Breads—fresh, hot; rye with seeds; coarse whole-grain; pretzels

Cereals—bran; coarse whole-grain

Cheese—strongly flavored

Desserts—rich cakes and cookies; any with chocolate, coconut, dried or glazed fruit, nuts; doughnuts; pastries; pies; tarts

Eggs—fried

Fats—salad dressings

Foods allowed:

Fruits—raw: avocado, banana, grapefruit and orange sections or juice; canned or cooked: baked apple without skin, apricots, peaches, pears; strained plums or prunes

Meat, fish, poultry—TENDER baked, broiled, creamed, roasted, or stewed: beef, chicken, fish, lamb, liver, sweetbreads, turkey, veal
Note: mince or grind unless very tender

Milk—in any form

Sauces—mild cheese, cream, tomato without hot seasonings or onion

Seasonings—in moderation: salt, sugar, flavoring extracts

Soups—strained cream with allowed vegetables

Sweets—jelly, sirup, or sugar in moderation

Vegetables—canned or cooked: asparagus tips, beets, carrots, peas, white potatoes, spinach, string beans, sweet potatoes, winter squash

Foods to avoid:

Fruits—raw except those listed; berries; figs; pineapple

Meat, fish, poultry—all fatty meats; tough meat with gristle; salted or smoked: bacon, bologna, corned beef, frankfurters, ham, herring, sardines, sausage; spiced luncheon meats; fresh pork

Sauces—catsup, chili, meat gravies, or meat sauces such as Worcestershire, A-1, etc.

Seasonings—horse-radish, meat extracts, mustard, pepper, vinegar

Soups—made with meat or chicken stock

Sweets—candy containing chocolate, coconut, nuts, glazed fruit; jam with seeds, marmalade

Vegetables—all raw; strongly flavored: broccoli, Brussels sprouts, cabbage, cauliflower, cucumber, onion, pepper, radish, turnip; dried beans, corn, tomatoes

Miscellaneous—chewing gum; fried foods; nuts; olives; pickles

MEAL PATTERN

Breakfast

Fruit without fiber or seeds, juice, or banana
Strained whole-grain cereal
Milk and sugar
Egg
Toast with butter
Beverage

Midmorning

Milk—1 glass
Soda crackers

SAMPLE MENU

Canned apricots without skin

Strained oatmeal with milk and sugar

Soft-cooked egg
Enriched toast with butter
Coffee with half milk

Milk—1 glass
Soda crackers

MEAL PATTERN	SAMPLE MENU

Luncheon or supper

Cream soup, if desired	Cream of asparagus soup
Egg, or substitute of mild, soft cheese, or tender meat, or fish	Scrambled egg
White potato (without skin), rice, noodles, spaghetti, or macaroni	Buttered rice
Enriched bread with butter	Enriched bread with butter
Fruit without fiber	Applesauce
Milk	Milk
Citrus juice—4 ounces	Orange juice

Midafternoon

Milk—1 glass	Milk shake—1 glass
Plain cake or cookies	Angel food cake

Dinner

Tomato or citrus fruit juice—4 ounces	Tomato juice
Tender meat, fish, or fowl	Broiled lamb chop
White potato without skin	Mashed potato
Cooked vegetable	Diced beets
Enriched bread with butter	Dinner roll with butter
Dessert	Vanilla ice cream
Milk	Milk—1 glass

Evening nourishment

Milk—1 glass	Eggnog—1 glass
Plain cake, cookies, or crackers	Arrowroot cookies

Liberal diet for peptic ulcer. On the basis of clinical observations, many physicians have noted that rigid dietary restriction results in no more rapid healing of the ulcer than does a liberal diet. Moreover, restricted regimens are more likely to be nutritionally inadequate and are poorly accepted by the patient.

Wolf [150] observed the effects of various foods on two patients with a fistula, one having an active ulcer and one having a normal gastric mucosa. He found no irritation of the gastric mucosa even though chemicals and strong condiments were applied. He has stated:

Certainly, before prescribing limitations to the diets of persons with peptic ulcer, we need better evidence that ordinary foods are either stimulating or irritating to the stomach.*

* Wolf, S.: "A Critical Appraisal of the Dietary Management of Peptic Ulcer and Ulcerative Colitis," *J. Clin. Nutrition,* **2:**3, 1954.

Schneider and his associates [151] tested the possible irritant effects of many spices and herbs on patients with active and with healing ulcers. They noted subjective reactions of the patients and made gastroscopic observations of the gastric mucosa. The patient's reactions, the rate of healing of the ulcer, and the appearance of the mucosa were not altered by allspice, caraway seeds, cinnamon, mace, paprika, thyme, or sage when they were given with foods. Slight reddening of the mucosa and some symptoms of gastric discomfort were noted with chili powder, cloves, mustard seeds, nutmeg, and black pepper.

Shull [152] has suggested that toleration for foods is best determined by trial with the individual. He states further:

It is highly improbable that 'coarse' or 'rough' foods, such as fruit skins, lettuce, cabbage, kale, nuts, celery, and endive when subjected to proper mastication or mixture with saliva could ever actually traumatize a peptic ulcer. The emphasis, therefore, should be placed upon the proper preparation of food for gastric digestion. Ordinarily this is done satisfactorily in the mouth by mastication and mixture with saliva. Only when the teeth are poor or absent is artificial grinding or puréeing necessary.*

The recommendation for a liberal diet, however, does not mean the patient can eat just as he pleases. Physicians are agreed that an adequate diet, neutralization of acid by frequent feedings and suitable medications, and moderation in the choice of foods are necessary. Bland Diet V represents a typical regimen for a patient for whom a liberal diet may be used.

BLAND DIET V

Characteristics and general rules:

This diet includes all foods permitted for Bland Diet IV, page 420. Additional selections from the various food groups are indicated below.

Three meals of moderate size and three between-meal feedings should be used. Meal patterns for Bland Diet IV may be used.

Food should be chewed well and eaten slowly.

Foods known to produce intolerance in the individual should be omitted.

Foods allowed in addition to Bland Diet IV:

Breads—graham crackers
Cereals—all cooked without straining; Puffed Wheat and other cereals without coarse bran
Fats—mayonnaise and cooked salad dressing
Fruits—raw: apple, cherries, peaches, pears, plums, prunes, tangerine

* Shull, H. J.: "Diet in the Management of Peptic Ulcer," *J.A.M.A.*, **170**:127, 1959.

Meat—duck, fresh pork
Seasonings—allspice, caraway seeds, cinnamon, mace, paprika, sage, thyme
Vegetables—lettuce and other tender salad greens; celery; tomatoes

Modification of diet in bleeding ulcer. The use of food in the treatment of bleeding ulcers is based on the principle of reducing the number and violence of stomach contractions by providing small, frequent feedings of easily digested foods. The gastric juice is given something other than the ulcer on which to act, thus permitting a clot to form.

Just how soon food may be given cannot be exactly stated. If the patient complains of nausea, or is vomiting, nothing can be gained by immediate feeding; but if the patient has a desire for food and has no gastric distress, he may benefit from prompt feeding.

Meulengracht [153] and others [154] have reported a marked reduction in mortality when patients were fed promptly at 2-hour intervals with milk, eggs, puréed fruits and vegetables, bread and butter, and pudding. After the first 2 days, ground meats are allowed.

Another regimen by Andresen [155] consists of 6-ounce feedings of a milk-cream-gelatin mixture given at 2-hour intervals. Selected foods are added at the beginning of the fifth day. By the ninth day the patient is receiving a bland diet without meat, fish, or poultry.

Bland Diets II and III described earlier in this chapter are similar to the Meulengracht and Andresen regimens and may be used in early stages following hemorrhage. Bland Diet IV with six meals daily may be used subsequently.

Instruction of the patient. Regardless of the regimen prescribed, careful instruction of the patient is essential. The emphasis should be placed on foods which may be used rather than on foods to avoid. A consideration of the patient's cultural pattern in planning the diet to be followed at home will help to ensure adherence to a desirable diet.

While a rigid diet which does not consider individual likes will not be followed for any length of time, there is, on the other hand, value in recommending dietary discipline with respect to nutritive adequacy, regularity of mealtimes, frequent feedings, and moderation in the amounts of food eaten.

Emphasis must always be given to the importance of eating meals in a pleasant environment with a calm, happy frame of mind. Rest before and after meals—even a few minutes—is conducive to greater enjoyment of meals. Foods should be properly chewed and eaten slowly, rather than with haste. Family problems or any irritating subjects should not be discussed at mealtime.

Ulcers have a tendency to flare up even after complete healing has taken place. Alvarez [156] has emphasized the importance of prompt and strenuous treatment after psychic strain in order to avoid flare-ups. The stomach tends to be empty of food but full of highly acid gastric juice from 10 P.M. to 3 A.M., and it is likely that this is the period when the greater part of the injury to the gastric and duodenal mucosa occurs. Following any emotional strain such as grief or worry, it is advisable to use a continual antacid drip during the night for 1 or 2 nights, according to Alvarez. In place of the continuous drip the patient may partake of food every 2 hours from dinnertime until 2 or 3 o'clock in the morning.

INDIGESTION

Nausea, regurgitation, heartburn, abdominal pain, a feeling of fullness and distention, and flatulence are frequent complaints by many people. These symptoms may occur in organic disorders or they may be related to dietary errors.

Many an incident of indigestion has been brought about by poor cookery: too long cooking of vegetables, especially those which are strongly flavored; too low a temperature for frying food so that the food has absorbed a lot of excess fat; too high a temperature for frying so that the fats break down to produce irritating substances; excessive heat and prolonged cookery for protein foods such as meat and cheese. In addition, long-continued use of an unbalanced diet, too many rich and fatty foods, an overabundance of fibrous foods, excessive amounts of concentrated sweets, too much food for one's habits, hasty eating, and irregularity of meals will all contribute to discomfort. Fatigue and emotional upsets such as worry, fear, anger, and grief will also contribute to the symptoms of indigestion.

Modification of the diet. The correction of indigestion rests upon the removal of the cause, and providing appropriate instruction for the patient. Guidance in the use of a normal diet (see p. 338) or a soft diet (see p. 341) is sufficient for many. Others will find Bland Diet IV (p. 420) to be more suitable.

GASTRITIS

Gastritis is an acute or chronic inflammation of the mucous membrane of the stomach.

Acute gastritis. This condition may be caused by the ingestion of poisons such as strong alkali, acid, or drugs, alcohol, or dietary excesses. When it occurs, the stomach should be freed of the offending substance as soon as possible by lavage or by induced vomiting. No food is given for 1 or 2 days in order to permit adequate rest for the stomach. Even water is restricted to small amounts of hot water, or bits of cracked ice. After 24 to 48 hours, feeding may be started by giving teaspoonful amounts of foods allowed on a full-fluid diet every half hour as tolerated (p. 344). Foods are increased in amount and variety very gradually until the patient is able to take a full soft diet. The latter may need to be continued for a week or more.

Chronic gastritis. Like acute gastritis, chronic gastritis may be the result of toxic drugs, excessive alcohol, or dietary errors such as overeating, rapid eating, large amounts of fibrous foods, or highly seasoned foods. It may also accompany such disorders as carcinoma, ulcers, cirrhosis, nephritis, myocardial failure, and tuberculosis, to mention but a few. The usual symptoms include poor appetite, distention, gastric distress, and hypoacidity, although hyperacidity occasionally is found.

The cause must be determined before chronic gastritis can be treated. Any dietary indiscretions must first be corrected, after which the Bland Diet (p. 420) is suitable. It is usually necessary to restrict fats since they depress further the secretion of the already deficient acid, but when hyperacidity is present particular emphasis should be placed on protein foods such as milk and eggs.

CANCER OF THE STOMACH

If a diagnosis of cancer is made early enough, surgery may lead to complete cure. Unfortunately, symptoms such as poor appetite, indigestion, fatigue, nausea, vomiting, and weight loss which bring the patient to the doctor may not appear until the cancer is moderately far advanced. Moreover, these symptoms are common to many disorders, and a positive diagnosis can be established only with x-ray, and sometimes surgical exploration is necessary.

Modification of the diet. Following gastrectomy the postoperative regimen (see p. 403) should be used. Meals, of necessity, must be small and easily digested. A certain proportion of patients may have the dumping syndrome following surgery and should be given the diet recommended on page 405.

When operation is inadvisable for one reason or another, the prime consideration is the comfort of the patient. Anorexia is such a common finding that every effort should be made to comply with the patient's inclinations. In general, the diet should consist of soft, low-fiber, bland foods given in small frequent feedings. Since hypochlorhydria is usually present, fats are preferably kept at a minimum.

PROBLEMS AND REVIEW

1. List some of the nutritional disturbances which may develop when the stomach and intestinal tract are impaired.

2. Give examples of gastric disorders of functional origin; of those which are organic in nature.

3. Name at least eight dietary factors which might lead to the development of indigestion.

4. Which classes of foods are most likely to stimulate acid secretion? Which ones depress acid secretion? Which are most effective in the neutralization of acid? Which foods are likely to increase motility of the gastrointestinal tract?

5. The use of each of the following illustrates a principle in the dietary treatment of peptic ulcer. Identify the principles involved for each:

    a. milk and cream

    b. orange juice at the end of the meal, but not between meals

    c. tender meat, fish, poultry

    d. feedings at 2-hour intervals

    e. omission of coffee and tea

    f. omission of strongly flavored vegetables

    g. enriched, refined breads and cereals

6. *Problem.* Plan a diet for a man with a healed peptic ulcer who works from 7 A.M. to 3 P.M. in a factory. It is necessary for him to carry his meals to work. Show the hours at which he should plan to eat.

7. *Problem.* List five food combinations which would be suitable for between-meal feedings for an individual who must carry meals to work.

8. What possible role may diet play in causing or relieving the emotional stress to which some patients with peptic ulcer may be subjected?

9. It is sometimes said: "Once an ulcer; always an ulcer." What prophylactic measures can be taken to avoid recurrence?

10. What objections can you see to nomenclature such as this: progressive ulcer diet; ambulatory ulcer diet?

CHAPTER 31

Diet in Disturbances of the Small Intestine and Colon

Low-residue Diet; High-fiber Diet; Wheat-, Oat-, and Rye-free Diet

DIARRHEA

Classification. Diarrhea is characterized by a morbid frequency in bowel evacuation, the stools being fluid in nature. It may be acute or chronic in character. Diarrhea is only a symptom and may be classified as functional or organic in origin.

Kantor [157] has listed some of the functional diarrheas: the result of some irritant in the normal person; putrefactive or fermentative; allergic; nervous; a result of achlorhydria; associated with burns or uremia; the result of endocrine imbalance, such as hyperactivity of the thyroid gland or lowered activity of the adrenal cortex; or nutritive as associated with pellagra.

The organic diarrheas are those caused by bacteria as in bacillary dysentery or typhoid fever, Protozoa as in amebic dysentery, poisons, or certain unknown factors as in chronic ulcerative colitis or sprue. The role of food and water contamination in the incidence of diarrhea has been discussed in Chapter 21.

Modification of the diet. In acute diarrhea the entire digestive tract requires a rest. For 12 to 24 hours the patient is permitted nothing by mouth except cereal gruels without milk, weak tea, fat-free broth, toast, and water in abundance. Thereafter, a very low-residue diet and then a soft diet (p. 341) are used. The normal diet is modified as follows:

Fiber and residue. The use of the terms "fiber" and "residue" interchangeably is not necessarily correct, but no altogether satisfactory differentiation has yet been established. Fiber, as the term is used in dietetics, refers to "indigestible organic tissue, either plant or animal." * The plant fibers of im-

* Turner, D. F.: *Handbook of Diet Therapy*, 3rd ed. The University of Chicago Press, Chicago, 1959, p. 206.

portance would include the bran coatings of cereal grains, the skin and seeds of fruits, the structural fibers of vegetables.

The term residue refers specifically to the amount of bulk remaining in the intestinal tract following digestion. Obviously, this would include the indigestible fibers of plants, but many clinicians state that milk, while fiber free, leaves an appreciable amount of residue in the gastrointestinal tract. Experimental work [158] has indicated that tender beef, veal, chicken, hard-cooked eggs, boiled or steamed rice, strained fruit juices, and broth leave little if any residue in the intestinal tract.

Fluids. Because of the extensive loss of body fluids in the watery stools, it is imperative that the patient consume fluids in abundance.

Nutritive adequacy. In acute phases of diarrhea, the diet is necessarily so restricted that the nutritive needs cannot be met. In chronic diarrheas, liberal intakes of protein, calories, minerals, and vitamins must be provided.

VERY LOW-RESIDUE DIET

Characteristics and general rules:

This diet is essentially fiber-free and leaves a minimum of residue in the intestinal tract.

If the diet is used for more than a few days, it should be supplemented with calcium, iron, and multivitamin concentrates.

As improvement takes place, the diet is liberalized by gradually adding puréed vegetables and fruits, and milk.

Foods allowed:

Beverages—coffee in limited amounts, tea

Breads—enriched bread or toast, crackers, plain rolls, Melba toast, zwieback

Cereals—corn meal, farina, strained oatmeal; corn flakes, Puffed Rice, rice flakes; macaroni, noodles, rice, spaghetti

Cheese—cottage, cream, mild American in sauces

Desserts—plain cake, cookies, custard, gelatin, ice cream, puddings, rennet desserts

Eggs—cooked any way except fried

Fats—butter, cream, margarine, vegetable oils

Fruits—strained juices only. Occasionally applesauce is given to patients

Foods to avoid:

Beverages—milk and milk drinks

Breads—whole-grain breads or crackers

Cereals—whole-grain such as wheat flakes, wheat meal

Cheese—sharp

Desserts—with fruit or nuts; pies and pastries. Note: milk desserts are occasionally omitted

Fruits—all except juices

Foods allowed:

with diarrhea because of its pectin content

Meats—tender or minced lean meat, fish, or poultry

Soups—clear: bouillon or broth without fat

Sweets—hard candy, honey, jelly, sirup, sugar in moderation

Vegetables—tomato juice; white potato

Miscellaneous—salt; spices in moderation

Foods to avoid:

Meats—tough; fried; fatty meat, fish, or poultry such as pork, mackerel, goose

Soups—fatty; cream; spicy

Sweets—with fruit or nuts; jam, marmalade

Vegetables—all except tomato juice and potato

Miscellaneous—nuts, popcorn, pickles, excessive seasonings

MEAL PATTERN

Breakfast

Strained fruit juice
Refined cereal with cream and sugar
Egg
White toast with butter
Coffee with cream and sugar

Dinner

Strained citrus juice
Tender meat, poultry, or fish
Potato or substitute

White bread with butter
Plain dessert
Coffee or tea

Luncheon or supper

Broth
Tender meat, fowl, fish, or egg
Potato, rice, macaroni, or noodles
White bread with butter
Plain dessert
Coffee or tea

REGIONAL ILEITIS

Symptoms and clinical findings. Regional ileitis (regional enteritis) is an inflammatory disease of the lower ileum, although other parts of the intestine may be involved. All structures of the intestinal wall are affected by edema, cellular infiltration, fibrosis, and ulcerations.

The patient usually complains of anorexia, abdominal cramps, fever, weight loss, and diarrhea. Anemia and other signs of malnutrition are common. The disease is characterized by exacerbations and remissions. Acute ileitis may subside, but in chronic ileitis the intestinal lumen becomes narrowed, inelastic, and may, on occasion, be obstructed so that surgical intervention is necessary.

Modification of the diet. Since malnutrition is a prominent feature, it is important that the patient eat well. The acutely ill patient may be given the Very Low-residue Diet initially, followed by the Bland High-protein Diet (p. 432). Vitamin supplements are usually indicated.

DIVERTICULOSIS AND DIVERTICULITIS

Diverticulosis consists of the presence of diverticula or small, mucosal sacs which protrude from the intestinal lumen, usually the colon, through the bowel wall. Their presence does not produce symptoms until they become inflamed.

Diverticulitis is the inflammatory condition which is characterized by such symptoms as nausea, vomiting, fever, abdominal tenderness, distention, pain, and intestinal spasm. The inflammatory process may lead to intestinal obstruction or perforation, thus necessitating surgery.

During the acute episodes nothing except water and clear fluids is given by mouth. The Full Fluid Diet (p. 344) or Very Low-residue Diet (p. 429) may then be used. Patients with chronic diverticulitis should continue to use a diet moderately restricted in fiber. The selection of foods for Bland Diets IV and V (pp. 420 and 423) is appropriate.

ULCERATIVE COLITIS

Symptoms and clinical findings. Ulcerative colitis is a chronic inflammatory condition in which the whole or part of the large intestine is involved. The exact cause is unknown, but infections are frequent. There appears to be a close correlation between the severity of the disease and the presence of psychogenic factors. Many of the patients are nervous, irritable, apprehensive, introspective, and emotionally unstable. Food allergy may account for the occurrence in some patients.

The patient looks sick and is chronically ill. He has little appetite and has lost much weight. In fact, the poor appetite together with the persistent diarrhea may result in multiple deficiencies which constitute the major problem in treatment. The patient also complains of fever, mild to severe abdominal cramps, distention, flatulence, diarrhea which at times is severe, and the appearance of blood, pus, and mucus in the stools. The mucosa of the colon becomes hyperactive and fragile so that it bleeds easily; eventually it may ulcerate and perforate.

Modification of the diet. Customarily the diet is planned to supply sufficient nutrients to reinstate and maintain normal nutrition and to avoid injury to the colon. The following modifications are usually necessary:

Protein. About 100 to 150 gm protein are essential to replace losses which have occurred. Meat, eggs, and milk should be provided in abundance. Sometimes patients do not seem to tolerate pasteurized whole milk in which case homogenized, boiled, skim, or evaporated milk may be substituted. Some patients tolerate milk and cheese in prepared dishes such as creamed vegetables, cream soups, and puddings. If none of these forms of milk can be used, the diet must provide especially liberal amounts of meat, fish, poultry, and eggs.

Energy. About 3000 calories or more are necessary to compensate for the loss of nutrients in the stool and the consequent great weight loss.

Minerals. Anemia is a common finding in colitis so that supplements of iron salts may be prescribed. Whenever milk is not tolerated, it is also necessary to prescribe calcium salts.

Vitamins. Some of the deficiency symptoms seen in patients with ulcerative colitis are the result of poor dietary intake together with excessive gastrointestinal losses. When they occur, or whenever the diet itself is restricted, multivitamin supplements should be prescribed.

Fiber. The Very Low-residue Diet (p. 429) may be used initially with gradual transition to a bland high-protein diet.

Management of the diet. No factor in treatment is more important than that of diet. It requires the continuous individualized attention of the dietitian and nurse. Wolf [150] believes that it is more important to help the patient to adjust to his day-to-day problems than to prescribe a severely restricted dietary regimen. Patients receiving consideration in their adjustment to life but using a normal diet improved to a greater degree than did those who were treated with the usual dietary regimen unaccompanied by psychologic assistance. Wolf states further that undue restriction may lead to malnutrition and to resentment, but he also recognizes that a carefully balanced diet associated with a "certain amount of ritual" may be psychologically advantageous for the over-meticulous patient.

Bland Diets IV and V described on pages 420 and 423 are suitable for most patients with ulcerative colitis, but the protein and caloric levels should be augmented. Because many of these patients have poor appetites to begin with, the use of midmorning and midafternoon feedings may not be advisable because the meal intake would be further reduced. A bedtime feeding, however, should be included. The following meal pattern illustrates an adaptation of Bland Diet IV. It will be noted that broth, meat extractives, coffee, and tea are not restricted as they should be for the patient with peptic ulcer.

BLAND HIGH-PROTEIN DIET

MEAL PATTERN	SAMPLE MENU
Breakfast	
Fruit without fiber or seeds	Sliced bananas with milk
Fine-grain or strained cereal	Cream of Wheat with cream and sugar
Milk or cream and sugar for cereal	
Eggs—1 to 2	Soft-cooked eggs—2
Enriched toast with butter or margarine	Enriched toast with butter or margarine
Beverage	Coffee with cream and sugar

MEAL PATTERN	SAMPLE MENU

Luncheon or supper

Soup, clear or creamed	Strained cream of mushroom soup
Meat, fish, poultry, egg, or cheese— large serving	Broiled beef patties—2
Potato or substitute	Buttered noodles
Cooked vegetable	Julienne green beans
Enriched bread with butter or margarine	Enriched bread with butter or margarine
Fruit without fiber	Orange sections
	Sugar cookies
Milk	Milk

Dinner

Citrus fruit or tomato juice	Tomato juice
Tender meat, fish, or poultry—4 oz	Baked breast of chicken
Potato without skin	Mashed potato with butter
Vegetable	Buttered carrots
Enriched bread with butter or margarine	Dinner roll with butter or margarine
Dessert	Tapioca cream
Milk	Milk

Evening nourishment

Enriched bread-meat, egg, or cheese sandwich	Sliced roast beef sandwich
Milk beverage	High-protein eggnog
Custard or pudding	Chocolate pudding

ATONIC CONSTIPATION

Constipation is the infrequent or difficult passage of feces. However, it cannot be exactly defined, for certain variations in the frequency of bowel movement and completeness of evacuation are entirely physiologic. Most people have a bowel movement daily, but for some individuals an evacuation every second or third day is entirely normal. The most important factor for well-being is the maintenance of elimination at regular intervals according to the individual.

Constipation may be temporary because of lack of exercise as in illness, a change in habits of living, or nervous strain. The return to normal habits of living corrects such constipation without difficulty. On the other hand, it might be chronic with a change in the musculature of the intestinal tract. It might result from an organic disorder such as obstruction, tumor, or diverticulitis, or it might be functional in nature. The determination of the cause is obviously important so that appropriate treatment can be instituted. Attention to diet may be beneficial in *atonic* and *spastic* constipation (see Irritable Colon), but consideration of other factors in the pattern of living is also essential.

Causes. Some of the most important functional causes of constipation are:

1. Poor personal hygiene in which one neglects to respond to the urge for defecation, or fails to maintain regular habits of evacuation.

2. A diet containing too little fiber and consisting largely of concentrated and refined foods which leave little if any residue upon reaching the colon.

3. Irregular meals, too little rest and relaxation, and a hurried pattern of living.

4. Lack of exercise which leads to reduction in muscular tone of the intestine and inability to move the fecal mass into and along the colon at the normal rate.

5. Excessive and long-continued use of laxatives and enemas often resorted to by people who are unduly conscious about evacuation, with the result that in time the normal colon becomes irritated and sensitive.

6. Nervous disturbances of various sorts. Excitement developed by mental patients at times prevents the bowel from emptying itself for several days or more. Nervous contractions of the musculature may be caused by irritation and brought about by overstimulation.

Bed patients, invalids such as arthritics, the aged, and other sedentary individuals are most likely to be affected by atonic constipation. The intestinal walls lack muscle tone so that peristaltic action is impaired and the digestive wastes cannot move down the tract at a normal rate.

Treatment. In the correction of atonic constipation emphasis must be placed on good health habits; that is, a regular time for elimination, adequate rest and relaxation, exercise if possible, regular time for meals, adequate intake of fluids (8 to 10 glasses a day), and a diet providing a sufficient amount of fiber to stimulate the intestinal mucosa and to provide bulk to the intestinal contents.

The normal or house diet is suitable for the correction of atonic constipation. When the diet is planned to include the normal allowances of raw and cooked fruits and vegetables it will provide cellulose to equal or exceed the estimated requirement of 5 to 6 gm fiber per day. The fiber may be increased in the following ways without changing the diet from its normal pattern:

Use whole-grain cereals and breads instead of refined cereal foods.

Include one or two salads daily, emphasizing raw fruits and vegetables.

Eat whole fruits, including their skins, rather than peeling them or using juices only; for example, raw apple with skin, or orange with white membrane.

Use stewed fruits and juices such as stewed prunes, prune juice, apricots, figs.

Bran may be used occasionally. The possibility of excessive bran being irritating to the intestinal tract or causing an obstruction must not be overlooked.

Patients are often helped by taking a glass or so of water, hot or cold, with or without lemon, according to their preference, before breakfast.

The physician may sometimes prescribe agar-agar, a type of seaweed that is not affected by intestinal enzymes and that absorbs water thus giving the necessary bulk. It may be given as a special preparation or it may be sprinkled dry on the cereal at breakfast. Mineral oil is also prescribed quite frequently, usually to be taken at bedtime. The excessive use of mineral oil or its use in conjunction with meals as in salad dressings is undesirable because of the interference with the absorption of the fat-soluble vitamins.

IRRITABLE COLON

Irritable colon refers to abnormal motor activity of the colon in the absence of organic lesions and is characterized by abdominal distress and constipation or diarrhea. It is known by a variety of terms: [159] spastic, mucous, or cathartic colitis; functional, spastic, or unhappy colon; gastric or intestinal neurosis. This condition probably accounts for 50 to 70 per cent of all gastrointestinal complaints.

Etiology. Many factors contribute to this functional abnormality, among them being: [159] excessive use of laxatives and cathartics; excessive amounts of coffee and coarse, fibrous, or laxative foods; antibiotic therapy; enteric infections; and poor hygiene with respect to sleep, work, fluid intake, and evacuation. Emotional upsets are a frequent cause of this disturbance. It is well known that sudden fear will produce hypermotility, cramping, and diarrhea in many persons, but these symptoms disappear promptly. Some people, however, who have never learned to deal with the normal anxieties and frustrations of life, and others who may have tensions over many years are especially sensitive to gastrointestinal neurosis.

Symptoms and clinical findings. The patient may complain of belching, heartburn, a sense of fullness, distention, mild or severe cramping pain, and flatulence. Loss of appetite, nausea, vomiting, headache, palpitation, and nervousness are often encountered. The peristaltic movements are increased resulting in intermittent spasms and irregular movement of the food mass. The stools are usually dry, hard, small, and frequently combined with mucus.

Treatment. As in atonic constipation, emphasis must be placed on good habits of personal hygiene, rest, relaxation, freedom from nervous upsets, and ample intake of water. While some bulk in the diet is essential, the fiber should be soft and nonirritating. The Soft Diet (p. 341) or the more restricted Bland Diet (p. 418) are suitable for these patients.

INTESTINAL OBSTRUCTION

The movement of the intestinal contents may be impaired or prevented by many causes such as tumors, impaction of material in the intestine, or paralytic ileus following surgery. As a rule, the obstruction must be removed by surgical intervention before an adequate diet can be administered. The postoperative diet should be fiber-free (see p. 429) for a period of time, following which a soft diet may be ordered.

PANCREATIC DISORDERS

Acute pancreatitis. A high percentage of cases of acute pancreatitis are associated with biliary disease. The inflammation is associated with severe epigastric pain, nausea, vomiting, fever, decrease in peristalsis, increased pulse rate, and, in some instances, by circulatory collapse. Nothing is given by mouth until the acute symptoms have subsided. Then a clear fluid, full fluid, and bland diet may be used in sequence.

Chronic pancreatitis is usually caused by repeated attacks of acute pancreatitis. The episodes of severe pain occur as in the acute pancreatitis. The functioning of the pancreatic glands may be disturbed, leading to inadequate production of digestive enzymes. As a result, the stools become bulky and foul, and contain undigested fat (steatorrhea), increased amounts of nitrogen, and sometimes carbohydrate. Loss of weight follows and the decreased absorption of minerals and vitamins may lead to multiple deficiency signs.

During an exacerbation the patient is treated as for acute pancreatitis. Between attacks the diet should be high in carbohydrate and protein, and low in fat.[160] Pancreatin is administered with each meal to facilitate the absorption of fat. Bland Diets III, IV, and V (see pp. 418, 420, and 423) are suitable for patients with chronic pancreatitis except that the fat content must be reduced by the following measures:

Skim milk is substituted for whole milk.
Only lean meats, poultry, and fish are used.
All table and cooking fats are eliminated.
Foods prepared with fat are eliminated; creamed sauces and soups, cakes (except angel and sponge), cookies, fried foods, ice cream, pastries, pies, whole-milk puddings, etc.

Six small meals are usually preferable since the appetite is poor. Multivitamin supplementation is usually indicated.

In some patients with pancreatitis, the islet tissue is affected so that the typical symptoms of diabetes follow. In these instances the dietary considerations for diabetes are then followed (see Chap. 33) with suitable adjustments for fat and fiber content.

SPRUE

Etiology and incidence. The cause of sprue is not known. Tropical sprue which occurs abruptly and is endemic in certain tropical areas is considered by some to be a nutritional deficiency disease, a concept favored by the fact that the administration of folic acid or vitamin B_{12} produces remarkably rapid improvement. However, the disease not infrequently occurs in only one member of a family, all of whom are consuming the same diet. Nontropical sprue occurs sporadically in Europe, Africa, South America, and the United States and is rarely associated with a poor diet.

Symptoms and clinical findings. Sprue bears a number of similarities to celiac disease; in fact, celiac disease in children may disappear only to have the symptoms recur later in adult life. Diarrhea, steatorrhea (fatty stools), and abdominal distention are striking features of the disease. The usual symptoms and laboratory findings include:

1. Weakness, apathy, listlessness
2. Sore tongue (glossitis); anorexia
3. Impaired motility of the gastrointestinal tract; abdominal distention; occasional cramps
4. Muscle wasting and rapid weight loss to the point of emaciation as a result of the poor appetite and the faulty absorption
5. Diarrhea in which the stools are bulky, foul, frothy, with excessive excretion of fats and fatty acids
6. Macrocytic anemia; iron absorption often impaired also
7. Impaired absorption of all of the fat-soluble vitamins. Low prothrombin levels in the blood lead to the danger of severe hemorrhage
8. Excessive calcium loss together with impaired vitamin-D absorption results in hypocalcemia, occasionally tetany, bone pain, osteomalacia
9. Carbohydrate absorption is interfered with as evidenced by a flat glucose tolerance curve
10. Hypofunction of the adrenal cortex; increased pigmentation of exposed areas of the trunk and extremities.

Modification of the diet. Dramatic response is obtained in tropical sprue with folic acid, vitamin B_{12}, or liver extract, either alone or in combination with a diet such as described below. These specific therapeutic agents produce a rapid regeneration of hemoglobin and red blood cells, the glossitis and diarrhea quickly subside, absorption becomes more nearly normal, the appetite returns and may be even ravenous, and weight gain is marked.

For some unknown reason, the vitamins and liver extract are somewhat less effective in nontropical sprue. In refractory cases prompt remissions have been obtained with ACTH and cortisone,[161] but such therapy does not replace diet. For both tropical and nontropical sprue the following dietary considerations are important:

Protein. A high-protein intake—120 gm or more—is essential to replace the wasted tissues. The proteins of lean meat, poultry, fish, cottage cheese, egg whites, nonfat dry milk, and fresh skim milk are well utilized.

Fat. Most patients benefit by a restriction of fats to those which are easily digested, at least in the initial stages of treatment. Even though a level of 25 gm fat may be used initially, as a rule the patient can tolerate 50 to 100 gm fat after a short period of time.

Carbohydrate. Because of the faulty absorption of carbohydrate, it has been common practice in the past to restrict carbohydrates to those from fruits, fruit juices, low-starch vegetables, simple sugars, and Melba toast. However, the elimination of gluten from the diet, as described below, has resulted in marked improvement without the drastic restriction in sugars and starches.

Gluten. When certain protein fractions—gluten and gliadin—are eliminated many patients show striking improvement. The gluten-rich sources include wheat, oats, rye, and barley.

Minerals. In addition to a liberal allowance of milk, calcium salts are sometimes prescribed to overcome the excessive loss which has occurred in the stools. Iron salts are necessary if there is an hypochromic anemia. Potassium deficiency may be present when the patient has been eating poorly, in which event the physician makes an appropriate prescription.

Vitamins. In addition to folic acid or vitamin B_{12}, it is necessary to prescribe supplements of the fat-soluble and water-soluble vitamins.

Texture and flavor. The reduction in gastrointestinal motility and the ever-present distention usually require that strongly flavored vegetables and other gas-forming foods be avoided, at least initially. The fiber content may be reduced by using only cooked fruits and vegetables at first, and eliminating the skins and seeds of foods.

The following diet is adapted from the plan described by Mike: [162]

WHEAT-, OAT-, AND RYE-FREE DIET

Characteristics and general rules:

This diet excludes all products containing wheat, rye, oats, and barley. Read all labels carefully.

Aqueous multivitamins are usually prescribed in addition to the diet.

The diet may be progressed gradually; that is, small amounts of unsaturated fats may be used at first, adding harder fats later. Fiber may be reduced initially by using only cooked fruits and vegetables. Strongly flavored vegetables may be poorly tolerated at first.

Include these foods, or their nutritive equivalents, daily:

4 cups milk
6–8 ounces (cooked weight) lean meat, fish, or poultry
1 egg
4 vegetables including:
    1 dark green or deep yellow
    1 potato
    2 other vegetables
    One to be served raw, if tolerated
3 fruits including:
    1–2 servings citrus fruit or other good source ascorbic acid
    1–2 other fruits
4 servings breads and cereals: corn, rice, soybean
    NO WHEAT, RYE, OATS, BARLEY
2 tablespoons fat
Additional calories are provided by using more of any of the foods listed, desserts, soups, sweets

Nutritive value of listed foods: protein, 105 gm; fat, 110 gm; carbohydrate, 200 gm; calories, 2200. Minerals and vitamins in excess of recommended allowances.

Foods allowed:

Beverages—carbonated, cocoa, coffee, fruit juices, milk, tea

Breads—corn bread, muffins, and pone with no wheat flour; breads made with corn meal, cornstarch, Lima bean, potato, rice, soybean flours

Cereals—cooked corn meal, Cream of Rice, hominy or grits, rice; ready-to-eat: corn or rice cereals such as corn flakes, rice flakes, Puffed Rice

Cheese—cottage; later, cream cheese

Desserts—custard, fruit ice, fruit whips, plain or fruit ice cream (homemade), plain or fruit gelatin, meringues;

Foods to avoid:

Beverages—ale, beer, instant coffee containing cereal, malted milk, Postum, products containing cereal

Breads—all containing any wheat, rye, oats, or barley; bread crumbs, muffins, pancakes, rolls, rusks, waffles, zwieback; all commercial yeast and quick bread mixes; all crackers, pretzels, Ry-Krisp

Cereals—cooked or ready-to-eat breakfast cereals containing wheat,* oats; barley, macaroni, noodles, pasta, spaghetti, wheat germ

Desserts—cake, cookies, doughnuts, pastries, pie; bisques, commercial ice cream, ice cream cones; prepared

---

* A listing of trade products containing wheat is provided in Chapter 39, page 552.

Foods allowed:

homemade puddings—cornstarch, rice, tapioca; rennet desserts; sherbet; cakes and cookies made with allowed flours

Eggs—as desired

Fats—oil: corn, cottonseed, olive, sesame, soybean; French dressing, pure mayonnaise, salad dressing with cornstarch thickening
Later addition: butter, cream, margarine, peanut oil, vegetable shortening

Flour—corn meal, Lima bean, potato, rice, soybean

Fruits—all cooked, canned, and juices; fresh and frozen as tolerated, avoiding skin and seeds initially

Meat—all lean meats, poultry, fish: baked, broiled, roasted, stewed

Milk—all kinds

Soups—broth, bouillon, cream if thickened with cornstarch, vegetable

Sweets—candy, honey, jam, jelly, marmalade, marshmallows, molasses, sirup, sugar

Vegetables—cooked or canned: buttered; fresh as tolerated

Miscellaneous—gravy and sauces thickened with cornstarch; olives, peanut butter, pickles, popcorn, potato chips

Foods to avoid:

mixes containing wheat, rye, oats, or barley; puddings thickened with wheat flour

Fats—bacon, lard, suet, salad dressing with flour thickening

Flour—barley, oat, rye, wheat—bread, cake, entire wheat, graham, self-rising, whole-wheat, wheat germ

Fruits—prunes, plums, and their juices; those with skins and seeds at first

Meat—breaded, creamed, croquettes, luncheon meats unless pure meat, meat loaf, stuffings with bread, scrapple, thickened stew
Fat meats such as corned beef, duck, frankfurters, goose, ham, luncheon meats, pork, sausage
Fatty fish such as herring, mackerel, sardines, swordfish, or canned in heavy oil

Soups—thickened with flour; containing barley, noodles, etc.

Sweets—candies with high fat content, nuts; candies containing wheat products

Vegetables—creamed if thickened with wheat, oat, rye, or barley products
Strongly flavored if they produce discomfort: baked beans, broccoli, Brussels sprouts, cabbage, cauliflower, corn, cucumber, lentils, onions, peppers, radishes, turnips

Miscellaneous—gravies and sauces thickened with flours not permitted

MEAL PATTERN	SAMPLE MENU

Breakfast

Fruit, preferably citrus or good source of ascorbic acid	Tomato juice
Rice or corn cereal	Rice Krispies
Milk, sugar	Milk, sugar
Bread: rice or corn	Southern corn muffins
Butter or margarine	Butter or margarine
Jelly, if desired	Currant jelly
Eggs	Scrambled eggs
Beverage	Coffee, with cream, sugar

Luncheon or supper

Meat, poultry, or fish; or cheese; eggs (no thickened casserole dishes)	Beef stew (not thickened)
	Beef cubes
Potato, or substitute, or vegetable	Potato
	Carrots
	Onions
Salad—vegetable or fruit, if tolerated	Tossed green salad
	French dressing
Bread: rice or corn	Rice flour bread
Butter or margarine	Butter or margarine
Milk	Milk
Dessert or fruit	Vanilla cornstarch pudding with sliced frozen peaches

Dinner

Meat, poultry, or fish	Broiled lamb patties (all meat)
	Mint jelly
Potato or rice	Rice with saffron seasoning
Cooked vegetable	Buttered asparagus
Salad, if tolerated	Celery and olives
Bread, corn or rice, if desired	
Butter	
Milk	Milk
Dessert or fruit	Lemon meringue pudding (thickened with cornstarch)
Tea or coffee	Coffee with cream, sugar

PROBLEMS AND REVIEW

1. Discuss the role of diet in the incidence of diseases of the small intestine and colon.

2. What is the relationship of psychologic factors to the occurrence of gastrointestinal disorders? Cite examples.

3. What do the terms *fiber* and *residue* mean?

4. What are the characteristics of a very low-residue diet? In which respects is the diet inadequate? Name four situations in which it might be used.

5. Compare the Very Low-residue Diet with Bland Diet IV and the Soft Diet with respect to nutritive adequacy, fiber content, and food choices.

6. The physician has indicated that a patient with ulcerative colitis may select his diet according to his tolerance. As a nurse, what problems are you likely to encounter with such a patient? What dietary instruction is necessary when the patient goes home?

7. *Problem.* Plan a day's menu for a patient with chronic ulcerative colitis, allowing at least 125 gm protein. Restrict the milk to that used in prepared foods. What are the reasons for each modification you have made from the normal diet?

8. What are the outstanding characteristics of atonic constipation? What are the chief causes? What type of individual is likely to develop atonic constipation?

9. *Problem.* Write a menu for a normal diet for 1 day which places emphasis on fiber.

10. What factors, other than diet, must be considered in the treatment of constipation?

11. What diet would you recommend for a person with an irritable colon?

12. What is gluten? Gliadin? Why are these substances contraindicated for some patients with sprue? What changes would be necessary in the diet you ate yesterday to make it free of gluten and gliadin?

CHAPTER 32 /

Diet in Disturbances of the Liver and Gallbladder

High-protein, Moderate-fat, High-carbohydrate Diet; Moderately Low-fat Diet

Functions of the liver. No organ of the body is concerned with so many different functions as the liver. It manufactures vital body substances, stores, modifies, and dispatches food materials, protects the body from poisons, and performs a variety of other functions not fully understood.

Protein metabolism. The liver maintains appreciable protein reserves which are readily released for the maintenance of the serum protein level. Body proteins are synthesized from the amino acids brought to the liver. The blood concentration of amino acids is controlled by the liver in that excess amino acids not needed for tissue synthesis are deaminized and thus made available for energy. The resulting ammonia is converted to urea and the remainder of the amino acid molecule yields glucose or fatty acids.

Carbohydrate metabolism. The liver is the chief storehouse of carbohydrate in the body, with ¼ to ½ pound of glycogen representing a normal amount. When the various simple sugars reach the liver from the portal circulation, they may be converted to glucose for immediate use or they may be manufactured into glycogen. Thus, the liver plays an important role in the regulation of the blood sugar level.

Lipid metabolism. The liver does not normally store fat, but it plays an essential role in the continual and rapid turnover of fats. It converts fatty acids into phospholipids for the more ready transportation of fats in the circulation; it synthesizes fats from fatty acids, carbohydrates, and deaminized amino acids; it synthesizes cholesterol; it oxidizes fatty acids to provide energy; and it converts excess cholesterol into bile salts. The normal and rapid turnover of fats in the liver requires certain lipotropic factors such as choline and methionine (see pp. 40, and 156).

Mineral and vitamin metabolism. Relatively large reserves of iron and

443

copper exist in the liver. The worn-out red blood cells are broken down so that the iron can be used over again.

About 95 per cent of the body's store of vitamin A and a considerable proportion of vitamin D are kept in the liver. Lesser reserves of vitamin B_{12}, other B-complex vitamins, ascorbic acid, and vitamin K are likewise present. Vitamin K is converted to prothrombin in the liver, and to some extent carotene may be converted to vitamin A.

Manufacture of bile. Bile is manufactured continuously by the liver and is carried by the many bile ducts to the hepatic duct and thence to the cystic duct for concentration and storage in the gallbladder. Approximately 500 to 1000 ml of bile are secreted daily. Bile salts, bile acids, bile pigments, and cholesterol are the more important constituents of this secretion.

The bile salts possess the capacity to lower surface tension. This property accounts for the emulsification of fats and thus the more efficient action of lipase in the intestine. The bile salts also render fats and fat-soluble vitamins more soluble and thus aid in the absorption of these substances from the intestine. Bile salts are a stimulus to the further production of bile in the liver.

The bile is a channel for the excretion of waste products. The bile pigments, bilirubin and biliverdin, are the result of hemoglobin disintegration. Excess cholesterol is also disposed of in this manner.

Other functions. The liver plays a role in the regulation of blood coagulation in that it synthesizes fibrinogen, a protein essential for the clotting process, and heparin, an anticoagulant substance. Its function in converting vitamin K to prothrombin, another substance required for blood clotting, has been mentioned above.

The liver effectively detoxifies substances which are toxic end products of digestion because of bacterial action, and likewise protects the body from the toxic effects of certain drugs such as sulfa drugs, arsenic, mercury, and others providing the intake of carbohydrate and protein has been satisfactory. The ammonia resulting from bacterial decomposition in the intestine and from deaminization of the amino acids is a toxic substance to the body which is rendered harmless by the elaboration of urea by the liver.

DISEASES OF THE LIVER

Jaundice is a symptom common to many diseases of the liver and biliary tract and consists of a yellow pigmentation of the skin and body tissues because of the accumulation of bile pigments in the blood. *Obstructive jaundice* results from the interference of the flow of bile by stones, tumors, or inflammation of the mucosa of the ducts. *Hemolytic jaundice* results from an abnormally large destruction of blood cells such as occurs in yellow fever, pernicious anemia, etc. *Toxic jaundice* originates from poisons, drugs, or virus infections.

HEPATITIS

Hepatitis is an inflammation of the liver which may be caused by infectious agents such as viruses and bacteria, or toxic drugs such as arsenicals, or solvents such as carbon tetrachloride. Necrosis or rapid destruction of the liver cells occurs.

Infectious hepatitis, also known as viral hepatitis and formerly called catarrhal jaundice, assumed epidemic proportions in the armed forces of World War II. Outbreaks occur especially in young people from time to time. The infection is caused by a virus readily transmitted through contaminated food or water. Homologous serum jaundice is similar to infectious hepatitis and results from transfusions of blood from a donor who is a carrier of the virus, or from improperly sterilized needles used for inoculations.

Hepatitis is usually characterized by marked anorexia, fever, headache, rapid and often marked weight loss, loss of muscle tone, jaundice, and abdominal discomfort.[163] The disease may continue for 4 to 8 weeks.

Modification of the diet. The objectives of the diet are to avoid further injury and strain to the liver, and to aid in the regeneration of liver tissue. With a liberal diet and adequate rest permanent liver damage can be avoided.

Energy. About 3000 to 4000 calories daily may be required to counteract weight loss, and to assist in maximum utilization of protein.

Protein. A liberal protein intake is essential for the maintenance and repair of the liver tissue itself and to furnish lipotropic factors for the utilization of fat. Usually an intake of 1½ to 2 gm per kg body weight or 100 to 150 gm daily will prove to be a satisfactory allowance.

Carbohydrate. Large amounts of carbohydrate exert a protein-sparing effect and supply the bulk of the caloric need. Moreover, a liberal carbohydrate intake ensures a large reserve of glycogen which aids in the maintenance of hepatic function and the protection of the liver against injury. An intake of 300 to 400 gm daily should be encouraged.

Fat. The studies of Hoagland and his associates [164] show conclusively that patients on high-protein, high-carbohydrate diets with relatively liberal intakes of fat (150 gm) had better appetites, gained weight, and improved more rapidly than did patients on equally high-protein intakes but with limited amounts of fat (50 gm daily). The authors believe that the greater improvement was the result of the higher caloric intake and the consequent nutritional betterment rather than the result of fat intake as such. The liberal fat intake provided a more palatable diet as well as an increased caloric level without undue amounts of bulky foods.

It now appears that the total level of the fat is probably less important than the type of fat which is permitted. The fats of whole milk, cream, butter, and eggs are easily utilized and should be used in sufficient amounts to enhance the palatability of the diet. Thus, 100 to 150 gm fat daily may be incorporated.

Consistency. A liquid to soft diet may be used during the acute illness, progressing to a wider choice of foods with convalescence.

Management of the diet. Since anorexia is characteristic of the disease, good cookery and attractive food service must be emphasized. Three meals of small to moderate size may be offered to the patient when high-protein beverages are used as supplements between meals and at bedtime. A considerable amount of persuasion is often needed to get the patient to eat. Some years ago Berger [163] found that moderate amounts of spices, condiments, relishes, catsup, and pickles aided in stimulating the appetite.

HIGH-PROTEIN, MODERATE-FAT, HIGH-CARBOHYDRATE DIET

Characteristics and general rules:

The caloric level may be increased by adding high-carbohydrate foods. Small amounts of cream and ice cream may be used when tolerated.

Fat may be decreased to approximately 35–40 gm daily by selecting only lean meats, fish and poultry, by using skim milk, and by omitting the butter.

The protein intake may be increased by adding nonfat dry milk to liquid milk. See page 672 for high-protein beverages.

Modifications in fiber and consistency may be made by applying restrictions concerning the Soft Diet (p. 341) to the foods listed below.

Six or more small feedings may be preferred when there is lack of appetite.

When sodium restriction is ordered, all food must be prepared without salt. Low-sodium milk should replace part or all of the prescribed milk. See Sodium-restricted Diets, p. 507.

Include these foods daily:

1 quart milk
8 ounces lean meat, poultry, or fish
1 egg
4 to 5 vegetables including:
    2 servings potato or substitute
    1 serving green leafy or yellow vegetable
    1–2 servings other vegetable
    One vegetable to be raw each day
3 servings fruit including:
    1 serving citrus fruit or other good source of ascorbic acid
    2 servings other fruit
1 serving enriched or whole-grain cereal
6 slices enriched or whole-grain bread
2 tablespoons butter or fortified margarine

4 tablespoons sugar, jelly, marmalade, or jam
Additional foods to further increase the carbohydrate as the patient is able to
take them

Nutritive value of basic pattern above: protein, 135 gm; fat, 106 gm; carbohydrate,
236 gm; calories, 2590; calcium, 2.53 gm; iron, 18.3 mg; vitamin A, 18,770
I.U.; thiamine, 2.11 mg; riboflavin, 3.39 mg; niacin, 27.6 mg; ascorbic acid,
159 mg.

Foods allowed:

Beverages—carbonated beverages, milk
and milk drinks, coffee or substitute,
tea, fruit juices, cocoa flavoring
Breads and cereals—all kinds
Cheese—cottage, cream, mild Cheddar
Desserts—angel cake, plain cookies and
cake, custard, plain or fruit gelatin,
fruit whip, fruit pudding, Junket,
milk and cereal desserts, sherbets,
ices, plain ice cream
Egg—1 only
Fat—butter, fortified margarine, cream,
in amounts stated above
Fruits—all except avocado

Meat—lean beef, veal, lamb, liver, non-
fatty fish, chicken

Potato or substitute—hominy, macaroni, noodles, rice, spaghetti, sweet
potato
Seasonings—salt, spices, vinegar in
moderation
Soup—clear without fat
Sweets—honey, jam, jelly, sugar, sugar
candy, sirup
Vegetables—all except olives

Foods to avoid:

Beverages—chocolate; alcohol

Cheese—strong
Desserts—rich cake, cookies, doughnuts, pie, pastries

Egg—fried
Fat—all except butter, cream; visible
fat on meat; salad dressing
Fruits—avocado; if melons, raw apple,
and berries cause distress, they are
omitted
Meat—fat meat or fish such as bacon,
duck, goose, ham, pork, sausage, sardines
Potato—fried, potato chips

Seasonings—excessive use; pepper

Soup—with fat
Sweets—candy with chocolate or nuts

Vegetables—if strongly flavored vegetables give distress omit broccoli,
Brussels sprouts, cauliflower, cabbage, cucumber, onion, peppers, radish, turnips, legumes
Miscellaneous—chocolate, fried foods,
nuts, peanut butter, salad dressings,
gravies

MEAL PATTERN	SAMPLE MENU

Breakfast

Fruit	Half grapefruit
Cereal with milk and sugar	Wheatena with milk and sugar
Egg—1	Scrambled egg
Whole-grain or enriched toast—2 slices	Whole-wheat toast
Butter or margarine—2 teaspoons	Butter
Marmalade—1 tablespoon	Orange marmalade
Beverage with cream and sugar	Coffee with cream and sugar

Luncheon or supper

Lean meat, fish or poultry—4 ounces	Broiled whitefish
Potato or substitute	Escalloped potatoes
Cooked vegetable	Buttered asparagus
Salad	Celery and carrot strips
Whole-grain or enriched bread—2 slices	Whole-wheat bread
Butter or margarine—2 teaspoons	Butter
Jelly—1 tablespoon	Grape jelly
Fruit	Sliced banana
Milk	Milk

Midafternoon

Milk with nonfat dry milk	High-protein milk with strawberry flavor

Dinner

Lean meat, fish, or fowl—4 ounces	Roast beef, trimmed of all fat
Potato	Mashed potato
Vegetable	Baked acorn squash
Whole-grain or enriched bread—2 slices	Dinner rolls
Butter or margarine—2 teaspoons	Butter
Jelly—1 tablespoon	Apple jelly
Fruit, or dessert	Raspberry sherbet
Milk—1 glass	Milk
Tea, if desired	

Evening nourishment

Milk beverage	High-protein milk flavored with caramel
	Bread and jelly sandwich

CIRRHOSIS OF THE LIVER

Cirrhosis is a chronic disease of the liver in which increased fibrous connective tissue replaces the functioning liver cells. Among the causes are infectious hepatitis, chronic alcoholism, hepatotoxic agents, and prolonged stasis of the biliary tract from gallstones. Patients with portal cirrhosis (Laennec's cirrhosis; "alcoholic" cirrhosis) respond most favorably to diet. Alcoholism accounts for a large proportion of these patients. Although the alcohol consumed furnishes the bulk of the caloric intake, other nutrients are seriously lacking in the extremely poor food intake. The malnutrition which ensues, rather than the alcohol, per se, is believed to be responsible for the accumulation of fat in the liver, destruction of the liver cells, and the proliferation of fibrous tissue.

Symptoms and clinical findings. The onset of cirrhosis may be gradual with gastrointestinal disturbances such as anorexia, nausea, vomiting, pain, and distention. As the disease progresses, jaundice and other serious changes occur.

Ascites is the accumulation of fluid in the abdominal cavity and results when the portal circulation is impaired and portal hypertension is present. Low blood protein levels, especially a lowered albumin level, may also contribute to ascites and peripheral edema.

Esophageal varices (varicose veins) and distended abdominal veins may follow impairment of the portal circulation. Hemorrhage is then an everpresent danger and may be provoked by roughage of any kind. The hemorrhage itself may be fatal, or the blood may provide for the accumulation of ammonia and subsequent hepatic coma.

Modification of the diet. If diet therapy is initiated early in the course of the disease, and if alcohol is withheld, regeneration of liver cells occurs with considerable subjective improvement. The diet outlined above for infectious hepatitis is satisfactory for such patients. When cirrhosis is more advanced, the following further considerations must be given to dietary planning.

Protein. While a liberal protein intake may be advantageous to most patients, considerable caution should be exercised since hepatic coma is a possible danger in advanced cirrhosis. A diet providing the recommended allowances of protein—1 gm per kilogram body weight—is considered suitable by some clinicians, while 1½ to 2 gm protein per kilogram are recommended by others. Protein should be immediately and drastically curtailed if the patient has signs of impending coma.

Vitamins. The diet itself, when well taken, includes a liberal allowance of all vitamins (see p. 447). When malnutrition has been present for some time, multivitamin supplements may be prescribed for a few weeks.

Sodium. A sodium-restricted diet is prescribed together with other measures to improve sodium excretion if ascites and peripheral edema are present. A diet restricted to as little as 200 mg sodium has been shown to be effective; [165] however, such restriction necessitates the substitution of low-sodium milk for regular milk, and careful planning of the protein intake. See pages 506–19 for full details concerning the planning of such a diet.

Consistency. In early stages of cirrhosis no change in fiber content is usually necessary, but a smooth or even liquid diet is essential if esophageal varices are present.

HEPATIC COMA

Hepatic coma is a neurologic disorder which may occur as a complication in acute hepatitis or in cirrhosis. It may be initiated by a variety of factors such as an acute infection, a gastrointestinal hemorrhage, trauma or surgery, a transfusion reaction, acute alcoholism, or following paracentesis. While it is undoubtedly a complex syndrome, one common explanation given is that of ammonia intoxication. If liver cells are sufficiently damaged, as in severe hepatitis, or if the portal circulation by-passes the liver cells, as in advanced cirrhosis, ammonia gains access to the general circulation.

Symptoms. The brain tissue is especially sensitive to ammonia. The patient with impending coma shows signs of drowsiness, confusion, and disorientation and may have a flapping tremor of the arms and legs when they are extended. He lapses into sleep, fails to respond to stimuli, and may have convulsions. The breath has a fecal odor—*fetor hepaticus.* Death rapidly ensues unless prompt treatment is initiated.

Modification of the diet. The fundamental principle in the dietary management of hepatic coma is to restrict protein metabolism to a minimum thereby reducing the amount of ammonia produced. This means that catabolism of tissue proteins must also be avoided.

Energy. About 1500–2000 calories daily are sufficient to keep body tissue breakdown to a minimum. Carbohydrates and fats provide all of the energy at first.

Protein. A protein-free diet is recommended at first by some, while others permit 20–30 gm protein daily. When improvement occurs, the protein intake is increased by 10–20 gm daily until a normal allowance of 1 gm per kilogram is reached. With each addition the patient is carefully watched; any signs of returning coma must be met with continued curtailment of protein.

Levels of 40–50 gm protein daily may be used for long periods of time without detriment to nutritional status if the diet is otherwise adequate. Davidson states that protein intakes as low as 30 gm daily will permit nitrogen balance if the quality of the protein is good and if the caloric intake is adequate.[165]

Management of the diet. These patients are usually difficult to feed because of anorexia and widely varying patterns of behavior ranging from irritability and sometimes hyperexcitability to drowsiness and confusion. The protein-free diet consisting of commercial sugar-fat emulsions, a butter-sugar mixture, or glucose in beverages or fruit juices may be used initially through oral or tube feeding. The details of such a regimen are described in Chapter

37, page 525. With improvement the diets providing 20, 40, and 60 gm protein may be gradually introduced.

DISEASES OF THE GALLBLADDER

Function of the gallbladder. The gallbladder concentrates bile from the liver and serves as a storehouse for it. The presence of fats in the duodenum causes the hormone, cholecystokinin, to be released to the blood stream. The hormone brings about the contraction of the gallbladder and the consequent emptying of bile into the common duct and thence into the small intestine.

Symptoms and clinical findings. Cholecystitis is an inflammation of the gallbladder, while cholelithiasis consists in the formation of stones which may block the ducts and thus impede the flow of bile. It is understandable that the ingestion of fatty foods would lead to pain, sometimes very severe, because of the contraction of the gallbladder in these circumstances. The patient experiences a sense of fullness and often complains of distention, especially after eating certain strongly flavored vegetables, legumes, melons, and berries. The diminished flow of bile to the small intestine leads to impairment of fat digestion and absorption.

Modification of the diet. The objectives in diet therapy of gallbladder disease are to provide adequate nutrition and to reduce the discomfort by giving a low-fat diet, bland in flavor, and restricted in very coarse fiber.

Energy. Many patients with gallbladder disease are overweight and should be given a low-calorie diet (see Chap. 27). With restriction of fat, carbohydrates are used liberally to provide the needed calories.

Fat. Most patients tolerate small amounts of easily digested fats such as those of butter or margarine, whole milk, and egg yolk. Thus, a diet restricted to approximately 60 gm fat daily may include sufficient amounts of these foods to enhance the palatability of the diet. When fat must be reduced to 20–25 gm daily, only skim milk is used, butter and margarine are omitted, only very lean meats may be used, and egg yolk is omitted.

Cholesterol. Gallstones contain appreciable amounts of cholesterol, and in the past it has been customary to employ low-cholesterol diets for patients with cholelithiasis. However, restriction of dietary cholesterol alone is of doubtful value since the endogenous production of cholesterol is 10 to 20 times as high as that contained in the diet. Probably the restriction of dietary fat and the reduction of caloric level are of greatest benefit because fewer acetate building units are thus available for cholesterol formation. The sources of cholesterol are given in Table 7 in the Appendix, page 780.

MODERATELY LOW-FAT DIET

Characteristics and general rules:

The fat content of this diet may be reduced to approximately 25 gm daily by:
(1) using skim milk; (2) omitting butter, margarine, and other visible
fats; (3) selecting lean meats, poultry, and fish and using them in restricted
amounts.

A higher protein content may be obtained by using skim milk, cottage cheese
made from skim milk, and egg white.

The caloric level may be adjusted by using more or less of potato, bread, cereals,
sweetened fruits and fruit juices, and sugars and other sweets.

A vitamin-A supplement is desirable when the fat is reduced below 50–60 gm
daily.

Individual tolerances to foods vary widely. While strongly flavored vegetables,
legumes, melons, and berries are included among foods to avoid, some
patients experience no discomfort and should then be permitted to use
these foods.

If a bland diet reduced in fiber is desirable the regimen described on pages
420–24 should be consulted, applying appropriate modifications for fat
content.

Include these foods daily:

2 cups whole milk—skimmed if very low fat level is desired
4 ounces lean meat, fish, poultry, or cottage cheese
1 egg
4 servings vegetables including:
    1 serving deep green leafy or deep yellow vegetable
    1–2 servings potato or substitute
    1–2 servings other vegetable
    One vegetable to be served raw, if tolerated
3 servings fruit including:
    1 serving citrus fruit
    2 servings other fruit
1 serving enriched or whole-grain cereal
3 slices enriched or whole-grain bread
1 tablespoon butter or fortified margarine—omit on very low-fat diet
2 to 4 tablespoons sugar, or other sweets
Additional foods such as bread, cereal, hard candy, potato, jelly, and sugar
should be used except in obesity.

Nutritive value—allowing whole milk, egg, butter: protein, 75 gm; fat, 56 gm;
carbohydrate, 191 gm; calories, 1540.

Foods allowed:

Beverages—whole milk, only 2 cups; skim milk as desired; coffee, coffee substitute, tea; fruit juices

Breads—all kinds except those with added fat

Cereals—all cooked or dry breakfast cereals, except possibly bran; macaroni, noodles, rice, spaghetti

Cheese—cottage only

Desserts—angel cake; fruit whip; fruit pudding; gelatin; ices and sherbets; milk and cereal puddings using part of milk allowance

Eggs—1 only

Fats—1 tablespoon butter or fortified margarine

Fruits—all kinds when tolerated

Meats—broiled, baked, roasted, or stewed without fat: lean beef, chicken, lamb, liver, veal, sweetbreads, fish

Seasonings—in moderation: salt, pepper, spices, herbs, flavoring extracts

Soups—clear

Sweets—all kinds: hard candy, jam, jelly, marmalade, sugars

Vegetables—all kinds when well tolerated; cooked without added butter, or cream

Foods to avoid:

Beverages—with cream; soda-fountain beverages with milk, cream, or ice cream

Breads—griddle cakes; sweet rolls with fat; French toast

Cheese—all whole-milk cheeses, both hard and soft

Desserts—any containing chocolate, cream, nuts, or fats: cookies, cake, doughnuts, ice cream, pastries, pies, rich puddings

Eggs—fried

Fats—cooking fats, cream, oil, salad dressings

Fruits—raw apple, berries, melons may not be tolerated

Meats—fatty meats, poultry, or fish: bacon, corned beef, duck, goose, ham, fish canned in oil, mackerel, pork, sausage

Smoked and spiced meats if they are poorly tolerated

Seasonings—sometimes not tolerated: pepper; curries; meat sauces; excessive spices; vinegar

Soups—cream, unless made with milk and fat allowance

Sweets—candy with chocolate and nuts

Vegetables—strongly flavored may be poorly tolerated: broccoli, Brussels sprouts, cabbage, cauliflower, cucumber, onion, peppers, radish, turnips; dried cooked peas and beans

Miscellaneous—fried foods; gravies; nuts; olives; peanut butter; pickles; popcorn; relishes

MEAL PATTERN	SAMPLE MENU

Breakfast

Fruit	Stewed apricots
Cereal with milk and sugar	Corn flakes with milk and sugar
Egg—1 only	Poached egg
Enriched or whole-grain toast	Whole-wheat toast with butter
Butter—1 teaspoon only	
Beverage with milk and sugar	Coffee with milk and sugar

Luncheon or supper

	Tomato bouillon
Lean meat, fish, poultry, or cottage cheese	Fruit salad plate:
	Cottage cheese
Potato or substitute	Sliced orange
Vegetable	Tokay grapes
Salad; no oil dressing	Pear
	Romaine
Enriched or whole-grain bread	Sliced chicken sandwich, with 1 tea-
Butter or margarine—1 teaspoon only	spoon butter
Dessert or fruit	Vanilla blanc mange (using milk allow-
	ance)
Milk—½ cup	Tea with milk, sugar

Dinner

Lean meat, poultry, or fish	Roast lamb, trimmed of fat
Potato or substitute	Boiled new potatoes; no added fat
Vegetable	Zucchini squash
Enriched or whole-grain bread	Parkerhouse roll, buttered
Butter—1 teaspoon	
Dessert or fruit	Angel cake with sliced peaches
Milk—1 glass	Milk—1 glass

Diet following cholecystectomy. Following removal of the gallbladder, the low-fat diet described above may be used for a number of months. When the irritation has subsided, the individual is able to consume a normal diet.

PROBLEMS AND REVIEW

1. Discuss in detail the functions of the liver in digestion, metabolism, storage, manufacture, regulation, and detoxication.

2. What are the functions of bile?

3. Of what importance is the gallbladder?

4. What reasons can you give for the use of a high-protein, high-carbohydrate, moderate-fat diet in hepatitis?

5. What additional considerations apply in the planning of diet for a patient with cirrhosis of the liver?

6. *Problem.* For a patient with cirrhosis of the liver plan a soft diet which includes 100 gm protein, 120 gm fat, and 350 gm carbohydrate.

7. Under what circumstances would sodium restriction be required? What changes would be necessary to adapt the diet in Problem 6 to 250 mg sodium daily?

8. What is hepatic coma? Why is a protein-free or low-protein diet ordered? Why is an adequate caloric intake so essential?

9. *Problem.* Write menus for 1 day for a patient with impending hepatic coma, keeping the protein restricted to 20 gm.

10. What is the rationale for the use of a low-fat diet in gallbladder disease?

11. If cholesterol restriction is ordered for a patient with gallbladder disease, what foods should be omitted?

12. Why are these foods often contraindicated for patients with gallbladder disease: cabbage, raspberries, baked beans, chile con carne?

13. *Problem.* Plan a diet for 1 day which is suitable for a patient who is overweight, who has gallbladder disease, and for whom a 25-gm fat level has been ordered.

UNIT IX /
Diet in Metabolic and Nervous Disorders

CHAPTER 33 /

Diabetes Mellitus

Nature of diabetes. Diabetes mellitus is a disease of metabolism the outstanding characteristic of which is the lessened ability, or the complete inability, of the tissues to utilize carbohydrate. Abnormal fat and protein metabolisms are associated with the disorder. Excessive urination, glycosuria, and hyperglycemia are cardinal findings.

Insulin, one of the hormones manufactured by the cells of the islands of Langerhans in the pancreas, is intimately concerned with the metabolism of carbohydrate. On the stimulus of carbohydrate, insulin is released into the blood stream and functions in the conversion of glucose to glycogen in the liver and for the later oxidation of glucose by the tissues. In diabetes mellitus too little insulin is produced.

To ascribe diabetes simply to a defect in the production of insulin is an oversimplification. The anterior pituitary and adrenal cortical hormones exert an effect on carbohydrate metabolism which is antagonistic to that produced by insulin (see Fig. 33-1). An overproduction of these hormones results in hyperglycemia, glycosuria, and ketosis and may thus produce the diabetic state just as a deficiency of insulin will produce diabetes.

The anterior pituitary also produces hormones that govern the action of the adrenal and thyroid glands, and thus carbohydrate metabolism is indirectly influenced. Therefore, it appears that the balance of several hormones produced by the pancreas, the pituitary, the adrenal, and the thyroid glands may be disturbed in diabetes mellitus. These relationships are poorly understood at the present time.

Incidence and predisposing factors. Conservative estimates place the incidence of diabetes mellitus in the United States at more than 2 million; more than 25,000 deaths occur annually. Diabetes is essentially a disease of middle age, the highest incidence occurring at 50 to 60 years of age. However, no age is free of it, for even infants may have it. The illness is much more severe as a rule in children and is considerably more difficult to treat. Heredity and obesity are the most important predisposing factors in the development of diabetes. A predisposition to diabetes is inherited as a Mendelian recessive character; that is, if two diabetic persons marry, all of their children will be diabetic if they live long enough. If a diabetic marries a diabetic carrier, half of the children will be potential diabetics, while if a diabetic marries one who is neither a diabetic nor a diabetic carrier, none of the children will have diabetes.

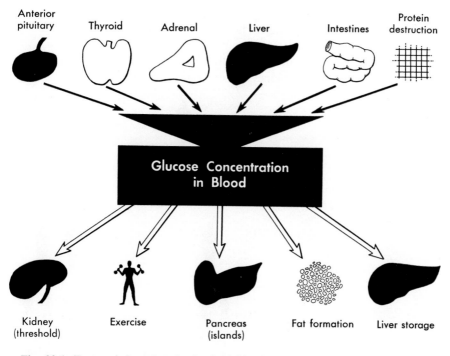

Fig. 33-1. Factors influencing the level of blood sugar. Excessive secretory activity of anterior pituitary, adrenal cortex, or thyroid may, by stimulating glucose formation and reducing glucose utilization, raise the blood sugar to levels that increase greatly the demands on the pancreas. Should such hyperfunction persist or be unduly prolonged, the islands of Langerhans may fail and permanent diabetes may result. The pathogenic influence of a high blood sugar level may be interrupted when hyperglycemia is controlled by insulin. (*Courtesy, the Lilly Research Laboratories, Indianapolis.*)

The percentage of obese individuals showing diabetes is far greater than that of individuals who are of normal weight or slightly underweight (see Fig. 33-2). Approximately 80 per cent of the adults in Joslin's diabetic clinic had previously been overweight by 5 per cent or more. On the contrary, children and adolescents have been more commonly underweight than overweight.

The disease is more prevalent among sedentary workers than manual laborers and is more frequent among people who have a bountiful supply of food and plenty of leisure. The Jewish people have been subject to diabetes more often than other racial groups, but this may be related to their food habits rather than to any racial characteristics.

Hundley [166] believes that the avoidance of obesity at all times during life would significantly reduce the incidence of diabetes, just as it is well known that correction of obesity in the diabetic improves the state of health in the patient.

Symptoms and clinical findings. The disturbed metabolism in diabetes brings about the following characteristic symptoms of the disease.

Polyuria, or a frequent and abnormally large outflow of urine, results when glucose passes through the kidneys in excessive amounts.

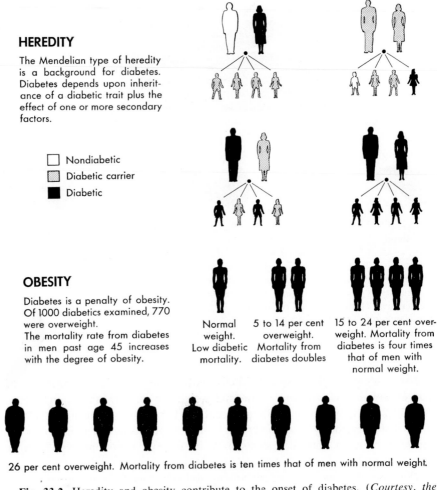

HEREDITY

The Mendelian type of heredity is a background for diabetes. Diabetes depends upon inheritance of a diabetic trait plus the effect of one or more secondary factors.

☐ Nondiabetic
▩ Diabetic carrier
■ Diabetic

OBESITY

Diabetes is a penalty of obesity. Of 1000 diabetics examined, 770 were overweight.
The mortality rate from diabetes in men past age 45 increases with the degree of obesity.

Normal weight. Low diabetic mortality.

5 to 14 per cent overweight. Mortality from diabetes doubles

15 to 24 per cent overweight. Mortality from diabetes is four times that of men with normal weight.

26 per cent overweight. Mortality from diabetes is ten times that of men with normal weight.

Fig. 33-2. Heredity and obesity contribute to the onset of diabetes. (*Courtesy, the Lilly Research Laboratories, Indianapolis.*)

Polydipsia, or excessive thirst, is explained by the great loss of body fluids in the urine and the need for replacement in the tissues.

Dehydration is occasioned by the excessive urinary output and the failure to balance it by water intake.

Polyphagia, or increased appetite, results from failure to utilize the food for nourishment of the body cells.

General weakness and loss of weight follow the inability to use foods and the subsequent breakdown of body tissues.

Decreased resistance to infection, especially staphylococcal infection and tuberculosis, becomes apparent in untreated and poorly regulated cases of diabetes.

Decreased ability of the tissues to heal occurs with a high blood sugar and poor fluid balance.

Degenerative changes such as peripheral neuritis, retinitis, atherosclerosis with disease of the coronary arteries, and vascular changes in the kidneys are evident in advanced cases, especially those which have been poorly controlled.

Ketosis, or acidosis, is the accumulation of lower fatty acids in the blood and may ultimately lead to *coma* and even death.

The diagnosis of diabetes is based on the above symptoms and findings plus results of the following laboratory tests on the urine and blood (see pp. 575–77).

Glycosuria, or the occurrence of sugar in the urine, should be regarded as evidence of diabetes until proved otherwise. Situations in which sugar is present in the urine of nondiabetics include pentosuria as the result of the body's failure to use the carbohydrate known as pentose; lactosuria in nursing mothers; alimentary glycosuria from extra dietary loads of carbohydrate; and renal glycosuria because of a reduction of the ability of the tubules to reabsorb glucose. The latter condition is seen in some cases of hyperthyroidism and occasionally in pregnancy.

Hyperglycemia may be detected by determination of the concentration of sugar after a fast of 12 hours. A fasting blood sugar of more than 140 mg per 100 ml is suggestive of diabetes.

Ketonuria, or the excretion of ketones, occurs when fatty acids are incompletely oxidized in the body. The detection of acetoacetic acid is a simple and routine test.

The *glucose tolerance test* is a measure of the ability of the body to utilize a known amount of glucose. Under the conditions of the test, a normal individual shows a rise in blood sugar about ½ hour after ingestion of the sugar, but the blood sugar value returns to the normal level in 2 hours. If the blood sugar rises above 140 to 150 mg per 100 ml and fails to return to normal fasting levels within 3 hours, diabetes is presumed to be present.

Metabolism in diabetes. The basal metabolic rate in diabetes is essentially normal, except in those severe, uncontrolled patients who may have become extremely undernourished because of their inability to utilize glucose. In the latter group one may find a reduction of the basal metabolism by as much as 30 per cent. In order to adequately understand the disordered carbohydrate, fat, and protein metabolism in diabetes, the reader first should review carefully the normal metabolism of these nutrients (pp. 40, 60, and 71).

Carbohydrate metabolism. The normal fasting glucose concentration in the blood is 70 to 90 mg per 100 ml. If there is too little insulin being produced, glucose will not be converted to glycogen in the liver and tissues, and glucose will be inadequately utilized in the tissues. Consequently, the glucose concentration in the blood increases markedly as the sugars are absorbed from the intestine or may be derived from the breakdown of dietary or body proteins and fats. Sugar begins to spill over into the urine when the renal threshold is reached. This point varies in different individuals but is approximately 170 mg per 100 ml. In severe diabetes, the fasting blood sugar may reach 400 mg per 100 ml or even more.

Fat metabolism. In diabetes, with the failure to synthesize glycogen and to utilize glucose, the glycogen stores of the liver are rapidly depleted. In such a circumstance the metabolic needs are met by breaking down of an increased quantity of fatty acids, and the liver releases into the blood stream larger amounts of the ketone bodies (acetone, beta-hydroxybutyric acid, and acetoacetic acid). The acid-base equilibrium is disturbed with the release of these compounds in larger than normal amounts, since acetoacetic acid and beta-hydroxybutyric acid are fairly strong acids. When the kidneys attempt to dispose of them in the urine, significant amounts of basic elements are lost from the body. The depletion of body base leads ultimately to acidosis.

Atherosclerosis appears at an early age in diabetics and progresses more rapidly than in nondiabetic individuals. This condition and the attendant cardiovascular diseases are associated with high blood lipid levels, of which cholesterol is one. The reasons for these changes in the diabetic are not understood, although there is undoubtedly some relationship to the faulty fat and carbohydrate metabolism.

Protein metabolism. Protein tissues, as well as fatty tissues, are broken down when carbohydrate is not being normally metabolized. The resulting amino acids are deaminized and the nonnitrogenous part of the molecule would normally be utilized as glucose or fatty acids. In the diabetic, the breakdown of protein leads to a further increase of glucose in the circulation and of incompletely oxidized fatty acids. About 58 per cent of the amino acids are potential sources of glucose, but so high a rate of conversion is not usually realized.[167] It should be evident that the excessive breakdown of either protein or fatty tissue leads to progressive weight loss.

Modifications of the diet. While the importance of the dietary regimen for the diabetic individual is universally accepted, viewpoints differ somewhat concerning the degree of dietary control that is necessary. Three points of view have been summarized by Cohen.[168]

Chemical control. A measured diet and insulin dosage are carefully regulated so that the blood sugar is kept within normal limits and the urine is free or nearly free of sugar at all times. Such control is believed to reduce the incidence and severity of degenerative complications. One criticism sometimes leveled against it is that the treatment may tend to be directed to the diabetes and not to the person as a whole.

Clinical control. Hyperglycemia and glycosuria are disregarded, and insulin is used to control ketosis. The diet differs little if any from that of normal persons and is controlled only to the point of maintenance of normal weight. Some physicians use these so-called "free" diets in the most liberal sense, but others restrict concentrated carbohydrate foods, especially those from sources contributing no other nutrients. Those who favor clinical control believe that the patient has an increased sense of well-being and that the degenerative complications are not more frequent.

Intermediate control. The majority of physicians adopt a regimen which falls between the preceding two. The objectives are: (1) to treat the patient as an individual and not on the basis of his diabetes alone; (2) to provide adequate nutrition for the maintenance of normal weight, a sense of well-being, and a life of usefulness; (3) to keep the blood sugar almost at normal levels for a large part of the day by using insulin as needed but avoiding hypoglycemia; (4) to keep the urine sugar-free or with only traces of sugar for most of the day.

Daughaday[167] cites three arguments for a controlled diabetic diet: (1) its educational value in helping the patient to understand his disease and the need for optimum nutrition; (2) 30 to 40 per cent of all diabetic patients do not need insulin if their diets are controlled; and (3) dietary control with insulin permits correlation of the diet with the type of insulin so that a normal blood sugar is achieved without too much risk of insulin shock.

The diabetic patient must observe dietary restriction for the remainder of his life. Such regulation, when properly made, permits the patient to lead an essentially normal life. However, great care must be taken that this diet always provides the elements of good nutrition. Each diabetic diet is specific for the individual concerned.

Energy. It is no longer believed necessary, or even desirable, to maintain undernutrition. Appreciable loss of weight must be avoided, and the patient must not be permitted to lose his sense of well-being. If the patient is greatly undernourished, efforts are made to increase his weight. On the other hand, obesity is by all means to be avoided. Obese individuals should be placed on a low-calorie diet until the ideal weight for height and age is attained. Such weight loss in middle-aged, obese patients very often leads to return to normal glucose tolerance. An allowance of 8 to 12 calories per pound of desirable body weight is suitable.

The caloric allowance is essentially the same as that for normal individuals of the same activity, size, and sex. The following is a convenient guide for calories based on normal body weight.*

	CALORIES PER KILOGRAM	CALORIES PER POUND
For a bed patient	25	11.5
For light work	30	13.5
For medium work	35	16
For heavy work	40	18

These levels can be increased or decreased as necessary to maintain the optimum weight.

Protein. About 1 to 1½ gm of protein per kilogram (½ to ⅔ gm per pound) of desirable body weight is a satisfactory allowance. The higher level of protein gives greater satiety value to the diet. Somewhat higher protein levels are in order for growing children, in pregnancy and lactation, or when there has been extensive loss of weight and associated hypoproteinemia.

Carbohydrate and fat. The distribution of the nonprotein calories between carbohydrate and fat is a much discussed subject. Physicians ordinarily recommend a moderate reduction of carbohydrate from the normal level. Generally, the carbohydrate should not be less than 150 gm, this being approximately one-half of the normal carbohydrate level of the diet. Somewhat greater restriction may occasionally be used for those patients who are mild diabetics and who may be able to avoid taking insulin. Sample diet plans developed by a committee of the American Dietetic Association [169] at calorie levels ranging from 1200 to 3500 include 125 to 370 gm carbohydrate. The so-called "high-carbohydrate" diets for diabetics are essentially normal carbohydrate intakes. The carbohydrate level of most diabetic diets will be found to fall within 40 to 60 per cent of the nonprotein calories.

When the protein and carbohydrate levels have been established, the fat is calculated to supply the remainder of the calories. Some physicians arbitrarily set the fat level at 90 to 120 gm per day, since this amount of fat will provide a palatable diet without an excess of fat. In this instance, the carbohydrate level is calculated to make up the needed calories.

The kind and amount of fat in the diet have been implicated in the incidence of atherosclerosis (see p. 498). While it cannot be stated with certainty

* Pennock, L. L.: "Simplification of the Treatment of Diabetes," *J. Lab. & Clin. Med.,* **29,** 1944, p. 168.

what modification of fat will be most effective in the diabetic diet with respect to reducing the degenerative complications, these possibilities should be kept in mind: (1) a very low fat diet—20 to 50 gm daily—would necessitate additional carbohydrate to maintain the caloric balance and would thus increase the insulin requirement; and (2) the usual level of fat may be prescribed, but the unsaturated fatty acids derived chiefly from vegetable oils may be recommended with a corresponding restriction of the saturated fatty acids. The latter course would permit maintenance of a fat level consistent with American diet patterns and would also help to keep insulin requirements to a minimum.

Calculation of the diabetic diet prescription. The diabetic diet is individualized for each patient and so planned that it is physiologically correct. The physician calculates the prescription basing his allowances on:

1. The history of both the patient and his family
2. Sex, age, weight, height, and activity of the patient
3. Type of diabetes—mild or severe
4. Type of insulin, amount, and when administered
5. Nutritional requirements as based on the above data

An illustration is here given of the manner in which a diabetic prescription may be calculated. Let us assume that a diet is to be planned for a secretary who is 25 years old and 66 inches tall. According to the table of heights and weights in the Appendix (p. 785), her desirable weight is 128 pounds (medium frame).

1. *Calories:* 13.5 calories per pound of desirable body weight
   $128 \times 13.5 = 1728$ calories per day
2. *Protein:* 0.5 to 0.67 gm per pound of desirable body weight
   $128 \times 0.6 = 77$ gm protein per day
3. *Nonprotein calories:* $1728 - 308 = 1420$ calories to be divided between carbohydrate and fat
4. *Carbohydrate:* 40 to 60 per cent of nonprotein calories
   50 per cent of 1420 calories $= 710$ calories
   $710 \div 4 = 177.5$ gm carbohydrate per day
5. *Fat calories:* total calories − calories from protein and carbohydrate
   $1728 - (308 + 710) = 710$ calories
   $710 \div 9 = 78.9$ gm fat per day

By rounding off the numbers the prescription thus becomes: carbohydrate, 180 gm; protein, 75 gm; and fat, 80 gm.

If the fat had been restricted to 50 gm per day, the prescription for the above patient would be completed as follows:

Carbohydrate calories: total calories — calories from protein and fat
1728 — (308 + 450) = 970
Carbohydrate: 970 ÷ 4 = 242.5 gm

The prescription would become: carbohydrate, 245 gm; protein, 75 gm; and fat, 50 gm.

Distribution of carbohydrate. The meal distribution of carbohydrate is determined according to the type of insulin being used and is modified according to each patient's needs in order to achieve the best possible regulation of carbohydrate utilization. Whenever no insulin is being given, the carbohydrate is divided, as a rule, into three equal parts. In many patients the blood sugar tends to be higher in the morning, in which case a smaller amount of carbohydrate—⅕ to ¼ of the total—may be given for breakfast with larger amounts at noon and night.

Regular insulin is now rarely used alone except for emergencies such as diabetic coma and surgery. It is sometimes given together with one of the more slowly acting insulins. When it is used alone, the larger amounts of carbohydrate will be included at the meal or meals immediately following the insulin injection.

Several slowly acting insulins are now widely used. Because the duration of action is prolonged for 18 to 24 hours or longer, a portion of the carbohydrate—usually 20 to 40 gm—is reserved for a bedtime feeding. This carbohydrate must be in slowly available form, and should be accompanied by a portion of the day's protein. After the bedtime carbohydrate has been subtracted from the day's allowance, the remainder of the carbohydrate is distributed to correspond to the peak activity and the duration of the activity of the insulin that is being used (see p. 471). The table which follows illustrates approximately how the carbohydrate might be divided with the several types of insulin.

TYPICAL MEAL DISTRIBUTIONS OF CARBOHYDRATE

TYPE OF INSULIN	BREAKFAST	NOON	MID-AFTERNOON	EVENING	BEDTIME * gm
None	⅓	⅓		⅓	Usually
	⅕	⅖		⅖	none
Regular (before breakfast and dinner)	⅖	⅕		⅖	Usually none
Protamine zinc	⅕	⅖		⅖	20–40
Protamine zinc with regular at breakfast	⅓	⅓		⅓	20–40
Isophane (NPH); or lente	⅓	⅓		⅓	20–40
	⅕	⅖		⅖	20–40
Globin	²⁄₁₀	³⁄₁₀	¹⁄₁₀	⁴⁄₁₀	

* The bedtime carbohydrate is subtracted from the day's total allowance. Then the meal fractions are applied to the remainder of the carbohydrate.

Planning the meal pattern. The calculation of the diet prescription and the distribution of the carbohydrate are the physician's responsibility. The dietitian and the nurse must translate these factors into terms of common foods which will also assure the patient of a sufficient amount of the essential minerals and vitamins. There are a number of points to keep in mind while planning the diet.

1. The diet should be planned with the patient so that it can be adjusted to his pattern of living. This requires consideration of the patient's economic status, the availability and cost of food, national, religious, and social customs, personal idiosyncrasies, occupation, facilities for preparing or obtaining meals, and so on.

The diabetic diet need not be an expensive one, and, ideally, it should be so planned that it fits in with the menus of the rest of the family. However, if the family dietary pattern is a poor one, the entire family will benefit when

CALCULATION OF A DIABETIC DIET *

Carbohydrate: 180 gm   Protein: 75 gm   Fat: 80 gm

LIST	FOOD	MEASURE	WEIGHT gm	CARBO-HYDRATE gm	PROTEIN gm	FAT gm
1	Milk	3 cups	720	36	24	30
2	Vegetable					
	group A	up to 1 cup	—	—	—	—
	group B	½ cup	100	7	2	—
3	Fruit	3 exchanges	varies	30	—	—
				73		
4	Bread	7 exchanges	varies	105	14	—
					40	
5	Meat	5 exchanges	varies	—	35	25
						55
6	Fat	5 exchanges	varies	—	—	25
				178	75	80

180 gm carbohydrate prescribed total
 73 gm carbohydrate from milk, vegetables, and fruit
107 gm carbohydrate to be supplied from bread exchanges
          $107 \div 15 = 7$ bread exchanges

75 gm protein prescribed total
40 gm protein from milk, vegetable, and bread exchanges
35 gm protein to be supplied from meat exchanges
          $35 \div 7 = 5$ meat exchanges

80 gm fat prescribed total
55 gm fat from milk and meat exchanges
25 gm fat to be supplied from fat exchanges
          $25 \div 5 = 5$ fat exchanges

* The composition of food groups and lists of food exchanges are given in Table 4 of the Appendix, page 768.

the basic food groups become the center about which the meals are planned. Every effort should be made to regard the patient as a "normal" individual who does not require many special foods and who does not deprive other members of the family.

2. Adequacy of the diet for minerals and vitamins is most easily assured if one includes the minimum amounts of the Four Food Groups (see p. 178).

3. The foods selected must satisfy the demands of the normal appetite. Most diabetic diet prescriptions today are sufficiently liberal that this is not a major problem. However, the lack of satiety value in a diet often leads patients to break their diets. Including some of the protein and fat into each of the meals helps to provide more satisfying meals.

4. The exchange lists of foods (Table 4, p. 768) recommended by the joint committee of the American Dietetic Association, the American Diabetes Association, and the U.S. Public Health Service are used in the majority of hospitals in this country. The use of these lists for dietary calculation permits reasonable dietary constancy from day to day and considerable flexibility in meal planning. See page 362 for further description of these lists.

5. The calculated daily totals for carbohydrate, protein, and fat should be within 2 to 3 gm of the prescribed totals. The meal allowance for carbohydrate can be adjusted to within 7 or 8 gm. It is not advisable to use fractions of any of the exchanges since awkward amounts of food may be involved.

6. The meal distribution of protein and fat should be arranged for maximum flexibility in menu planning. To illustrate, the inclusion of milk at breakfast permits either cereal or bread to be selected from the bread exchanges; meat exchanges are wisely divided among the three meals with somewhat larger amounts being allocated to the dinner.

7. For greatest ease in planning the dietary pattern follow these steps: Include the necessary amounts of milk, vegetables, fruit, and bread so that the carbohydrate total for the day is correct; subtract the protein value of the milk, vegetables, and bread from the day's protein allowance; calculate the number of meat exchanges required to fill the prescribed protein total; subtract the fat value of the milk and meat exchanges from the day's fat allowance; calculate the number of fat exchanges required to fill the prescribed fat total. These steps are illustrated in the calculation on page 467.

8. Patients frequently ask about the use of dietetic foods. They will find water-packed fruits to be useful in meal planning when fresh fruits are unavailable or may be expensive. These fruits are now available in most groceries and are not much more expensive than the usual sweetened canned fruits. Many of these products are now packed with artificial sweeteners added.

Other dietetic foods are not necessary in the diabetic diet of today which

MEAL PATTERN AND SAMPLE MENU

Carbohydrate division: breakfast, 50 gm; luncheon, 50 gm; dinner, 50 gm; bedtime, 30 gm

MEAL PATTERN	EXCHANGES	CARBO-HYDRATE gm	SAMPLE MENU	MEASURE	WEIGHT gm
Breakfast			*Breakfast*		
Fruit, list 3	1	10	Orange	1 small	100
Meat, list 5	1	—	Egg, poached	1	
Bread, list 4	2	30	Whole-wheat toast	1 slice	25
			Wheat flakes	¾ cup	20
Milk, list 1	1	12	Milk	1 cup	240
Fat, list 6	1	—	Butter	1 teaspoon	5
Coffee or tea			Coffee; *no sugar*		
		52			
Luncheon			*Luncheon*		
Meat, list 5	1	—	Cheese sandwich		
Bread, list 4	2	30	Cheese	1 ounce	30
Fat, list 6	2	—	Rye bread	2 slices	50
			Butter	1 teaspoon	5
Vegetable, group A, list 2		—	Sliced tomatoes on lettuce	medium salad	
			French dressing	1 tablespoon	15
Milk, list 1	1	12	Milk	1 cup	240
Fruit, list 3	1	10	Fresh blackberries	1 cup	150
		52			
Dinner			*Dinner*		
Meat, list 5	2	—	Chopped round steak	2 ounces	60
Bread, list 4	2	30	Potato, mashed	½ cup	100
			Roll	1, 2 inch diameter	30
Fat, list 6	1	—	Butter	1 teaspoon	5
Vegetable, group B, list 2	1	7	Parsley carrots	½ cup	100
Fruit, list 3	1	10	Cantaloupe	¼, 6 inch diameter	200
Coffee or tea			Tea with lemon		
		47			
Bedtime			*Bedtime*		
Milk, list 1	1	12	Milk	1 cup	240
Bread, list 4	1	15	Saltines	5	20
Meat, list 5	1	—	Peanut butter	2 tablespoons	30
Fat, list 6	1	—	Butter	1 teaspoon	5
		27			
TOTAL CARBOHYDRATE		178			

follows so closely the selection of foods for the general population. Many of these foods are expensive, they add little by way of palatability, they emphasize that the patient is "different," and their composition is variable. For example, gluten bread is lower in carbohydrate than regular bread, but its protein finally is broken down to provide appreciable quantities of available glucose. Dietetic candies, cookies, and cakes likewise must be evaluated in the dietary pattern if they are used.

9. Patients who find it difficult to adjust to a diabetic diet without sugar may find the artificial sweetening agents to be useful. Saccharin is about 400 times as sweet as sugar, while Sucaryl has about 30 times the sweetening power of cane sugar. Both products are available in pill or liquid form. Individuals usually show marked preference for one or the other.

INSULIN

When the body does not manufacture enough insulin, it must be supplied by injection. Insulin, which has revolutionized the treatment of diabetes, was discovered by Banting and Best of Toronto, Canada, in 1921. It is protein in nature and identification of its chemical structure has established that it contains most of the naturally occurring amino acids. It is now prepared from beef, pork, and sheep pancreas.

Insulin unitage. Insulin is measured in units, 1 unit being the activity of 0.125 mg of the international standard. The assay of insulin is based on the lowering of the blood sugar of a fasting rabbit weighing 2 kg from the normal level to 45 mg per 100 ml. One unit of insulin will oxidize approximately $1\frac{1}{2}$ to 2 gm of glucose, but there is wide variability.

Insulin comes in solutions of various strengths, such as U-40 and U-80 (see Fig. 33-3). This means that 1 ml of U-80 contains twice as many units as 1 ml of U-40. Insulin must be injected since the digestive juices would attack the protein molecule if it were taken by mouth.

Types of insulin. *Unmodified or regular insulin* is infrequently used alone because several injections are necessary each day, but it is the insulin of choice for emergency use. It is also used in conjunction with the more slowly acting insulins in order to effect smoother control of the diabetic.

Protamine zinc insulin, developed by Hagedorn of Denmark, *isophane insulin* (also known as NPH—neutral protamine Hagedorn), and *globin insulin* are relatively insoluble by virtue of the presence of the basic proteins, protamine or globin, and of the zinc salt. Consequently, the insulin is slowly absorbed and the action more nearly approaches that of the insulin normally secreted in the body. *Lente insulin* is a newer insulin which is relatively insoluble, thus being slowly absorbed—the name is derived from the Latin, meaning slowly. It possesses the advantage of containing no foreign protein.

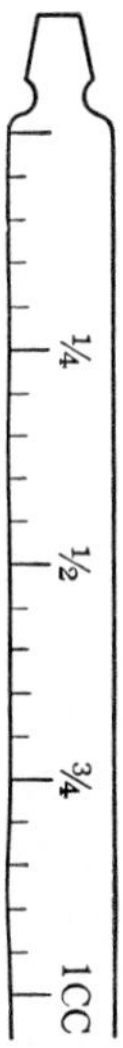

	Units of Insulin			
	U20	U40	U80	U100
	1	2	4	5
	2	4	8	10
	3	6	12	15
	4	8	16	20
¼	5	10	20	25
	6	12	24	30
	7	14	28	35
	8	16	32	40
	9	18	36	45
½	10	20	40	50
	11	22	44	55
	12	24	48	60
	13	26	52	65
	14	28	56	70
¾	15	30	60	75
	16	32	64	80
	17	34	68	85
	18	36	72	90
	19	38	76	95
1CC	20	40	80	100

Fig. 33-3. (*Courtesy, Dr. Russell M. Wilder, The Mayo Clinic, Rochester, Minn.*)

Isophane and lente insulins are most widely used today. The following table describes the activities of the various kinds of insulin.

TIME OF ACTION OF VARIOUS INSULIN PREPARATIONS
AFTER INJECTION *

TYPE OF INSULIN PREPARATION	EFFECTIVE ONSET hr	PEAK hr	DURATION hr
Regular crystalline or amorphous	1–2	3–4	4–6
NPH (neutral protamine Hagedorn)	4–5	12–16	20–24
PZI (protamine zinc insulin)	6–10	16–20	20–30
Globin	2–4	10–16	16–20
Lente (insulin zinc suspension)	4–5	12–16	20–24

* Cohen, A. S.: "Current Concepts in Diabetes Mellitus," *J. Am. Dietet. A.*, **32**:104, 1956.

Oral compounds. Since 1954 a number of drugs known as sulfonylureas have been intensively studied in the United States and in Europe with respect to their effectiveness in controlling blood sugar levels in diabetes. Sobel and Levine [170] have described the current status of tolbutamide (Orinase *). While the mode of action is by no means clearly understood, these clinicians and others suggest that the drug stimulates the islet cells of the pancreas to release insulin and is not a substitute for insulin itself.

* The Upjohn Company, Kalamazoo, Michigan.

On the basis of clinical experience to date, the drug is believed to be most useful for adults whose diabetes has started after maturity and in whom the diabetes is mild but requires more than just dietary control. It may be especially useful for elderly persons who cannot be relied upon to give the insulin to themselves, or who may have visual difficulties in measuring their insulin. Patients who are using tolbutamide require dietary control just as do those who are receiving insulin; the drug must not be substituted for dietary control.

Tolbutamide is not recommended for: (1) juvenile diabetics; (2) adults who have had diabetes a long time and who require large amounts of insulin; (3) patients who go into acidosis easily; (4) patients with severe infections; (5) patients who are being well controlled with insulin, although it may reduce the amount of insulin required; and (6) patients in whom the diabetes can be controlled by weight reduction and diet alone. In the first two categories, it will be recognized that the drug is without effect when there is little or no functioning islet tissue to stimulate.

One must keep in mind the possibility that long-time use of tolbutamide might have toxic effects on the liver, although current studies do not show this; continued stimulation of the pancreas might lead to eventual exhaustion of the insulin supply; patients may exercise less dietary control and may gain weight too easily. Continued investigation of this and similar drugs will be awaited with great interest.

EDUCATION OF THE PATIENT

The ultimate success of the treatment of diabetes is dependent upon the intelligent cooperation of the patient himself. The better informed the patient is with regard to the nature of his disease, its treatment, and possible complications, the greater are the chances that the given patient will enjoy a normal span of life with gainful occupation and enjoyable leisure. The education of the patient requires patience and skill on the part of physician, nurse, and dietitian. Each has a role to play in providing instruction that is adequate but not overwhelming.

The new diabetic who is initially stabilized while in a hospital has an opportunity to learn a great deal about his treatment providing that professional personnel accept responsibility for instruction. Every meal illustrates the use of the exchange lists, and the patient should be guided by the nurse and dietitian to see how each food item fits into his dietary plan.

Dietary instruction. The patient should be taught (1) the reasons for a specified diet, (2) the size of portions which may be used, and (3) the substitutions which are possible on the diet. He must be convinced of the importance of maintenance of normal weight, and that foods should be eaten in the kinds and amounts prescribed.

Standardization of portions in the hospital is exceedingly important and weighing of diabetic diets may be the only way to achieve this. However, it is neither necessary nor desirable for the patient to weigh his food at home. Standard measuring cups and spoons are sufficiently accurate for measuring the diet at home; in time the patient learns to judge the correct size of serving portions.

Nothing favors breaking diet so much as serving the same foods over and over again. Patients need to learn to select the correct foods from the exchange lists so that their menus may be varied. At the beginning of dietary instruction, it is not advisable to select foods which require recipe computation. Later on, they may be able to adapt simple recipes from a cookbook or to use cookbooks written for the diabetic. A number of teaching aids are listed in the references in the Appendix, page 819.

Other factors requiring emphasis. In addition to dietary instruction, the patient needs to be taught (1) the method of insulin administration and the regulation of dosage, (2) the method of testing the urine, (3) the importance of adequate rest, well-regulated exercise, and good hygiene with special emphasis on foot care, and (4) the dangers, symptoms, and necessary procedures for the control of diabetic coma or insulin shock. Diabetics should make every effort to maintain a calm, contented life, learning how to cope with daily stresses without undue emotional strain.

COMPLICATIONS OF DIABETES

Insulin shock. The symptoms of hypoglycemia or insulin shock are caused by an overdose of insulin, a decrease in the available glucose because of delay in eating, omission of food, or loss of food by vomiting and diarrhea, or an increase in exercise without accompanying modification of the insulin dosage.

The patient going into insulin shock becomes uneasy, nervous, weak, and hungry. He is pale, his skin is moist, and he perspires excessively. He may complain of trembling, dizziness, faintness, headache, and double vision. His movements may be uncoordinated. Emotional instability may be indicated by crying, by hilarious behavior, or by belligerency. Occasionally, there may be nausea and vomiting or convulsions. Without treatment stupor follows and death is impending. Laboratory studies show a blood sugar below 70 mg per 100 ml for mild symptoms and below 50 mg for stupor. The second urine specimen is negative for sugar and acetone.

Orange juice or other fruit juices, sugar, candy, sirup, honey, or any readily available carbohydrate may be given. If absorption is normal, recovery follows in a few minutes. If there is stupor, intravenous glucose is necessary. Most patients are now using one or another of the slowly acting insulins, in which case reactions may recur after a few hours. To avoid such subsequent reactions, it is necessary to follow the initial carbohydrate therapy in 1 or 2 hours and at later intervals with foods containing carbohydrate which is slowly absorbed—such as in milk and bread.

The patient must be impressed with the importance of balance between his diet and insulin dosage and the importance of close adherence to the physician's orders. He should always carry some sugar or hard candy to avert symptoms when they are still mild.

Diabetic acidosis and coma. A dreaded complication in diabetes is the state of coma which is brought about by acidosis. Diabetic coma often originates because the patient consumed additional foods for which his insulin did not provide, or because he failed to take the correct amount of insulin or omitted it entirely. The presence of diabetes is first detected in some persons who were not aware of the disease until coma occurred. Infection is an especially sinister influence since even a mild infection reduces the carbohydrate tolerance and severe acidosis may sometimes occur before the insulin dosage has been appropriately increased. Trauma of any kind, whether an injury or surgery, aggravates the diabetes so that acidosis is more likely.

Some of the signs of diabetic acidosis and coma are similar to those of insulin shock, and a differentiation cannot be made without information concerning the patient prior to the onset of the symptoms, together with blood and urine studies. The patient complains of feeling ill and weak; he may have a headache, anorexia, nausea and vomiting, abdominal pain, and aches and pains elsewhere. His skin is hot, flushed, and dry; his mouth is dry and he is thirsty. An acetone odor on the breath, painful, rapid breathing, and drowsiness are typical signs. Symptoms of shock, unconsciousness, and death follow unless prompt measures are taken. Sugar, acetone, and acetoacetic acid are present in the urine, the blood glucose is elevated to very high levels, and the blood carbon dioxide content is decreased.

When early signs of ketosis are present, small repeated doses of insulin are given together with small carbohydrate feedings. Diabetic coma, however, is a medical emergency best treated in a hospital where close nursing care can be given. The physician directs the therapy which includes large doses of regular insulin with smaller doses repeated as needed every hour or so until the urine sugar is reduced and the blood sugar is lowered to less than 200 mg per 100 ml; saline infusions for the correction of dehydration; gastric lavage if the patient has been vomiting; and alkali therapy for the correction of the severe acidosis.

When the urine sugar decreases and the blood sugar begins to fall, glucose is given by infusion in order to avoid subsequent hypoglycemic reactions. As soon as fluids can be taken orally, the patient is given fruit juices, gruels, ginger ale, tea, and broth. All of these are useful for their fluid content; fruit juice, ginger ale, and gruels provide carbohydrate; broth and gruels contain sodium chloride; and fruit juices, broth, and gruels contribute potassium.

These fluids may be given in amounts of 100 ml, more or less, every hour or so during the first day. By the second day, the patient is usually able to take a soft diet which is calculated to contain 100 to 200 gm carbohydrate, and by the third day he may take the diet which meets his particular requirements.

Diabetes and surgery. The diabetic patient as well as the nondiabetic individual should have a good store of glycogen in order best to withstand surgical procedures. That reserve can be assured only (1) if sufficient foods of high carbohydrate content are given up to 12 hours before operation and (2) if insulin is supplied in great enough amounts to oxidize the carbohydrate. It is advisable to give fluids in abundance. In emergency operations where coma and acidosis impend, it is usually necessary to give parenteral glucose and saline.

Carbohydrate feedings should begin within 3 hours after operation, as a rule. These may be in the form of glucose and saline infusions. When liquids may be taken by mouth, orange juice, ginger ale, and oatmeal water gruel with glucose may be used at first. As soon as full liquids are permitted, the diet may be calculated to meet the protein and fat as well as carbohydrate allowances.

Infection. Any infection intensifies diabetes, because the carbohydrate tolerance is lowered. A mild diabetic may become a severe case, and in untreated diabetes infections may precipitate coma. If a patient who is not taking insulin develops an infection, the physician usually orders insulin, at least temporarily, until the infection subsides. The diet may be changed to a fluid and soft consistency as the situation demands.

Diabetes in pregnancy. The diabetic woman who is pregnant requires an increase in her diet during the last half of pregnancy and corresponding adjustment of insulin dosage. The nutritive requirements are similar to those of the nondiabetic woman who is pregnant. Diabetes increases the hazards of pregnancy because of dangers of glycogen depletion, hypoglycemia, acidosis, and infection. The diabetic mother, as a rule, is not able to produce enough milk for her baby and should not be encouraged to nurse her infant because of the additional strain on her body.

Diabetes in childhood. See Chapter 40, page 555.

PROBLEMS AND REVIEW

1. What is diabetes mellitus?
2. Name the important predisposing factors in diabetes.
3. What are the outstanding symptoms of diabetes? What laboratory tests may aid in diagnosis?
4. How is the metabolism of each of these factors altered in diabetes: total energy metabolism; protein; carbohydrate; fat?
5. On the basis of the modified metabolism in diabetes, what should be the

objectives for treatment? What changes would you make in the diet with respect to each nutrient?

6. List eight points to observe in the planning of the diabetic diet.

7. Compare the types of insulin commonly used for treatment of diabetes.

8. What is meant by U-40? U-80?

9. What are the characteristic symptoms of overdosage of insulin?

10. What treatment is effective for insulin shock?

11. When is tolbutamide desirable in diabetic therapy? When is its use contra-indicated?

12. What features distinguish insulin shock from acidosis?

13. How is acidosis treated?

14. What factors are important for reducing the incidence of acidosis and of insulin shock?

15. What dietary modification would be necessary for each of the following circumstances: for a child of 7 years; for a patient who has hyperthyroidism; for a woman who is 5 months pregnant; for a patient who is to have an operation in 2 days; for a patient who has just had a cholecystectomy?

16. Be able to define or explain each of the following: hypoglycemia; hyperglycemia; glycosuria; renal threshold; glucose tolerance; available glucose of a diet; ketogenic factors in a diet; ketone body; carbohydrate classification of fruits and vegetables; clinical control; chemical control; free diet.

17. *Problem.* Plan a prescription and a diet for a man who works in a factory and who must carry his lunch. He is 69 inches tall and weighs 220 pounds. He is 45 years old.

18. *Problem.* Outline a plan of instruction for a patient such as the one described in Problem 17.

19. *Problem.* Show how 200 gm of carbohydrate might be distributed for the various meals, using each of the following kinds of insulin: regular; protamine zinc; globin; lente; isophane.

20. Give some reasons why sugar is omitted or restricted in most diabetic diets.

CHAPTER 34

Various Metabolic Disorders

Low-purine Diet

Many diseases for which dietary modification is an effective part of treatment are deviations of normal metabolic pathways in the body. They occur because of abnormal production of one or more hormones, a deficiency of an enzyme, or a modification of excretion. Those which are discussed in this chapter fall into one or another of these categories but otherwise bear little, if any, relation to each other.

SPONTANEOUS HYPOGLYCEMIA

Types of hypoglycemia. Spontaneous hypoglycemia is a symptom of disordered carbohydrate metabolism which may be of functional or organic origin. The symptoms are characteristic of those described for insulin shock (see p. 473). The patient becomes weak, nervous, extremely hungry, perspires freely, trembles, and may even lose consciousness. Convulsions occur occasionally.

On the basis of dietary management, Conn [171] has classified hypoglycemias in two groups, namely, (1) stimulative and (2) fasting. Tumors of the islet cells of Langerhans also lead to overproduction of insulin, but surgery rather than dietary management is essential.

FUNCTIONAL HYPERINSULINISM

Nature of hypoglycemia. Functional hyperinsulinism is a stimulative type of hypoglycemia in which there is no known organic lesion. Under the stimulus of carbohydrate the islet cells respond to a greater than normal degree with the following characteristics of the blood sugar: (1) a normal fasting blood sugar; (2) hypoglycemia 2 to 4 hours after meals, especially in the forenoon and late afternoon; (3) no hypoglycemia following fasting or the omission of meals; and (4) a glucose tolerance curve (see p. 577) which shows a

477

normal fasting sugar, initially elevated glucose level after taking the glucose, and a sharp fall to very low sugar levels.

A condition similar to functional hyperinsulinism occurs when nutrients are absorbed at an extremely rapid rate, for example, following gastroenterostomy or gastrectomy. In such situations the food reaches the small intestine much more rapidly than is normal, is very quickly absorbed, and the sudden elevation of the blood sugar serves as an extra stimulus to the islet cells and a subsequent hypoglycemia. See page 405 for description of the dumping syndrome.

Modification of the diet. A diet prescription to meet each patient's needs is calculated according to the following principles.

Carbohydrate. Because the carbohydrate serves as a stimulus to further insulin secretion and is provocative of the hypoglycemic attack, it is usually restricted to levels below 100 gm. Beeuwkes [172] suggests that the initial diet contain 75 gm carbohydrate with further reduction to 50 gm if the patient shows no improvement.

Protein. A high-protein diet, 120 to 140 gm, has been advocated,[173] since there is no appreciable increase in the blood sugar level following high-protein meals even though protein furnishes approximately 50 per cent of its weight in available glucose. This available glucose is released to the blood stream so gradually that there is no stimulation to the islands of Langerhans.

Fat. When the levels of carbohydrate and protein have been established, the remaining calories are obtained from fat. Because the carbohydrate is so severely restricted, the fat level is, of necessity, high.

Planning the diet. The exchange lists (see p. 768) may be used for calculation of the diet prescription. Since carbohydrates are drastically restricted, it becomes apparent that the bread exchanges will usually be omitted. In order to include adequate amounts of fruits and vegetables, milk is limited to 2 or 3 cups; children should receive calcium supplements. Vegetables from the 2A list are calculated to provide 2 gm protein and 3 gm carbohydrate per 100 gm.

In order that absorption from the intestine will be gradual, the daily allowances of protein and fat, as well as carbohydrate, are divided into three approximately equal parts. Midmorning, midafternoon, and bedtime feedings are often desirable, in which case part of the food planned for the preceding meal can be used for the interval feeding. Carbohydrate-containing foods must be carefully measured.

FASTING HYPOGLYCEMIA

In many circumstances hypoglycemia is most marked in the fasting condition (blood sugar levels below 60 mg per 100 ml before breakfast) and becomes more severe if carbohydrate is restricted. This is in contrast to the functional hyperinsulinism described above. Fasting hypoglycemia may occur in adrenal cortical deficiency (Addison's disease), liver disease, hypopituitarism, and other conditions. The appropriate diet in these disturbances is one high in carbohydrate and protein to provide a constant source of available glucose. Between-meal feedings and a late feeding (10 P.M. or thereafter) help to minimize hypoglycemia. These patients should carry some carbohydrate food with them to avert the insulin shock.

ADDISON'S DISEASE

Addison's disease is a comparatively rare condition resulting from an impairment of the functioning of the adrenal cortex. The successful use of hormone therapy has practically eliminated the need for dietary modification of sodium, potassium, and carbohydrate. However, a discussion of the underlying disturbances of metabolism in this disease is useful in understanding the role of the adrenal gland in nutrition.

Symptoms and clinical findings. The disease is characterized by a loss of appetite, particular dislike for fatty foods, extreme weakness, fatigue, occasional hypoglycemia, and a tan to bronze pigmentation of the skin. Gastrointestinal disturbances, such as vomiting and mild to severe diarrhea, lead to dehydration and loss of weight. Hypochlorhydria is almost always present. Cardiovascular manifestations such as syncope, palpitation, and dyspnea are often seen. The blood pressure is low, and secondary anemia is present in varying degree. These patients may experience mild to severe prostration associated with the disturbances in mineral balance.

Metabolism. The electrolyte balance is upset in that sodium chloride is excreted in the urine in excessive quantities while there is a decreased ability to excrete potassium. This imbalance results because of inadequate production of the sodium-retaining hormone by the affected adrenal gland. Concomitant with the sodium loss, water excretion increases and severe dehydration follows. These changes may progress to the point where the abnormally low blood sodium levels and the high potassium levels lead to severe prostration, known as Addisonian crisis. A diet high in potassium, low in sodium, and restricted somewhat in fluid has been used by some as a diagnostic aid in studying these metabolic changes. (See Chap. 41 for additional details.)

The intermediary metabolism of carbohydrate is also affected in Addison's disease. Many patients show a low fasting blood sugar and a flat glucose tolerance curve indicating impaired carbohydrate absorption (see p. 577). On the other hand, in these same patients, carbohydrate may be burned so rapidly that glycogen stores are quickly depleted. Symptoms of hypoglycemia may develop after only 5 to 6 hours of starvation. These patients seem to be unable to convert protein to carbohydrate.

Modification of the diet. Hormone therapy provides effective control of the metabolic disturbances so that the diet is planned for maintenance of optimum nutrition. Because weight loss has frequently occurred, a high-protein (100 gm), high-calorie diet (3000 calories) is usually indicated. Three meals with interval feedings, all of which include both protein and carbohydrate, help to maintain the blood sugar above hypoglycemic levels.

Excessive hormone therapy may lead to retention of sodium and water. While the dosage is being adjusted, it may be necessary to use a diet mildly restricted in sodium (see p. 508). On the other hand, some clinicians increase the intake of sodium chloride somewhat, thereby reducing the requirement for the hormone.

METABOLIC EFFECTS OF ADRENOCORTICAL THERAPY

The adrenocorticotropic hormone of the anterior pituitary gland (ACTH) and the steroids of the adrenal cortex are used for the treatment of a wide variety of diseases such as arthritis, allergies, skin disturbances, adrenal insufficiency, many gastrointestinal diseases, and others. While the various products used may vary somewhat in the degree of their effects on metabolism, it is important to be aware of possible nutritional implications of long-continued use of these hormones.

Water and electrolyte metabolism. Adrenocortical steroids in excess lead to retention of sodium and water and loss of potassium. Some sodium restriction is necessary for many patients. Usually, it is sufficient to avoid salty foods and to use no salt at the table, but a 1000 mg sodium diet may occasionally be required (see p. 508). When the patient is eating well, the amounts of potassium in the diet are liberal. Foods especially high in potassium include broth, fruit juices, fruits, vegetables, whole-grain cereals, and meats.

Protein metabolism. A negative nitrogen balance may result when large doses of cortisone are used. This can be prevented when the diet is sufficiently liberal in carbohydrate to exert maximum protein-sparing effect and when high-protein intakes are emphasized.

Carbohydrate metabolism. Cortisone therapy increases the storage of glycogen by increasing the amount of glycogen formation from protein. There also appears to be an insensitivity to insulin, as indicated by hyperglycemia and glycosuria. In diabetic patients who are also receiving cortisone, additional insulin may be required.

Gastrointestinal system. Hydrochloric acid secretion is increased following adrenocortical steroid therapy, and peptic ulceration may develop. In such a situation, the dietary modification described for peptic ulcer should be used (see Chap. 30).

HYPERTHYROIDISM

Symptoms and clinical findings. Hyperthyroidism is a disturbance in which there is an excessive secretion of the thyroid gland with a consequent increase in the metabolic rate. The disease is also known as exophthalmic goiter, thyrotoxicosis, Graves' disease, or Basedow's disease. The chief symptoms are weight loss sometimes to the point of emaciation, excessive nervousness, prominence of the eyes, and a generally enlarged thyroid gland. The appetite is often increased, weakness may be marked, and signs of cardiac failure may be present.

Metabolism. All of the metabolic processes in the body are accelerated in hyperthyroidism.

Energy. The basal metabolic rate may be increased by as much as 50 per cent, and frequently more. Serum protein-bound iodine values are elevated. Moreover, the patient tends to be restless so that the total energy metabolism is further increased.

Protein. The increased rate of nitrogen metabolism may lead to destruction of tissue proteins. Unless both protein and caloric levels are adequate, loss of weight may be rapid.

Glycogen. When the level of calories is insufficient, the liver store of glycogen is rapidly depleted. This is specially serious just prior to surgery since postoperative shock is more likely.

Minerals. The excretion of calcium and phosphorus is greatly increased in hyperthyroidism. Osteoporosis leading to osteomalacia and fractures has been observed.[174]

Vitamins. The B-complex vitamins are used at an accelerated rate in accordance with the increased energy metabolism. The utilization of vitamin A and ascorbic acid is also speeded up.

Modification of the diet. Antithyroid compounds are now widely used to relieve the symptoms of hyperthyroidism, and in more severe instances to prepare the patient for surgery. These drugs reduce the basal metabolic rate to normal, but a liberal diet is still indicated because patients have usually experienced severe malnutrition prior to therapy.

Until normal nutrition is restored, approximately 4000 to 5500 calories and 100 to 125 gm protein should be allowed (see High-calorie Diet, p. 387). Calcium intakes of 2 to 3 gm daily are desirable together with supplements of vitamin D.[174] The calcium may be provided as calcium salts in addition to the liberal use of milk. The diet itself will include generous allowances of vitamin A, the B complex, and ascorbic acid, but supplements are often prescribed.

HYPOTHYROIDISM

Hypothyroidism, or decreased production of the thyroid hormone, is known as myxedema when severe in the adult, or cretinism when its symptoms become apparent shortly after birth (see p. 102). Myxedema is characterized by a lowered rate of energy metabolism—often 30 to 40 per cent below normal, muscular flabbiness, puffy face, eyelids, and hands, sensitivity to cold, marked fatigue with slight exertion, and a personality change including apathy and dullness. The patient frequently responds to therapy with desiccated thyroid.

Obesity is an occasional problem in patients with hyperthyroidism since they may continue in their earlier patterns of eating even though the energy metabolism has been significantly reduced. In other patients the appetite may be so poor that undernutrition results.

JOINT DISEASES

Many joint diseases are grouped under the common terms "arthritis" and "rheumatism." They are characterized by inflammation of the joints, stiffness, pain, and, in some diseases, by deformities. They may be acute or chronic in nature. Some of them are progressive, but there are frequent spontaneous remissions and exacerbations. Others run a self-limiting course.

Rheumatic fever is a special threat to the child or young adult because inadequate treatment may permanently damage the heart (see p. 392). The metabolic error in gout, sometimes referred to as acute or gouty arthritis, has been identified as an abnormal uric acid utilization and will be discussed later in this chapter. For other forms of chronic joint disease, of which rheumatoid or atrophic arthritis and osteoarthritis or degenerative arthritis are the most common, the etiology is poorly understood.

One would suspect some metabolic aberration in the connective tissue of patients suffering with rheumatoid arthritis or osteoarthritis. Probably few diseases have had more theories offered concerning their cause and treatment. Controlled studies on the effects of high and low levels of protein, fat, carbohydrate, acid-producing foods, ascorbic acid, and vitamin D have failed to provide any basis for explaining the cause or the treatment of patients with these diseases. Many fad diets which have been not only ineffective but also harmful have been unethically promoted for persons looking for some miraculous cure. That nutritional factors are concerned with either the causation or the treatment of the arthritis itself has not yet been established.

The supportive role of diet. While no specific nutrients are implicated in the treatment of arthritis, the over-all care of the patient should include emphasis on the importance of adequate nutrition. When patients are of normal weight and in good nutritional status, the normal or house diet is suitable.

Many patients with rheumatoid arthritis have lost weight and are obviously malnourished. For them, a high-protein, high-calorie diet (see p. 373) is indicated until a normal nutritional status has been achieved. Such a diet will provide the desired liberal levels of minerals and vitamins, although supplements are sometimes also prescribed.

Obesity, a more common problem in osteoarthritis than in rheumatoid arthritis, must be avoided inasmuch as extra weight places additional stress on the weight-bearing joints (see p. 384 for low-calorie diets).

Adrenocortical therapy is widely used for the treatment of these diseases, and as a consequence some restriction of sodium may be needed. See page 480 for discussion of adrenocortical therapy.

In severe forms of arthritis, the amount of exercise may be so reduced that constipation becomes a problem. The diet should be planned to include whole-grain cereals and breads, fresh and cooked fruits and vegetables, and an abundance of liquids to maintain normal elimination (see also Chap. 31).

GOUT

Gout is a hereditary disease occurring especially in males and characterized by a disturbed purine metabolism which leads to the deposition of sodium urate (tophi) in and about the joints. Painful attacks recur from time to time. Overeating and excessive drinking of alcoholic beverages are no longer accepted as etiologic factors. Allergy has been suggested as a predisposing factor, since certain individuals have been found to develop acute attacks of gout upon eating certain foods regardless of their purine content.[175]

Nature and occurrence of uric acid. Cellular material of both plant and animal origin contains *nucleoproteins.* Glandular organs such as liver, pancreas, and kidney are among the richest sources, while meats and the embryo or germ of grains and legumes, together with the growing parts of young plants, also furnish appreciable amounts. During digestion nucleoproteins are first split into proteins and nucleic acid. Further cleavage of nucleic acid leads to several products, one group of which are the purines. The latter in turn are oxidized to uric acid, probably by the liver.

In addition to the uric acid available from the metabolism of nucleic acid, the body can synthesize purines from the simplest carbon and nitrogen compounds such as carbon dioxide, acetic acid, and glycine. Thus any substance from which these materials originate, namely carbohydrate, fat, and protein, gives rise to a considerable production of uric acid. Even in the fasting state there is a constant production of uric acid from cellular breakdown.

The liver and tissues store uric acid and its precursors for variable lengths of time and release them later. As a normal constituent of urine, uric acid represents a part of the daily nitrogenous excretion. Some uric acid is also excreted via the bile into the intestinal tract.

Symptoms and clinical findings in gout. Purine metabolism in gout is disturbed for some reason not clearly understood, with the result that the levels of uric acid in the blood are much larger than in the normal individual. The gouty patient converts a greater proportion of dietary components to uric acid, whereas the normal person would convert the same nitrogenous constituents to urea. Instead of being excreted, the uric acid is deposited as urates in the cartilage, kidneys, and soft tissues.

Gout occurs in both acute and chronic forms, the acute attacks being sometimes referred to as acute arthritis. The chief symptom of acute gout is the inflammation of the joint which occurs suddenly with pain which is frequently severe. The metatarsal, knee, and toe joints are most frequently affected. The joint becomes red and tender, and the swelling increases rapidly. In acute gout the attacks are usually of short duration but recur at varying intervals of time. In chronic gout, deformity is often present, and inflammation of the joints is more or less constant.

Modification of the diet. Drugs such as colchicine are used for the joint pain, while others such as probenecid are given to increase the excretion of uric acid. The effectiveness of drug therapy, together with the realization that uric acid can be formed from simple carbon and nitrogen compounds, has minimized the emphasis on exogenous purine restriction. Some individuals progress equally well without dietary modification when appropriate drug therapy is used. Moreover, drastic dietary restrictions have little possibility of being adhered to over the course of years.

In full recognition of the limitations of dietary effectiveness, it is, nevertheless, pertinent to give consideration to the following principles in considering the individual patient.

Purines. Although drugs are effective in bringing about the elimination of uric acid, many physicians prescribe a diet practically free of purines during an acute attack. This requires a selection of foods from group I of the lists below. During interval treatment, 2 to 3 ounces of fish, poultry, or meat, other than glandular meats, may be permitted three to five times a week.

Coffee and tea contain methylated purines which are oxidized to methyl uric acid. The latter is apparently excreted in the urine and not deposited in the tissues. Hence, the customary omission of coffee and tea on low-purine diets may impose an unnecessary hardship.

Energy. Since obesity has adverse effects on general health as well as on the gout, the overweight individual should gradually lose weight. A 1200- to 1500-calorie diet, rather than more restricted levels, is desirable so that weight loss will not result in too rapid metabolism of fatty tissues.

Protein. Because the nitrogen for the purine nucleus is supplied by protein, the intake of proteins may be restricted to maintenance levels, that is, to 1 gm per kilogram of body weight.[176]

Fat. The incidence of acute attacks of gout seems to increase with increased metabolism of fats.[176,177] Such attacks have been quite generally observed when considerable amounts of adipose tissue were being used during periods of too rapid weight reduction or during inadequate food intake as in acute illness. Gradual weight reduction, as pointed out above, is important. During any illness when food intake is poor, it is essential that high-carbohydrate fluids be given in order that adipose tissue is not excessively metabolized.

A high dietary level of fat could also provoke the attacks, but it is improbable that the amount of fat in a well-balanced diet is great enough to have such an effect. Some physicians limit fat to 60 gm per day.

Carbohydrate. When the appropriate fat and protein levels have been established, the caloric balance is maintained through the use of carbohydrate.

Planning the diet. Foods are classified according to their richness in purine content as shown in the accompanying table. The Low-purine Diet given below meets the specifications for maintenance of nutrition, but it may need to be restricted in calories for some individuals.

PURINE CONTENT OF FOODS PER 100 GRAMS *

GROUP I (0–15 milligrams)	GROUP II (50–150 milligrams)	GROUP III (150 milligrams and over)
Vegetables	Meats	Sweetbreads
Fruits	Poultry *	Anchovies
Milk	Fish	Sardines
Cheese	Sea food	Liver
Eggs	Beans, dry	Kidney
Breads and cereals	Peas, dry	Meat extracts
Fish roe *	Lentils	Gravies *
Caviar *	Spinach	Brains *
Gelatin *	Oatmeal *	
Butter and other fats *		
Nuts *		
Sugar, sweets *		

* Adapted from Turner, D.: *Handbook of Diet Therapy,* 3rd ed. University of Chicago Press, Chicago, 1959, p. 100. Starred items are additions to Turner's list.

LOW-PURINE DIET

General rules:

For a diet essentially free of exogenous purines, use foods only from Group I.
For a low-purine level, allow 3 to 5 small servings of lean meat, poultry, and fish from Group II each week.
If a low-fat regimen is ordered, the butter may be omitted, and skim milk may be substituted for the whole milk.

Include these foods daily:

3 cups milk
2 eggs
1–2 ounces cheese; allow 2 to 3 ounces lean beef, veal, lamb, poultry, or fish 3 to 5 times a week during interval therapy
3–4 servings vegetables including:
    1 medium potato
    1–2 servings green leafy or yellow vegetable
    1 serving other vegetable

2–3 servings fruit including:
    1 serving citrus fruit
    1–2 servings other fruits
1 serving enriched cereal
4–6 slices enriched bread
2 tablespoons butter or fortified margarine

Additional calories are provided as needed by increasing the amount of potato, potato substitutes such as macaroni, rice, noodles, bread, sugars, sweets, fruits, and vegetables.

Nutritive value of basic foods above: Calories, 1850; protein, 68 gm; fat, 80 gm; carbohydrate, 220 gm; calcium, 1400 mg; iron, 11.3 mg; vitamin A, 11,350 I.U.; thiamine, 1.3 mg; riboflavin, 2.3 mg; niacin, 10 mg; ascorbic acid, 145 mg.

Foods to avoid:

All foods high in purines (see Group III, p. 485)
Condiments and excessive seasoning
Alcohol
For low-fat diets:
    Pastries and rich desserts
    Cream and ice cream
    Fried foods
    Eggs not to exceed 2 daily; hard cheese not to exceed 1 ounce. Severe restriction may require the omission of eggs, whole milk, cheese, and butter. Skim milk and cottage cheese must then be used in ample amounts to provide the necessary protein.

MEAL PATTERN	SAMPLE MENU
Breakfast	
Fruit	Half grapefruit
Cereal (except oatmeal) with milk and sugar	Rice Krispies with milk and sugar
Enriched white toast	Buttered toast
Butter—1 teaspoon	
Egg	Scrambled egg
Beverage	Coffee with milk and sugar
Luncheon or supper	
Egg or cheese	Jelly omelet
Potato, macaroni, spaghetti, rice, or noodles	Boiled rice
Vegetable	Broiled tomato
Salad	Half peach with cottage cheese on lettuce

MEAL PATTERN	SAMPLE MENU

Luncheon or supper (*continued*)

Bread with butter	Bread with 1 teaspoon butter
Fruit	
Milk	Milk—1 glass

Dinner

Egg or cheese; small serving meat, if allowed	Cheese soufflé
Potato	Baked potato
Vegetable	Beets
	Green celery strips
Bread with butter	Bread with 1 teaspoon butter
Dessert	Apple snow
Milk	Milk—1 glass

Bedtime

| Milk—1 glass | Milk—1 glass |

PROBLEMS AND REVIEW

1. Differentiate between the hypoglycemia in functional hyperinsulinism, Addison's disease, and liver diseases. What modification of carbohydrate level of the diet is required for each?

2. What is the advantage of a high-protein and high-fat intake in hyperinsulinism?

3. *Problem.* Calculate a diet for a patient with functional hyperinsulinism who requires 2400 calories, 130 gm protein, and 75 gm carbohydrate. Use the exchange lists for the calculation. Divide the day's allowance into three equal meals.

4. What modifications of mineral and water metabolism are present in Addison's disease? In what way is this corrected by hormone therapy?

5. Why is a sodium-restricted diet occasionally ordered for a patient receiving hormone therapy in Addison's disease? Under what circumstances would an increase in sodium intake be used?

6. On the basis of your understanding of the metabolism in Addison's disease, what are some of the functions of the adrenal gland in the normal individual? What is the effect of the activity of the pituitary?

7. What are the characteristic symptoms of hyperthyroidism?

8. Compare the diet which might be used in a hyperthyroid patient who is well controlled with antithyroid drugs, and one who has an elevated metabolic rate.

9. Suggest five ways in which the calories of a diet for a patient with hyperthyroidism might be increased.

10. Why does a surgeon so frequently insist that a patient gain weight before an operation on the thyroid?

11. What is myxedema? What is its chief cause? How can you explain the frequent occurrence of overweight?

12. Diet is neither causative nor curative in arthritis. On this basis, outline briefly the principles of dietary consideration in arthritis.

13. What are the dietary implications of long-term use of cortisone in arthritis or other diseases?

14. What are the sources of uric acid to the body? In what ways is uric acid metabolism disturbed in gout?

15. How can you explain the fact that a person who has gout may have an acute attack following surgery or during an acute infection?

16. What is the basis for restricting the protein intake to 1 gm per kilogram in the dietary planning for a patient with gout?

17. What problems are entailed when a purine-free diet is ordered for a patient, insofar as nutritional adequacy is concerned?

18. *Problem.* Plan a menu for 1 day for a low-purine diet.

CHAPTER 35

Diet in Nervous Disturbances

Ketogenic Diet

Nutrition and the functioning of the nervous system. The response of man to his food under varying circumstances has been discussed in Chapter 15. But it is also likely that food, or its lack, could have an effect on the behavior of man. Commonly understood is the irritability experienced when one is hungry. It is also a well-accepted fact that poorly fed individuals are poor workers.

Carbohydrate is the chief, if not the only, nutrient oxidized by the brain for energy; and when any factor interferes with its normal utilization functional disorders will occur. When deficiency is prolonged, structural changes may take place in the peripheral nerves, the spinal cord, or the brain. If these changes are sufficiently extensive, they may become irreversible. Since certain B-complex vitamins are specially associated with carbohydrate metabolism, it is not surprising that deficiency of these vitamins may have an adverse effect on the nervous system.

The polyneuritis of beriberi or associated with chronic alcoholism and the therapeutic effects of thiamine supplementation are well known. Brozek [178] studied the effect of thiamine deprivation of 10 healthy young men who had diets restricted in thiamine for 168 days, and who then received no thiamine whatsoever for an additional 15 to 27 days. The period of acute deprivation led to severe nausea, general weakness, elevated blood pyruvic acid levels, incoordination of the legs, paresthesias, and muscle tenderness. The subjects complained increasingly of such symptoms as inability to concentrate, loss of appetite, muscle and joint pains, irritability, lack of a sense of well-being, and many others. The steadiness of the hand, the coordination of eye-hand movements, and the speed of motion were adversely affected. The psychoneurotic scales—hypochondriasis, depression, and hysteria—indicated deterioration of personality. Thiamine supplementation provided consistent improvement.

The studies of Jolliffe [179] and Williams [180] showed the regular occurrence of symptoms when thiamine-depleted diets were fed to human beings. Such depleted individuals failed to perform their usual tasks, were suspicious, and fearful. They had numerous complaints concerning gastrointestinal disturbances, increased sensitivity to pain, shortness of breath, palpitation, and burning of the feet. When thiamine was administered without the subject's knowledge of any change in routine, the symptoms quickly and dramatically disappeared. It would be quite incorrect to try to explain all neurasthenic complaints of patients on a nutritional basis, but, unquestionably, deficient food intake or utilization does play a role.

The use of niacin in the treatment of the psychotic pellagrin represents an outstanding advance in neuropsychiatry as well as in nutrition. Some years ago convulsions were observed in infants whose formulas were deprived of vitamin B_6.[62] Tuberculous patients treated with isoniazid, which is antagonistic to the action of vitamin B_6, experience a polyneuritis which can be prevented by including vitamin B_6 supplements. Although no pantothenic acid deficiency has been observed in man with customary food intakes, the experimental production of deficiency of this vitamin in man resulted in apathy, numbness and tingling of the extremities, dizziness, irritability, and sullenness. The neurologic manifestations resulting from lack of vitamin B_{12} as in pernicious anemia (Chap. 38) are well known.

Mental retardation is characteristic of certain metabolic disorders. For example, a deficiency of iodine sufficient to produce severe hypothyroidism in children results in such retardation and apathy. Two inborn errors of metabolism which become apparent shortly after birth lead to severe mental retardation if dietary treatment is not promptly instituted. One of these, phenylketonuria, is a failure to utilize the amino acid phenylalanine, while the other, galactosemia, results from the inability to utilize galactose. These conditions are discussed more fully in Chapter 40.

Diet for the mentally ill. Diet is an important part of the total program of rehabilitation for the psychiatric patient. Aside from its nutritional necessity, food provides basic security and pleasurable satisfaction. It helps the patient to feel that someone is concerned about his welfare and cares for him. Eating meals with others helps the withdrawn patient toward the goal of resocialization.

To plan a nutritionally adequate diet is obviously not enough. The service of food which is attractive to the eye, tempting of odor, and satisfying to the palate is just as important in the psychiatric hospital as in any other feeding situation. The mentally ill may express marked irritability when given foods which they dislike. Food service in a cafeteria permits the patient to exercise some choice in his food selection, and thus helps to eliminate some of the irritations.

Patients react favorably and are less destructive when an attractive dining environment is provided. A well-planned dining room with a cheerful color scheme, curtains or draperies at the windows, small attractive tables, and suitable background music is conducive to food acceptance and contributes to the therapy of the patient. Attention to birthdays, holidays, and other special events provides additional evidence that the patient is cared for.

Psychiatric patients frequently eat inadequate or excessive amounts of food. A regular schedule of weighing of patients—about once a month—will help to detect such changes, and correction can be started before marked weight change has occurred. Marked weight gain is not uncommon. It would seem easy to control this in a hospital by providing a diet designed for weight maintenance. However, the privileges of food purchases from a canteen and food gifts from relatives and friends must be taken into consideration. Patients are often known to eat food left by other patients.

Refusal to eat is a problem presented by other psychiatric patients. Hussar [181] recommends that the nurse or attendant should note any patient who refuses more than half of a meal. A 4- or 5-day simple check list helps to identify whether the refusal follows a pattern with respect to a particular food or meal. Refusal of food sometimes denotes an underlying physical illness about which the patient who is withdrawn or mute does not complain. Those who need to gain weight may require close supervision in taking small, frequent feedings; some may be helped if butter is spread on the bread, milk and sugar are put on the cereal, the milk container is opened, the meat is cut, and so on; sincere words of encouragement should be offered when progress is made. Tube feeding (see Chap. 29) may be resorted to when all attempts to achieve satisfactory intake of food fail.

Feeding the mentally retarded presents many problems which may be especially acute in the child. The management of the diet for these patients is discussed in Chapter 40.

EPILEPSY

The nature of epilepsy. Epilepsy is a disease of the central nervous system characterized by loss of consciousness which may last for only a few seconds, as in petit mal attacks, or which may be accompanied by convulsions, as in grand mal attacks. It occurs more frequently in children than in adults.

Treatment. During recent years various drugs (phenobarbital, diphenylhydantoin sodium, and others) have been employed with considerable success in the treatment of epilepsy, and have largely replaced the ketogenic diet, once so widely used.[182,183] As a rule, a normal diet for the individual's age and activity is prescribed when drug therapy is used. Fluid restriction is considered to be effective by some.[183,184]

The ketogenic diet finds occasional use today when a patient shows poor tolerance to drug therapy. When properly administered, approximately one-third of the patients may be expected to show considerable improvement, while another third are benefited to some degree.

Regardless of the drug or diet therapy ordered, it is important that the patient maintain his normal interest and participation in school, work, or other activities. The disease in no way affects the individual's mental ability, but unthinking relatives and friends sometimes attach an entirely unwarranted stigma to the disease, and thus may increase the tension states in the patient.

Modification of the diet. The purpose of the diet is to produce an acidosis by curtailing very severely the amount of available glucose and increasing markedly the intake of fat so that complete combustion of fats cannot take place. The following modifications of the diet are necessary.

Energy. Sufficient calories for normal weight and for the maintenance of normal growth are necessary. An allowance of 16 calories per pound of body weight is usually adequate for adults, while 25 calories per pound of body weight are necessary for children.

Protein. An allowance of ⅔ gm protein per kilogram body weight (0.3 gm per pound) is suitable for the adult, while 1–2 gm per kilogram (0.5–0.9 gm per pound) of body weight is advised for the child.

Carbohydrate and fat. The nonprotein calories are so divided that a ketogenic to antiketogenic ratio of approximately 3 to 1 is maintained. Ketogenic factors (fatty acids) in the diet include 90 per cent of the fat and about 50 per cent of the protein. The antiketogenic factors (available glucose) are derived from 100 per cent of the carbohydrate, plus approximately 50 per cent of the protein and 10 per cent of the fat. Obviously, to achieve a 3 to 1 ratio, the carbohydrate intake must be sharply restricted and the fat intake greatly increased. The level of carbohydrate usually needs to be less than 30 gm if ketosis is to be produced, but should never be less than 10 gm daily.

The diet for a child weighing 100 pounds illustrates the calculation of a diet prescription.

1. Calories: $100 \times 25 = 2500$
2. Protein: 0.5 to 0.9 gm per pound
   $100 \times 0.7 \text{ gm} = 70 \text{ gm}$
3. Calories from protein: $70 \times 4 = 280$
4. Calories from carbohydrate and fat: $2500 - 280 = 2220$

If we allow 30 gm carbohydrate, the fat intake will need to be 233 gm as noted in the following calculation:

5. Calories from carbohydrate: $30 \times 4 = 120$
6. Calories from fat: $2220 - 120 = 2100$
7. Grams of fat: $2100 \div 9 = 233$

The fatty acid to glucose ratio of this diet is as follows:

$$\frac{\text{Fatty acids}}{\text{Available glucose}} = \frac{0.50\,(70) + 0.9\,(233)}{0.50\,(70) + 0.1\,(233) + 1.0\,(30)} = \frac{245}{88} \text{ or about } \frac{3}{1}$$

The maintenance of a constant state of acidosis is evident when the urine shows the presence of acetoacetic acid. The amount of carbohydrate may need to be further decreased, and the fat correspondingly increased to bring about this result.

Minerals and vitamins. It is essential that supplements of calcium, iron, and the water-soluble vitamins be provided.

Fluids. The intake of fluids is usually restricted to 600 ml or less daily at the beginning of treatment, and is kept low for several months according to the condition of the patient.

Management of the diet. It is not advisable to make too sudden a change from the regular diet because nausea and vomiting may result. With adults a period of starvation for 3 to 4 days initiates the acidosis which is subsequently maintained with the ketogenic diet. During this period only 8 ounces of orange juice, tea, broth, and noncaloric bran wafers are given daily.

The starvation regimen is not advisable for children. It has been found practical to place the patient on a diet containing 75 gm of carbohydrate on the first day, reducing this to 50 gm on the second day, and to the diet prescription by the third or fourth day. As the carbohydrate level is reduced, the caloric level is kept constant by correspondingly increasing the fat intake. If nausea develops at any stage during the reduction of carbohydrate, small amounts of orange juice are given, and the diet is not further reduced until nausea has disappeared.

KETOGENIC DIET

Characteristics and general rules:

For best results this diet should be weighed.

Three meals equal in protein, fat, and carbohydrate are given in order to maintain a constant ketosis.

Cream may be used with cocoa shells for a beverage, in ice cream, in custards, or with vegetables.

Saccharin may be used for sweetening.

One ounce of Cheddar cheese may be substituted for 1 ounce of meat.

Vegetables should be restricted to those low in carbohydate (group A).

The fruit exchange list may be used, but selection should be restricted to those fruits providing the most bulk.

Bran wafers with little if any food value add bulk and serve as a vehicle for the butter.

Foods to avoid:

Beverages: all containing sugar

Breads and cereals

Desserts such as cake, cookies, ice cream, pastries, pie, puddings
Milk
Sweets such as candy, sugar, jellies, preserves
Vegetables and fruits high in carbohydrate

Progression of the diet. The diet is one which requires a great deal of fortitude and cooperation on the part of the patient. It is an expensive diet, it lacks bulk, and, because so few foods can be used, it becomes monotonous.

SAMPLE CALCULATION FOR KETOGENIC DIET

	MEASURE	WEIGHT gm	PROTEIN gm	FAT gm	CARBOHYDRATE gm
Breakfast					
Eggs, whole	2	100	12	12	—
Bacon, cooked	3 slices	24	7	12	
Butter	4 teaspoons	19	—	15	—
Cream, whipping	½ cup	120	3	39	4
Fruit	½ exchange	varies	—	—	5
			22	78	9
Luncheon or supper					
Meat, with fat	2½ ounces	75	18	19	—
Vegetable, group A	1 cup	200	4 *	—	6 *
Mayonnaise	1 tablespoon	15	—	12	—
Cream, heavy	½ cup	120	3	39	4
Butter	3 teaspoons	14	—	11	—
Cellu wafers					
			25	81	10
Dinner					
Meat, with fat	2½ ounces	75	18	19	—
Vegetable, group A	½ cup	100	2	—	3
Cream, heavy	½ cup	120	3	39	4
Butter	2 teaspoons	10	—	8	—
Mayonnaise	1 tablespoon	15	—	12	—
Fruit	½ exchange	varies	—	—	5
Cellu wafers					
			23	78	12
TOTAL FOR THE DAY			70	235	31

* The protein value for group A vegetables is estimated to be 2 gm per 100 gm of vegetable, and the carbohydrate 3 gm per 100 gm vegetable.

If no improvement occurs within 6 months, there is nothing to be gained by further continuance of the diet. If improvement does occur, the diet must be continued rather strictly for a year after the seizures are entirely overcome. No change is made in the initial diet until 3 to 4 months after the last seizure. Then a gradual return to the normal diet is accomplished by a monthly increase of 5 gm of carbohydrate, and an increase every third month of 5 gm of protein, reducing the fat in proportion if the child is gaining properly. By the end of a year after the last seizure, the diet will have approached nearly normal proportions.

PROBLEMS AND REVIEW

1. Vitamin deficiencies are known to precipitate certain nervous disturbances. List some of the disorders which may occur and the particular vitamin lack which is primarily responsible.

2. Proper feeding of the mentally ill can be of great psychologic value as well as of nutritional importance. What are some factors which may be kept in mind in feeding such patients?

3. What is meant by a ketogenic diet? What is the relative importance of the ketogenic diet in the treatment of epilepsy?

4. What foods are stressed in the planning of a ketogenic diet? Which ones are restricted or omitted?

5. The ketogenic diet is not nutritionally adequate. What nutrients are especially deficient? How can provision be made for adequacy?

6. *Problem.* Plan a ketogenic diet for a child weighing 65 pounds. Use 15 gm of carbohydrate daily.

7. *Problem.* Outline the instructions you would give to the mother of an epileptic child for careful control of the diet. Include a number of suggestions or recipes for the use of the fat in the diet.

UNIT X /
Diet in Cardiovascular and Renal Disorders

CHAPTER 36

Diet in Diseases of the Cardiovascular System

Modified-fat Diet; Sodium-restricted Diet

In the United States, diseases of the heart and of the blood vessels account for more than half of all deaths in any given year. In addition, millions of persons are more or less restricted in their activities, or even incapacitated, as a result of such illness. While there are many kinds of heart and circulatory disorders, coronary disease, hypertension, and rheumatic disease account for most of the incidence.

The discussion of symptoms and pathologic findings in this chapter is limited to those aspects which require specific dietary consideration. For a complete description of a particular condition the student should consult a textbook of medicine. The physician, nurse, and dietitian are especially concerned with: (1) the possible role of diet in the etiology of diseases of the heart, with particular emphasis at present on the quantity and nature of the fat; (2) the dietary modification necessitated by inadequate functioning or failure of the heart; (3) the use of a sodium-restricted diet when there is fluid and sodium retention, or when blood pressure is elevated. Each of these will be discussed in this chapter.

DIET AND THE INCIDENCE OF ATHEROSCLEROSIS

Atherosclerosis is a disease primarily concerned with the intimal layer of the artery and is characterized by thickening and loss of elasticity of the arterial wall. The atheromatous lesions contain free cholesterol and cholesterol esters, triglycerides, a highly insoluble lipid material not found in the circulating plasma known as *ceroid,* deposits of calcium and iron, red blood cells, and fibrous tissue. The lesions may ulcerate with the result that the clot which forms partially or completely occludes the lumen of the artery; when the coronary artery is affected the outcome may be near-fatal or fatal. Coronary occlusion is by no means attributed only to the ulcerations, however.

Multiple influences in atherosclerosis. No field of medicine or of nutrition is being more widely investigated at present than the relation of diet to the incidence, treatment, or prevention of atherosclerosis and coronary disease. However, many factors undoubtedly are interrelated in the susceptibility of individuals to atherosclerosis, including: (1) age, specially in the fifth and sixth decades; (2) males more frequently affected; (3) obesity as a predisposing element; (4) lack of physical activity; (5) stress; (6) a family susceptibility; (7) endocrine imbalance; (8) long-standing diabetes; (9) long-standing hypertension; (10) deviations in lipid transport and metabolism in the body; (11) abnormal clotting mechanisms; (12) diet, and others. Obviously, to implicate any aspect of diet alone as the culprit is not justified; likewise, to expect universal improvement of all patients by dietary manipulation is unrealistic.

Diet and atherosclerosis. The relation of diet to atherosclerosis and coronary disease may be stated thus:

$$\text{diet} \xrightarrow{\;A\;} \text{abnormal blood lipids} \xrightarrow{\;B\;} \text{atherosclerosis} \xrightarrow{\;C\;} \text{coronary disease}$$

In this scheme it seems well established that certain factors of the diet have been found to increase the concentration of blood lipids (A), especially the β-lipoproteins, while others will decrease them. Cholesterol, an important constituent of the β-lipoproteins, generally increases or decreases in the blood parallel with the lipoproteins; since the blood cholesterol is more readily determined in the laboratory, its concentration is commonly used as a basis for evaluation of progress made under various regimens. Although the hypothesis has not been proven, the present evidence strongly suggests that abnormal lipid patterns lead to atherosclerosis (B), and in turn to coronary disease (C).

Numerous investigations have led to general acceptance of the following statements concerning the effect of the amount and nature of the fat in the diet:

1. Epidemiologic studies show that populations who consume low-fat diets generally have lower blood serum cholesterol levels than those consuming high-fat diets. Some association also exists between the total caloric intake, the animal protein level, and the level of blood cholesterol. There appears to be a strong correlation between high-fat consumption and death rates from coronary heart disease.

2. The blood cholesterol level is lowered, at least temporarily, during weight loss.

3. The blood cholesterol level is lowered when the diet is changed to one very low in total fat—e.g., 25 to 30 gm daily.

4. The blood cholesterol level is lowered when fats containing a high proportion of polyunsaturated fatty acids (especially linoleic acid) are sub-

stituted for the more saturated fats. Conversely, a high intake of fats containing saturated fatty acids results in an increase in the blood cholesterol. A reduction of dietary butterfat, for example, by 1 gm, or an increase of dietary vegetable oils high in linoleic acid by 3 gm, appears to have approximately equal effect in lowering the blood cholesterol.[185]

5. Within the ranges found in normal diets (up to 1 gm daily), the cholesterol level of the diet has little if any effect on the blood cholesterol level.

6. A fatty meal induces hypercoagulability of the blood for some hours.[185] Following major surgery thromboembolic complications are more frequently observed in people who have a high-fat intake.

Modification of the diet. Any dietary regimen intended to bring about reduction of atherosclerosis must be regarded as tentative at the present time. There is insufficient evidence to warrant widespread change in the intake of fat by the general public, but many physicians are now advising a diet in line with the regimen described below for those patients who may have a proneness to coronary disease on the basis of their heredity and the elevated blood cholesterol.

Nutritive adequacy. If Modified-fat Diets are to be effective in lowering

VERY LOW-FAT DIET

FOOD	MEASURE	WEIGHT gm	ENERGY calories	PRO-TEIN gm	CARBO-HYDRATE gm	TOTAL FAT gm	FATTY ACIDS Sat. gm	Oleic gm	Lin-oleic gm
Milk, skim	2 cups	492	180	18	26	tr			
Egg, whole	1	50	80	6	tr	6	2	3	tr
Lean meat, fish, poultry *	4 ounces (cooked)	120	300	33	tr	16	6	7	2
Potato	1 medium	120	90	3	21	tr			
Leafy green or yellow vegetable	½–⅔ cup	100	30	2	6	tr			
Other vegetable	½–⅔ cup	100	40	2	8	tr			
Citrus fruit	1 serving	100	45	1	12	tr			
Other fruit	2 servings	200	120	2	32	tr			
Cereal	1 serving	20 (dry)	75	2	16	tr			
Bread	3 slices	69	180	6	36	3	1	2	tr
Sugar, sweets	1 table-spoon	12	50	0	12	0			
TOTAL			1190	75	167	25	9	12	2

* Values based on average consumption in America, including each week about: 10 ounces beef, 9 ounces pork, 2½ ounces lamb and veal, 1 ounce liver, 1½ ounces fish, 6 ounces poultry. In this diet, only *lean* cuts of each meat selected may be used; all visible fat is removed.

the blood cholesterol, they must be used for an indefinite length of time. Therefore, it is essential that the recommended allowances for protein, minerals, and vitamins be fully met. The Four Food Groups serve as a basis for dietary planning in the calculation of the diet on page 500.

Energy. Sedentary patients may be kept in caloric balance, as a rule, at 2000 calories or less, while a 1200-calorie diet or less is desirable for the obese. See also Low-calorie Diets, Chapter 27.

Fat. The calculation on page 500 indicates the food allowances for a diet containing no more than 25 gm fat. This diet also contains only a small amount of linoleic acid.

The very low-fat diet may be modified for its caloric level and its content of polyunsaturated fatty acids according to the following plan. The calculations are based on the use of corn oil and would be somewhat higher in linoleic acid if safflower oil, for example, were used. An important increase in the level of linoleic acid is not possible when the calories are restricted inasmuch as the addition of each ounce of oil represents approximately 270 calories.

MODIFIED FAT DIETS

Include these foods each day:	1200 calories		2000 calories	
	LOW FAT	ADDED LINOLEIC ACID	LOW FAT	ADDED LINOLEIC ACID
Milk, skim, cups	2	2	2	2
Egg	1	1	1	1
Lean meat, fish, poultry, cooked, ounces	4	4	4	4
Potato, medium	1	1	2	1
Dark green or deep yellow vegetable, cups	½–⅔	½–⅔	½–⅔	½–⅔
Other vegetable, cups	½–⅔	½–⅔	½–⅔	½–⅔
Citrus fruit, servings	1	1	1	1
Other fruit, servings	2	2	2	2
Cereal, servings	1	0	1	1
Bread, slices	3	1	8	3
Sugar, sweets, tablespoons	1	0	4	2
Corn, cottonseed, or soybean oil, tablespoons	0	2	2	6
Nutritive values				
Calories	1190	1195	1980	1990
Protein, gm	75	69	88	75
Carbohydrate, gm	167	115	284	179
Total fat, gm	25	51	58	109
Saturated, gm	9	10	12	15
Oleic acid, gm	12	19	24	36
Linoleic acid, gm	2	16	16	44
Percentage calories from fat	19	39	26	49

Food preparation for low-fat diet. When the diet is drastically restricted in fat, the following measures should be taken:

1. Select only very lean cuts of meat, poultry, and fish. Trim off any visible fat. Cook meats by baking, broiling, or stewing. Meats that are broiled or roasted until well done will have somewhat greater fat loss in the drippings. For greater moisture retention, very lean cuts may be wrapped in metal foil and then roasted.

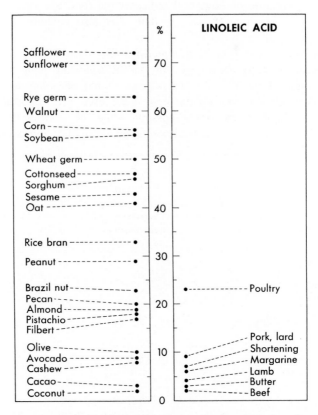

Fig. 36-1. Percentage of linoleic acid in fats and oils of plant and animal origin. (*Courtesy, Dr. Callie M. Coons and the* Journal of the American Dietetic Association.)

2. Eliminate all fat in cooking or baking. No foods may be fried, nor is fat used in the flavoring of vegetables.

3. Use only skim milk. Eliminate butter, cream, ice cream, whole-milk cheeses, margarine.

4. Herbs, spices, lemon juice, vinegar, and tomato sauce may be used for flavor variety in meats and vegetables. See page 709 for suggestions.

5. The egg may be soft cooked, poached, scrambled in a double boiler

with skim milk, or incorporated into skim milk puddings. Egg white may be used as desired.

6. Jelly, jam, marmalade, and honey may be used on bread instead of butter, but the allowance for the caloric level must be watched.

7. Desserts are limited to those low in fat. They may include fruit of all kinds, gelatin plain or with fruit, fruit whips, fruit puddings, puddings made with skim milk and the egg allowance, angel food cake, and meringues.

8. A tomato-juice fat-free dressing is well accepted for vegetable salads and is also useful for marinating meats before they are cooked.

Food preparation with added vegetable oils. Safflower, corn, cottonseed, and soybean oils contain high concentrations of linoleic acid (see Fig. 36-1, and also Table 1, Appendix). These polyunsaturated oils may be used in cookery in place of fats high in saturated fatty acids. The basis for selection of foods is that of the low-fat diet, but measured amounts of oil are used as follows:

1. Oil may be substituted in many recipes for an equivalent amount of solid fat: muffins, griddle cakes, waffles, yeast breads. Special recipes are also available for pie crust, cake, and biscuits made with oil.

2. Meat, fish, poultry, and other foods may be fried in oil. Meat and fish may be brushed with oil before broiling and roasting.

3. Oil may be added to cooked vegetables for flavoring, together with other seasonings.

4. Oil may be blended with skim milk and flavored for a beverage.

5. A number of plastic margarines that contain a high proportion of poly-unsaturated fatty acids and a low proportion of hydrogenated fat are now available on the market. The label should be read carefully for correct inter-pretation.[186]

A meal pattern and sample menu for the 2000-calorie diet with added linoleic acid-rich oils are illustrated below. It should be emphasized that oils in the daily food allowance must be completely consumed in order that the proper ratio of polyunsaturated to saturated fatty acids may be maintained. This means that any oil remaining in pans after foods have been cooked, should be poured over the food before service.

MEAL PATTERN   SAMPLE MENU

(2000 calories, high in polyunsaturated fatty acids)

Breakfast

Citrus fruit or other good source of   Orange and grapefruit slices
  ascorbic acid
Cereal—1 serving   Whole-wheat cooked cereal with brown
Milk, skim—½ cup   sugar, skim milk
Egg—1   Egg, fried in oil (1½ teaspoons)

MEAL PATTERN

SAMPLE MENU

Breakfast (*continued*)

Enriched or whole-grain bread—1 slice
Sugar or sweets—2 teaspoons
Corn, cottonseed, or soybean oil—2 tablespoons

Whole-wheat toast—1 slice with oil spread, 1 tablespoon
Coffee with sugar

Luncheon or supper

Lean meat, fish, poultry, or cottage cheese—2 ounces

Broiled minute steak—2 ounces, brushed with oil
Ripe tomato slices fried in oil

Dark green or yellow vegetable—1 serving
Bread—1 slice

Tossed green salad with French dressing—1 tablespoon
Muffin, made with oil and skim milk
Grape jelly

Milk, skim—1 cup
Fruit—1 serving
Sugar or sweets—2 teaspoons
Corn, cottonseed, or soybean oil—2 tablespoons

Milk, skim—1 cup
Baked apple

Dinner

Lean meat, fish, poultry—2 ounces

Breaded veal cutlet—2 ounces, braised in oil
Cranberry sauce—1 tablespoon

Potato—1

Baked potato with oil spread and chopped chives

Vegetable—1 serving
Bread—1 slice
Milk, skim—½ cup
Fruit—1 serving
Sugar or sweets—2 teaspoons
Corn, cottonseed, or soybean oil—2 tablespoons

Asparagus with pimento, oil
Hard roll with oil spread
Milk, skim—½ cup
Sliced peaches
Tea with lemon, sugar

DIETARY MANAGEMENT OF ACUTE AND CHRONIC DISEASES OF THE HEART

Role of nutrition in cardiac efficiency. The heart muscle is dependent upon an adequate supply of essential amino acids for continuous tissue replacement, of carbohydrate for easily available energy, of mineral elements in balanced concentrations for normal contraction, and of B-complex vitamins for enzyme systems which regulate metabolism. The markedly malnourished peoples of the world frequently manifest cardiac impairment such as dyspnea and palpitation on exertion, enlargement of the heart, and systolic murmurs. Inadequate thiamine has been shown to be especially responsible for these conditions which are common manifestations of beriberi.

Semistarvation diets given to 36 young men in controlled studies at the University of Minnesota [187] resulted in loss of weight, lower metabolic rate, decrease in blood pressure, pulse rate, and heart size. There was a general depression of circulatory function in these previously normal individuals which must not be confused with circulatory failure. When these men were again given normal diets, the blood pressure returned to normal. The increase in body weight and the total daily metabolism placed a temporary strain on the cardiovascular system which resulted in the frequent occurrence of moderate tachycardia and dyspnea.

Similar observations were made in a survey of the population in Leningrad during and following the siege of World War II.[187] During the period of semistarvation the incidence of hypertension and of associated cardiac disease decreased very markedly, but the rate and severity of hypertensive disease increased so alarmingly during recovery as to constitute a major medical problem.

Clinical findings related to dietary management. The diseases of the heart may be functional or organic, and acute or chronic. The parts affected may be (1) the pericardium or outer covering of the organ, (2) the endocardium or membranes lining the heart, and (3) the myocardium or the heart muscle. In addition, the blood vessels within the heart or leaving the heart, or the heart valves may be diseased.

The heart may be only slightly damaged so that nearly normal circulation is maintained; this is a period of "compensation." On the other hand, in severe damage or "decompensation," the heart is no longer able to maintain the normal circulation to supply nutrients and oxygen to the tissues, or to carry away wastes; and prompt, drastic measures are essential to relieve the strain.

Impairment of the heart may be manifested by dyspnea on exertion, weakness, and pain in the chest. In severe failure there is a marked dilatation of the heart with enlargement of the liver. The circulation to the tissues and through the kidney is so impaired that sodium and water are held in the tissue spaces. Edema fluid collects first in the extremities and, with increasing failure, in the abdominal and chest cavities.

Infections, obesity, hypertension, and constipation complicate and make the treatment of diseases of the heart more difficult. Moreover, the heart is located close to several other organs, especially the stomach and intestines, and distention taking place in either of these organs is likely to press against and interfere with the functioning of the heart. Loss of appetite and digestive disorders are common symptoms of heart disease. These in turn may bring about a limitation of food intake resulting in malnutrition to further aggravate a damaged heart.

Modification of the diet. Vital objectives in the dietary management of cardiac patients include (1) maximum rest for the heart, (2) prevention or elimination of edema, (3) maintenance of good nutrition, and (4) acceptability of the program by the patient. The following modifications of the diet are necessary to achieve these goals.

Energy. Loss of weight by the obese leads to considerable reduction in the work of the heart because the imbalance between body mass and strength of the heart muscle is corrected. There are a slowing of the heart rate, a drop in blood pressure, and thereby improved cardiac efficiency. Some physicians recommend a mild degree of weight loss even for the cardiac patient of normal weight. Usually a 1000- to 1200-calorie diet is suitable for an obese patient in bed; rarely is it necessary to reduce calories to a level below this.

Those patients whose weight is at a desirable level are permitted a maintenance level of calories during convalescence and their return to activity. Usually 1600 to 2000 calories will suffice, with slight increases as the activity becomes greater.

Protein. A protein intake of 1 gm per kilogram of body weight or about 60 to 70 gm daily is satisfactory for maintenance of body tissues.

Carbohydrate and fat. The relative proportions of carbohydrate and fat are adjusted according to the caloric level and the nature and amount of fat to be included. See discussion on page 501.

Minerals. Normal allowances of all mineral elements, except possibly sodium, should be provided. The elimination of salt may reduce the iodine intake below desirable levels in certain parts of the country. Thus, when a sodium-restricted diet is prescribed, the physician may also advise a source of iodine other than salt, especially for children and for pregnant women.

Vitamins. The allowances for vitamins are those of the normal individual. However, the omission of carrots and some deep green vegetables that are high in sodium could reduce the vitamin-A intake to undesirable levels. Likewise, a modified-fat diet in which no butter, whole milk, and margarine are permitted would also be low in vitamin A. The inclusion of a small serving of liver weekly, or a vitamin-A supplement, would correct this lack.

Sodium. The prophylactic and therapeutic value of sodium restriction in congestive heart failure is generally accepted. The degree of restriction is dependent upon the severity of the illness in the individual patient. Many patients improve satisfactorily when the daily sodium intake is kept to 500 mg, others require further restriction, and some may be allowed somewhat more sodium. Those who have associated renal disease are unable to retain sodium in a normal fashion and do not require as severe restriction; in fact, too little sodium in the diet of such patients may lead rapidly to the sodium-deficiency syndrome. Once edema has disappeared most patients may be permitted an intake of sodium ranging between 1000 to 1500 mg.

Fluid. The formation of edema fluid can be prevented when the sodium intake is carefully limited, since the mechanisms which usually regulate the sodium concentration in extracellular fluid do not permit the retention of water without sodium. Therefore, when sodium is not available for such fluid formation, water will be excreted by the kidney.

Newburgh [188] emphasized the fact that patients with a restricted fluid intake experience discomfort and great thirst, and that in case of a damaged kidney there is less ability to excrete wastes so that the latter accumulate in the blood stream. It was found that the consumption of 2 liters of fluid daily entailed less work for the kidney than 1 or 3 liters.

Amount of food. Small amounts of food given at frequent intervals are preferable, since bulky, large meals may result in an excessive strain on the heart during digestion. Part of the food normally allowed at mealtime may be saved for between-meal feedings.

Consistency. When decompensation occurs, it is especially important that soft, bland, easily digested foods which require little chewing be used. During this stage the patient must not even be permitted to feed himself. When the patient's condition improves, he may be given foods which are not strained but which are easy to chew and to digest.

Choice of food. Constipation, which must be avoided, can be relieved through judicious use of fruits and vegetables. The choice of foods must be restricted to those which are nondistending. Vegetables of the cabbage family, onions, turnips, legumes, and melons are generally contraindicated although there is much variation in individual tolerance.

Progression of the diet. During severe decompensation, as in coronary occlusion, rest is the primary consideration, and all attempts to feed the patient are avoided for the first few days. Then small feedings of bland, easily digested foods are given as tolerated. At this stage, sodium is restricted to 500 mg or less daily. The foods may be selected from those permitted for the Soft Diet, page 341, giving only small amounts at each of six feedings. Initially, the foods may be puréed to eliminate the need for chewing.

The *Karell* diet has been a widely used regimen of undernutrition during the initial stages of treatment. It consists of only 800 ml of milk daily in four feedings of 200 ml each given at 4-hour intervals. This amount of milk provides 32 gm protein, 680 calories, and 480 mg sodium. After 3 or 4 days this routine is liberalized to include toast, eggs, cream soups, and fruit. A diet of regular consistency is allowed only when the patient is able to feed himself and can chew without too much strain on the heart.

SODIUM-RESTRICTED DIETS

Levels of sodium restriction. Sodium-restricted diets are used for the prevention, control, and elimination of edema in many pathologic conditions, and occasionally for the alleviation of hypertension. Since sodium is the ion of importance, it is incorrect to designate a diet as salt-free, salt-poor, or low-salt. Moreover, to call a diet low-sodium or sodium-restricted is misleading, since any amount of sodium below the normal sodium intake would satisfy such a description, but would not necessarily be at therapeutic levels. Sodium-restricted diets should be prescribed in terms of milligrams of sodium; e.g., 500-mg sodium diet.

The normal diet contains about 3 to 6 gm of sodium daily, although a liberal intake of salty food results in considerably higher sodium levels. The normal diet may be modified for its sodium content as follows:

250-mg sodium diet (very low sodium): cirrhosis of the liver with ascites; occasionally for hypertension; for congestive heart failure when higher levels are ineffective.

500-mg sodium diet (strict sodium restriction): congestive heart failure; occasionally in renal diseases with edema, or in cirrhosis with ascites.

1000-mg sodium diet (moderate sodium restriction): for prevention of edema in cardiac and renal diseases; edema occurring during pregnancy; ACTH therapy.

Mild sodium restriction (variable sodium level—from 2400 to 4500 mg): to prevent recurrence of edema in cardiac and renal diseases.

Sources of sodium. The sodium-restricted diet must be planned with respect to the amount of naturally occurring sodium in foods and the sodium added in food preparation and processing.

Naturally occurring sodium in foods. A table of estimated best sodium values for common foods is given in the Appendix (p. 773). The natural sodium content of animal foods is relatively high and reasonably constant. Thus, meat, poultry, fish, eggs, milk, and cheese are the foods which, while nutritionally essential, must be used in measured amounts. Organ meats contain somewhat more sodium than muscle meats. Shellfish of all kinds are specially high in sodium, but other salt-water fish contain no more sodium than fresh-water fish. A few plant foods, especially greens like spinach, chard, and kale, contain significant amounts of sodium and are omitted in the more severely restricted diets.

Fruits, cereals, and most vegetables are insignificant sources of sodium. In some localities the water may contain appreciable quantities of sodium, either naturally or through the use of water softeners. In such a situation it is necessary to purchase bottled water for the use of the patient.

Sodium added to foods. Table salt is by far the most important source of sodium in the diet. It is used not only in cooking and at the table but it also finds its way into many foods through manufacturing processes: as a preservative for numerous foods such as ham, frozen and dried fish; in the brining of pickles, corned beef, sauerkraut; in koshering of meat; as a rinse to prevent the discoloration of fruit prior to canning; as a means of separating peas for quality before canning.

Baking powder and baking soda are widely used in food preparation. Potassium bicarbonate may be used in place of sodium bicarbonate, and sodium-free baking powder may be purchased or formulated in a drugstore (see p. 707).

Numerous sodium compounds are used in food manufacture, and their presence in foods may nullify the best efforts in restricting salt, baking powder, baking soda. It is, therefore, essential to read labels carefully to note whether compounds such as sodium benzoate, sodium alginate, sodium propionate, sodium acetate, sodium sulfite, monosodium glutamate, sodium citrate, and many others have been used (see Fig. 36-2). Dietetic foods intended for

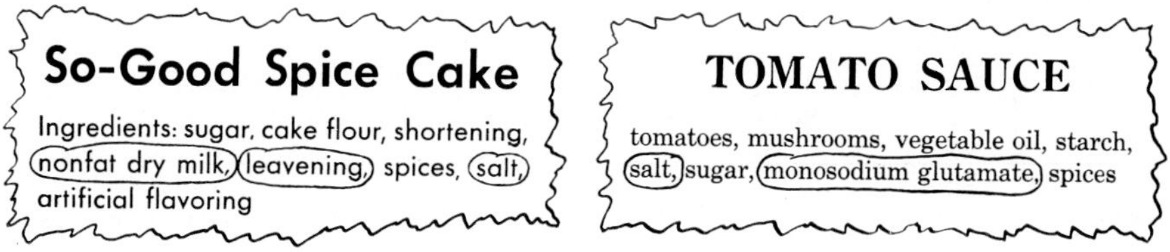

So-Good Spice Cake

Ingredients: sugar, cake flour, shortening, nonfat dry milk, leavening, spices, salt, artificial flavoring

TOMATO SAUCE

tomatoes, mushrooms, vegetable oil, starch, salt, sugar, monosodium glutamate, spices

Fig. 36-2. Watch for the words *salt* and *sodium* on labels when selecting foods for sodium-restricted diets. Leavenings and nonfat dry milk also contribute significant amounts of sodium.

sodium-restricted diets are required to carry a statement indicating the sodium content in an average serving of the food and in 100 gm of the food (see Fig. 36-3).

Incidental sources of sodium. Many drugs contain enough sodium to nullify the effects of the most carefully observed diet. Substitutes should be planned for sodium salicylate, sodium penicillin, and others. The patient needs to be

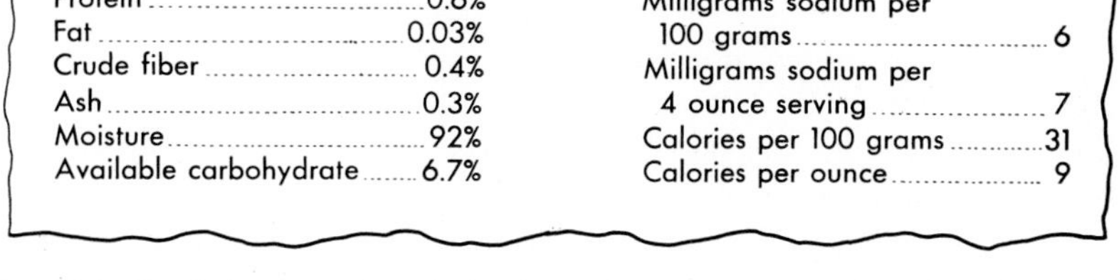

Dietetic Peaches

Packed in water without added sugar

PROXIMATE ANALYSIS
(including liquid in this can)

Protein	0.6%	
Fat	0.03%	
Crude fiber	0.4%	
Ash	0.3%	
Moisture	92%	
Available carbohydrate	6.7%	

Milligrams sodium per 100 grams ... 6
Milligrams sodium per 4 ounce serving ... 7
Calories per 100 grams ... 31
Calories per ounce ... 9

Fig. 36-3. Foods intended for use in therapeutic diets must be labeled with information concerning their nutritive values. The sodium content per 100 gm and per average serving is included.

warned against self-medication with antacids. Some dentrifices contain sodium, and the patient should be warned to rinse the mouth well after their use.

Unit lists for sodium-restricted diets. A joint committee of the American Dietetic Association, the American Heart Association, and the United States Public Health Service has grouped foods for sodium-restricted diets in *Unit Lists*. Each list corresponds closely to the meal exchange lists (Table 4, Appendix), but foods which are not to be used are also listed. It will be noted that the Group C vegetables of the unit lists are those included in the bread exchange lists. In addition, a "Free Choice" list providing 75 calories per unit permits somewhat more flexibility in menu planning.

NUTRITIVE VALUES OF FOOD LISTS FOR PLANNING
SODIUM-RESTRICTED DIETS *

LIST	AMOUNT	ENERGY calories	PROTEIN gm	FAT gm	CARBO-HYDRATE gm	SODIUM mg
1. Milk, whole	1 cup, regular	170	8	10	12	120
	1 cup, low-sodium	170	8	10	12	7
Milk, nonfat	1 cup, regular	85	8	—	12	120
	1 cup, low-sodium	85	8	—	12	7
2. Vegetables						
Group A	½ cup	—	—	—	—	9
Group B	½ cup	35	2	—	7	9
Group C	varies with choice	70	2	—	15	5
3. Fruits	varies with choice	40	—	—	10	2
4. Low-sodium breads, cereals	varies with choice	70	2	—	15	5
5. Meat, poultry, fish, eggs, or cheese	1 ounce meat or equivalent	75	7	5	—	25
6. Fats	1 teaspoon butter or equivalent	45	—	5	—	tr
7. Free choice	varies with choice	75	See list; depends on selection made.			

* Arranged from: *Your 500 Milligram Sodium Diet,* American Heart Association, New York, 1958.

LIST 1. MILK UNITS

Each unit whole milk: sodium, 120 mg (7 mg when low-sodium milk is used); calories, 170; protein, 8 gm; fat, 10 gm; carbohydrate, 12 gm.

Each unit fresh skim or nonfat dry milk: sodium 120 mg (7 mg when low-sodium milk is used); calories, 85; protein, 8 gm; fat, negligible; carbohydrate, 12 gm.

Foods to avoid:

Milk, whole	1 cup	Commercial foods made
Milk, evaporated whole	½ cup	with milk: ice cream,
Milk, nonfat dry	3 to 4 tablespoons	sherbet, milk shakes,
	(Read label for exact	chocolate milk, malted
	amount to make 1 cup)	milk, milk mixes, con-
Milk, fresh skim or non-		densed milk.
fat reconstituted	1 cup	

Note: Nonfat dry or fresh skim milk are equal to whole milk in caloric and fat value when 2 fat units are added to each milk unit.

LIST 2. VEGETABLES

Fresh, frozen, or dietetic canned vegetables only

Group A, each unit: sodium, 9 mg; calories, protein, fat, and carbohydrate, negligible. Each unit is a ½ cup serving.

Foods to avoid:

Asparagus	Escarole	Squash, summer	Canned vegetables or
Broccoli	Green beans	(yellow, zuc-	juices except low-
Brussels sprouts	Lettuce	chini, etc.)	sodium dietetic
Cabbage	Mushrooms	Tomato juice	Beet greens
Cauliflower	Okra	(low-sodium	Celery
Chicory	Peppers, green or	dietetic)	Chard, Swiss
Cucumber	red	Tomatoes	Dandelion greens
Endive	Radishes	Turnip greens	Kale
		Wax beans	Mustard greens
			Sauerkraut
			Spinach

Group B, each unit: sodium, 9 mg; calories, 35; protein, 2 gm; fat, negligible; carbohydrate, 7 gm. Each unit is a ½ cup serving.

Foods to avoid:

Onions	Beets
Peas (fresh or low-sodium dietetic	Carrots
canned)	Frozen peas if processed
Pumpkin	with salt
Rutabaga (yellow turnip)	Canned vegetables except
Squash, winter (acorn, butternut, Hub-	dietetic
bard, etc.)	

Note: Two units of vegetables from Group A may be substituted for one unit from Group B.

LIST 2. VEGETABLES (*continued*)

Group C, each unit: sodium, 5 mg; calories, 70; protein, 2 gm; fat, negligible; carbohydrate, 15 gm.

Foods to avoid:

Beans, dried, Lima or navy	½ cup cooked	Frozen Lima beans if
Beans, Lima, fresh	⅓ cup cooked	processed with salt
Beans, baked (no pork)	¼ cup	Canned vegetables except
Corn	⅓ cup or ½ small ear	dietetic low-sodium
Lentils, dried	½ cup cooked	Potato chips
Parsnips	⅔ cup	
Peas, split green or yellow, or cowpeas	½ cup cooked	
Potato, white	1 small or ½ cup mashed	
Potato, sweet	¼ cup or ½ small	

Note: One unit from the bread list may be substituted for one unit of Group C vegetable.

LIST 3. FRUITS

Unsweetened: fresh, frozen, canned, or dried

Each unit fruit: sodium, 2 mg; calories, 40; protein, negligible; fat, negligible; carbohydrate, 10 gm.

Foods to avoid:

Apple	1 small	Grapefruit	½ small	Crystallized or
Apple juice or apple cider	⅓ cup	Grapefruit juice	½ cup	glazed fruit
Applesauce	½ cup	Grapes	12	Maraschino cherries
Apricots, dried	4 halves	Grape juice	¼ cup	Dried fruit
Apricots, fresh	2 medium	Honeydew		with sodium
Apricot nectar	¼ cup	melon	⅛ medium	sulfite added
Banana	½ small	Mango	½ small	
Blackberries	1 cup	Orange	1 small	
Blueberries	⅔ cup	Orange juice	½ cup	
Cantaloupe	¼ small	Papaya	⅓ medium	
Cherries	10 large	Peach	1 medium	
Cranberries, sweetened	1 tablespoon	Pear	1 small	
Dates	2	Pineapple	2 slices or ½ cup diced	
Fig	1 medium			
Fruit cup or mixed fruit	½ cup	Pineapple juice	⅓ cup	
		Plums	2 medium	

Prunes	2 medium	Strawberries	1 cup
Prune juice	¼ cup	Tangerine	1 large
Raisins	2 tablespoons	Tangerine	
Rhubarb,		juice	½ cup
sweetened	2 tablespoons	Watermelon	1 cup

Note: Use as desired: fresh lemons and limes and their juices; unsweetened cranberries and cranberry juice; unsweetened rhubarb.

LIST 4. BREAD

Low-sodium breads, cereals, and cereal products

Each bread unit: sodium, 5 mg; calories, 70; protein, 2 gm; fat, negligible; carbohydrate, 15 gm.

Foods to avoid:

Breads and rolls (*yeast*) *made without salt*

Bread	1 slice	Yeast bread, rolls, or Melba
Melba toast, unsalted	4 pieces (3½″ x 1½″ x ⅛″)	toast made with salt or from commercial mixes
Roll	1 medium	

Breads (*quick*) *made with sodium-free baking powder or potassium bicarbonate and without salt, or made from low-sodium dietetic mix*

Biscuit	1 medium	Quick breads made with bak-
Corn bread	1 cube (1½″)	ing powder, baking soda,
Griddle cakes	2 three-inch	or salt, or made from com-
Muffin	1 medium	mercial mixes

Cereals, cooked, unsalted

Farina	½ cup cooked	Quick-cooking and enriched
Grits	½ cup cooked	cereals which contain a so-
Oatmeal	½ cup cooked	dium compound. Read the
Rolled wheat	½ cup cooked	label.
Wheat meal	½ cup cooked	

Cereals, dry

Puffed Rice	¾ cup	Dry cereals except as listed
Puffed Wheat	¾ cup	
Shredded Wheat	1 biscuit	

Any for which the label indicates the sodium content is less than 6 mg sodium per 100 gm cereal.

Barley	1½ tablespoons, un-cooked	
Corn meal	2 tablespoons	Self-rising corn meal
Cornstarch	2½ tablespoons	

LIST 4. BREAD (*continued*)

Foods to avoid:

Crackers, low-sodium	5 two-inch squares	Graham crackers or any other except low-sodium dietetic
Flour	2½ tablespoons	
Macaroni	½ cup cooked	
Matzo, plain, unsalted	1 five-inch square	
Noodles	½ cup cooked	
Popcorn, unsalted	1½ cups	Salted popcorn
		Pretzels
Rice, brown or white	½ cup cooked	
Spaghetti	½ cup cooked	
Tapioca	2 tablespoons uncooked	
Waffle, yeast	1 three-inch square	Waffles containing salt, baking powder, baking soda, or egg white

Note: One unit from the vegetable list, Group C, may be substituted for one bread unit.

LIST 5. MEAT

Meat, poultry, fish, eggs, and low-sodium cheese and peanut butter

Each meat unit: sodium, 25 mg; calories, 75; protein, 7 gm; fat, 5 gm; carbohydrate, negligible.

Foods to avoid:

Meat or poultry: fresh, frozen, or canned low-sodium
One ounce cooked is a unit.

Beef	Liver (only once in 2 weeks)	Tongue, fresh	Brains or kidneys
Chicken		Turkey	Canned, salted, or smoked meat: bacon, bologna, chipped or corned beef, frankfurters, ham; kosher meats, luncheon meat, salt pork, sausage, smoked tongue, etc.
Duck	Pork	Veal	
Lamb	Quail		
	Rabbit		

Fish or fish fillets, fresh only
One ounce cooked is one unit.

Bass	Eels	Salmon	Frozen fish fillets
Bluefish	Flounder	Sole	Canned, salted, or smoked fish: anchovies, caviar, salted and dried cod, herring, canned salmon (except dietetic low-sodium), sardines, canned tuna (except dietetic low sodium)
Catfish	Halibut	Trout	
Cod	Rockfish	Tuna	

Salmon, canned low-sodium dietetic   1 ounce

		Foods to avoid:
Tuna, canned low-sodium dietetic	1 ounce	Shellfish: clams, crabs, lobsters, oysters, scallops, shrimp, etc.
Cheese, cottage, unsalted	¼ cup	
Cheese, processed, low-sodium dietetic	1 ounce	Cheese, except low-sodium dietetic
Egg (limit, 1 per day)	1	
Peanut butter, low-sodium dietetic	2 tablespoons	Peanut butter unless low-sodium dietetic

LIST 6. FAT

Each fat unit: negligible sodium; calories, 45; fat, 5 gm.

		Foods to avoid:
Avocado	⅓ of four-inch	
Butter, unsalted	1 teaspoon	Salted butter
Cream, heavy, sweet or sour	1 tablespoon	
Cream, light, sweet or sour	2 tablespoons	
Fat or oil, cooking, unsalted	1 teaspoon	Bacon and bacon fat
		Salt pork
		Olives
French dressing, unsalted	1 tablespoon	Commercial French or other dressing, except low-sodium
Margarine, unsalted	1 teaspoon	Salted margarine
Mayonnaise, unsalted	1 teaspoon	Commercial mayonnaise, except low-sodium
Nuts, unsalted	6 small	Salted nuts

LIST 7. FREE CHOICE

Each free choice unit: 75 calories, and small amount of sodium. Other nutrients depend upon the choice which is made.

Bread list	1 unit
Candy, homemade, salt-free, or special low-sodium	75 calories
Fat list	2 units
Fruit list	2 units
Sugar, white or brown	4 teaspoons
Sirup, honey, jelly, jam, or marmalade	4 teaspoons
Vegetable list, Group C	1 unit

MISCELLANEOUS FOODS

Foods to avoid:

Beverages
Alcoholic with doctor's permission
Cocoa made with milk from diet   Instant cocoa mixes
Coffee, instant   Prepared beverage mixes, including
                                          fruit-flavored powders
Coffee, regular   Fountain beverages
Fruit juices (but count as fruit units)
Lemonade, using sugar from diet, or calcium
  cyclamate, or saccharin
Milk (but count as milk units)   Malted milk and other milk prep-
                                          arations
Postum
Tea

Candy, homemade, salt-free, or special low-   Commercial candies
  sodium

Gelatin, plain, unflavored (use fruit allow- Commercial sweetened gelatin des-
  ance)   serts

Leavening agents
Cream of tartar
Sodium-free baking powder   Regular baking powder
Potassium bicarbonate   Baking soda (sodium bicarbonate)
Yeast

Rennet dessert powder (not tablets)   Rennet tablets
Tapioca (count as bread unit)   Pudding mixes

                                        Molasses

FLAVORING AIDS

Avoid these flavoring aids:

Allspice	Cloves	Bouillon cube, regular
Almond extract	Cocoa (1–2 teaspoons)	Catsup
Anise seed	Cumin	Celery salt, seed, leaves
Basil	Curry	Chili sauce
Bay leaf	Dill	Garlic salt
Bouillon cube (low-sodium)	Fennel	Horse-radish prepared with salt
	Garlic	
Caraway seed	Ginger	Meat extracts, sauces, ten-derizers
Cardamom	Horse-radish (prepared without salt)	
Chives		Monosodium glutamate
Cinnamon	Juniper	Mustard, prepared

Lemon juice or extract
Mace
Maple extract
Marjoram
Mint
Mustard, dry
Nutmeg
Onion, fresh, juice or sliced
Orange extract
Oregano
Paprika
Parsley
Pepper
Peppermint extract
Pimento
Poppy seed
Poultry seasoning
Purslane
Rosemary

Saccharin
Sucaryl (calcium salt only)
Saffron
Sage
Salt substitutes (with physician's approval)
Savory
Sesame seeds
Sorrel
Sugar
Tarragon
Thyme
Turmeric
Vanilla extract
Vinegar
Wine, if allowed by physician
Walnut extract

Olives
Onion salt
Pickles
Relishes
Salt
Soy sauce
Worcestershire sauce

Meal planning with unit lists. The 500-mg sodium diet at three caloric levels is as follows:

500-MILLIGRAM SODIUM DIET

Food List	1200 Calories	1800 Calories	Unrestricted Calories
	units	units	units
Milk	2 (skim)	2 (whole)	2 (whole)
Vegetables, A	1	1	1 or more
B	1	1	1 or more
C	1	1	1 or more
Fruit	4	4	2 or more
Bread	5	7	4 or more
Meat	5	5	5 only
Fat	0	4	as desired
Free choice	1	2	as desired

The 500-mg sodium diet may be adjusted for lower or higher levels of sodium as follows:

250 mg sodium: substitute low-sodium milk for regular milk

1000 mg sodium: substitute 2 slices ordinary salted bread (contains 400 mg sodium) and 2 teaspoons salted butter (contains 100 mg sodium) for 2 slices unsalted bread and 2 teaspoons unsalted butter; *or* use $\frac{1}{4}$ teaspoon salt each day at the table to salt the food.

Mild sodium restriction: use foods lightly salted and allow ordinary salted bread and butter, regular milk. Omit the salting of food at the table; salty foods such as potato chips, salted popcorn and nuts, olives, pickles, relishes, meat sauces, smoked and salted meats.

MEAL PATTERN	SAMPLE MENU
(500 mg sodium, 1800 calories)	

Breakfast

Fruit—1 unit	Baked apple with sugar
Egg—1 only	Soft-cooked egg
Bread—2 units	Puffed Wheat
	Low-sodium toast—1 slice
Butter—1 unit	Butter, unsalted—1 teaspoon
Milk—$\frac{1}{2}$ cup whole	Milk—$\frac{1}{2}$ cup
Coffee or tea	Coffee with sugar (Note: 2 teaspoons
Sugar—4 teaspoons	sugar used in apple)

Luncheon or supper

Meat, fish, or poultry—2 ounces	Broiled fresh flounder
Vegetable, A group	Stewed tomatoes
Bread—3 units	Baked potato—1 small
	Low-sodium muffins—2 medium
Butter, unsalted—1 unit	Butter, unsalted—1 teaspoon
Jelly—2 teaspoons	Grape jelly—2 teaspoons
Milk—1 cup	Milk, whole—1 cup
Fruit—1 unit	Bing cherries

Dinner

Meat, fish, or poultry—2 ounces	Broiled breast of chicken
Vegetable, B group—$\frac{1}{2}$ cup	Fresh green peas
Vegetable, C group—$\frac{1}{2}$ cup	Steamed rice (from bread list)
Bread, unsalted—2 units	Low-sodium rolls—2
Butter, unsalted—2 units	Butter, unsalted—2 teaspoons
Jelly—2 teaspoons	Currant jelly—2 teaspoons
Fruit—2 units	Sliced banana
Milk—$\frac{1}{2}$ cup	Milk—$\frac{1}{2}$ cup
	Tea with lemon

Preparation of food. Ingenuity is required in the preparation of foods for sodium-restricted diets so that they may be accepted by the patient. A number of salt substitutes are available, but they should be used only upon the recommendation of the physician since some of them contain potassium which may be contraindicated when there is renal damage.

Numerous flavoring aids are available (see p. 516 for list) to provide taste appeal. Herbs and spices are especially useful, but they should be used with a light touch. Suggestions for suitable combinations are provided on page 709.

Delicious yeast breads, muffins, waffles, and doughnuts may be prepared using part of the milk and egg allowance of the diet. Low-sodium baking powder must be substituted for regular baking powder. Low-sodium milk is prepared by passing milk through an ion exchange resin in the cold. The sodium is replaced by an equivalent amount of potassium, and the resultant milk is similar in flavor to whole milk. The calcium value of low-sodium milk is about 80 per cent of that of whole milk, the thiamine content is about half as great, and the potassium level is almost twice as high. In other nutrients low-sodium milk compares favorably with whole milk.[189] When diets are restricted to low-sodium milk, recipes requiring milk may be prepared successfully by substituting low-sodium milk.

Dangers of sodium restriction. Diets that are very low in sodium must be used with caution since there is occasional danger of depletion of body sodium. Hot weather may bring about great losses of sodium through the skin, while vomiting, diarrhea, surgery, renal damage, or the use of mercurial diuretics also increases the amounts of sodium lost from the body. Sodium depletion is characterized by weakness, abdominal cramps, lethargy, oliguria, azotemia, and disturbances in the acid-base balance. Patients must be instructed to recognize the symptoms of danger and to consult a physician immediately when they occur.

Instruction to patients. Some instruction should be provided to the patient when the sodium-restricted diet is first prescribed so that he may understand the reasons for the diet. Far too many patients have assumed that the salt was omitted in the hospital cookery and have eaten forbidden foods brought in by well-meaning but uninformed relatives and friends. When a sodium-restricted diet is to be continued in the home, the patient should be instructed concerning the foods that are permitted on his diet, what foods are too high in sodium to be allowed, where he may purchase low-sodium bread and rolls, and how to prepare palatable foods with flavoring aids. The booklets for patient instruction of the American Heart Association are valuable in guiding the patient. They provide most of the answers to questions that patients may raise, but like any educational material these booklets will be most helpful when the dietitian or nurse explains the essential features of the diet.

HYPERTENSION

Hypertension, or elevation of the blood pressure above normal, is a symptom which accompanies many cardiovascular and renal diseases. It may occur at any age but is found most frequently in people over 40 years of age. Hypertension may be caused temporarily by emotional disturbances or by excessive smoking. Certain kidney disturbances or tumor of the adrenal are responsible for a small proportion of the instances of hypertension. However, about 85 to 90 per cent of patients belong to the group known as essential hypertension, for which the cause is unknown.

Symptoms and clinical findings. Many persons with hypertension have no symptoms, and the condition is discovered in the course of a routine physical examination as for life insurance. Among the symptoms which are frequently observed when the blood pressure is rising are headache, dizziness, impaired vision, failing memory, shortness of breath, pain over the heart, and gastro-intestinal disturbances such as gastritis and diarrhea. The extent of the symptoms depends on the height of the pressure and on the length of time it has been present.

Modification of the diet. The discovery of antihypertensive drugs has increased the interest in low-sodium regimens for the treatment of hypertension. When a low-sodium regimen is ordered, it must be strictly observed for at least 4 to 6 weeks before noticeable improvement may be seen. A diet containing not more than 200 to 250 mg is prescribed (see p. 507). The rice-fruit diet successfully used by Kempner [190] some years ago is probably efficacious because of its low-sodium content rather than its low-protein level. The characteristics of this diet are:

1. Allow 200 to 300 gm dry rice daily. Boil or steam rice without the addition of salt, milk, or fat. The rice may be cooked in plain water or in combination with fruits and fruit juices. The rice will provide 700 to 1050 calories.

2. Allow fresh or canned fruits. If substances other than sugar are used for the preservation of fruits, such fruits must not be used. Dates, avocados, and dried fruits are to be avoided.

3. Allow brown or white sugar, honey, molasses, or Karo sirup.

4. Allow about 1000 ml of fruit juices, but no additional water.

5. Prescribe supplements of iron and vitamins.

6. Continue this diet for 6 weeks or longer.

7. This diet provides for each 2000 calories about 15–30 gm protein, 5 gm fat, 460 gm carbohydrate, and 100–150 mg sodium. It is practically free of cholesterol.

PROBLEMS AND REVIEW

1. Explain each of these terms: atherosclerosis; β-lipoproteins; polyunsaturated fatty acid; hydrogenated fat; saturated fat.

2. List at least eight factors which have a bearing on the blood cholesterol level.

3. What relationship exists between the amount and nature of the dietary fat and the blood cholesterol level?

4. Why is it inadvisable at the present time to recommend that all Americans modify the kind and amount of fat they ingest?

5. In what circumstances is a modified-fat diet recommended?

6. What is the effect of a high-fat meal on the blood clotting time?

7. *Problem.* Plan a normal diet for 1 day. Calculate the total fat, the saturated fat, and the linoleic acid content. Revise the diet so that the linoleic acid level is three times as high as the saturated fat. What measures can you suggest for making such a change acceptable to the patient?

8. Examine advertising and labeling for food fats. Evaluate the statements made according to your understanding of the relationship of fat to the change in blood cholesterol level.

9. What reason can you give for a sodium-restricted diet in the treatment of cardiovascular disease? When is a 250-mg diet likely to be recommended? A 500-mg sodium diet? A 1000-mg sodium diet? A mild restriction?

10. For a patient with congestive heart failure, what modifications of diet are required with respect to: (a) caloric level; (b) protein; (c) fluid intake; (d) number of meals; (e) choice of food?

11. In what circumstances is a sodium-restricted diet dangerous?

12. *Problem.* Plan a 500-mg sodium diet for 1 day, restricting calories to 1800. What are some of the problems you are likely to encounter in getting the patient to follow this diet? How would you meet them?

13. How does low-sodium milk compare with regular milk in its nutritive value? When should it be used?

CHAPTER 37

Diet in Diseases of the Kidney

Low-protein Diets; Calcium- and Phosphorus-restricted Diet

Functions of the kidney. The kidneys are highly selective filters and excretory organs the chief function of which is the maintenance of a constant blood composition and volume. The functioning unit of the kidney is the *nephron,* of which there are more than one million in each kidney. Each nephron consists of a *glomerulus,* or tuft of capillaries, surrounded by a capsule and attached to a long winding *tubule* (see Fig. 37-1). The glomeruli behave as filters; the glomerular filtrate is of essentially the same composition as blood except that it contains practically no protein. It has been estimated that the glomeruli of the normal kidney in the adult filter about 125 ml of fluid per minute or about 180 liters in 24 hours. About 99 per cent or more of the fluid entering the tubules is reabsorbed into the blood circulation, thus leaving a urine volume of 1 to 2 liters daily.

Not only is water returned to the circulation, but the tubules also maintain appropriate concentrations of certain essential substances in the blood; thus, all of the glucose, most of the phosphate, amino acids, and sulfate, and some of the sodium chloride, and urea are returned to the blood. For example, it has been estimated that almost ½ pound of glucose and over 3 pounds of sodium chloride must be reabsorbed in 24 hours.[191] The wastes are emptied by means of collecting tubules into the pelvis of the kidney. This fluid waste then enters the bladder by means of the ureters and is finally eliminated from the body as urine.

Urinary solids account for about 5 per cent of the urine, the rest being water which holds them in solution. By means of the antidiuretic hormone secreted by the posterior pituitary gland, the amount of water reabsorbed from the tubules can be controlled. Urea is the chief excretory product of nitrogen metabolism, while much smaller amounts of uric acid and creatinine are excreted. Sodium chloride is the chief inorganic salt of the urine, but other salts are also eliminated.

The kidneys play an important role in helping to maintain the normal pH of body fluids by excreting an acid urine and by synthesizing ammonia whenever necessary. Foreign substances which cannot be utilized by the body are eliminated in part by the kidney. One example of such a foreign substance is hippuric acid, which is synthesized by the liver from the benzoic acid occurring in certain foods.

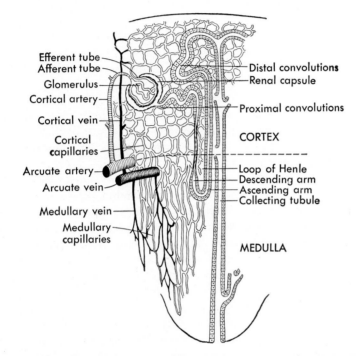

Fig. 37-1. Nephron and its blood supply. Length of tubule approximately 35 to 40 mm, diameter about 0.02 mm; diameter of capsule about 0.2 mm. (Kimber, D. C.; Gray, C. E.; Stackpole, C. E.; and Leavell, L. C.: *Anatomy and Physiology,* 14th ed. The Macmillan Company, New York, 1961.)

Disturbances of kidney function. Nephritis, or Bright's disease, is an inflammation of the kidney, involving the parenchyma and interstitial tissues. If there is serious interference with the functioning of the kidney, waste products accumulate in the blood so that eventual acidosis and uremia occur. Edema may be initiated if the proteins in the circulation and in the tissues have been depleted because of inadequate protein intake or excessive loss in the urine. An accumulation of sodium in the body may likewise result in edema. It may be expected, then, that the diet will be modified with respect to its protein level and its mineral content. The dietary regimens for acute and chronic glomerulonephritis, nephrosis, nephrosclerosis, acute anuria and uremia, and urinary calculi will be discussed in this chapter.

ACUTE GLOMERULONEPHRITIS

Symptoms and clinical findings. Acute glomerulonephritis, also known as hemorrhagic nephritis, is primarily confined to the glomeruli. It occurs mostly in children and young adults as a frequent sequel to streptococcic infections such as scarlet fever, tonsillitis, pneumonia, and respiratory infections. It is usually characterized by a diminished urinary volume (oliguria), hematuria, some albuminuria, slight generalized edema, varying degrees of hypertension, and some nitrogen retention (azotemia). Nausea and vomiting may be especially annoying symptoms.

The acute phase of the illness lasts for several days to a week, but renal function returns to normal much more slowly. Full recovery is the rule, providing treatment is prompt and appropriate. The length of time for recovery may vary from 2 or 3 weeks to several months, as determined by function tests rather than subjective impressions.

Modification of the diet. Diet assumes secondary importance during the acute phase of the illness since nausea and vomiting make it unrealistic to provide an adequate intake. During this period an effort should be made to provide sufficient fluid to maintain water balance, and to provide nonprotein calories to avoid excessive tissue catabolism. Initially, carbohydrate may be provided as fruit juices sweetened with glucose if the patient is able to take them; or it may occasionally be necessary to give glucose intravenously or by tube feeding. As the patient improves, the following dietary modifications are appropriate.

Energy. An adequate intake of carbohydrate and fat reduces the nitrogen metabolism to a minimum and thus reduces the work required of the kidney. Moreover, a reduction in tissue breakdown slows down the release of potassium from the cells into the extracellular fluid.

Protein. Marked restriction of protein—about 0.2 gm per kilogram—is recommended by some clinicians [192] for all patients during the acute phase, while others prescribe such restriction only when the blood nitrogen levels are elevated. During recovery the protein may be increased to 0.5 gm per kilogram for adults and 0.75 gm per kilogram for the child. However, if there is marked albuminuria, the protein intake should be increased by the amount of protein lost in the urine.

Three levels of protein are outlined on page 526. The 20-gm protein diet should be used for only a few days. If the patient does not consume sufficient food to meet his energy needs, the work of the kidney will not be appreciably diminished since excessive tissue breakdown will also result in nitrogenous wastes to be excreted.

The 40-gm and 60-gm levels of protein will maintain nitrogen equilibrium in the adult and may be used for longer periods of time providing that (1) the patient has not been previously malnourished, (2) the caloric intake satisfies energy needs, (3) some complete protein is included at each meal, and (4) there are no protein losses in the urine.

Sodium. When edema and hypertension are present, sodium restriction of 500 to 1000 mg is generally indicated. Danowski [193] recommends some sodium restriction in all patients because of the danger of hypertension, congestive failure, and pulmonary edema. Rigid restriction of sodium may seriously interfere with an already poor appetite.

Fluid. During the oliguric stage, fluids are usually limited to 500 to 700 ml daily; this approximately replaces the fluid losses by insensible perspiration. Larger amounts of fluid are given when there has been vomiting or other gastrointestinal losses, or excessive perspiration.

Management of the diet. When nausea and vomiting have subsided, the patient is given easily digested foods with emphasis on a liberal carbohydrate intake. Between-meal feedings are desirable to provide a continuous source of calories, thus minimizing tissue catabolism.

Sugars, sirups, jelly, and hard candy contribute effectively to the carbohydrate intake without increasing the protein intake, but excessive amounts may be irritating and nauseating to some patients so that the appetite is impaired. Sweetened fruits and fruit juices may be used between meals to provide carbohydrate; fruit ices are especially refreshing while contributing carbohydrate. Breads, cereals, rice, macaroni, spaghetti, noodles, and potato provide liberal levels of carbohydrate; each serving of these foods also contains 2 to 3 gm protein.

Cream and butter usually may be included to advantage.

VERY LOW TO MODERATELY LOW PROTEIN DIETS *

Characteristics and general rules:

Milk, eggs, meat, poultry, and fish are restricted (or omitted) depending upon the desired protein level. When they are allowed, some of these complete protein foods should be included at each meal to provide the most effective mixture of amino acids.

Calcium, riboflavin, and iron levels are below the Recommended Dietary Allowances for the 20-gm and 40-gm protein diets. If the diets are used for more than a few days, supplements should be prescribed.

For a soft diet in the initial stages, select breads, cereals, fruits, and vegetables from the list of foods allowed on page 341.

When sodium restriction is ordered, the food selection should be based on the unit lists in Chapter 36, page 510.

The allowance of sugars and sweets may be used in fruit juices, as carbonated beverages, hard candy, fruit ices, sirups, or jellies.

* Adapted from regimen described by Agnes Wallsten, unpublished research report, Drexel Institute of Technology, 1959.

When fluids are restricted, fruit juices may be used instead of water. However, the meal pattern below may also require some restriction in beverages and other fluids.

Include these foods daily:

	Prescribed Protein Level		
	20 gm	40 gm	60 gm
Milk, cups	0	½	2
Cream, cups	½	½	0
Lean meat, poultry, or fish, ounces	0	1	2½
Eggs	0	1	1
Vegetables, including one raw:			
Potato or substitute, servings	2	2	2
Green leafy or deep yellow, servings	1	1	1
Other vegetable, servings	1–2	1–2	1–2
Fruits, including one citrus:			
Fresh, canned, or frozen, with sugar, servings	3	3	3
Fruit juice, cups	2	1	0
Cereal, enriched or whole-grain, servings	1	1	1
Bread, enriched or whole-grain, slices	3	4	4
Butter or margarine, tablespoons	3	3	3
Sugar, jelly, jam, tablespoons	7	4	4

Nutritive values:

Calories	1990	2025	2020
Protein, gm	20	40	60
Fat, gm	70	85	80
Carbohydrate, gm	320	275	265
Sodium—using regular milk; all foods processed and prepared without added sodium, mg	150	300	500

MEAL PATTERN
(20 gm protein)

SAMPLE MENU

Breakfast

Fruit	Stewed figs
Cereal with cream, sugar	Cooked Ralston with cream and sugar
Enriched or whole-grain toast—1 slice	Enriched toast
Butter—2 teaspoons	Butter
Jelly—1 tablespoon	Grape jelly
Sugar—1 tablespoon	
Beverage	Coffee with cream and sugar

Midmorning

Fruit juice with glucose	Grapefruit juice with glucose

Luncheon or supper

Potato or substitute	Baked macaroni with tomato
Cooked vegetable	Buttered broccoli
Salad with dressing	Tossed green salad; French dressing
Bread with butter	Rye bread with butter
Fruit	Canned apricots
Beverage with sugar	Tea with sugar

Midafternoon

Fruit juice	Grape juice and ginger ale

Dinner

Potato or substitute with butter	Baked potato with butter
Vegetable with butter	Pimento wax beans
Salad with dressing	Grapefruit, apple, and avocado salad
	Fruit salad dressing
Bread with butter—1 slice	Dinner roll with butter
Dessert	Lime ice
Beverage with sugar	Tea or coffee, if desired

Evening nourishment

Fruit juice with glucose	Orange juice with glucose

MEAL PATTERN FOR 40 gm PROTEIN

Follow pattern for 20-gm protein level, with these additions:

Breakfast

Milk—$\frac{1}{2}$ cup

Luncheon

Egg—1
Bread—1 slice

Dinner

Meat—1 ounce

MEAL PATTERN FOR 60 gm PROTEIN

Follow pattern for 20-gm protein level, with these additions:

Breakfast

Milk—1 cup; omit cream

Luncheon

Egg—1
Milk—1 cup
Bread—1 slice

MEAL PATTERN FOR 60gm PROTEIN (*continued*)

Dinner

Lean meat, poultry, fish—2½ ounces

CHRONIC GLOMERULONEPHRITIS

Nephritis may be of short duration, subacute or latent, or chronic as illustrated in the following diagram: *

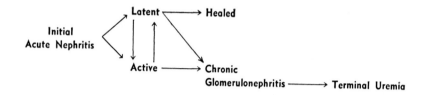

During latent periods, the patient appears to be in good health and is asymptomatic. The nephritis may be detected only by laboratory tests. As the disease progresses, there is gradually increasing involvement: proteinuria, hematuria, hypertension, and vascular changes in the retina. The kidneys are unable to concentrate urine, and there is both frequent urination and nocturia. The nephrotic syndrome characterized by massive edema and severe proteinuria may develop (see p. 530). Malnutrition characterized by a persistent anemia and depletion of plasma proteins is often marked. Eventually the symptoms of renal failure occur (see Uremia, p. 530).

Modification of the diet. Good nutritional management can prolong life and enhance the sense of well-being. The objectives of dietary management are: (1) to maintain the patient in a state of good nutrition to afford better resistance to infection; (2) to control and correct protein deficiency; (3) to prevent edema; (4) to avoid unnecessary harm to the kidneys; and (5) to provide attractive, easily digested meals adjusted to the individual patient's requirements. A rigid dietary program may be so poorly accepted by the patient that the principles upon which the regimen is based cannot be put into practice.

Protein. Many clinicians recommend moderate to severe restriction of protein in chronic nephritis, while others believe that no good purpose is served by limiting protein below normal levels of intake. A number of factors must be considered in determining the protein level for a given patient.

Some breakdown of body tissues continues as long as life exists, but this can be minimized when the carbohydrate and fat intakes are fully adequate. Superimposed upon the wear-and-tear quota of protein, there may be a

* Duncan, G. G.: *Diseases of Metabolism,* 2nd ed. W. B. Saunders Company, Philadelphia, 1947, p. 954.

variable loss of protein in the urine. The end result of too much restriction of dietary protein is an accompanying reduction of tissue and plasma proteins followed by edema and progressive weakness. On the other hand, excessive dietary intake of protein leads to an additional load of nitrogenous constituents to be excreted by the kidney.

During the latent stage, the normal daily allowance of protein—60 to 70 gm for the adult—plus the amount of protein lost in the urine suffices. When nitrogen retention becomes more marked, further restriction of protein to 40 to 50 gm daily is recommended. Patients who are malnourished, edematous, and who lose much protein in the urine may require as much as 80 to 100 gm protein daily to replenish the tissues and correct for urinary losses.

Energy. Sufficient carbohydrate and fat should be provided so that the body's energy needs may be met without the breakdown of body protein. A carbohydrate intake of 300 gm and fat intake of 80 gm would provide 1900 nonprotein calories; this level is sufficient for the sedentary patient. The fats should be chosen from those that occur in highly emulsified form.

Sodium. Levels of sodium ranging between 500 and 1000 mg daily are often used during edema, while the reformation of edema fluid may be prevented with less rigid sodium restriction.

It will be noted that the sodium restriction is usually less severe than that recommended for cardiovascular diseases. The diseased kidney has less ability to reabsorb sodium so that varying amounts of sodium are excreted regardless of the dietary restriction. Thus, too marked a restriction may actually lead to body depletion of sodium with its attendant weakness, nausea, and symptoms of shock. Some patients are "salt wasters," that is, they excrete large amounts of sodium.

Potassium. As kidney damage becomes more severe, the ability to excrete potassium is diminished. Most foods contain considerable amounts of potassium (see Table 6). Salt substitutes should be used with caution if they contain potassium.

Fluid. The inability of the kidney to concentrate urine makes it undesirable to restrict fluids. Usually 1 to 2 liters of liquids will suffice to satisfy thirst. This amount permits the excretion of solid wastes with a minimum of work by the kidney. Additional fluid may be necessary in the presence of a fever, vomiting, or nitrogen retention.

Management of the daily diet. The normal diet, page 338, may serve as the basis during the latent stages of nephritis. If mild sodium restriction is desired, the patient should be instructed concerning the foods which are high in salt content and should avoid use of salt at the table. Cooked foods should be lightly salted.

Diets restricted in protein to 40 gm and 60 gm daily are described on pages 526–27. Frequent small feedings of high-carbohydrate foods should be encouraged so that tissue catabolism may be minimized.

DEGENERATIVE BRIGHT'S DISEASE (NEPHROSIS)

Degenerative Bright's disease is distinguished clinically from glomerulo-nephritis by the consistent absence of hypertension and hematuria and the usual absence of anemia and nitrogen retention. Like glomerulonephritis, it is characterized by proteinuria, but to an even more marked degree. The serum proteins are more seriously depleted than in glomerulonephritis, and this characteristic, which often results in massive edema, presents a primary problem in treatment. There is usually no associated cardiovascular disease.

The primary dietary factor requiring consideration is the replacement of protein, since urinary losses may be very large. A high-protein diet with sodium restriction is suitable.

NEPHROSCLEROSIS (ARTERIOSCLEROTIC BRIGHT'S DISEASE)

Nephrosclerosis, or hardening of the renal arteries, occurs in adults after 35 years of age as a rule, and is associated with arteriosclerosis. The disease may run a benign course for many years. During late stages there is some albuminuria, nitrogen retention, and retinal changes. Death usually results from circulatory failure. In a small number of younger persons nephrosclerosis runs a stormy, rapid course leading to uremia and death. This is called malignant hypertension.

Modification of the diet. Weight reduction of the obese is desirable. A 200-mg sodium diet has been used successfully in some instances. The protein intake may be kept at a normal level until marked nitrogen retention indicates that the kidney is no longer able to eliminate wastes satisfactorily. The diet on page 525 may be used, with or without sodium restriction, when a lower level of protein becomes necessary.

ACUTE ANURIA

Anuria refers to the suppression of renal secretion. It may occur as the result of obstruction of the urinary pathways, following a disturbance of the general circulation with a depression of renal flow, or in terminal nephritis. Acute renal failure may occur in acute glomerulonephritis (see p. 524), following the ingestion or inhalation of poisons (carbon tetrachloride, mercury), or subsequent to extensive burns or severe injuries. The chief metabolic derangements include: (1) elevation of the nitrogenous constituents of the blood (uremia); (2) water and sodium imbalance; and (3) an elevated potassium level (hyperkalemia) unless there are concomitant losses due to vomiting and diarrhea.

Uremia. The symptoms of uremia appear when kidney function has decreased to such an extent that waste products are no longer excreted from the body. The patient may complain of headache, visual disturbances, weakness, nausea, and vomiting. Drowsiness, lethargy, and finally coma take place. Edema, hypertension, and cardiac failure may be present. In addition to the marked retention of nitrogenous constituents, there are usually an accompanying acidosis and water imbalance.

Modification of the diet. Any planned dietary regimen may prove to be disappointing because the patient may have marked anorexia or severe vomiting. Treatment should be directed toward: (1) reducing the production of nitrogenous waste products and avoiding their accumulation in the blood insofar as possible; (2) preventing hyperkalemia; and (3) avoiding sodium and water retention.

Calories. As little as 100 to 200 gm carbohydrate is effective in reducing tissue catabolism and the consequent accumulation of phosphates, sulfates, and potassium in the serum. When both fat and carbohydrate can be used, the daily caloric requirement can be more nearly met.

Protein. During anuria protein is avoided, but when diuresis occurs protein is gradually added. A diet providing 20 gm protein (see p. 526) may be used initially, with progression to the 40-gm and 60-gm levels.

Fluid. Daily fluid losses and the fluid intake must be skillfully balanced. See discussion of water balance, page 162. The fluid losses include those in the urine, from the skin and lungs (600 to 800 ml when there is no sweating), and from vomiting, diarrhea, or drainage. Before the level of fluid intake is recommended, it is necessary to subtract the water made available to the body by the oxidation of foodstuffs—about 400 to 500 ml daily. When there are no severe losses from sweating or from the gastrointestinal tract, the intake of fluid usually should be about 500 to 700 ml.

Potassium. Increased serum potassium levels constitute a threat to life. No potassium should be given in the diet. Moreover, an adequate intake of calories is imperative if tissue breakdown and its consequent addition of potassium to the circulation are to be avoided.

Sodium. Little if any sodium is given except when there are extra losses through sweating or through abnormal gastrointestinal losses.

Management of the daily diet. A protein-free, electrolyte-free diet permits little food choice. Moreover, the patient is likely to be anorexic or may be vomiting. Glucose or lactose (100 to 200 gm daily) may be added to the daily water ration. The patient sips this solution throughout the day. Hard candy may also be eaten.

The butter-sugar diet recommended by Borst,[194] when taken as prescribed, meets the caloric need of the bed patient. It consists of:

¾ cup sugar
¾ cup butter

2 tablespoons flour
2 cups water

Mix flour and sugar. Add water and butter. Cook to consistency of soup. Flavor with vanilla or other extract. Chill before serving.
Serve as six equal feedings.

Another variant of the butter-sugar diet consists of liberal servings of rice with butter and sugar; tea with sugar; and butter balls rolled in sugar and chilled.

Commercial sugar-fat emulsions are frequently used.* These may be taken orally or as a tube feeding.

Diet in the polyuric stage. With the onset of diuresis, the 20-, 40-, and 60-gm protein diets described on page 525 may be used in sequence. The food must be bland and easily digested. Since sodium and fluid losses may be great at this time, dietary restriction of sodium is not necessary. In fact, sodium, potassium, and fluid depletion must be guarded against.

URINARY CALCULI

Urinary calculi (kidney stones) may be found in the kidney, ureter, bladder, or urethra. They consist of an organic matrix with interspersed crystals and may vary in size from fine gravel to large stones. They constitute a symptom of other disorders, rather than a distinct disease entity.

About 90 per cent of all stones contain calcium as the chief cation. More than half of these are mixtures of calcium, ammonium, and magnesium phosphates and carbonates, while oxalate constitutes the anion in the remainder.[195] Uric acid and cystine stones represent about 4 per cent and 1 per cent of the total incidence of calculi.

The formation of stones is more probable in the presence of urinary tract infections, during periods of high urinary excretion of calcium, and in disorders of cystine or uric acid metabolism. High urinary excretion of calcium occurs in hyperparathyroidism, following overdosage with vitamin D, in long periods of immobilization, in osteoporosis, or following excessive ingestion of calcium and of absorbable alkalies as in the Sippy regimen for peptic ulcer. While vitamin-A deficiency has been cited as contributing to the formation of calculi, this is not believed to be an important factor in the United States.

Rationale of treatment. When the cause of urinary calculi is known, the physician can effectively direct treatment toward the correction of the disorder. For example, this might entail the treatment of an infection, or modification of the regimen for peptic ulcer, or avoidance of long immobilization.

---

* Ediol (Schenley Laboratories, Inc., New York, N.Y.); Lipomul^R oral (Upjohn Company, Kalamazoo, Michigan).

However, in a large percentage of urinary calculi, the cause is not known or the disorder is not easily corrected.

The solubility of salts may be increased and the tendency to stone formation minimized by means of acidifying or alkalinizing agents which increase or decrease the pH of the urine. Such treatment implies that the nature of the stones has been determined by laboratory analyses of the stones themselves or by appropriate urine and blood studies.

A liberal fluid intake is essential—3000 ml or more daily—to prevent the production of a urine at a concentration where the salts precipitate out. The patient should be impressed with the importance of fluids throughout the day, so that the urine dilution is maintained.

Binding agents are often used to reduce the absorption of calcium and phosphorus from the gastrointestinal tract.

Modification of the diet. No diet of itself is effective in bringing about solution of stones already formed. However, for the predisposed individual it is thought that diet may be of some value in retarding the growth of stones or preventing their recurrence, although the effectiveness of such prophylaxis has not been fully established.

Calcium and phosphorus restriction. The diet on page 534 is planned to provide maintenance levels of calcium and phosphorus. Such a diet serves as the starting point for the prevention of calcium phosphate stones. Aluminum hydroxide gel is sometimes prescribed since it combines with phosphate to

ACID-PRODUCING, ALKALI-PRODUCING, AND NEUTRAL FOODS

ACID-PRODUCING	ALKALI-PRODUCING	NEUTRAL
Bread, especially whole-wheat	Milk	Butter
Cereals	Fruits	Candy, not chocolate
Cheese	Vegetables	Coffee
Corn		Cornstarch
Crackers	*Especially these:*	Fats, cooking
Cranberries	Almonds	Honey
Eggs	Apricots, dried	Lard
Lentils	Beans, Lima, navy	Salad oils
Macaroni, spaghetti, noodles	Beet greens	Sugar
Meat, fish, poultry	Chard	Tapioca
Pastries	Dandelion greens	Tea
Peanuts	Dates	
Plums	Figs	
Prunes	Molasses	
Rice	Olives	
Walnuts	Peas, dried	
	Parsnips	
	Raisins	
	Spinach	
	Watercress	
	Foods prepared with baking powder or baking soda	

form an insoluble aluminum phosphate and thus diminishes the absorption of phosphorus and the subsequent formation of insoluble precipitates in the urinary tract.[196] Sodium acid phosphate or sodium phytate similarly reduces the absorption of calcium.[195]

Modification of urine pH. When stones are composed of calcium and magnesium phosphates and carbonates, therapy is directed toward maintaining an acid urine. On the other hand, if oxalate and uric acid stones are being formed, the urine should be kept alkaline. Acidifying or alkalinizing agents are more effective than dietary modification, although the diet should support the therapy by medications.

When an acid-ash diet is prescribed, acid-producing foods (see list, p. 533) would be emphasized. Only 1 pint milk, 2 servings fruit, and 2 servings vegetables would be permitted.

On the other hand, for an alkaline-ash diet fruits and vegetables are used liberally, and the acid-producing foods are restricted to the amounts necessary for satisfactory nutrition.

Oxalate restriction. Some oxalate is produced in the body during the metabolism of foodstuffs. Dietary restriction of oxalates may be tried when calculi contain oxalate, but such restriction has not been shown conclusively to be of value. Oxalate-rich foods include: green and wax beans, beets and beet greens, chard, endive, okra, spinach, sweet potatoes; currants, figs, gooseberries, Concord grapes, plums, rhubarb, raspberries; almonds, cashew nuts; chocolate, cocoa, tea.

Reduction of uric acid metabolism. The formation of uric acid stones may be minimized by using a Low-purine Diet (see p. 485) and restricting the protein intake to 1 gm per kilogram body weight.

Cystine stones. A low-protein diet reduces the intake of sulfur-containing amino acids, but has not been shown to be effective in the prevention of cystine stones.

CALCIUM- AND PHOSPHORUS-RESTRICTED DIET *

Characteristics and general rules:

The diet provides maintenance levels of calcium and phosphorus. Milk constitutes the main source of calcium in the diet, and milk, eggs, and meat are the principal sources of phosphorus.

When further restrictions of calcium and phosphorus are desired, the milk and egg may be eliminated. The calcium level is then reduced to 170 mg, the phosphorus level to 740 mg, and the protein level to 64 gm.

* Modification of regimen described by Mary Alice White, unpublished report, Drexel Institute of Technology, 1958.

INCLUDE THESE FOODS DAILY: *		PROTEIN gm	FAT gm	CARBO-HYDRATE gm	Ca mg	P mg
Milk	1½ cups	12	15	18	430	340
Egg	1 whole	7	5	—	25	105
Meat, fish, or poultry	6 ounces	42	30	—	20	375
Vegetables:						
Potato	1 small	2	—	15	15	65
Leafy or yellow	½ cup	2	—	7	25	35
Other	½ cup	2	—	7	25	45
Fruits:						
Citrus	½ cup	—	—	10	30	20
Other	2 servings	—	—	20	25	40
Cereal, refined, without added calcium	2 servings	4	—	30	5	30
Bread, refined, without added calcium	6 slices	12	—	90	20	115
Fats	2 tablespoons	—	30	—	—	—
Sugars, sweets	2 tablespoons	—	—	30	—	—
		83	80	227	620	1170

* Protein, fat, and carbohydrate values on the basis of Meal Exchange Lists, page 768. Calcium and phosphorus values have been rounded off to the nearest 5 mg. Values for vegetables, fruits, cereals, and breads are averages of those permitted. Individual selections vary somewhat from these averages.

Foods allowed:

Beverages: milk in allowed amounts; coffee, tea

Breads: French or Italian without added milk; pretzels; saltines, matzoth; water rolls

Cereals: corn flakes, corn grits, farina, rice, rice flakes, Puffed Rice; macaroni, noodles, spaghetti; corn meal, cornstarch, tapioca, white flour

Cheese: ½ ounce Cheddar or Swiss cheese may be used instead of ½ cup milk

Desserts: angel cake, white sugar cookies, gelatin, fruit pies, fruit tapioca, fruit whip, pudding with allowed milk and egg, shortbread, water ices

Eggs: 1 whole. Whites as desired

Foods to avoid:

Beverages: chocolate; cocoa; fountain beverages; proprietary beverages containing milk powder

Breads: biscuits; breads: brown, corn, cracked wheat, raisin, rye, white with nonfat dry milk, whole-wheat; rye wafers; muffins; pancakes; waffles

Cereals: bran, bran flakes, corn and soy grits, oatmeal, wheat flakes, wheat germ, Puffed Wheat, Shredded Wheat; rye flour, soybean flour, self-rising flour, whole-wheat flour

Desserts: cakes and cake mixes, custard, doughnuts, ice cream, Junket, pies with cream filling or milk and eggs, milk puddings—except when daily allowance is used

Foods allowed:

Fats: butter, cooking oils and fats, lard, margarine, French dressing

Fruits: all, but restricting dried fruits to: dates (3), prunes (2), raisins (1 tbsp)

Meats: beef, ham, lamb, pork, veal; chicken, duck, turkey; bluefish, cod, haddock, halibut, scallops, shad, swordfish, tuna

Milk: 1½ cups daily

Soups: broth of allowed meats; consommé; vegetable; cream soups using allowed milk

Sweets: sugar, sirup, jam, jelly, preserves, hard candy, marshmallows, mints without chocolate

Vegetables: artichokes, asparagus, beans —green or wax, Brussels sprouts, cabbage, carrots, cauliflower, corn, cucumber, eggplant, escarole, lettuce, onions, peppers, potatoes—white and sweet, pumpkin, radishes, romaine, squash, tomatoes, turnips

Miscellaneous: pickles, mustard, salt, spices

Foods to avoid:

Fats: mayonnaise, sweet and sour cream

Meats: clams, crab, herring, lobster, mackerel, oyster, fish roe, salmon, sardines, shrimp; brains, heart, kidney, liver, sweetbreads

Soups: cream in excess of milk allowance; bean, lentil, split pea

Sweets: caramels, fudge, milk chocolate, molasses, dark brown sugar

Vegetables: dry beans—kidney, Lima, navy, pea, soybean; beet greens, broccoli, chard, collards, chickpeas, dandelion greens, kale, okra, parsnips, peas—fresh and dried, rutabagas, soybeans, soybean sprouts, spinach, turnip greens, watercress

Miscellaneous: chocolate, cocoa, nuts, olives, brewers' yeast

MEAL PATTERN

Breakfast

Fruit, preferably citrus
Cereal, refined
Milk—½ cup
Egg—1 only
Bread, Italian or French
Butter or margarine
Jelly
Beverage with sugar, if desired

Luncheon or supper

Meat, poultry, or fish—3 ounces
Potato or substitute
Vegetable
Salad

Bread, Italian or French

SAMPLE MENU

Fresh raspberries
Corn flakes
Milk—½ cup
Soft-cooked egg
Toasted Italian bread
Butter or margarine
Apple jelly
Coffee

Cold sliced turkey
Potato salad (potato, diced cucumber, minced green pepper and onion, French dressing) on lettuce; tomato wedges
Italian bread

MEAL PATTERN	SAMPLE MENU

Luncheon or supper (continued)

Butter or margarine	Butter or margarine
Dessert	Angel cake with fresh strawberries
Milk—1 cup	Milk—1 cup only
Tea or coffee, if desired	

Dinner

Meat, poultry, or fish—3 ounces	Roast pork
Potato or substitute (use potato only once daily)	Buttered noodles
Vegetable	Zucchini squash
Bread or rolls, without added milk	Hard rolls, made without milk
Butter or margarine	Butter or margarine
Fruit or dessert	Fruit gelatin
Coffee or tea	Tea with lemon

PROBLEMS AND REVIEW

1. What are the parts of the nephron? How do these parts function?

2. What are the chief wastes excreted by the kidney?

3. In addition to excreting wastes, what other functions are performed by the kidney?

4. What are the characteristic symptoms of acute glomerulonephritis? In what way do these symptoms affect dietary planning?

5. In what way do the abnormal excretion products in renal diseases affect dietary planning?

6. *Problem.* Outline the principles for a dietary regimen for a patient with acute glomerulonephritis, showing the progression of diet from time to time.

7. *Problem.* On the basis of the principles outlined in Problem 6, write a menu for a patient for 1 day. Assume that the diet order restricts protein to 40 gm and sodium to 1000 mg.

8. What reasons can you give for using a protein-free, high-carbohydrate, high-fat diet in acute renal failure? Why are frequent small feedings preferable to three meals?

9. Prepare a list of foods which are high in calcium; in phosphorus. Why are such foods avoided in the diet of certain patients with urinary calculi?

10. When is an acid-ash diet used? Name six specific foods to emphasize on such a diet.

11. When is an alkaline-ash diet used? Name at least six foods to emphasize on such a diet.

CHAPTER 38 /

Anemias

Blood is a constantly changing, highly complex tissue which is concerned with the transport of cell nutrients, the elimination of wastes, and the maintenance of chemical equilibrium. Its intricate functions and composition suggest the need for a considerable variety of nutrients. This chapter is especially concerned with deficiencies arising in the framework of red blood cells and in the hemoglobin within these cells.

Normal blood regeneration. Hemoglobin is a protein which is composed of an organic iron compound, *heme,* and the protein, *globin,* the latter being a sulfur-bearing protein which makes up 96 per cent of the molecule. The formation of hemoglobin is dependent principally on adequate dietary supplies of iron and of protein. It has been demonstrated that a generous intake of iron results in poor hemoglobin regeneration if the supplies of protein are inadequate. Copper is known to be essential for the utilization of iron in the building of hemoglobin, but dietary deficiency does not occur except when an exclusive milk diet in infancy is used overly long. Chapter 8 should be consulted for a more detailed discussion of iron metabolism.

The framework of the red blood cells is constructed in the bone marrow. The synthesis of nucleoproteins and the subsequent development and maturation of the young blood cells are dependent upon the presence of a number of vitamins, especially vitamin B_{12}, Folacin, and folinic acid. When these vitamins are unavailable, large immature cells are released into the circulation; moreover, the total number produced is reduced. Vitamin B_{12} is identical with the "extrinsic" factor, or the "erythrocyte maturation" factor described in earlier literature. Diets which provide an adequate level of protein contain sufficient amounts of vitamin B_{12} to meet body requirements. The absorption of vitamin B_{12} from the gastrointestinal tract depends upon the presence in gastric juice of an unidentified principle designated by Castle [197] as the "intrinsic" factor. Ascorbic acid appears to be essential for the conversion of Folacin to folinic acid.

Studies on experimental animals lend support to the importance of other vitamins, in addition to those heretofore mentioned, for the building of the cells: riboflavin, vitamin B_6, niacin, and pantothenic acid. It has not been

538

demonstrated that these vitamins have been sufficiently deficient in the diet of human beings to affect adversely the formation of red blood cells. The secretion of the thyroid gland and other hormones appear to be involved in blood regeneration.

The values for hemoglobin and red cells may be affected by age, sex, and geographic location. As a rough approximation, the following may be given as normal blood values:

Red blood cell count	4.5 to 5.0 million per cu mm
Hemoglobin	14 to 15 gm per 100 ml
Packed cell volume	45 per cent

Anemias. This is a condition in which there is a reduction of the number or size of the red blood cells, or of the quantity of hemoglobin, or both. It results in a decreased ability of the blood to carry oxygen to the tissues. This in turn brings about skin pallor, loss of skin tone, weakness, headache, loss of appetite, gastrointestinal disturbances, nervousness, palpitation, and shortness of breath. The various types of anemia are often accompanied by additional symptoms.

Anemias may be caused by blood loss, decreased production of blood, or by increased destruction of blood. Faulty nutrition either occasioned by failure to provide essential nutrients, such as iron and protein, or by poor utilization of dietary constituents (for example, failure to absorb vitamin B_{12}) may lead to anemia, the type being dependent upon the initiating defect. Exposure to x-ray or radium, bone tumors, cirrhosis of the liver, carcinoma, and leukemias are examples of conditions which may interfere with red-cell formation by the bone marrow. Increased destruction of the blood may be the result of the action of intestinal parasites, hemolytic bacteria, chemical agents such as coal-tar products and sulfonamide compounds, or abnormal red cell structure (sickle cells).

The treatment of all anemias must be based, first of all, upon the elimination of the cause, and, secondly, upon the restoration of normal nutrition with respect to blood formation.

IRON-DEFICIENCY ANEMIA

Factors in causation. Iron-deficiency anemia is frequently designated as "hypochromic," which means low color, and "microcytic," which means that the cells are of small size. The chief lack is in the amount of hemoglobin present within the cells. The number of cells may also be reduced, but not as markedly as is the hemoglobin content. This type of anemia is often referred to as "secondary" or "nutritional" anemia, but the term "nutritional" may also be applied to other types of anemia and is thus confusing. While depletion of the iron stores is the chief causative factor, hypochromic anemia may occasionally occur coincident with marked protein deficiency. Hypochromic anemias may be grouped as below, depending upon the factor primarily responsible for initiating the deficiency.

    I. Due to blood loss (most common cause in adults)
        A. Accidental hemorrhage
        B. Chronic diseases, such as tuberculosis, ulcers or intestinal disorders, when accompanied by hemorrhage
        C. Excessive menstrual losses
        D. Excessive blood donation
   II. Deficiency of iron in the diet during period of accelerated demand
        A. Infancy—rapidly expanding blood volume
        B. Adolescent girls—rapid growth and onset of menses
        C. Pregnancy and lactation
  III. Inadequate absorption of iron
        A. Diarrhea, as in sprue, pellagra
        B. Lack of acid secretion by the stomach
  IV. Nutritive deficiencies such as severe protein depletion

Whenever hypochromic anemia occurs in adult males or in women past the menopause, blood loss, as from a bleeding ulcer or other cause, must always be suspected. Menstrual losses by some women may be sufficiently great to result in anemia, especially if the diet is poorly selected. The range of such losses has been found to be 2.28 to 78.96 mg.[198] The repeated donation of blood likewise could be a significant factor in anemia causation unless a liberal diet relatively rich in protein and iron were taken.

Whenever there is a loss of blood, fluid is quickly drawn in from the tissues to maintain the blood volume. The hemoglobin level and red cells are thus reduced in concentration, but the individual with adequate stores quickly replenishes the levels so that anemia is not evident unless hemorrhage is prolonged or repeated.

Anemia during infancy is of frequent occurrence and is closely related to the body store of iron at birth. It occurs especially in premature infants and twins, because the body reserves of iron in such circumstances cannot be built up to desirable levels. In babies whose mothers had a deficient intake of iron, such stores will likewise be low. As the body increases in size, the blood volume also increases, so that the supply of iron will be depleted and anemia will result unless adequate provision is made for the inclusion of foods such as iron-enriched cereals, egg yolk, and strained meats in early infancy. On the other hand, the early inclusion of such foods cannot be expected to prevent an anemia in which body stores were initially low, and iron supplementation thus becomes necessary.

Improved dietary measures have resulted in a decreased incidence of anemia in girls during adolescence. Many girls at this age even today select a poor diet, satisfy the whims of a freakish appetite, or maintain ill-advised reduction regimens with a resultant anemia. Continual emphasis is necessary on the fact that during adolescence there is an accelerated demand for iron to satisfy the still-increasing blood volume as well as to compensate for losses through menstruation. When pregnancy occurs during these years, it is indeed difficult for the young woman to meet the additional demands of the fetus.

Modification of the diet. Anemia is much more easily prevented than corrected. During periods of growth continual emphasis on the importance of a liberal intake of iron can do much to prevent the occurrence of iron-deficiency anemia. Once hypochromic anemia is present, diet alone is only slowly effective in restoring normal hemoglobin levels. However, the importance of improving the general nutritive state cannot be overemphasized since anemia, especially if long-standing, is usually accompanied by poor appetite and failure to maintain adequate nutrition. An optimum diet, plus supplements of iron prescribed by the physician, are considered as primary therapy for hypochromic anemia.

Iron. Usually, even with good planning, the iron level of the diet will range between 12 and 15 mg. When special emphasis is given to the inclusion of liver, dried fruits, dark green leafy vegetables, and enriched or whole-grain cereals, it may be possible to increase the iron intake to approximately 20 mg. Regeneration of hemoglobin with dietary iron alone is thus bound to be too slow; hence, iron salts such as ferrous sulfate and ferrous gluconate are given orally. However, it is essential that the diet be corrected with respect to its adequacy in iron so that the patient may maintain adequate hemoglobin levels once his anemia has been treated. Whipple's extensive study [199] on the effectiveness of various foods in hemoglobin regeneration grouped foods as follows in descending order of potency.

I. Liver (except fish liver), kidney, gizzard
II. Peaches, apricots, prunes
   Raisins, apples, grapes
   Skeletal meats, sweetbreads, brains
III. Common vegetables
   Whole-grain cereals, eggs
   Cheese, milk, cream

Protein. The diet should be adequate in proteins of high biologic value such as milk, cheese, eggs, and meat. Whenever there is any evidence of protein insufficiency in the body, a daily intake of 100 gm or more of protein is advisable.

Ascorbic acid. The absorption of iron is facilitated with a liberal intake of ascorbic acid.[200] At least 2 servings of citrus fruits and other ascorbic-acid rich foods are desirable daily.

PERNICIOUS ANEMIA

Pernicious anemia is a disturbance in which the red blood cells cannot be supplied by the bone marrow at a rapid enough rate to replace worn-out cells. The cause of the disease is inadequate formation of the intrinsic factor in the gastric juice. When the intrinsic factor is absent, vitamin B_{12} cannot be absorbed from the gastrointestinal tract.

Symptoms and clinical findings. Pernicious anemia occurs chiefly in middle-aged to elderly persons. It is characterized by a deficiency in the blood-forming system, gastrointestinal disturbances, and nervous manifestations. Lack of vitamin B_{12} results in an increasing proportion of immature large cells (macrocytes) in the circulation, while the total count decreases markedly. One of the outstanding symptoms is the characteristic lemon-yellow pallor of the patient. This is rarely seen when the red blood cell count is above 2,500,000 per cu mm, and it has been seen to disappear rather quickly after vitamin B_{12} or liver extract has been introduced.

There is invariably a lack of hydrochloric acid in the gastric juice. Digestion and absorption are retarded, the appetite is poor, and general weakness is manifested. The mouth may become sore; the membranes of the tongue, gums, and entire gastrointestinal tract may become dry and glazed; diarrhea occurs frequently.

A large proportion of untreated patients complain of coldness of the extremities, numbness in the limbs, and difficulty in walking. As the condition progresses, there may be loss of the sense of position of the feet, ataxia, or spasticity.

Modification of the diet. Until Minot and Murphy [201] introduced liver therapy in 1926, pernicious anemia was invariably fatal. Their use of large amounts of liver started the search for the factor in liver which was responsible for the improvement observed in patients. Liver extract replaced the liver diet and was in turn superseded by vitamin B_{12}. When given parenterally, vitamin B_{12} produces marked hematopoietic response in doses as small as 1 to 5 mcg. The vitamin is ineffective when given orally; however, the addition of a preparation of intrinsic factor promotes absorption, although oral therapy cannot be used exclusively. True pernicious anemia is a permanent defect and must be adequately treated for the duration of the patient's life.

The patient who has pernicious anemia usually presents a picture of general nutritional deficiency. While the anemia itself is controlled with injections of vitamin B_{12} or liver extract, the dietary management is directed toward maintaining the patient in good nutrition and in improving the general sense of well-being. The following considerations may be applied to the planning of the diet:

Protein. The protein allowance may be increased from 100 to 150 gm depending on the degree of deficiency (see High-protein Diet, p. 373).

Fat. The absence of acid in the stomach retards digestion. Therefore, fats are preferably kept at moderate or low levels, with emphasis on their selection from highly emulsified sources.

Energy. Calories are usually increased to facilitate utilization of the protein and to restore weight to normal.

Minerals and vitamins. Since general nutritional deficiencies occasioned by poor dietary intake in the past are prevalent, the diet should be planned to include a liberal intake of minerals and vitamins. Supplements of iron and sometimes of the vitamins, especially the B-complex, are sometimes ordered. They improve the general nutritional status but do not substitute for therapy with vitamin B_{12} or liver extract, nor do they affect the course of the anemia itself.

Consistency. A sore mouth, anorexia, or irritation of the gastrointestinal tract may necessitate a soft or even liquid diet until the symptoms diminish or disappear. Special care must be taken that such diets are nutritionally adequate.

OTHER MACROCYTIC ANEMIAS

Macrocytic anemias occur in a number of situations. In each instance it is first essential to determine the cause before effective therapy can be instituted.

1. Following gastrectomy, the absence of intrinsic factor impairs the absorption of vitamin B_{12}. This anemia responds to parenteral therapy with vitamin B_{12}.

2. The so-called pernicious anemia of pregnancy is caused by a folic acid deficiency and may be treated orally with this vitamin. It is not a permanent defect.

3. Macrocytic anemia of infancy is believed to be caused by inadequate conversion of folic acid to folinic acid as a result of an insufficient intake of ascorbic acid. It is likely to be observed in scurvy, and is treated with liberal amounts of ascorbic acid and folic acid.

4. Gastrointestinal disorders such as celiac disease in children or sprue in adults interfere with the absorption of many nutrients including folic acid and vitamin B_{12}. Correction of the malabsorption and folic acid therapy combined with a suitable diet are essential. See page 437 and page 558 for further discussion of these conditions.

PROBLEM AND REVIEW

1. What is the normal red blood cell count?
2. What is hemoglobin? What is its normal value?

3. What food factors are necessary for the production of hemoglobin and cells?

4. What is meant by anemia? What are some of the etiologic agents?

5. Hypochromic anemia is characterized primarily by a lack of hemoglobin. What nutrients are especially involved? Under what circumstances is it likely to occur?

6. Iron is the most important nutrient in the treatment of hypochromic anemia. What factors may interfere with its efficient use?

7. What foods are good sources of iron?

8. Why are high-iron diets impractical?

9. What other food factors require consideration in the diet for iron-deficiency anemia?

10. Pernicious anemia is due to the absence of the intrinsic factor in the gastric juice. What symptoms are usually present which may complicate dietary treatment?

11. What is the most effective treatment for pernicious anemia?

12. List the dietary principles for feeding a patient with pernicious anemia.

13. *Problem.* Plan a diet for a patient with hypochromic anemia including 15 mg or more of iron (without the use of liver) and 100 gm of protein.

UNIT XI /
Diet in Miscellaneous Disorders

CHAPTER 39

Diet in Allergic and Skin Disturbances

Elimination Diets

Definitions, common allergens. Allergies represent the abnormal reaction of an individual to the food he eats, the air he breathes, or the substances he touches. Anything which produces an allergic reaction is known as an *allergen*. *Food allergies* may be defined as a sensitivity occurring in certain parts of the body to one or more specific foods. Usually the allergen is of a protein nature, but it is thought by some that carbohydrates, lipids, and various chemicals may also be sensitizing agents on occasion.

The discussion in this chapter is confined to food allergies. Any food may produce reactions in some individuals, but the most frequent offenders are generally stated to be eggs, milk, wheat, grapefruit, orange, corn, tomato, chocolate, potatoes, fish and shellfish.

Foods unlike in flavor and structure but belonging to the same botanic group may result in allergic manifestations. For example, buckwheat is not of the cereal family but in a group which includes rhubarb. The sweet potato is not related to the white potato but is a member of the morning-glory family. Spinach, a frequent reactor, is in the same family with beets. The following botanic classification of a few common foods illustrates the relation of foods which at first thought appear to be dissimilar.

Cereal—wheat, rye, barley, rice, oats, malt, corn, sorghum, cane sugar
Lily—onion, garlic, asparagus, chives, leeks, shallots
Gourd—squash, pumpkin, cucumber, cantaloupe, watermelon
Cabbage and mustard—turnips, cabbage, collards, cauliflower, broccoli, kale, radish, horse-radish, water cress, Brussels sprouts

Manner of induction. Allergic reactions may be brought about by various means, as:

1. By ingestion of food or drugs
2. By contact with foods, pesticides, drugs, adhesive, fur, hair, feathers, molds, fungi, etc.

3. By inhalation of pollens, dust, cosmetics, perfumes, molds, fungi

4. By injection of vaccines, serums, antibiotics, hormones

Some characteristics of allergies. Some individuals are only mildly sensitive and can eat a particular food for several days before characteristic symptoms develop, while others have violent reactions within 1 or 2 hours. Allergies appear to be closely related to one's physical and emotional status; reactions to a substance may occur in a stress situation, but may not occur at another time. It has been observed that many food allergies tend to disappear during the course of psychiatric treatment.[202]

Heredity appears to play a role in allergy, but one does not inherit a sensitivity to a specific substance nor to an identical manifestation of the allergy. For example, a child born of a parent who suffers from asthma may not develop asthma, but may have eczema or some gastrointestinal disturbances. The parent may be sensitive to wheat and the child to eggs, and so on.

The skin and mucous membranes are particularly sensitive to the offending substances. Since the substances may be carried by the circulation to all parts of the body, it is reasonable to expect that the manifestations will be many and varied.

1. Skin lesions such as urticaria, nettle rash, and eczema are among the most frequent symptoms of allergy.

2. Nausea, vomiting, and diarrhea are common gastrointestinal manifestations. Symptoms suggestive of colitis, appendicitis, ulcers, and even gallbladder disease may be of allergic origin, and confusion in diagnosis results.

3. Head colds, asthma, and headaches may be caused by allergens.

4. Redness, swelling, burning, and itching of the eyes may occur independently or may accompany irritation of the nasal passages.

5. Canker sores and fever blisters occur when the individual eats certain foods to which he is sensitive.

Diagnosis of allergies. No single test is wholly reliable for the establishment of a diagnosis of allergy to any given food or foods. The procedures used include a careful history of the patient; skin testing; and dietary testing programs.

History. A complete history of the patient is clearly indicated. It must include the physical status, and conditions and events preceding the attack. A carefully kept record of food eaten and of the occurrence of symptoms is in many instances sufficient to establish what the offending factor may be. Individual likes and dislikes must be taken into consideration. One patient may dislike an important food and claim to be allergic to that food in order not to be called upon to eat it. Another may like a food sufficiently to be willing to risk an attack in order to eat it. Obviously, in any dietary testing one must eliminate the psychologic factors which may interfere with a correct interpretation.

Skin tests. These are: (1) the *scratch test,* in which a bit of suspected solution is dropped onto a scratch made on the back or arm of the patient; (2) the *intradermal test,* in which the suspected solution is injected underneath the skin; and (3) the *patch test,* in which the suspected powder or liquid is put on a filter paper which is placed on the skin, covered with cellophane, and held in place with adhesive. Readings are made at the end of 10 to 20 minutes, except in the patch test, where readings are made after 48 hours or more. If a red inflammation or hivelike wheal appears at the site of the scratch or point of contact, the material is suspected as an allergen. The tests are suggestive but not conclusive. A positive skin test does not necessarily mean that the patient is sensitive at the time to the material; it may represent a past sensitivity. Individuals who have intestinal manifestations of allergy may not react positively to skin tests.

Provocative diets and intentional feeding. The use of a diet consisting exclusively of milk, egg, wheat, beef, orange, and potato has been described by Lee and Squier.[203] This diet is given for 1 week unless the patient's previous history definitely contraindicates its use. Since the foods are commonly involved in allergies, any disturbances are likely to show up within the week. If no symptoms occur, foods are added to this regimen, one at a time, as described on page 549. If symptoms do occur, other tests must be used.

The intentional feeding procedure[204] consists in completely eliminating the test food from the diet for a week, following which it is eaten by the patient in substantial amounts three or four times a week. The test is repeated for 2 consecutive weeks. A food is not considered to be positive if it produces reactions only once in the 3-week testing period. Intentional feeding helps to confirm positive skin tests, and also helps to detect sensitivities where skin reactions were negative.

Synthetic diets. Food allergies may sometimes be diagnosed quickly by means of synthetic diets.[205,206] Such diets are made up of amino acids, sugar, salt mixtures, vitamin concentrates, water, and in some cases emulsified fats; none of the constituents of the feeding will produce allergy. The feeding is given by mouth or through a tube inserted into the stomach. The formulas are unpalatable, so that only patients with major allergic manifestations are likely to have the fortitude to give the regimen the necessary trial.

Patients who are allergic to food show marked improvements with the synthetic diet in a few days, while those who are sensitive to other materials than food will not improve. If it has been ascertained that food is responsible for the allergy, the feeding can be continued over a longer period of time, adding first one and then another of the important foods to determine which ones may be safely included and which ones should be omitted.

Elimination diets. Various systems of elimination diets, one of which is quoted on pages 549–50, have been successful in the diagnosis of food allergies. Each group of diets is so planned that common allergens are eliminated from one or more of the diets. The successful use of the diet depends on a strict adherence to the prescribed list of foods.

ELIMINATION DIETS *

DIET 1	DIET 2	DIET 3	DIET 4
Rice	Corn	Tapioca	Milk †
Tapioca	Rye	White potato	Tapioca
Rice biscuit	Corn pone	Breads made of any	Cane sugar
Rice bread	Corn-rye muffins	combination of	
	Rye bread	soy, Lima bean,	
	Ry-Krisp	and potato starch	
		and tapioca flours	
Lettuce	Beets	Tomato	
Chard	Squash	Carrot	
Spinach	Asparagus	Lima beans	
Carrot	Artichoke	String beans	
Sweet potato or		Peas	
yam			
Lamb	Chicken (no hens)	Beef	
	Bacon	Bacon	
Lemon	Pineapple	Lemon	
Grapefruit	Peach	Grapefruit	
Pears	Prunes	Peach	
	Apricot	Apricot	
Cane sugar	Cane or beet sugar	Cane sugar	
Sesame oil	Mazola oil	Sesame oil	
Olive oil ‡	Sesame oil	Soybean oil	
Salt	Salt	Salt	
Gelatin, plain or	Gelatin, plain or	Gelatin, plain or	
flavored with	flavored with	flavored with	
lime or lemon	pineapple	lime or lemon	
Maple sirup or	Karo corn sirup	Maple sirup or	
sirup made with	White vinegar	sirup made with	
cane sugar fla-		cane sugar fla-	
vored with maple		vored with maple	
Royal baking	Royal baking	Royal baking	
powder	powder	powder	
Baking soda	Baking soda	Baking soda	
Cream of tartar	Cream of tartar	Cream of tartar	
Vanilla extract	Vanilla extract	Vanilla extract	
Lemon extract		Lemon extract	

* Rowe, A. H.: *Elimination Diets and the Patient's Allergies,* 2nd ed. Lea & Febiger, Philadelphia, 1944.

† Milk should be taken up to 2 to 3 quarts a day. Plain cottage cheese and cream may be used. Tapioca cooked with milk and milk sugar may be taken.

‡ Allergy to it may occur with or without allergy to olive pollen. Mazola oil may be used if corn allergy is not present.

SAMPLE MENUS FOR ELIMINATION DIETS

DIET 1	DIET 2	DIET 3
Breakfast	*Breakfast*	*Breakfast*
Half grapefruit with or without sugar Rice Krispies with pear juice or maple sirup Lamb patties Lemonade, hot or cold; or grapefruit juice *	Sliced peaches on corn flakes or corn-meal mush Bacon Rye toast or rye muffins (whole rye flour only) Pineapple or apricot jam Prune, pineapple, or apricot juice *	Half grapefruit with or without sugar Bacon Muffins, using soybean, Lima bean, or potato flour Apricot, peach, or grapefruit marmalade or maple sirup Tomato juice, grapefruit juice or lemonade *
Luncheon or supper	*Luncheon or supper*	*Luncheon or supper*
Sautéed lamb liver (using sesame oil) Boiled rice Carrots Rice bread or biscuits Grapefruit marmalade or maple sirup Molded pear in lemon gelatin Grapefruit juice or lemonade	Baked or fried chicken (using Mazola) Harvard beets (white vinegar, sugar, cornstarch) Rye-corn muffins Pineapple or apricot jam Sliced pineapple Pineapple, apricot, or prune juice	Beef broth Beef patties Baked white potato Sliced tomatoes French dressing (soybean oil, lemon juice, salt) Biscuits made of Lima bean, potato, or soybean flour Apricot or peach preserves Tomato juice, grapefruit juice or lemonade
Dinner	*Dinner*	*Dinner*
Lamb chop or roast lamb Baked sweet potato or yam Spinach Lettuce with French dressing (sesame oil, lemon juice, salt) Rice bread or biscuit Grapefruit marmalade or maple sirup Fresh pear Lemonade or grapefruit juice	Sliced chicken Baked squash Asparagus Ry-Krisp or rye bread Pineapple or apricot preserves Stewed apricots or prunes Pineapple, apricot, or prune juice	Roast beef Carrots and peas (no cream sauce) String beans Grapefruit with French dressing (no lettuce) Lima bean, soybean, or potato bread Grapefruit marmalade Apricot tapioca Tomato, grapefruit, or apricot juice, or lemonade

* If the patient remains symptom-free on the diet being used for 5 to 7 days, tea may be added as a beverage. In the same manner coffee may be added.

The patient is first placed on the diet which, on the basis of skin tests and a dietary history, is least likely to produce allergic reactions. The diet will be used from 1 to 3 weeks, unless severe reactions have occurred in the meantime. A second diet is then tried for a similar period. Two to 3 weeks is usually necessary to give time for previous allergic manifestations to wear off, and for any possible new reactions to appear. If there has been no adverse reaction to two or more diets, all foods on the combined lists may be used. On the other hand, when untoward symptoms appear, another diet is used until all diets have been tried. If the patient shows no improvement on any of the diets of a given regimen, the allergy is probably not of food origin.

Treatment of food allergy. Restricted diets or desensitization may be used in the treatment of food allergy. For severe allergic manifestations, adreno-corticotropic hormone or cortisone is sometimes used for relief of symptoms.

Restricted diet. If improvement has occurred on an elimination diet, foods may be added, one at a time, to the allowed list of foods. Several days must elapse between the addition of each new food. Moreover, a given food should be tested on at least two, preferably three, occasions before it is permanently added to, or eliminated from, the diet.

If a single food such as strawberries or grapefruit is implicated, it is easy to omit this food from the diet. On the other hand, common foods like milk, eggs, and wheat may be hidden in a great variety of dishes. The successful treatment of the allergy thus necessitates a knowledge of the exact composition of any foods that are eaten. It is advisable to set up lists of foods that may contain the offending factors. Such lists are given on page 552 for milk, eggs, and wheat.

Dietary adequacy becomes a matter of great concern when important foods are eliminated for a long period of time. For example, if milk cannot be used, additional amounts of meat may be included to provide the necessary amounts of protein; calcium and riboflavin supplements will be indicated in such a situation.

The allergy to major food groups also poses a problem in food preparation. If wheat must be eliminated, soy, potato, rye, and rice flours may be used, but they do not possess the gluten characteristics which result in light-textured breads. A publication by the American Dietetic Association, "Allergy Recipes," is useful for its suggestions on food preparation.

Desensitization consists in decreasing the sensitivity to a given substance by giving minute doses of the allergen in gradually increasing amounts. This procedure is useful in those instances where a major food, such as eggs or milk, is involved; it is a tedious routine and is usually not practical for minor allergies.

No hard and fast rules can be given, but the initial doses are extremely minute and are determined by the degree of reaction. If severe reactions occur at any time during the hyposensitization, the next dose should not be increased, and the progression to larger amounts must be more gradual. Once hyposensitization is begun, the intervals between doses must not be too long lest the hyposensitivity be lost.

For the treatment of allergies in children, see page 571.

DIET WITHOUT WHEAT *

Foods to avoid:

Beverages—Cocomalt, malted milk, Mellin's food, Nestlé's food, Postum; beer, gin, whisky

Bread—all breads, including rye and oatmeal, hot breads and muffins, corn bread, baking-powder biscuits, etc.; gluten bread; matzoth, pretzels, and zwieback. Note: 100 per cent rye bread, crackers, and wafers may be used. Bread may be made from soy, rice, corn, potato flours.

Cereals

All-bran	Grape-Nuts	New oats	Wheat flakes
Beemax	Grape-Nuts	Pablum	Wheat germ
Bran flakes	flakes	Pep	Wheaties
Cheerios	Kix	Pettijohn's	Wheatsworth
Crackels	Krumbles	Puffed Wheat	Wheat Chex
Cream of	Maltex	Ralston cereals	
Wheat	Mellow-wheat	Shredded Wheat	
Farina	Muffets	Wheatena	

Crackers and cookies

Desserts—cakes, cookies, doughnuts, pies, ice-cream cones

Flour in any form, including graham, white, or whole-wheat

Griddle cakes, waffles; either homemade or commercially prepared mixes

Gravies or sauces thickened with flour

Macaroni, noodles, spaghetti, or vermicelli

Meat prepared with flour, bread or cracker crumbs, such as croquettes and meat loaf or stews thickened with flour or made with dumplings

Meats prepared commercially, such as frankfurters, sausages, or meat loaf in which wheat may be used as a filler

Salad dressings in which flour is used for thickening

DIET WITHOUT EGGS *

Foods to avoid:

Eggs in any form	Cookies
Bread and rolls containing egg, such as sweet rolls, griddle cakes, waffles	Cocomalt
	Custard
Cakes	Eggnogs or other egg drinks
Candy as chocolate, fondant, nougat	Hollandaise sauce

* Adapted from *Diet Manual,* Nutrition Department, The Presbyterian Hospital, New York City, 1957.

Foods to avoid (*continued*)

Ice cream
Mayonnaise
Marshmallows
Meringue
Meat prepared with egg as meat loaf,
    breaded meat
Muffins

Noodles
Ovaltine
Pies such as coconut, cream, custard,
    lemon, pumpkin
Pretzels
Puddings containing eggs
Zwieback

DIET WITHOUT MILK *

Foods to avoid:

Milk in all forms including fresh, evap-
    orated, dry, malted, buttermilk
Bread with milk added (includes most
    commercial breads)
Butter
Cake or cookies made with milk
Caramels
Cheese
Chocolate candy
Cocomalt
Cream
Cream of Rice
Cream sauces
Cream soups

Custards
Gravy made with milk, cream, butter,
    or margarine
Ice cream
Margarine
Mashed potatoes
Ovaltine
Piecrust made with butter or margarine
Pies, soft or cream type
Puddings made with milk
Sherbets
Vegetables seasoned with butter or mar-
    garine, or creamed
Zwieback

DISEASES OF THE SKIN

The quality of the diet is a determining factor in skin health. Deficiency of one or more vitamins is known to produce various cutaneous disorders. For example, there are the dermatitis associated with pellagra and resulting from lack of niacin, the eruptions which accompany severe vitamin-A deficiency, and the cheilosis of riboflavin lack, to mention but a few. Some individuals may be allergic to certain substances and thus manifest skin disorders such as eczema or urticaria.

Many bizarre diets have been prescribed for skin diseases. Needless restrictions often are made when there is no proven association between the disorder and the ingestion of the food. Adolescent boys and girls who are especially prone to *acne vulgaris* are particularly likely to eliminate nutritionally important foods in a vain attempt to correct a skin condition.

* Adapted from *Diet Manual,* Nutrition Department, The Presbyterian Hospital, New York City, 1957.

The best diet which can be prescribed in skin disorders is one which is nutritionally adequate; that is, it should include sufficient milk, eggs, meat, fruits, vegetables, enriched or whole-grain cereals and breads, and butter or margarine. The consumption of these foods will usually accomplish a great deal more than the hit-or-miss elimination of certain foods.

Whenever allergy is suspected as a cause for cutaneous diseases, it is essential to determine the offending agent as described in the preceding part of this chapter. No single food or group of foods predominates in producing allergic skin disorders.

High-fat and concentrated carbohydrate diets have been considered to have unfavorable effects in certain skin diseases, but the evidence is not conclusive. There is no harm in the exclusion of candies and sweets, fried foods, chocolate, and rich desserts from the diet, but improvement through such limitation is by no means assured. As a matter of fact, when the Four Food Groups are eaten in the needed amounts, there is less desire to consume these rich foods.

Attention should be directed to improving the general hygiene, including regular meal hours, sufficient fluid intake, adequate rest, proper elimination, and psychologic support.

PROBLEMS AND REVIEW

1. Name some of the characteristic symptoms of allergy.

2. Name five foods to which a great number of allergies are due. Name some foods which rarely cause sensitivity.

3. What is meant by skin test; elimination diet; provocative diet; intentional feeding?

4. What are the principles for the construction of elimination diets? What are some of the shortcomings of many of these diets?

5. *Problem.* Plan a day's menu for a patient who is sensitive to wheat, potatoes, and grapefruit.

6. *Problem.* Prepare a list of foods which a patient should avoid if he is allergic to corn.

7. What recommendations could you make to a 15-year-old girl who has *acne vulgaris?*

CHAPTER 40

Nutrition in Children's Diseases

Starch- and Fat-restricted Diets; Galactose-free Diet; Low-phenylalanine Diet

Although the principles of normal and therapeutic nutrition that apply to the adult are also applicable to the sick child, additional factors that must be carefully considered for the child are: (1) growth needs; (2) stage of physical, emotional, and social development; (3) the presence of physical handicaps in some; and (4) the more rapid nutritional deterioration which occurs.

Earlier discussions in this text pertaining to the normal nutritional needs of children (see Chaps. 18 and 19), the factors influencing food acceptance (see Chap. 15), and the nutritional care and rehabilitation of sick people (see Chap. 23) provide the basis for the feeding of sick children. Those dietary regimens for diseases that are common to adults and children may be adjusted according to the child's needs by consulting programs described in preceding chapters. This chapter will include a description of problems pertaining especially to children, and to certain metabolic disorders seen primarily in children.

Feeding problems of the sick child. Like adults, children face many obstacles in illness. Eating a satisfactory diet may be difficult because of fatigue, nausea, lack of appetite occasioned by the illness and by drugs, and pain. Children often regress to an earlier stage of feeding; for example, the child who has learned to accept chopped foods may refuse them, or the child who can feed himself may refuse to eat unless someone feeds him. Older children especially may experience a sense of failure and express it by excessive eating or refusal to eat. Illness produces emotional tensions in the child as well as in the adult. When the child must be placed in a hospital, he is also faced with the separation from his home and his parents. The principles of feeding the normal child apply in even greater degree to the child who is ill.

Insofar as possible the feeding program should establish a pattern of continuity with that to which the child is accustomed. A record of the child's feeding history is a first requisite so that the normal or therapeutic diet makes allowances for individual likes and dislikes. The period of a child's illness is no time in which to introduce new foods or to provide equipment which the child does not know how to handle.

Even though careful menu planning takes into consideration the usual likes of children, and includes variations in both flavor and texture, foods may be refused. The illness itself and the strange environment are sufficient cause for such refusal; sometimes portions are a bit too large, or there may be a slight change in the flavoring or texture of a familiar food. Regardless of the reason for refusal, nothing can be gained by trying to force a child to eat. If the personnel responsible for the care of the child maintain a consistently relaxed and pleasant atmosphere, the child will sooner or later respond favorably to the care which is given him.

For preschool and school children who are not confined to bed, group feeding is particularly useful since children, like adults, enjoy companionship at meals, learn to get along with one another, and may show improvement of appetite.

WEIGHT CONTROL

Obesity. Children, like adults, become overweight because they eat in excess of their daily requirements. The first step toward the correction of the obesity is a determination of the reason for overeating.[207] Many children are fat because their mothers have assumed an overprotective attitude and have fed their children large quantities of food in the mistaken notion that it was necessary. For example, a child may have been ill at one time and eaten poorly; the extra amounts of high-calorie foods which were fed during convalescence may not have been reduced so that as a result the child continued to gain weight. Then again, large amounts of concentrated foods, such as candy, have frequently been used by the mother as a bribe. The mother thus retains an intimate hold on her child who craves more and more sweets. The fat child is often an unhappy child who may be eating simply for the solace which he obtains from food.

Because the energy requirements of children are relatively high, their diet is usually less restricted than that for adults. About 1200 to 1800 calories may be included, depending upon the stature and activity of the child. Liberal protein, mineral, and vitamin allowances are essential so that tissue and stature development are not adversely affected. The Low-calorie Diet described in Chapter 27 may be used as a basis for planning the child's diet. To this diet should be added 1 cup of milk daily so that the child receives his quota of 1 quart. Vitamin-D concentrates are usually prescribed.

It is vital that the child (and his mother) be so approached that he will realize what a loss of weight may mean to him. For some children this means emphasis on good appearance, poise, and gracefulness; for others it means greater participation in sports; and for still others it implies the approbation of fellow playmates and schoolmates. The physician, nurse, and dietitian who are guiding the child's weight reduction program must show understanding of the child's problems and must maintain interest through a careful follow-up of the progress which is being made.

Underweight. The child who fails to show normal gains in weight and height usually tires easily, is irritable and restless, and more susceptible to infections. As in the correction of obesity, the cause for underweight must first be sought so that treatment may be properly directed. The diet is corrected with respect to its adequacy of the essential nutrients, after which increases in the caloric level may be made gradually. A reasonable amount of outdoor exercise and regulated rest are important elements of the weight-gaining program. For high-calorie diets see Chapter 27.

DIARRHEA IN INFANTS AND CHILDREN

Diarrhea occurring in infants and children may be functional or organic and is caused by the same factors as in adults. Probably most acute diarrhea is accounted for by improper handling of the food supply, especially milk. The incidence is several times as high in bottle-fed as in breast-fed infants and is greatly increased during the summer months when it is traceable to unsanitary preparation or inadequate refrigeration of food, including infant formulas. Greater emphasis on education of parents in the preparation, sterilization, and storage of formulas has resulted in a markedly decreased incidence and mortality.

Serious consequences follow diarrhea in infants under 1 year of age if treatment is not prompt. The large loss of fluids and electrolytes quickly leads to dehydration, fever, loss of kidney function, and severe acidosis if electrolyte loss is chiefly through the intestinal tract. There may also be marked vomiting with a loss of acid, in which case there may be no acidosis but a lowering of total body anions and cations.

Modification of the diet. When mild diarrhea occurs in breast-fed infants, it is usually sufficient to discontinue breast feeding entirely for 12 to 24 hours and to provide weak tea or 5 per cent glucose at 3- or 4-hour intervals. At the end of the first 12 hours, the infant is permitted to nurse for a few minutes after taking the tea or glucose. The time of nursing is gradually increased as improvement occurs.

Artificially fed infants are given only weak tea or glucose solution until the diarrhea appears to be lessening—usually about 24 to 48 hours—after which skim milk or skim lactic acid milk may be given at half strength. Since adequate intake of fluid is important, the glucose solution or water should be continued until the infant can tolerate the full volume of formula. Both the quantity and concentration of the formula should be increased only gradually so that diarrhea will not become more severe.

When diarrhea in infants is severe, it is essential to correct the dehydration and acidosis by the administration of alkali, fluids, amino acids, glucose, and vitamins in water-soluble preparations by parenteral means. Only water, weak sweetened tea, glucose solution, or amino acid solutions are permitted by mouth. Convalescence may be prolonged, and the diet must be increased cautiously. Skim and then whole lactic acid milk (p. 252) is especially useful.

Scraped apple or apple powder has been useful in the treatment of diarrhea in infants and older children. The apple powder may be mixed with water or with milk, if milk is tolerated. A thick paste is prepared using 4 level teaspoons of apple powder and a small quantity of boiled and cooled water. When the paste is smooth, it is gradually diluted with liquid until the volume equals 8 ounces. This quantity is taken every 3 to 4 hours, as directed by the physician.

The treatment of diarrhea in older children is similar to that for adults, namely, the omission of food during the first day or two, the gradual introduction of low-residue foods (Chap. 31), and progression to a bland diet (Chap. 30).

CELIAC DISTURBANCES

The celiac syndrome includes several disturbances, all of which are characterized by intolerance to dietary starch or fat or both. True or idiopathic celiac disease may be mild (starch intolerance) or severe. Cystic fibrosis of the pancreas presents many of the symptoms of celiac disease as a result of inadequate or absent secretion of pancreatic juice. Kwashiorkor (Chap. 4) or severe dietary deficiency bears many similarities to the syndrome, as does also sprue in adults (Chap. 31).

Mild celiac disease (starch intolerance). This condition is characterized by abdominal distention, chronic diarrhea, and growth failure. It occurs more frequently than severe celiac disease. The amylase concentration in the duodenum is low, thus resulting in considerable amounts of undigested starch in the stools. Fat is present in abnormal amounts in the feces but disappears after varying periods of treatment. The diet must be restricted for years as described below for celiac disease, but more liberal amounts of fat may be permitted than in the initial stages of treatment for severe celiac disease.

Severe celiac disease. Classic celiac disease occurs in children as early as 6 months of age but is seen more frequently during the second year of life. It may occur up to the age of 5 years. The many instances of multiple cases in a family point to a hereditary factor. Celiac disease is chronic in character and presents these symptoms: (1) a marked enlargement of the abdomen; (2) wasting of the tissues, particularly about the buttocks and groin; (3) severe loss of weight and retardation of growth; (4) loss of muscle tone;

(5) loss of appetite, vomiting, and the development of secondary anemia; (6) behavior changes ranging from irritability and evidences of fatigue to hysterical outbursts; (7) pale, foul, excessively bulky stools which may be semifluid in character.

Consistently, the absorption of carbohydrate is impaired in celiac disease, accounting for the presence of large amounts of undigested starch in the stools. Fat digestion is normal because there is sufficient bile and pancreatic lipase, but the absorption of fat is reduced to from 65 to 85 per cent of the ingested fat.[208] The normal rate of absorption is about 90 to 95 per cent.

Poor absorption of fat interferes with the absorption of the fat-soluble vitamins and also of calcium and iron. Tetany, osteoporosis, rickets, or hypochromic anemia has been observed in some patients. The excessive loss of sodium and potassium in periods of severe diarrhea may lead to dehydration, shock, and acidosis. Protein deficiency is of common occurrence probably because dietary protein is used in large part to meet the energy needs of the body.

Cystic fibrosis. This congenital disturbance affects the exocrine glands, that is, the glands which discharge their secretions to the outside of the body. Large amounts of mucus may obstruct the bronchi, the nasal passages, and the ducts leading to the gastrointestinal tract. The sweat contains an excessive amount of salt. Lack of pancreatic enzymes in many, but not all, patients interferes seriously with the utilization of protein, fat, and carbohydrate. As much as 50 per cent of protein and fat of the diet may be present in the feces. The chief signs noted in the patient are slow growth in spite of a large appetite, bulky stools, chronic bronchitis, and frequently signs of deficiency of fat-soluble vitamins. Death may occur from malnutrition or bronchopneumonia.

Modification of the diet in celiac disturbances. The principles and stages for diet in the celiac syndrome have been fully described by Mike and are given in part below:

BASIC PRINCIPLES OF DIET IN THE CELIAC SYNDROME *

CELIAC DISEASE	FIBROCYSTIC DISEASE
CALORIES	
Acute phase: 120 to 200/kg body weight; an excess to compensate for past and present fecal loss and failures in absorption; formula calories may cover the entire caloric needs in crisis, and be two-thirds of the	All ages and conditions: 50 to 75 per cent above normal requirements Newborn period: 150 to 200/kg body weight; the same as the celiac patient in the acute phase Older child: 120 to 150/kg body weight;

* Arranged from Mike, E. M.: "Practical Management of Patients with the Celiac Syndrome," *Am. J. Clin. Nutrition,* **7:**463, 1959.

CELIAC DISEASE

FIBROCYSTIC DISEASE

CALORIES (*continued*)

total as the patient improves; *a very ill child requires frequent feedings,* every 2 to 3 hours day and night; soon after the acute phase of the disease, even for the very young, solids are added

After acute phase: About 20 per cent above normal calculated requirements; gradual return to normal requirements

between meal feedings are needed, especially for the older child, to prevent fatigue and excessive hunger; it may be necessary to use six small meals for some individuals

PROTEIN

Acute phase: 6 to 8 gm/kg body weight daily

After acute phase: Gradual return to normal calculated requirements; allergies are not uncommon; therefore the use of fish, particularly shellfish, should be restricted

All ages and phases: 6 to 8 gm/kg body weight daily; an excess is required at all times to compensate for the great loss; additional amino acids are required as part of the protein for infants under one year; this can be achieved by using *Probana* formula

SIMPLE CARBOHYDRATES AND STARCHES

Planned to make up the remaining calories

Acute phase: Use only formula initially, then increase the use of well-tolerated, relatively simple carbohydrates; avoid the use of starch; patients originally having the severe phase should not have starch liberalized for six months to one year after the last severe bout of diarrhea

Mild phase (starch intolerance): After about 14 months of age, more liberal use of cane sugar is tolerated; *gradual* introduction of selected starch follows; there may be an intolerance to gluten in which case wheat, rye, oats, and barley would be avoided; the effect of new foods should not be judged until they have been given one week *or longer,* since the intolerance may not be manifested immediately; during an infection and in very hot weather, relapses may occur, requir-

Planned to make up the remaining calories

Acute phase and under one year of age: As outlined under the acute phase of celiac disease

Over one year of age if not acutely ill: Gradually introduce starch; the selection is to be governed by the ability to chew as well as the socioenvironmental needs; the quantity is limited to assure an adequate intake of other important foods. This will vary with the age and appetite of the individual child; in this phase there is no intolerance to starch

NOTE: The quantity of foods should never be restricted by the adult's attitudes, but foods should be offered to the point of satiety of the patient

CELIAC DISEASE

FIBROCYSTIC DISEASE

SIMPLE CARBOHYDRATES AND STARCHES (*continued*)

ing a return to a more restricted diet for a week or more; some restrictions may be required for years, as influenced by the clinical picture of the child and laboratory data; gluten-containing foods are poorly tolerated; there is individual variation, and they should be introduced on a trial and error basis

FAT

Acute phase: Steatorrhea is present; the fat content of the diet is to be low; avoid visible fats and restrict to fat in the formula and a few selected foods; skim and whole milks, raw or pasteurized, and evaporated milks are not tolerated; however, protein milk, boiled skim and some types of dried skim milks are taken well; the fat in egg yolk and lean meat is not considered excessive and should be included in the diet

Mild phase (starch intolerance): The tolerance varies; utilization is generally increased if the gluten content of the diet is initially kept low and the added fats are unsaturated (corn, cottonseed, soybean, sesame, and olive oils); progression to other fats, and a more liberal use of all fats and oils is made with clinical improvement of the patient

The fat content of the diet is to be low; limited absorption and tolerance is present; restrict intake to fats contained in the natural foods which help to provide the optimal dietary essentials as well as aid in planning a varied and practical menu; *if the patient is doing well and* is near adolescence, limited amounts of creamy peanut butter, mild cheese, lean ham, and crisp bacon (drained) can be used; homogenized milk may be used when away from home, as in school; some older patients may tolerate homogenized milk instead of skim milk

Patients with normal duodenal enzymes: Fats are not restricted unless increased stools and digestive disturbances are produced

ROUGHAGE

Acute phase: Excessive roughage is not tolerated; the residue of puréed foods is not excessive

Mild phase: Puréed foods are used for a longer period than for the well child. It is not uncommon to find undigested foods and colored foods excreted; do not restrict the offending foods; raw vegetables and additional

Acute phase: Same as in celiac disease. Over two years of age: There is no intolerance; the use is governed by the ability to chew

CELIAC DISEASE   FIBROCYSTIC DISEASE

ROUGHAGE (*continued*)

raw fruits are added when there has
been a marked clinical improvement
—about three to four years of age

VITAMINS

Aqueous multivitamin preparation;   About 20 drops or 2 capsules daily;
about 20 drops (1.2 ml), or 2 cap-   (vitamin A to be between 10,000 to
sules daily; (vitamin A to be between   20,000 units)
10,000 to 20,000 units); in mild
phase about 10 drops or 1 capsule
may be adequate

B complex (Lederplex): 2 to 4 tea-   Same, depending on formula
spoons daily, or 2 to 4 capsules

Vitamin K: given when evidence of   Same
bleeding exists (prolonged prothrombin time)

SALT

Normal intake   All age groups: increased intake up to
                                         6 gm daily, in warm or hot weather;
                                         salt may be added to food or bever-
                                         age or given as NaCl tablets after
                                         meals

IRON

When indicated, use 10 mg of ele-   Usually not indicated
mental iron per kilogram body
weight; give with food other than
milk

PANCREATIN

Not required   Required for all patients with pancreatic
                                         deficiency; dosage varies with age and
                                         the number of meals scheduled

                                         Powder: $\frac{1}{2}$ to 1 gm ($\frac{1}{2}$ teaspoon) in
                                         each bottle or 1 to 2 gm (1 teaspoon)
                                         with each meal on a three-meal-a-
                                         day plan

                                         Tablets: 325 mg each. Give 1 to 3 tab-
                                         lets with each meal; older patients
                                         may require only 1 to 2 tablets as
                                         determined by the fat in the stools

                                         Granules: $\frac{1}{4}$ to $\frac{1}{2}$ teaspoon with each
                                         meal on a three-meal-a-day plan

The following stages are a suggested guide for planning the diet, but it must be emphasized that individual needs must receive first consideration. In addition to suitable modification for the celiac syndrome, the age and growth needs of the child must be constantly considered.

Formula: Probana * to provide ⅔ to ¾ or all of the calories. The *Probana*-to-water ratio should never be more concentrated than 1:4 by volume.

Hi Pro * or *Protein Milk* * to supply ⅔ to ¾ of the formula calories may be used. The remaining formula calories are provided by glucose and/or banana flakes or powder.

I. Two to 4 months of age. In addition to the formula, introduce the following foods gradually. This diet is known as the *strict no-starch, high-protein, low-fat diet.* See meal plan on page 565.

Cheese: cottage, uncreamed with jelly or honey
Dessert: plain gelatin
Egg: yolk
Fruit: scraped raw apple, apple juice, applesauce; banana or banana flakes; strained grapefruit or orange juice
Meat: beef or liver, strained or finely ground
Vegetables, all puréed: green beans, carrots, squash, tomato juice

II. Four to 14 months of age. This diet is known as *no-starch, high-protein, low-fat diet.* See meal plan on page 565.
Continue the formula and all foods from stage I. Add the following:

Desserts: fruit ices, fruit whips with egg white, rennet desserts, meringues
Eggs: whole, not more than three each day
Fruit: scraped raw pear; puréed apricots, cranberries, peaches, pears, pineapple; strained juices of apricot, cranberry, grape, lemon, lime, pear, pineapple, tangerine
Meat: lean chicken, heart, kidney, lamb, turkey, veal; fresh boneless fish (add with caution for celiacs), low-fat canned salmon, tuna
Sweets: honey, clear jelly, marshmallow, sugar, sirup, hard candy
Vegetables: puréed asparagus, beets, peas, spinach, Swiss chard
Miscellaneous: salt, flavoring extracts

III. Fourteen months to 2 years of age. This diet is known as *low-starch, high-protein, low-fat diet.* For patients with cystic fibrosis, a formula made of double-strength nonfat dry milk may be used. Those patients with celiac disease may be given a formula of boiled skim or homogenized milk. Selected foods with starch are allowed in restricted amounts if the gluten intake is not restricted. See meal plan on page 565.
Allow all foods from stages I and II, with the following additions or modifications:

---

* *Probana* and *Protein Milk* by Mead Johnson & Co., Evansville, Indiana; *Hi Pro* by Jackson-Mitchell Pharmaceuticals, Inc.

Cereal foods: 1 serving three times daily of any *one:* puffed cereals, 2 to 3 table-spoons; arrowroot crackers or social tea biscuits, 2 to 3; zwieback; Melba toast; crisp toast, ½ slice. If gluten is restricted, all wheat cereals and breads must be avoided. (See Chap. 31.)

Fruits: seedless grapes; cooked or canned apricots, peaches, pears need not be puréed at this stage

Meat: shellfish

Milk: skim or homogenized as tolerated

Vegetables: all cooked, but need not be puréed; add broccoli tops and cauliflower tops

Miscellaneous: cocoa

IV. Two to 4 years of age. This diet is known as *moderate-starch, high-protein, low-fat diet.*

Allow all foods permitted on stage III, with the following additions:

Cereal foods: cooked cereals; plain bread, saltines, soda crackers; macaroni, noodles, spaghetti, rice

Desserts: angel food or sponge cake, lady fingers, puddings

Fats: for celiac patients only—corn, cottonseed, olive, sesame, and soybean oils

Milk: homogenized for celiac patients; skim for pancreatic deficiency

Soups: cream

Vegetables: potato

V. Three to 6 years of age. At this stage raw fruits and vegetables may be gradually introduced by trial and error. Those foods which cause discomfort should be avoided. Celiac patients, but not those with pancreatic deficiency, may be given creamy peanut butter, vegetable shortening, and finally ice cream and butter.

VI. Over 6 years of age. The nutritional needs of the celiac patient are about the same as those of the normal child, and all foods of the family may be introduced gradually. The B-complex vitamins should be continued, and aqueous multivitamins should be given at the same levels as for the well child.

The patient with pancreatic deficiency needs a high-protein, high-calorie, moderately low-fat diet with additional vitamin-B complex, and aqueous multivitamins. Pancreatin must be continued. Some of those patients must continue to use a rigidly restricted fat diet.

Low-gluten diet. Several Dutch workers [209] and others in England [210,211] observed that the gluten of wheat was closely correlated with the amount of fat excreted in the feces. When wheat was omitted from the diet of celiac patients, there was improvement in the appetite, stools became more nearly normal, and the patient gained weight. The Wheat-, Oat-, and Rye-free Diet described in Chapter 31 may be adapted to the celiac patient when it is evident that gluten is the offending agent.

SUGGESTED MEAL PLANS FOR FIRST THREE STAGES OF DIET

STRICT NO-STARCH HIGH-PROTEIN LOW-FAT	NO-STARCH HIGH-PROTEIN LOW-FAT	LOW-STARCH HIGH-PROTEIN LOW-FAT
Breakfast		
Citrus or apple juice (strained)	Citrus juice (strained)	Citrus juice (strained)
Ripe banana, banana flakes or applesauce	Ripe banana or other fruit from list	Ripe banana or other fruit from list
Eggs—no added fat	Eggs—no added fat	Eggs—no added fat
Uncreamed skim milk cottage cheese or meat, if desired	Uncreamed skim milk cottage cheese or meat, if desired	Uncreamed skim milk cottage cheese or meat, if desired
Formula	Formula	Starch—1 serving
		Milk or formula
Dinner and supper		
Finely ground or strained canned beef or liver (2 or more tablespoons)	Finely ground or strained canned lean meat, poultry (or fish); *cut off all visible fat;* broil, boil, or roast	Finely chopped or ground lean meat, poultry or fish; *cut off all visible fat;* broil, boil, or roast
Cheese from list may be used for *one* meal	Cheese from list or egg may be used for *one* meal	Cheese from list or egg may be used for *one* meal
Puréed string beans, carrots or squash (1 or more tablespoons)	Puréed cooked vegetable	Cooked, fresh, frozen, or canned vegetable (puréed or chopped, dependent on age)
Dessert: gelatin desserts, applesauce, scraped raw apple, ripe banana, or banana flakes	Dessert: puréed fruit should be used for *one* meal	Dessert: fruit should be used for *one* meal
Formula	Formula	Starch—1 serving
		Milk or formula
Evening		
Formula	Formula	Milk or formula
Between-meal feedings		
Dependent on appetite	Dependent on appetite	Any foods on diet list, except starch in excess of allowance, if they do not interfere with the appetite at mealtime
		NOTE: These feedings should always be planned for those with cystic fibrosis

DIABETES

The first patient treated with the insulin prepared by Drs. Banting and Best in January, 1922 was a 14-year-old diabetic boy. Marble [212] estimates that approximately one of every 2000 children under 15 years of age are diabetic.

Comparison with adult diabetes. The disease in children differs in a number of important respects from that in adults. The onset of symptoms is usually more sudden and violent, and the disease tends to increase in severity during the period of growth. In contrast to the adult, obesity is uncommon; in fact, most diabetic children have a history of underweight. All diabetic children need insulin, since there appear to be few if any functioning cells of the islands of Langerhans. The maintenance of control between acidosis on the one hand and hypoglycemia on the other is often difficult because of the greater frequency of infections and the erratic physical activity. The additional nutrient needs for growth and the varying activity from time to time necessitate frequent dietary adjustments.

While the life span of diabetic children has improved greatly, the incidence of degenerative diseases is unusually high after 10 to 20 years. The possibilities of diminished vision and even blindness, of coronary artery disease, and of kidney disease during the prime of life are serious, and as yet unsolved, problems.

Psychologic considerations. Too often the child and his parents as well feel that he is somehow different from other children and that there is a certain stigma attached to the diabetic state. If the child experiences insulin reactions, he will be afraid to participate in the activities of other children, and he may become more dependent upon his parents. The diabetic adolescent is likely to be especially difficult to control. Like other adolescents he may rebel against authority, and one of the ways in which he may show his independence is through breaking diet.

The guidance of the child in all aspects of his development, not only in the treatment of the diabetes, requires great patience, forbearance, and understanding on the part of the parent and physician. The child and the parent must recognize the interrelationship of diet, insulin, and activity and the importance of regulation. It is equally important that the child learn—and his parents understand—that he can take his place in the family and society just as does the nondiabetic child. Nelson states: "The child who is not physically, mentally and socially able to compete with his colleagues cannot be considered an adequately treated diabetic child." *

Modification of the diet. The principles of dietary modification for the

---

* Nelson, W. E.: *Textbook of Pediatrics,* 7th ed. W. B. Saunders Company, Philadelphia, 1959, p. 1208.

diabetic child are similar to those for the adult (see Chap. 33). The nutritive requirements are the same as those for the normal child of the same age, size, and activity (see Chap. 19). Briefly, these needs are as follows:

Calories: to maintain desirable rate of growth; usually about 35 to 40 calories per pound desirable weight.

Protein: 1.5 gm per pound if under 3 years of age; 1 gm per pound for older children.

Carbohydrate and fat: 40 to 45 per cent of the calories from carbohydrate with the remaining calories from fat. Some clinicians restrict carbohydrate to 225–250 gm per day, or even less, in which case the fat level is proportionately higher to ensure adequate caloric intake.

The additional calcium requirements are easily met when 3 to 4 cups of milk are included daily. Other minerals and vitamins are provided in satisfactory amounts when the exchange lists are used as the basis of meal planning. Children should receive vitamin D either in milk or as a supplement.

The diet prescription should be adjusted periodically to make allowances for satisfactory growth. A reasonable meal constancy from day to day is desirable. Between-meal snacks should be included. It is better that a child receive a snack before activity to forestall the possibility of insulin reaction.

Opinions differ as to the degree of control which shall be exercised. Some clinicians maintain that chemical control is important if degenerative complications are to be avoided. Others use the "free" diet, allowing the child to eat all family foods, but usually restricting concentrated sweets and high-carbohydrate desserts. Enough insulin is given to metabolize food for normal growth and to avoid ketosis, but hyperglycemia and glycosuria are disregarded.

Insulin. The slowly acting insulins, especially lente and isophane, are most commonly used. For many children a small dose of insulin is needed before dinner or in the evening, as well as before breakfast, in order that morning hyperglycemia may be controlled. In addition, regular insulin is sometimes included with the morning injection. The oral sulfonylurea compounds are not suitable for juvenile diabetics.

Education of the child and his parents. When the child is old enough to accept instruction, he should always he included in the planning of his diet and his care. Regardless of opinions concerning clinical or chemical control, most pediatricians agree that close adherence to a diet at the beginning provides security and guidance for the child and the parent during the period of adjustment to the disease. Jackson [213] recommends that the initial diet provide few substitutions until the patient is thoroughly accustomed to it; then the diet is gradually liberalized with respect to food choice until the meal exchange lists are used with ease.

A diet planned within the scope of the meal exchange lists possesses the advantages of including nutritive essentials, keeps the child reasonably well controlled with respect to a normal blood sugar and the usual absence of urine sugar, and yet is not so restrictive that the child breaks diet too frequently. Some pediatricians recommend that the diet be weighed initially until the parent and the patient are accustomed to portion sizes and that weighing of food be practiced from time to time as a check on the amounts of food. Otherwise, the use of household measurements suffices.

Diabetic camps in many areas of the country have provided an unusual educational opportunity for children to learn more about the care of themselves with respect to their disease, and also to learn the important social adjustments with other children. Such camps are well staffed with recreational leaders, nurses, dietitian, physicians, and laboratory technicians.[212,214]

OTHER METABOLIC DISORDERS

Phenylketonuria. Mental retardation which may become apparent in infancy as early as 4 months of age is the outstanding characteristic of phenylketonuria. It is a hereditary disease in which the amino acid phenylalanine cannot be converted to tyrosine because of the lack of the hepatic enzyme, phenylalanine hydroxylase. As a result the phenylalanine in the blood serum increases from a normal level of 1–2 mg per 100 ml to 20–90 mg per 100 ml. Abnormal phenylketone bodies are excreted in the urine giving a musty, wild-game odor to the urine and to the unwashed body.

Phenylketonuria is believed to account for about 1 per cent of mental defectives in institutions. The intelligence quotient is below 25 in 60 to 80 per cent of the cases.[215] The children are extremely irritable and difficult to manage, often have eczema, and may experience convulsions. They are usually blond, fair, and blue-eyed even though they may come from dark-skinned families. This is explained by the deficiency of tyrosine, which is essential for the formation of the pigments.

Defective phenylalanine metabolism may be ascertained during the first few weeks of life before mental deficiency has become evident by using simple laboratory tests of the blood and urine. When treatment is instituted early enough, mental retardation can be averted. Children who are 3 or 4 years of age before treatment is begun may show some improvement of the personality, but the damage to the central nervous system cannot be reversed. Effective treatment, therefore, is directed to the young infant and consists in providing a low-phenylalanine diet.

Since phenylalanine constitutes about 5 per cent of the protein of the diet, it becomes evident that a normal milk formula—as well as other protein-containing foods—will contribute excessive amounts of phenylalanine. Two commercial preparations, Lofenalac,* and Ketonil,† are suitable substitutes

* Mead Johnson & Company, Evansville, Indiana.
† Merck and Co., Rahway, New Jersey.

for milk formulas. Lofenalac is a combination of low-phenylalanine casein hydrolysate, fat, carbohydrate, and the minerals and vitamins comparable to the usual milk formulas, requiring only dilution with water. Vitamin C and a multivitamin supplement are recommended. Ketonil contains the necessary amino acids and minerals, but is mixed with an oil, such as cottonseed, and sugar to meet the caloric requirements of the child. Vitamin supplements are prescribed. The manufacturers of both products have developed complete descriptions for the use of the amino acid preparations and for supplementary feeding.

Since phenylalanine is an essential amino acid, it must be provided in sufficient amounts for normal growth as soon as the initial formula has brought the serum level of phenylalanine within normal limits. The daily phenylalanine need for the infant has been variously estimated to range between 15 and 40 mg per kilogram body weight.[215] Because infants vary somewhat in their tolerance as well as in their needs for growth, the maintenance of chemical control is determined by periodic testing of the blood and the urine.

The protein needs of the infant are essentially met by the use of the amino acid formulas, but supplementary foods such as fruits, fruit juices, vegetables other than legumes, and cereals are added at appropriate intervals in the infant's diet. Approximately 5 per cent of the protein value of these foods may be considered as phenylalanine. More exact values are available from the publication *Amino Acid Content of Foods.*[216] It is essential that the phenylalanine intake from the amino acid formula and from the supplementary foods not exceed the daily requirements. For older children the amino acid powders may be better accepted if they are mixed with foods, or if they are served as beverages flavored with fruit juices, chocolate, or other nonprotein flavorings.

Just how long diet therapy must be continued is not known. It is quite possible that a normal diet may be used once the central nervous system has developed fully.

Galactose disease. The hereditary disorder, galactose disease, is caused by the absence of an enzyme (galactose-1-phosphate uridyl transferase—sometimes abbreviated P-Gal-transferase) which is needed in the liver for the conversion of galactose to glucose. Galactose results from the hydrolysis of lactose in the intestine. It is absorbed, but must be converted in the liver to glucose before the body can utilize it.

The disease becomes apparent within a few days after birth by such symptoms as anorexia, vomiting, occasionally diarrhea, drowsiness, jaundice, puffiness of the face, edema of the lower extremities, and weight loss. The spleen and liver enlarge, and in some there may be evidences of liver failure within a short time leading to ascites, bleeding, and early death. Mental retardation becomes evident very early in the course of the disease, and cataracts develop within the first year. Urine tests show the presence of galactose, albumin, and amino acids. A galactose tolerance test helps to establish the diagnosis.

The important dietary source of galactose is the lactose of milk, human milk being especially high in it. The substitution of a nonmilk formula leads to rapid improvement, as a rule. All of the symptoms disappear except that mental retardation which has already occurred is not reversible. Damage to the central nervous system is greatest during the first few weeks and months of life when the growth rate is rapid, so the importance of prompt therapy can scarcely be overemphasized.

A number of nonmilk formula products are available. A casein hydrolysate is the basis for Nutramigen,* soybeans are the basis for Sobee * and Mul-Soy,† and a meat base is used in another.‡ The formulas require supplementation with calcium gluconate or chloride, vitamins, and iron. Since milk is the only food which provides lactose, all other food may be introduced into the infant's diet at the appropriate times. These include breads, crackers, and cereals made without milk, eggs, meat, poultry, fish, fruits, vegetables, and gelatin desserts. All foods that contain any milk must be rigidly excluded: most commercial breads, cookies, cakes, puddings, pudding mixes, some ready-to-eat cereals, all cheeses, cream, ice cream, butter, margarine churned in milk, and others. The list of foods to be avoided in allergy to milk is helpful in the planning of a galactose-free diet (see p. 553).

Epilepsy. The ketogenic diet occasionally used for epilepsy has been fully described in Chapter 35.

NEPHROTIC SYNDROME

The nephrotic syndrome includes so-called pure lipoid nephrosis and the nephrotic phase of glomerulonephritis. This rare syndrome occurs in young children at an average age of $2\frac{1}{2}$ years. Its onset is usually insidious and is characterized by marked edema, heavy proteinuria, serious depletion of plasma proteins, especially the albumin fraction, and elevated blood cholesterol. In lipoid nephrosis hematuria, hypertension, and azotemia are absent. Some children after months or even years may recover completely, but many progress to the terminal stages of nephritis or succumb to infections.

The persistent edema is often so marked that it seems as if the skin would break. It may mask a severe state of undernutrition which becomes apparent only as diuresis takes place. The administration of ACTH or of cortisone has resulted in a great reduction of edema in most instances where it has been tried.

* Nutramigen and Sobee by Mead Johnson & Co., Evansville, Indiana.
† Mul-Soy by the Borden Company, New York City.
‡ Meat base formula by Gerber Products Company, Fremont, Michigan.

Modification of the diet. Patients with nephrosis have a particularly poor appetite, and every attempt must be made to serve foods which are acceptable to the child. Foods concentrated in protein and in energy value must be emphasized.

Energy. Unless the caloric intake is great enough to supply the body's energy needs, effective tissue regeneration will not take place. The needs should be based on the child's desirable weight rather than on his actual weight.

Protein. About 3 to 4 gm protein per kilogram body weight is suitable for the preschool child and 2 to 3 gm per kilogram for school-age children.

Sodium. When there is excessive edema, the sodium may be restricted (see Chap. 36). Unsalted foods are poorly accepted so that prolonged restriction is usually undesirable.

ALLERGY

Foods are responsible for the majority of allergies in children under 3 years of age. The chief offending foods are milk, eggs, wheat, white potato, chocolate, and oranges. When the child is young, it is relatively simple to determine which food is responsible by allowing only milk and crystalline vitamins. If a food other than milk is responsible, the symptoms, such as eczema, will be relieved in a few days; but if milk or nonfood allergy is responsible for the disturbance, no improvement will take place.

If milk is the allergen, it is sometimes only necessary to change the form of the milk; that is, boiled, powdered, acidulated, or evaporated milk may be satisfactory while fresh, unaltered milk is not. In other instances goat's milk may be an effective substitute for cow's milk, but occasionally the child will tolerate no milk whatsoever. Many infants have been fed on soybean "milk" or protein hydrolysates and have experienced normal growth and development.[217] A formula containing cooked rice, strained beef, Dextri-maltose, lard, salt mixture, and vitamins has been recently described.[218] The majority of infants gain tolerance to milk and need not continue on a milk-free diet indefinitely. Others may be desensitized to milk (see p. 551).

Where the symptoms of allergy are mild, one must always consider the relative importance of the allergic disturbance and the diet of the child. It is better management, for example, to treat a mild case of eczema locally than to subject the child to the dangers of an inadequate diet with its far more serious consequences.

For older children, the diagnosis of allergy is accomplished by means of skin tests and the usual elimination diets, and treatment is planned as for adults (see Chap. 39).

FEEDING HANDICAPPED CHILDREN

Cerebral palsy. Various crippling conditions occur as the result of brain damage. The feeding problems depend upon the type of crippling which is present.[219]

Reverse swallowing wave. When the motor system of the tongue and throat is affected, food is not pushed back to the throat, but the tongue motion pushes the food forward. Initially such children must be tube fed, but in time they learn to put food at the back of the tongue and by tilting the head backwards learn to swallow. These children often become severely undernourished because feeding is such a prolonged process. Concentrated foods with maximum protein and caloric value should be emphasized to keep the volume which must be taken to a minimum. Vitamin and mineral supplements are usually required.

Athetoids are those who are constantly in motion and who thus burn up a great deal of energy. They require a high-calorie diet but even so they may fail to gain weight. The high-caloric requirement also accelerates the vitamin requirement.

Spastics are very limited in their activity, and they may also be indulged in eating by their parents. Consequently they gain excessive amounts of weight, and the obesity in turn further restricts the ability to get around. These individuals require marked restriction of caloric intake without jeopardizing the intake of protein, minerals, and vitamins.

Cleft palate. Surgery for cleft palate is often not completed for several years. In addition to the needs for normal development, the infant and child must build up reserves for surgery, the promotion of healing, and the development of normal healthy gums and teeth. According to Zickefoose [220] the major problems of feeding these children may be met in the following ways:

1. Infants may have difficulty in sucking but most of them learn to use chewing movements to get the milk out of the nipple. An enlarged nipple opening is helpful. Some babies may be fed with a medicine dropper or a Brecht feeder.

2. To counteract the tendency to choke, liquids should be taken in small amounts and swallowed slowly.

3. More frequent "burpings" are necessary because of the large amount of air which may be swallowed.

4. Spicy and acid foods often irritate the mouth and nose and should be avoided. If orange juice is not well taken, ascorbic acid supplement should be prescribed.

5. Among the foods which may get into the opening of the palate are peanut butter, peelings of raw fruit, nuts, leafy vegetables, and creamed dishes. Some children have no difficulty with any foods.

6. Puréed foods may be diluted with milk, fruit juice, or broth and

given from a bottle with a large nipple opening. Some babies accept purées well if they are thickened with vanilla wafer or graham-cracker crumbs.

7. The time required for feeding may be long and requires much patience on the part of parent and nurse. For the older child, five or six small meals may be better than three.

When surgery has been performed, a liquid or puréed diet is offered until healing is complete.

Mental retardation. Some five million persons in the United States are estimated to be mentally retarded. Of these, about 75 per cent have an I.Q. between 51 and 75 (educable) and are designated as "high-grade." Approximately 20 per cent of the mentally retarded are "middle-grade," that is, they have an I.Q. between 21 and 50 (trainable). The "low-grade" individual with an I.Q. below 20 is believed to account for 5 per cent of the mentally retarded and presents the problems in feeding.

The nutritional requirements of the mentally retarded child and adult are like those of the individual of normal mental development. The nurse can help parents to understand the problems of feeding by giving encouragement and support.

The mentally retarded child may be kept on the bottle too long, thus increasing the difficulties of introducing other foods. The child may eat very slowly, and feeding may be messy. Hand sucking and vomiting are not uncommon.[221] To obtain adequate food intake for growth may require frequent, small feedings, and certainly an abundance of patience and ingenuity. One must strike a balance between overprotectiveness and lack of caring.

The retarded individual, like the normal person, has an active emotional life. He feels the shunning of others and his failure to achieve, but will respond to loving attention.[222] He resists new foods, has definite likes and dislikes, and finds it difficult to manage eating. He responds to the color of foods and like all children is fond of sweets.

When the individual is able to feed himself, he should be permitted to do so even though feeding may be messy. Food must be presented in a form that can be easily managed. Foods may be eaten with the fingers for a long time until simple utensils can be managed. The child unable to support himself should be held in a sitting position while he is being fed.

PROBLEMS AND REVIEW

1. What dietary problems may be anticipated in children who must be hospitalized? How can these problems be overcome?

2. How can a school child be helped to adjust to a prolonged therapeutic diet?

3. *Problem.* Adjust a 1500 calorie diet of an adult so that it will be suitable for a 12-year-old boy. In what ways would you try to effect acceptance of this diet?

4. What dietary considerations would apply for a 7-year-old child with scarlet fever?

5. *Problem.* List a number of ways in which you could encourage a boy with rheumatic fever to take an adequate diet.

6. *Problem.* Plan six high-calorie afterschool and bedtime snacks which could be added to the regular diet of a teen-age girl who is 20 pounds underweight.

7. What changes in diet might be indicated for an infant who is constipated? A 4-year-old child?

8. What are the similarities between celiac disease and cystic fibrosis? What differences are there?

9. *Problem.* Plan a day's meals for a 3-year-old child with celiac disease who is receiving a moderate-starch, high-protein, low-fat diet. How would you modify this diet for the child with pancreatic deficiency?

10. List the differences between diabetes in children and in adults.

11. What arguments can you give for, and against, chemical control in childhood diabetes?

12. Enumerate the points which are essential in the instruction of the child and/or his parent with respect to diabetes.

13. What is the effect of physical activity on the control of diabetes in the child?

14. Prepare a plan for the organization of a diabetic club for children. Include suggestions for meetings for such a group.

15. A diabetic child is invited to a birthday party. What plans can be made so that the child may eat at this party?

16. What is meant by phenylketonuria? What are the sources of phenylalanine in the diet?

17. *Problem.* Assuming that the patient might receive 500 mg phenylalanine in addition to his calculated formula, plan for the inclusion of typical foods which would supply this amount. Show how you arrived at this plan.

18. *Problem.* Prepare a list of foods which must be omitted on a galactose-free diet.

19. *Problem.* Examine the label information on *Sobee, Mul-Soy,* and *Nutramigen.* What foods must be added to formulas from these products for satisfactory nutrition of the infant?

20. *Problem.* Plan a diet suitable for a 2-year-old child with nephrosis containing 50 gm protein and 1200 calories. How would you modify this for 500 mg sodium?

CHAPTER 41 /

Diets and Tests for Diagnostic Purposes

There are many conditions in which certain dietary procedures must be used in order to make a diagnosis. In some cases it is necessary to omit or greatly reduce certain nutrients in the diet before starting the test. It may be necessary to use one food substance only, as in testing the patient for glucose tolerance. To illustrate such conditions, a few representative test diets and procedures have been included here, though the list is by no means complete.

URINE TESTS FOR SUGAR
BENEDICT QUALITATIVE TEST

Procedure. Urine samples for testing are collected at about 7 and 11 A.M., and 4 and 9 P.M. Place exactly 8 drops of the urine in a test tube and add exactly 5 ml of Benedict's qualitative solution. Place the tube in a vessel of bubbling boiling water, and allow it to remain there exactly 5 minutes. Permit to stand until cool. If an abnormal or pathologic amount of sugar is present, a greenish yellow, reddish brown, or red turbidity or precipitate results, which renders the solution opaque. (See Fig. 41-1.) If the urine and reagent are not accurately measured, or if the test tube is held over an open flame, the accuracy of the test may be impaired. Do not use Benedict's quantitative solution for this test.

Significance. The changes in color due to the presence of sugar in urine, as in diabetes mellitus, may be interpreted as follows:

1. The turbid green represents a trace of sugar; if the specimen is clear blue or green, sufficiently to allow print to be read through it, this specimen is considered negative.

2. A change to yellow and orange indicates the presence of about 0.5 to 1.0 per cent.

3. A change to brick red or chocolate brown indicates the presence of 2 or more per cent.

COMMERCIAL TESTS FOR URINE SUGAR

Two commercial preparations greatly simplify the detection of sugar in the urine. One of these, Clinistix[R],* consists of an enzyme-impregnated strip which is dipped into the sample of urine. One minute later, the color on the strip is compared with a standard color guide and the presence of small or large amounts of glucose can be detected.

Clinitest[R] * reagent tablets employ the principle of copper reduction, but heating is not required. Five drops of urine are placed in a test tube and 10 drops of water are added. The test tablet is dropped into the test tube, and allowed to stand for 15 seconds after the boiling reaction in the tube has ceased. The contents are then shaken, and the color compared with a color guide provided with each bottle of tablets (see Fig. 41-1B). This test provides a more quantitative estimation than that with the Clinistix[R].

URINE TEST FOR ACETOACETIC ACID (GERHARDT'S FERRIC CHLORIDE TEST)

Procedure. Pour 1 teaspoon (5 ml) of freshly voided urine into a clean test tube and add, drop by drop, a 10 per cent solution of ferric chloride, noting the change of color during the process. In the presence of acetoacetic acid the color of the specimen changes to a wine red. Ferric chloride solution is added until there is no further deepening of the color. One-half of the specimen just tested is then poured into a second tube which is heated over the flame 3 minutes or in boiling water 5 minutes. If acetoacetic acid is present, the color will fade to a lighter color. If the patient has been taking aspirin or antipyrine, the color will be a bluish red and remain so when the specimen is heated.

Significance. Acetoacetic acid is one of the ketones which may be present in urine when fat is incompletely oxidized. If it is present, it is a serious symptom and may indicate approaching diabetic coma. The patient should immediately take a specimen to his physician.

GLUCOSE TOLERANCE TEST

Test diet. For 3 days prior to the test the patient should eat a diet which contains at least 300 gm of carbohydrate. To prepare glucose for the test: dissolve glucose in water, using about 10 ml of water for each 4 gm of glucose. Some physicians specify 1.75 gm glucose per kg of body weight, while others use an arbitrary amount—50 to 100 gm. Lemon juice may be used for flavoring, if desired.

Procedure. The test is performed after a fast of 12 hours or more. Obtain

* Ames Company, Inc., Elkhart, Indiana.

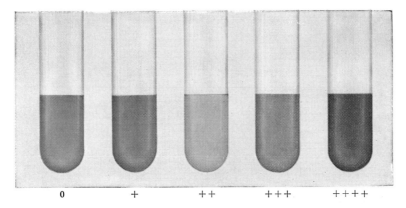

0   +   + +   + + +   + + + +

FIG. 41-1A. The Benedict color scale for sugar in urine. Eight drops of urine are added to a test tube containing exactly 5 ml of Benedict's solution. The test tube is then placed in boiling water and left there exactly 5 minutes. Permit to stand until cool. The color of the solution, when compared with the color scale, will indicate the presence and amount of sugar in the urine. *(Courtesy, Eli Lilly and Company, Indianapolis, Ind.)*

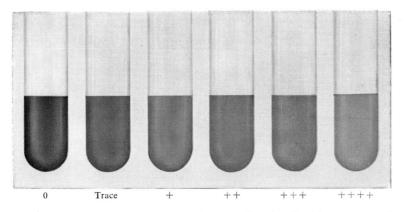

0   Trace   +   + +   + + +   + + + +

FIG. 41-1B. The Clinitest color scale for sugar in urine. In this test, external heat has been eliminated, as the reagent tablet generates heat inside the test tube. See page 576. *(Courtesy, The Ames Company, Inc., Elkhart, Ind.)*

a blood sample just before giving the prescribed amount of glucose, and again at the end of ½, 1, 2, and 3 hours after giving the glucose. Collect urine samples and test them for sugar.

Significance. The blood sugar rises sharply at ½ to 1 hour after giving glucose to normal individuals. It falls to the original level by the end of the second hour, if the individual has a normal sugar tolerance (see Fig. 41-2). There is no glycosuria.

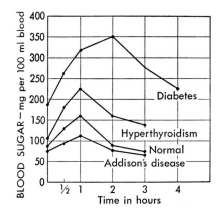

Fig. 41-2. Glucose tolerance curves.

In diabetes mellitus the maximum sugar concentration is reached at about the end of the second hour, and is slow in returning to the normal value. The elevated blood sugar levels are accompanied by an excretion of sugar in the urine.

The glucose tolerance curve is very flat in Addison's disease, in hypothyroidism, and in hyperinsulinism.

Elevation of the glucose tolerance curve is characteristic of hyperthyroidism.

GASTRIC ANALYSIS

Purpose. To examine the contents of the stomach in order to determine gastric acidity and emptying time of the stomach.

Test meals. There is an increasing tendency to omit test meals before gastric analysis. The purpose of giving meals is to stimulate the secretion of gastric juices.

Ewald test diet. The following meal is given on an empty stomach, usually in the morning.

1 shredded-wheat biscuit or 4 large soda crackers or arrowroot cookies
1½ glasses (300 to 400 ml) water or weak tea; no cream or sugar

Bread was formerly used in this test, but it has been found that the yeast or lactic acid may confuse the interpretation of results. The Ewald meal produces only mild stimulation and may indicate a high percentage of cases of achlorhydria.

Riegel meal.[223] This meal is used when hypoacidity is suspected. It consists of 200 ml of beef broth; 150 to 200 gm of broiled steak, well masticated; and 100 gm of mashed potato.

Alcohol test meal. Fifty ml of 7 per cent ethyl alcohol are injected into the fasting stomach through a small tube. The disadvantage of this method of stimulation is that it is somewhat unphysiologic.

Histamine. After the patient has fasted for 12 hours or more, a calculated dose of histamine is injected hypodermically. Histamine is a very powerful stimulant for the secretion of gastric juice and is used to test the ability of the stomach to secrete acid and pepsin. It helps to differentiate between a true and false achlorhydria.

Motor meal. Twelve hours preceding the examination the patient is given a meal consisting of such items as rice and raisins, a meat sandwich and 30 raisins, or a meal with stewed prunes. The fiber is readily recognized in the gastric contents of the morning of examination if there is decreased motility.

Barium or bismuth meal. It is customary to give the patient a bismuth or barium meal in order that an x-ray and fluoroscopic examination may be made to determine the character and extent of the disturbance. This meal consists of a pint of fluid, either buttermilk or malted milk, into which a certain amount of bismuth or barium chloride is mixed. The progress of this meal can be studied throughout the entire intestinal tract. It is possible to determine the emptying time, motility, and defects suggestive of disease.

Procedure. In the morning, before the patient has received food, a tube is passed into the stomach by way of the nose or pharynx so that the contents of the stomach may be withdrawn and examined. The test meal is then given, and a stomach tube reinserted. The tube is left in place and specimens of the stomach contents are obtained at stated intervals, usually at 15-minute intervals for about 2 hours. A single specimen taken at 45 minutes following the test meal is often used in place of the fractional method. The gastric contents are measured and examined for free and total acid, for the presence of bile, mucus, pus, and blood.

Significance. Many normal persons show a wide range of acid secretion so that the findings are not in themselves diagnostic but must be interpreted in the light of other findings. Amounts of fluid in excess of 50 to 100 ml for the first hour after an Ewald meal indicate hypersecretion or stasis, while volumes less than 20 ml are likely when emptying of the stomach is too rapid.

An increase of hydrochloric acid (hyperchlorhydria) may occur in peptic ulcers and in gastritis. A decrease of hydrochloric acid (hypochlorhydria) is significant in carcinoma in the early stages, chronic gastritis, and pellagra. Absence of hydrochloric acid (achlorhydria) is indicative of advanced carcinoma, pernicious anemia, some cases of pellagra, and occasionally of tuberculosis.

The diminution or absence of pepsin or rennin occurs in various organic stomach disorders. The presence of blood in the stomach contents usually indicates ulcers or carcinoma.

DUODENAL DRAINAGE

Purpose. To obtain duodenal contents for chemical, microscopic, or bacteriologic examination.

Procedure. Allow no food for 12 hours before and until after completion of the test. A flexible rubber tube is swallowed by the patient. It is carried into the duodenum after a time, and the fluid begins to siphon out. Tests may then be made on the collected contents.

Significance. Diminution or absence of amylopsin, steapsin, or trypsin indicates subnormal secretion of the pancreas or obstruction of the pancreatic duct. An excess of pus cells gives information on the possibility of inflammation of the duodenum. The presence of bile in the duodenal fluid rules out obstruction of the hepatic or bile ducts. An increase of urobilin is of significance in the diagnosis of hemolytic anemias.

GALACTOSE TOLERANCE

Purpose. To determine the ability of the liver to convert galactose to glycogen.

Procedure. Omit breakfast and hold lunch until test is completed. Give 40 gm of pure galactose in 500 ml of water flavored with lemon juice. Allow water as desired. Collect urine and blood hourly for 5 hours and test quantitatively for sugar.

Significance. An excretion of more than 3 gm of sugar may indicate intrahepatic jaundice.

HIPPURIC ACID TEST

Purpose. To determine the ability of the liver to synthesize hippuric acid from benzoic acid.

Test diet. A light breakfast consisting of toast and coffee is given.

Procedure. One hour after breakfast give 6 gm of sodium benzoate dissolved in 30 ml of water and follow with 100 ml of water. Collect urine specimens hourly for 4 hours, and determine the hippuric acid excretion.

Significance. Excretion of less than 3 gm of hippuric acid indicates liver impairment—catarrhal jaundice, hepatitis of various forms, cirrhosis.

GALLBLADDER SERIES

Purpose. To determine function of the gallbladder by x-ray.

Test meals. A low-fat supper is given at 5 P.M. followed by the dye at 6 P.M. No food or fluids are permitted after 10 P.M. The supper may consist of:

Fruit or tomato juice
Fruit or vegetable salad without dressing of any kind
Boiled vegetables without butter
Bread or toast with jelly; no butter
Canned fruit or plain gelatin without cream or milk
Tea with sugar; no milk

Some allow black coffee at breakfast the next morning, while others omit all fluid until after the x-ray which is taken about 10 A.M. The x-ray in some cases is repeated after a high-fat luncheon which may consist of:

2 slices bacon
2 eggs fried in butter
1 slice toast with a pat of butter
1 glass cream
Coffee or tea with cream and sugar
                  or
2 eggs with 1 pint cream, vanilla, and sugar

KIDNEY FUNCTION TESTS

DILUTION TEST

Purpose. To determine the ability of the kidney to excrete fluids.

Procedure. Omit breakfast. Discard the morning urine specimen and give 1500 ml of water at 8 A.M. Collect urine in separate containers at 8:30, 9, 9:30, 10, 10:30, 11, 11:30 A.M., 12 M., and as a single specimen from 12 M. to 8 A.M. Determine the specific gravity of each sample.

Significance. The total volume of urine excreted should be 80 to 120 per cent of the intake. The specific gravity of at least one sample should be as low as 1.003. A lower quantity than that indicated above and a consistently higher specific gravity are indicative of kidney impairment.

MOSENTHAL CONCENTRATION TEST FOR KIDNEY FUNCTION

Purpose. To measure the variations in specific gravity and volume of urine using the Mosenthal test-meal method.[224]

Test diet. Formerly, this test was performed with a diet prescribed by Mosenthal, but equally satisfactory results are obtained using a normal diet. On the day preceding the test and on the day of the test the patient is given at each meal, in addition to his regular diet, at least 1 pint of fluid in the form of water, tea, or coffee. No food or fluid is taken between meals, or until after 8 A.M. on the morning concluding the test.

Procedure. The patient is to empty the bladder at 8 A.M. and at each 2-hour interval thereafter. The specimens of urine are collected in separate, properly labeled bottles until 8 P.M. The 8 P.M. to 8 A.M. collection is kept in one container.

Significance. The volume of the night urine should be much less than that of the day collections. It will usually have a specific gravity above 1.018. Nocturnal polyuria (over 750 ml) suggests renal impairment. The maximal specific gravity of the day urine samples should exceed 1.018. The difference between the highest and lowest specific gravity should be at least 8 to 9 points; that is, if the most concentrated specimen has a specific gravity of 1.020, the most dilute will be 1.012 or less.

LOW-SODIUM, HIGH-POTASSIUM DIET FOR DIAGNOSIS OF ADRENOCORTICAL INSUFFICIENCY (CUTLER, POWER, WILDER DIET [225])

Purpose. To determine the concentration of chloride in the urine when a diet containing a low-sodium and high-potassium level is given.

Test meals. All food is prepared and served without salt. All foods are weighed.

Breakfast

	Grams
Orange	100
Salt-poor bread	50
Salt-poor butter	10
Jelly	20
Cream, 20 per cent	25
Coffee	300
Egg—1	

Luncheon or Supper

	Grams
Beef, raw weight	50
Baked potato	100
Canned peas	100
Lettuce	10
Grapefruit	100
Banana	100
Salt-poor bread	30
Salt-poor butter	10
Jelly	20
Cream, 20 per cent	75
Milk	200

Dinner

		Mineral Content	
Beef (raw weight)	75	Sodium	0.59
Baked potato	100	Chlorine	0.95
Canned tomato	90	Potassium	4.1
Lettuce	10		
Peaches	100		
Salt-poor bread	30		
Salt-poor butter	10		
Jelly	20		
Jell-O	150		
Cream, 20 per cent	25		
Coffee	200		

Procedure. A low-salt diet is given on the day preceding the test diet. The test diet is used for not more than 3 days. If any foods are refused, their potassium content is replaced with potassium citrate. In addition to the diet, potassium citrate is given on the afternoon of the first day at a level of 42 mg of potassium citrate per pound of body weight (33 mg potassium per kg of body weight). This dose is repeated on the morning of the second day. A fluid intake of 40 ml per kg of body weight is maintained. On the third day 20 ml of fluid per kg are given before 11 A.M. The tests end at noon of the third day. Urine is collected at 8 A.M. and 12 noon on the third day.

Caution. Because this diet may be dangerous in severe adrenal insufficiency, the patient must be watched carefully. Sodium chloride, glucose, and cortical hormone must be immediately available for intravenous therapy in the event of symptoms of Addisonian crisis.

Significance. Under the conditions of this test a urinary concentration of chloride above 225 mg per cent indicates poor function of the adrenal cortex, while a chloride concentration of 125 mg per cent or less indicates normal function. When glomerulonephritis or uncontrolled diabetes is present, the test is of limited value.

LOW-CALCIUM TEST DIET

Purpose. This is a diet providing a constant allowance of food for 1 week. It contains approximately 130 mg calcium, and 650 mg phosphorus, and yields a neutral ash.[226] It is used to study the metabolism of calcium under conditions of minimum intake.

Test diet. The following meal plan is used. No substitutions are made.

Breakfast

Orange juice	½ cup	Bread, Italian style		Crisp bacon	3 slices
Cooked farina		made without		Coffee or tea	
without added		milk	2 slices	Sugar; salt	
calcium	⅓ cup	Margarine			

Luncheon

Chicken	1 medium serving
Rice, cooked	⅓ cup cooked
Tomato, cooked or raw	1 serving
Bread	1 slice
Margarine	
Apple, raw or apple-sauce	1 serving
Tea or coffee	
Sugar; salt	

Dinner

Lean meat	1 serving
Potato	1 medium
Corn, not cream style	1 serving
Bread or crackers made without milk	1 slice
Margarine	
Banana	1 medium
Tea or coffee	
Sugar; salt	

PRACTICAL APPLICATIONS OF NUTRITION: ELEMENTARY FOOD STUDY /

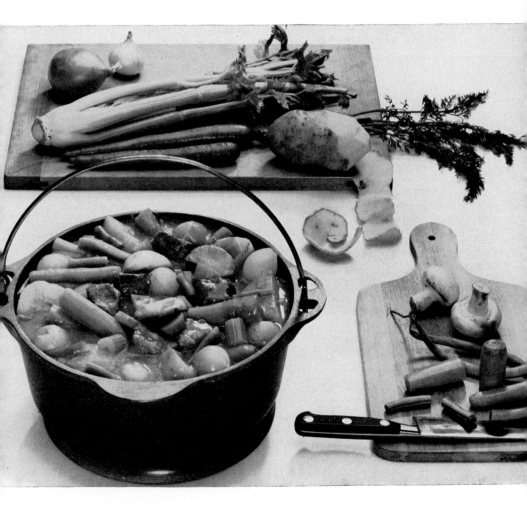

UNIT XII /
Foods—Their Characteristics and Preparation

CHAPTER 54 RECIPES (continued)

Desserts and Dessert Sauces

Eggs

Fruits

Meat, Poultry, and Fish

Salads and Salad Dressings

Sauces and Soups

Vegetables

Sodium-restricted Recipes

Introduction to the Study of Elementary Cookery

Knowledge concerning preparation and service of food is important. Good food is a fundamental physiologic and psychologic need of man. Only when the science and art of cookery are carefully interwoven is it possible to realize optimum utilization of food which has been produced and distributed at great cost in terms of time, money, and available resources. Good cookery implies a minimum waste of food because essential nutrients are retained during the preparation process and because the palatability score is so high that the food will be eaten.

The student nurse realizes that she must have the ability to apply the principles of nutrition in the daily selection of her own meals if she expects to enjoy good health and vitality in the pursuit of her profession. She knows that her attitudes toward food and her own radiant health are the best possible examples for better nutrition in others. She is aware of the fact that meals for the sick require special emphasis on many factors which influence palatability, since the appetite may be finicky even though nutritive needs may be greater than normal. A thorough knowledge concerning protein, calories, vitamins, etc., is of no avail if unappetizing food served to the patient arouses anger, resentment, and lack of cooperation.

The nurse of today is rarely expected to prepare food for her patient, but she should be able to plan, prepare, and serve simple nourishing meals when asked to do so. One of the important aspects of the plan for rehabilitation of every patient is consideration for diet—normal as well as therapeutic. Nurses, as well as dietitians, are assuming more responsibility for the nutrition education of the patient. This takes place in the hospital setting or in the out-patient clinic, and is not the sole responsibility of public health workers. The dietitian and nurse are normally expected to give instruction relating to therapeutic diets, but in order to make this teaching effective they must often give attention to the budgeting of the food dollar and include practical advice on food selection and preparation. Unless the dietitian and nurse have had some experience in these important areas of dietetics, it is improbable that

589

they will be able to command sufficient authority to be of assistance to the patient.

While the course in elementary cookery is designed primarily to acquaint the student with an appreciation, knowledge, and skill in simple food preparation for herself and for the patient, such training has lifelong value. In a short course in cookery one cannot expect to become truly skilled, but through continued observation and practice of procedures described in the text it is possible to achieve a high degree of accomplishment.

Reasons for cooking foods. The inclusion of some raw fruits and vegetables in the daily diet is considered essential. However, man's discovery of the cookery of food has greatly broadened the choice of edible foods as well as increased their palatability. One of the most important reasons for cooking food is to enhance the digestibility. Cooking softens the connective tissue of meat and the coarse fiber of fruits and vegetables so that the digestive period is shortened and the gastrointestinal tract is less subject to irritation. Cooking also bursts the starch granule of vegetables and cereals so that starch digestion is more rapid and complete.

The cooking of food is important to destroy microorganisms and parasites which may be present. It is well known that pork is safe to eat only after thorough cooking has destroyed Trichinella which may infest the meat. The limitations of cookery should be realized, however. Many foods are not subjected to a sufficiently high temperature to destroy microorganisms, and cookery should never be an excuse for permitting careless handling of food prior to its cookery. (See Chap. 21.)

Of equal importance are the psychologic benefits derived from the cooking of foods. Some foods such as meats are unappetizing in appearance when raw but achieve high desirability in their cooked form. The variety of uses to which foods may be put is greatly increased by the art of cookery, with the result that the diet becomes much more interesting.

Some considerations in the study of foods. Superior achievement in the preparation of foods is dependent upon adherence to sound scientific procedures and application of the principles of art in cookery.

The handling of foods from the producer to the consumer influences markedly their retention of nutrients and their safety. For example, vegetables which are crisp are better sources of vitamins than those which have not been properly hydrated. Storage, after purchase, is suited to the food. Perishable foods—milk, eggs, butter, meats, and many fruits and vegetables—require refrigeration not only to keep them safe but to keep them of high nutritive value. Other foods, such as cereals, sugar, and flour, do not spoil readily or change in value and are stored in a dry place in covered containers to exclude dust and insects.

Good sanitation requires observation of personal hygiene, proper cleanliness of dishes and utensils, and care in the preparation of the food itself. Fruits and vegetables should always be washed before they are cooked and served to rid them of dust, insects, sprays, and microorganisms.

Foods will be most palatable when these factors are emphasized.

1. *Color.* The first appeal of food is to the eye. Attractive combinations of color stimulate the appetite, just as vegetables which have retained their color not only look good to eat but actually taste better. For example, green broccoli served with hollandaise or cheese sauce is tempting, while over-cooked brown broccoli might well create a permanent dislike for this vegetable.

2. *Flavor.* Probably no class of foods is more frequently cooked poorly in public eating places than vegetables. The practice of overcooking, the use of too much or too little salt, or the flavor of baking soda mask or inhibit natural flavors of foods. Just as good color combinations are important, so good flavor combinations are necessary; that is, mild and strongly flavored foods, bland and acid foods.

3. *Texture.* No one likes monotonously soft foods, just as meals which require excessive mastication may be tiresome. Thus, a combination of textures is desirable. Cookery greatly affects texture, for meats may be tough or tender; vegetables may be crisp and tender, or soft and soggy; desserts may be smooth or lumpy. Overmature foods, for instance, peas or beans, may have poor texture in spite of the best efforts in cookery.

Standards for tray service. The observation of the above principles will go far in assuring good food for the patient. Satisfactory tray service requires consideration of these additional points. See Fig. 42-1.

1. The tray should be of a size suitable for the food to be served—small trays for liquid nourishment and large trays for full meals.

2. The tray cover and napkins, of linen or good quality paper, should be of suitable size for the tray, immaculately clean, and unwrinkled.

3. Everything on the tray must reflect cleanliness—sparkling glassware, shining silver, clean china. Salt and pepper shakers with finger marks, or soiled name cards detract markedly from good appearance.

4. The tray should be set with the most attractive china available.

5. The tray should be symmetrically arranged for the greatest convenience. All necessary silver and accessories should be included.

6. Foods should be attractively served, with the size of portions not being overlarge. Spilled liquid or sloppy serving of food is inexcusable. Garnishes help to make foods more appealing.

7. Foods should be served on time. This requires careful planning so that foods will be prepared in the proper sequence.

8. Foods should be served at the proper temperature. Hot foods should be served on hot plates, protected with a cover, while cold foods should be served on chilled dishes.

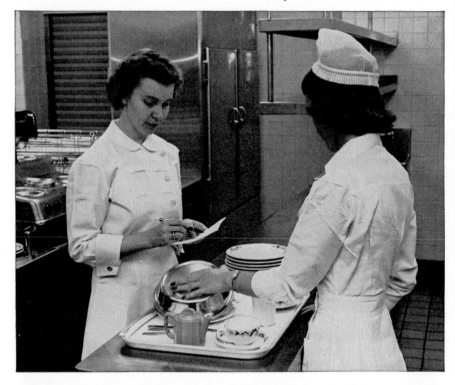

Fig. 42-1. Dietitian and nurse work closely together to assure satisfactory tray service to the patient. (*Courtesy, National Institutes of Health, U.S. Department of Health, Education, and Welfare.*)

Methods of cookery and definition of common terms. Foods may be cooked by moist heat, by dry heat, or by frying. Cookery by moist heat includes boiling, stewing, braising, and steaming.

Boiling is cooking in water at 212° F or 100° C. The bubbles break rapidly on the surface of the water.

Simmering is cooking at a temperature below the boiling point—approximately 200° F or 93° C. The bubbles of steam rise slowly to the surface of the vessel.

Stewing is cooking for a long time at about 200° F. It is used for tougher cuts of meat. The liquid is sometimes thickened.

Braising is cooking over direct heat or in an oven in a small amount of liquid at a low temperature with the pan tightly covered.

Steaming is cooking by the heat of direct steam or in a steam-jacketed vessel such as a double boiler or bain-marie. The pressure cooker employs increased pressure of steam, thus raising the temperature and shortening the cooking time.

Cooking by dry heat includes broiling, pan broiling, baking, and roasting.

Broiling is cooking by direct heat from a gas flame, electric wires, or live coals. It is usually used for tender cuts of meat, and the temperature is high enough quickly to sear the surface.

Pan broiling is cooking in a hot metal pan on the top of the stove with just enough fat to keep the food from sticking; fat is poured off as it accumulates.

Baking is cooking in an oven using an open or covered pan. The oven *roasting* of meats is really a baking process. The most commonly used oven temperatures are as follows:

Slow $= 250°$ to $350°$ F
Moderate $= 350°$ to $400°$ F
Hot $= 400°$ to $450°$ F
Very hot $= 450°$ to $500°$ F

Frying is cooking by immersion in hot fat at $350°$ to $400°$ F.

Sautéing is cooking in a small amount of fat in a frying pan, the food being turned frequently.

Fricasseeing is cooking in a small amount of fat and then serving with a sauce.

Many other terms are so frequently used in food preparation that an early understanding of them is helpful.

Basting is the process of pouring small amounts of liquid or fat over the surface of food to improve the flavor, prevent dryness, and avoid scorching. Roast fowl and meats may be basted, for example.

Beating is the turning of ingredients over and over with a rotary beater or whip to incorporate the maximum amount of air.

Creaming is the blending of sugar and fat by rubbing together with a wooden spoon or in an electric mixer.

Dicing is the cutting of food in small uniform cubes.

Dredging means to sprinkle flour and seasonings prior to browning, as in the preparation of Swiss steak or fried eggplant.

Folding is the combining of ingredients in such a way that air is retained. With a spoon, using a downward motion, one ingredient such as whipped egg white is cut into other ingredients and the entire mixture is then carefully turned over. This process is gently repeated, always in the same direction, until blending is just complete.

Marination is the coating of food with acid or oil to develop flavor or to tenderize the product. Thus, vegetable salads may be marinated with French dressing to improve the flavor, while meat may be coated with vinegar to tenderize it.

Mincing is the cutting of food into very fine pieces; for example, minced chives, parsley, or onion.

Parboiling is the partial cooking of food in liquid prior to other preparation.

Puréeing is the pressing of foods through a strainer to remove seeds and fiber. This is also referred to as *straining*.

Searing is browning of the surface of food such as meats in order to improve the color. Braised meats are often seared initially.

Stirring is the mixing of ingredients by using a circular motion with a spoon. A wooden spoon is preferable for many procedures.

How to measure ingredients. Accurate measurements are essential to successful food preparation. Correct measurements require a standard 8-ounce measuring cup divided into fourths and thirds, and standard measuring spoons. Nests of measuring cups—¼, ⅓, ½, and 1 cup—are ideal for measuring dry ingredients and soft fats.

All measurements in recipes are level. White flour and confectioner's sugar should be sifted once before measuring. Dry ingredients should be spooned lightly into the cup or measuring spoon until they are heaped over the edges, and then leveled off with the edge of a knife. Never dip the cup into the ingredient. Tapping the cup or shaking it to level it off should be avoided. Brown sugar is the only dry ingredient which is packed into the cup.

If standard measuring spoons are not available, to measure half a spoonful, fill spoon, level off with a knife, and divide contents lengthwise with a knife, removing the unnecessary portion.

Except for pastry, fat should be at room temperature. It is packed into the cup or spoon and leveled off with a knife. To measure ½ cup of cold fat, put cold water to the ½-cup mark, and add fat until the water rises to the 1-cup mark. Pour off the water and add the fat to the other ingredients. Likewise, to measure ¼ cup fat, bring water to the ¾-cup mark and add fat until the water rises to the 1-cup mark. Melted fat has the same volume as solid fat.

Liquids are more easily measured in a heat-resistant glass cup which has a space above the full-cup line to prevent spilling. One should be aware, however, of this extra space to avoid errors in measurement. When sirups or molasses are measured, a preliminary light greasing of the cup will facilitate emptying.

Instructions for work. It is required that the student learn to observe good working habits, such as:

1. Read directions for food preparation carefully before beginning work. Plan work in proper sequence in order to have all of the assignment completed on time.

2. Wash hands with soap and water before beginning food preparation. Keep nails short and manicured. Cover the hair with a net.

3. Assemble all materials and utensils before beginning work.

4. Always use a utility plate for carrying materials from the supply table to the desk.

5. Take from the supply table only the exact measure of food needed; do not waste materials!

6. Use gas, electricity, water, and cleaning supplies only as needed.

7. Use as few utensils and dishes as possible; measure dry ingredients first, then liquids to save time in washing dishes.

8. Put pans to soak as soon as they have been used; use cold water for dishes in which protein foods have been cooked and hot water for dishes which are greasy or which have been used for starch cookery.

9. Wash dishes with plenty of hot, soapy water or a detergent; rinse dishes with hot, clear water. Wash glassware first, then silver, china, serving dishes, and finally cooking utensils.

10. Check desks each day for cleanliness and proper placement of equipment.

11. Return equipment taken from cupboards.

12. Perform housekeeping duties as assigned by instructor:
    a. Clean refrigerator.
    b. Clean stoves.
    c. Clean sinks and drainboards.
    d. Put away food supplies and clean supply tables. Wash containers and clean cupboards as necessary.
    e. Distribute clean towels at beginning of period. Collect and count soiled towels at end of period.

13. Work quietly. Be considerate of others in every way.

14. Learn to judge the results of cookery critically for color, flavor, texture, correct temperature.

CHAPTER 43 /

Beverages

A beverage is any material used as a drink for the purpose of relieving thirst and introducing fluid into the body, nourishing the body, and stimulating or soothing the individual.

Classification. Beverages may be placed in these groups according to the functions they serve.

I. Refreshing; to relieve thirst
    A. Water, plain or carbonated
    B. Ginger ale and other bottled beverages
    C. Fruit juices and fruitades
    D. Iced tea or coffee
II. Nourishing
    A. Milk: pasteurized, skim, evaporated, dried, malted, buttermilk, acid, chocolate, cocoa; high-protein; low-sodium
    B. Eggnog made with whisky, rum, brandy, fruit juices, coffee, chocolate
    C. Fruit juices with egg white or whole egg
    D. Glucose lemonade or orangeade
    E. Tube feedings (see Chap. 29)
III. Stimulating
    A. Eggnogs made with whisky, rum, brandy, or coffee
    B. Coffee and tea
IV. Soothing
    A. Warm milk
    B. Hot tea

Ingredients in beverages. The ingredients, used singly or in combination for the preparation of beverages, are discussed below.

Milk is the most important of all the liquid foods since it gives more nutritive value than any other food for the money spent. Milk beverages add protein, calories, calcium, and other nutrients to the diet. The mild flavor of milk permits its use in a great number of ways. It may be served plain, malted, or acidulated; it may be reinforced with egg, nonfat dry milk, gelatin, yeast, or various sugars depending upon the type of nutrient needed; and it may be flavored with chocolate, coffee, and flavoring extracts. Milk is discussed in more detail in Chapter 44.

Eggs are especially useful for increasing the protein content of beverages. Eggnogs in which whisky or other alcoholic beverages are used constitute the most important of the stimulating beverages. Eggnog made with strong coffee is only mildly stimulating but lends variety to the general liquid diets. Fruit eggnogs contain egg, cream, and possibly milk and sugar in addition to fruit juice.

Fruit and vegetable juices in themselves are not only pleasantly refreshing but they are easily digested and especially useful in increasing the fluid intake. The citrus juices and tomato juice are excellent for their ascorbic acid content. Fresh, frozen, and canned juices may be served plain or, in the case of fruit juices, sweetened; they may be reinforced with egg white or whole egg. The following list includes the commonly used juices.

1. Citrus: oranges, lemons, grapefruit, limes, tangerines
2. Berries: blackberries, loganberries, raspberries, strawberries
3. Tree fruits: apple, apricot, peach, pear, plum, prune
4. Other fruits: grapes, pineapple
5. Vegetable: tomato, sauerkraut, mixed

Chocolate is the paste made by mashing the fermented and roasted *cacao bean*. The paste is molded and sold as bitter chocolate. It contains approximately 50 per cent fat and some protein and carbohydrate. A mild stimulant, theobromine, is present in chocolate. Sweet chocolate contains added sugar, while milk chocolate consists of chocolate, milk, and sugar. Chocolate is important primarily as a flavoring adjunct, but it does have food value as well. A double boiler should be used for melting it, since scorching occurs readily.

Cocoa is the ground product of the cacao bean after some of the fat has been removed. By government regulation "breakfast cocoa" must contain not less than 22 per cent fat, although cocoa not so labeled may contain as little as 8 per cent fat. Cocoa powder should be boiled with water before adding milk in order to cook the starch and develop the flavor.

Sweetening and flavoring agents. Cane sugar, glucose, corn sirup, molasses, and occasionally honey and lactose may be used to sweeten beverages and to supply additional calories. Vanilla, butterscotch, and maple extracts, various fruit flavorings, and nutmeg and cinnamon lend variety when appropriately used.

Coffee is the bean of the coffee plant which grows in tropical countries. As a rule, it is imported in the green form which is tasteless. Roasting develops the volatile oils, specially caffeol, which give the characteristic aroma and flavor to coffee. The typical flavors of individual brands of coffee depend upon the proportions of the various types of coffee—such as Java, Mocha—used and upon the length of time of roasting. Bitterness is increased if the coffee is combined with such substances as chicory.

Coffee alone has no food value, but it does furnish a certain amount of stimulation because of the caffeine which raises the blood pressure, stimulates renal activity, and momentarily masks fatigue. As a rule, a cup of coffee contains 1.5 to 2.5 grains of caffeine, depending upon the strength of the brew. Tannin, another alkaloid, may interfere with digestion. The amount of tannin in coffee also depends upon the method of preparation, since it is soluble in hot water; the longer coffee is brewed, the greater will be the tannin content. Coffee that is boiled a long time and left standing on the grounds will thus have a bitter flavor.

Coffee beans are ground to increase the surface area for maximum extraction of flavor. However, caffeol is rapidly lost, the loss being greater in finely ground coffee. Connoisseurs may purchase the whole coffee beans and grind them just before the beverage is brewed, but most people purchase coffee freshly ground or in vacuum-packed cans. Ground coffee should be kept in a tightly covered tin in a cool place and should be used promptly after purchase.

Several methods for the preparation of coffee are described on page 670. Drip and vacuum coffee contain the least amount of tannin and caffeine and the greatest amount of caffeol. Percolated coffee contains slightly more caffeine and less caffeol than drip coffee. "Boiled" coffee should be steeped instead of boiled. It contains more caffeine and tannin than either drip or percolated coffee.

Instant coffee is made from pure coffee which has been pulverized. The extraction of caffeine and tannin is high, but the amount in the finished beverage will depend upon the amount of coffee used. Some instant coffees are mixed with malted cereal.

Decaffeinated coffee sold under various brand names has about 95 per cent of the caffeine removed. It does not possess the stimulating properties of coffee and may often be used by patients who cannot have coffee as such. Coffee substitutes, or cereal coffees, are made from a combination of roasted grains. They furnish no stimulation save that which is derived from the heat of the beverage.

Tea is obtained from the leaves and flowers of the tea bush which grows in subtropical China, India, and Japan. Teas in great variety are available on the market, both in bulk and in individual bags. The top tiny leaves and buds or flowers at the end of the shoot furnish the choicest and most expensive brands, designated as "flowery pekoe." Orange pekoe, the most commonly marketed tea, consists of the first and second leaf just below the buds. Pekoe and Souchong teas are of poorer quality.

The kind of tea is determined by its treatment subsequent to picking. Green tea undergoes no fermentation process and is light in color and rich in tannin. Black tea is fermented, dark in color, and has lost some of its tannin. Oolong tea is an intermediate product between the black and the green teas.

A good cup of tea will contain a high proportion of volatile oils and a minimum amount of tannin. Theine is a stimulant like caffeine and has approximately the same physiologic effects as caffeine. However, the usual American brew of tea is such that the amount of theine extracted is much less than the amount of caffeine in a like amount of coffee. This explains the relatively greater stimulating effect of coffee.

Tea which is allowed to stand too long in contact with the leaves contains a considerable amount of tannin, which causes the finished beverage to be bitter and unpalatable. The cloudiness of some iced tea is due to the precipitation of tannin and is an indication of too long a period of steeping.

Alcoholic beverages. The dietitian and the nurse never include alcoholic beverages as part of the diet except when expressly ordered by the physician. However, when they are so ordered, it is necessary to make allowance for their caloric contributions in any diets which are calculated. Certain of these beverages, such as the liqueurs, which contain carbohydrate must be considered in the calculation of diabetic diets.

Pure alcohol, when oxidized, yields about 7 calories per milliliter; but the maximum quantity which can be oxidized in an hour is about 10 ml, the amount contained in about one ounce of whisky.[227] In addition to the alcoholic content, sweet wines, liqueurs, and beer contain carbohydrate as unfermented sugar or as malt.

Fermented beverages include malt liquors such as beer, which contains 3 to 6 per cent alcohol by weight; light wines, which contain 8 to 12 per cent alcohol; other wines, such as port and sherry, which contain as much as 20 per cent alcohol.

Distilled liquors—brandy, gin, rum, and whisky—contain 40 to 50 per cent alcohol. The alcohol, carbohydrate, and caloric values of typical alcoholic beverages are indicated in the table on page 768.

Preparation of beverages. In preparing and serving beverages the following points should be kept in mind.

1. Beverages should be served as soon as possible after preparation in order to retain fresh, natural flavor.

2. Fruit beverages must be sufficiently tart to be refreshing. The addition of a little lemon juice to the sweet fruit juices will give them character. Tart juices do not require this addition.

3. Hot beverages should be hot, and cold beverages ice cold. If fruit is chilled before juices are extracted, no ice is necessary. Glasses may be placed in a bowl of crushed ice at serving time.

4. Beverages must not be diluted too much with either water or ice.

5. The size of glass should be selected for the amount of juice to be served; that is, small glasses should be used if only 4 ounces are to be served, rather than using a large tumbler and half filling it.

6. If quantities of beverages are to be prepared it may be timesaving to prepare a standard sirup using sugar and water, which may be used for all beverages.

7. Beverages may be garnished with fresh uncrushed mint leaves, sliced orange, lemon, or pineapple, maraschino cherries, or ices.

Beverage recipes are found on pages 669–74.

PROBLEMS AND REVIEW

1. What are three important functions of beverages?

2. Name the foods commonly used in the preparation of beverages. State the purpose of each and its chief nutritive contributions.

3. List six different ways in which milk may be flavored or reinforced.

4. What is the essential difference between chocolate and cocoa? How does this affect the principle of cookery?

5. What stimulants are present in coffee? In tea? What is their physiologic action?

6. Caffeol, which gives aroma and flavor to coffee, is volatile. How is it possible to retain maximum caffeol content of coffee?

7. Prolonged boiling of water drives off some of the oxygen. How does this affect the flavor of coffee or tea?

8. Outline the steps in the preparation of coffee by the vacuum coffee maker, the percolator, and by "boiling." Discuss the merits of each.

9. What is the difference between black and green tea?

10. *Problem.* How much glucose would be required for 1 glass (200 ml) of lemonade with a 30 per cent carbohydrate concentration? How would you prepare this lemonade?

11. *Problem.* Calculate the protein and caloric value of 1 serving of the following beverages: high-protein milk (basic recipe, p. 672); pineapple eggnog (recipe, p. 674); high-protein eggnog (recipe, p. 672); and milk shake (recipe, p. 671).

12. *Problem.* Calculate the caloric value of the eggnog (recipe, p. 672) using ¼ cup milk and ½ cup light cream.

CHAPTER 44 /

Milk

Milk has served as the sole food of the young during the most critical period of life for some 8000 different species. In the United States milk and its products provide three-fourths of the calcium, one-half of the riboflavin, and one-fourth of the protein in the food supply. The milk of various mammals is used for food, depending upon the availability of the milch animal. Cow's milk is by far the most common and will be discussed here.

Composition. Milk is a complex substance in which over 100 separate components have been identified.[228] It is a fluid in spite of the fact that it contains more solids than many solid foods. For example, fresh cow's milk contains 87 per cent water and 13 per cent solids, while the solids in cabbage constitute 8 per cent, in strawberries 10 per cent, and in summer squash 5 per cent. The exact composition of milk varies with the breed of cattle, the feed used, and the period of lactation. However, the pooled milk sold by dairies has a uniform composition which may be varied slightly by local or state regulations for butterfat and solids content.

On the average, fresh cow's milk contains approximately 3.5 per cent protein; 3.9 per cent fat; 4.9 per cent carbohydrate; and minerals to make a total ash content of 0.7 per cent. One cup of whole milk provides 166 calories, while a cup of skim milk has 87 calories.

Importance of milk as a food. There is no adequate substitute for milk. No food has a wider acceptability or offers a greater variety of uses. It is recommended that adults of all ages include daily at least 2 cups of fluid milk or its equivalent as evaporated milk, dry milk, or hard cheese. This allowance should be raised to 3 to 4 cups for children and the pregnant woman, and to 6 cups for the nursing mother. Diets which contain little or no milk will almost certainly be inadequate in calcium and riboflavin.

Only the proteins of eggs are superior to milk protein for the support of growth (see Fig. 44-1). Casein, lactalbumin, and lactoglobulin are three important proteins in milk; of these, casein accounts for about three fourths in cow's milk. The essential amino acids present in these proteins are supplied in almost ideal proportions for maximum tissue structure. Milk supplements cereal proteins in an excellent fashion, for it supplies the amino acids lysine

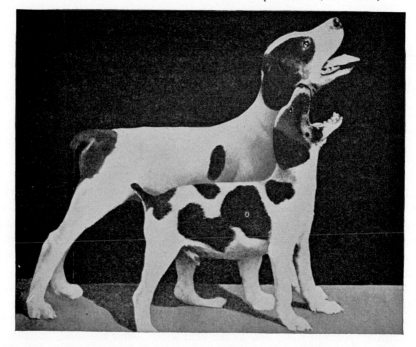

Fig. 44-1. Milk made the difference. These puppies from the same litter were of the same size at weaning time. After weaning, both were fed as much bread and cooked cereal as they would eat with some meat added. The big dog also received milk every day, but the small dog received none. (*Courtesy, the National Dairy Council, Chicago, Ill.*)

and tryptophan which are limiting in the cereals. Thus, the biologic value of proteins in white wheat flour, which is 50 per cent when used alone, is raised to 75 per cent when milk is used with it.[229] One quart of milk provides three-fourths of the recommended allowance of protein for a 2-year-old child, half of the allowance for an 8-year-old, and one-third of the allowance for a teen-age boy.

The fat of milk is highly emulsified and is easily digested. In the homogenization of milk the fat globules are still further reduced in size to give a perfect emulsion. Milk fat contains a high proportion of short-chain fatty acids which are specially well tolerated.

The lactose of milk is a carbohydrate which occurs nowhere else in nature. This sugar is peculiarly adapted to making milk the ideal food for the young because it is much less sweet, less soluble, and more stable than sucrose and other sugars. It gives to milk a bland flavor. Lactose favors the growth of acid-producing bacteria and thus probably helps to prevent intestinal putrefaction. It likewise favors the absorption of calcium and phosphorus.

While milk is not a good source of niacin, it is an excellent source of tryptophan which functions as a precursor of niacin; hence, milk was early recognized for its pellagra-preventive properties. Milk also supplies a liberal quota of vitamin A, vitamin B_{12}, and some thiamine. A large proportion of market milk today is fortified with vitamin-D concentrate to a level of 400 I.U. per quart—the recommended allowance for children.

That milk is not an entirely perfect food is indicated by the fact that it must be supplemented by other foods in the diet of the infant shortly after birth in order that dietary deficiencies may be avoided. It contains a limited amount of iron, although that which is present is readily available. It is low in manganese, copper, and ascorbic acid. It would provide a diet of excessive bulk if used as the sole source of calories.

Too many people become concerned about the caloric value of milk and sometimes eliminate milk from their diets for this reason. From Figure 44-2

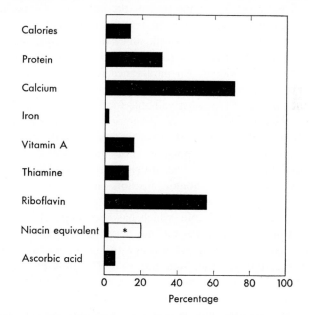

* Unshaded area represents niacin equivalent from tryptophan.

Fig. 44-2. Percentage contribution of 2 cups whole milk to the Recommended Dietary Allowances for a woman 25 years of age.

it will be noted that the percentage contribution of important nutrients from a pint of milk are greater than the percentage of calories toward the dietary allowance for a 25-year-old woman. By adjusting the fat levels in milk, caloric modifications can be made for low-calorie and high-calorie diets.

> 1 cup skim milk = 87 calories
> 1 cup whole milk = 166 calories
> ½ cup whole milk + ½ cup light cream = 328 calories

Digestion and utilization. Milk is easily and almost completely digested. The first step in digestion is the coagulation of the curd in the stomach by the enzyme rennin which is present in the infant's stomach and by hydrochloric acid in the adult. The size of the curd has an important effect on the ease of digestion. Homogenized, acidified, boiled, and evaporated milks produce finer and softer curd than raw or pasteurized milk, and this property of these milks is utilized in infant feeding and in certain patients who have an intolerance to some forms of milk.

Milk, in itself, is neither laxative nor constipating. Being fiber free it does not contribute to the stimulation of the gastrointestinal mucosa. Boiled milk is sometimes ordered for a patient who has a diarrhea, partly because the size of the curd is thereby reduced and partly because bacteria are destroyed.

Intolerance to milk. Many of the so-called "allergies" to milk are not allergies at all but a dislike on the part of the individual for the taste, color, or odor of milk. Other dislikes may be traced to prejudice of some member of the family who has refused to drink milk. It is a simple matter to prove whether a real allergy exists by introducing milk into the diet in a form not recognizable to the individual. An intolerance for milk is most unfortunate, because it is difficult to feed either a child or an invalid a diet which is adequate without the use of this most valuable food.

Types of milk used. Milk may be purchased as whole, fresh liquid milk; skim milk; buttermilk; evaporated milk; condensed milk; and dried whole, skim, or protein milk. It is also possible to obtain fermented or cultured milk by the addition of lactic or citric acid, Bulgarian or acidophilus bacteria. Fresh milk may be modified by homogenization, irradiation, acidification, or flavoring.

Homogenized milk is fresh milk which has been pasteurized and subjected to a process which breaks up the fat into very fine droplets and mixes them so completely as to make it impossible for the fat to rise as cream. It now accounts for three-fourths of all fluid milk sold. This milk has a "richer" taste but it is not different in food value from plain milk. It gives a softer curd and is more easily digested than a firm curd milk.

Vitamin-D milk is that milk to which a vitamin-D concentrate has been added to a level of 400 I.U. per quart. Almost all homogenized milk and other fresh milk is now fortified with this antirachitic vitamin, as is also evaporated milk.

Chocolate milk is whole milk to which chocolate sirup has been added, while *chocolate-flavored milk drink* or *chocolate-flavored dairy drink* is skim or partially skimmed milk to which the chocolate sirup has been added. The nutrients of milk are diluted in proportion to the amount of chocolate sirup which is used. The sirup adds caloric value without a corresponding addition of protective nutrients. These flavored milks are nutritious and wholesome, but they should not become the sole way in which milk is taken. Some children refuse to take white milk when they become accustomed to the sweetness of these forms of milk.

Cultured milks are prepared from pasteurized milk to which certain desirable microorganisms have been added. They have a nutritive value equal to that of the milk from which they were made. The most widely used of these cultured milks is *buttermilk,* which is a by-product in the manufacture of butter. Most buttermilk today is artificially produced by culturing skim milk, partly skimmed milk, or reconstituted nonfat dry milk with *Streptococcus lactis* and incubating it. Salt is usually added to bring out the flavor. *Acidophilus milk,* of very limited distribution, is cultured with *Lactobacillus acidophilus* under standard conditions. *Yogurt* is a pasteurized milk product of custardlike consistency which is fermented by using a mixed culture of organisms. It may be prepared from whole milk or from milk containing additional milk solids. The fermentation of the milk results in a formation of lactic acid from the lactose. Lactic acid, in turn, is believed to encourage a favorable intestinal flora. The consistency of the milk is less fluid, and the flavor is much desired by some people. These milks are sometimes referred to as soft curd milks.

Evaporated milk is the product obtained from fresh whole milk after a little more than half of the water has been removed. During processing the protein is so changed that a softer, finer curd results. Evaporated milk is fortified with vitamin-D concentrate. When diluted with water to its original volume, it has a composition like that of whole sweet milk. Evaporated milk is easily digested, free from bacteria until the can is opened, and lends itself particularly well to the preparation of infant formulas.

Condensed milk is prepared by adding sugar to milk and reducing its water content by evaporation. It owes its keeping qualities to its high-sugar content (42 per cent) rather than to the application of heat. It has found wide use in the preparation of desserts.

Dried milk results from the removal of 95 to 98 per cent of the water from fresh milk. *Nonfat dry milk* is made from skim milk and accounts for most dry milk on the market. Dried milks are made by passing milk in thin layers over heated surfaces in vacuo (roller process), or by spraying partially evaporated milk into warm dry air (spray process). It comes in finely divided form and may be easily reconstituted to its original composition. One pound of nonfat dry milk is about equivalent to 5 quarts fresh skim milk, and is therefore a concentrated source of protein, calcium, riboflavin, and other nutrients. Dried milks are easily stored and transported, for they require no refrigeration. Nonfat dry milk has excellent keeping qualities but whole dried milk is subject to rancidity.

Cream is the fat of milk which has been separated by centrifugation or by gravity. It is sold as light or "coffee" cream, which has a fat content of 18 to 20 per cent, and as heavy or "whipping" cream, which has a fat content of 35 to 40 per cent. *Half-and-half,* often used in high-calorie diets, consists of half milk and half light cream with a final fat content of about 11.5 per cent.

Production and care of milk for safety and quality. The Milk Ordinance and Code recommended by the United States Public Health Service [230] sets forth the types of regulations desirable for ensuring the safety and quality of milk. Most states and municipalities pattern their regulations after this code and require the inspection of cows for freedom from disease, and observation of rules for sanitation of utensils, barns, and personnel. The milk must be free from foreign material and disease-producing bacteria, low in bacterial count, high in nutritive value, and good in flavor. The safe production of milk is discussed in Chapter 21.

Even the best milk will not retain the highest nutritive value and be safe for consumption if it is not properly cared for after delivery. Riboflavin and ascorbic acid are easily destroyed by light. Moreover, milk exposed to sunlight for even an hour or two takes on a change in flavor because of the effects on riboflavin and methionine. Milk should be stored in the bottle or carton in which it was delivered, always keeping the bottle tightly covered and away from light. It should be kept in the coldest part of the refrigerator at 35° to 45° F and used within 4 or 5 days.

Ways of using milk in the diet. Milk is a basic food material for the preparation of both liquid and solid foods in the dietary. As a beverage, it furnishes one of the best carriers for the reinforcing agents since its mild flavor makes it easy to add egg white or whole egg, cream, chocolate, glucose or lactose, and bottled beverages. It is thus possible to vary the liquid diet acceptably. Milk soups made with a white sauce and puréed vegetables as well as chowders furnish important additions to the diet, while custards, milk puddings, rennet desserts, ice cream, and milk sherbets add materially to the palatability of the diet.

Nonfat dry milk may be used in a wide variety of cooked and baked dishes, in beverages, in the preparation of buttermilk of excellent flavor, and as an effective reinforcing agent when the protein intake must be increased above the normal level. In the latter capacity it may be used in the cookery of cereals, in bread, in mashed potatoes, meat loaf, and a host of other ways, as well as in the preparation of high-protein beverages.

Principles of cookery. The scalding of milk, as required in the preparation of many dishes, changes its flavor. Since albumin sticks to the sides and bottom of the pan, bringing down some calcium with it, scorching will occur readily, and therefore a double boiler is advisable in milk cookery. However, direct heat may be used when care is taken to adjust to a low heat and when the product is stirred continuously.

The soft curd of homogenized milk is easily broken and certain precautions should be taken when this milk is used in cookery. Since white sauces may show some separation, it is recommended that the salt be added at the end of the cooking period. Custards should be baked at slightly lower temperatures and somewhat longer than when plain milk is used; in fact, emphasis on low-temperature cookery is important for all milk products.

Nonfat dry milk may be reconstituted by putting a measured amount of water into a jar and adding the required amount of milk powder to the water. The "instant" dry milks dissolve readily with stirring. When reconstituted, dry milk should be handled exactly as fresh liquid milk since it will spoil readily. If nonfat dry milk is to be used in cookery, it is not necessary to reconstitute it before use. The measured amount of dry milk is mixed with the dry ingredients, and water is substituted for the milk in the recipe (see Fig. 44-3).

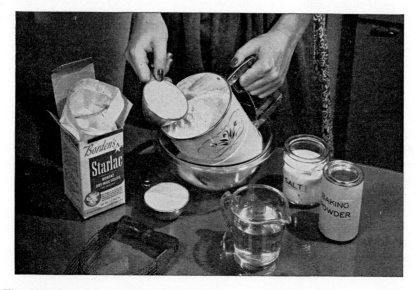

Fig. 44-3. In recipes, nonfat milk solids may be most conveniently used in the dry form by mixing with other dry ingredients listed in the recipe, then using water as the liquid. (*Courtesy, the Borden Company, New York, N.Y.*)

For example, if a recipe calls for 1 cup milk, 3 tablespoons nonfat dry milk are mixed with the dry ingredients, and 1 cup of water is added at the proper time in place of the cup of milk. The exact amount of dry milk to use varies with the brand, and the package labeling should be consulted for directions.

PROBLEM AND REVIEW

1. Define milk. Name some animals other than cows from which milk may be obtained.

2. Give the approximate composition of milk. Name the nutrients which make milk of outstanding importance in the diet of infants and children as well as that of adults.

3. Why is milk not a perfect food? Give three reasons.

4. How is milk made safe for human consumption? (See Chap. 21.)

5. Name the different types of milk which may be purchased in your community. Give the characteristics of each.

6. How much milk should a child of 1 year of age drink during the day? What are some effective ways of assuring this level of milk in the diet if the child is drinking only small amounts?

7. Name five ways in which milk may be used in the diet.

8. *Problem.* Assuming that a given family requires 3 quarts of milk per day, calculate the cost of milk for 1 month, using current prices and purchasing the milk in these ways: (1) as fresh, grade-A homogenized, irradiated milk; (2) as fresh grade-B plain milk—if available in your community; (3) as evaporated milk; (4) as half fresh milk and half nonfat milk solids. What supplementation, if any, is desirable with the nonfat milk solids?

9. Chocolate milk and chocolate flavored milk drink may not be sold in some school lunch programs. What reasons can you give for this prohibition?

of time so that a rapid turnover of this flour is essential. In view of these facts, it is of vast public health significance that refined cereals and breads be enriched with thiamine, riboflavin, niacin, and iron (see p. 315).

Ready digestibility and bland flavor are important factors in the wide use of cereals in both normal and modified diets. Cereals are usually, though not always, the first solid foods given to infants. They are also among the first foods allowed for patients who have been seriously ill.

When whole-grain cereals and breads are used, the amount of dietary fiber is increased, thus encouraging peristalsis in the gastrointestinal tract.

Cereal foods, it is well known, are the primary source of energy for much of the world's population. Many people imply from this fact that cereals per se are fattening, and so they omit this group of foods from their diets. By such omission they also lose the manifold benefits of other nutrients provided by the whole-grain or enriched product. Even in the United States, the bread-cereals group accounts for one-third of the thiamine, one-fourth of the energy, protein, iron, and niacin, and one-sixth of the riboflavin.[234] In other words the cereal foods contribute importantly to every nutrient need except vitamin A, ascorbic acid, and calcium. (See also Figure 46-2.)

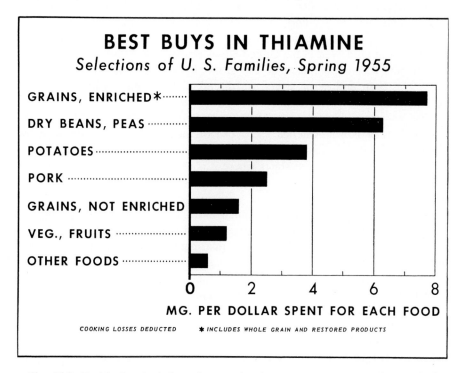

BEST BUYS IN THIAMINE
Selections of U. S. Families, Spring 1955

GRAINS, ENRICHED*
DRY BEANS, PEAS
POTATOES
PORK
GRAINS, NOT ENRICHED
VEG., FRUITS
OTHER FOODS

0   2   4   6   8
MG. PER DOLLAR SPENT FOR EACH FOOD

COOKING LOSSES DEDUCTED   * INCLUDES WHOLE GRAIN AND RESTORED PRODUCTS

Fig. 46-2. Enriched and whole grains are the cheapest sources of thiamine according to data from the 1955 household survey. (*Courtesy, Agricultural Research Service, U.S. Department of Agriculture.*)

Use of cereals in the diet. Wheat, rice, corn, oats, rye, and barley are the grains most commonly used for food. They are used for flours, of which bread is the single most important product, for breakfast cereals, for pastes, and a number of lesser purposes.

Flour. Wheat is superior to other flours in giving a light, porous quality to leavened products, and is consequently the grain of first importance in this country. Two proteins in wheat provide for the development of a high gluten content when moisture is added. The elasticity of the gluten permits the ready expansion by gas and consequent lightness of the finished product. The development of gluten depends upon the extent of mixing and the amount and type of liquid used. Long mixing tends to toughen gluten and makes the leavening process more difficult. Gluten develops more quickly in a batter than in a dough.

Hard winter wheat produces flour of a high gluten content and is ideally suited to the preparation of high-quality bread, since development of the gluten is an essential prerequisite for the porous quality of bread. Soft wheat gives flour of much lower gluten content and is utilized for cake flour. The tenderness of crumb desirable in cakes makes a limited development of gluten desirable. All-purpose flours combine the characteristics of hard and soft wheat, and such flours find widest usefulness in the multiple purposes for which flour is used in the home.

The wheat flour used in the United States is usually a 70 per cent extraction; this means that 70 per cent of the grain, namely the endosperm, is used, while the bran and germ layers are discarded for animal feeds. Practically all of the flour sold in retail markets is now enriched.

The ancient civilizations of the Incas in Peru, the Mayas in Mexico, and the Indians of North America used corn or maize—a food unknown to the Spanish adventurers and the English colonists. Even today corn meal is widely used in the southern states where it is prominent in corn bread as well as in spoon bread and mush, while in the Southwest corn is used for the preparation of tortillas.

Rye and barley flours are used much more extensively in Europe than in America. These flours produce a heavier loaf of bread than that of wheat.

The flours of potato, soybean, oats, rice, banana, and taro find some usefulness in specialty products; they are a great help to the individual who is allergic to wheat.

Bread. That bread is an important dietary constituent was convincingly demonstrated in a study reported by Widdowson and McCance.[235] These eminent British investigators observed the progress of 169 undernourished children, 4 to 15 years of age, for a year in a German orphanage at a time when food supplies were limited. The calories in the diets consumed by the children were distributed in these percentages: bread, 75; potatoes, 6; soups, vegetables, fruits, butter, margarine, 15; and milk, cheese, meat, fish, 4.

Whole-wheat, enriched, and unenriched white breads were tested. The diets were not low in protein, but only 8 to 9 gm were derived from animal sources. Supplements of vitamins A, D, and C were included.

At the end of 1 year the children had made more rapid gains in height and weight than would be expected of normal children at the same age level; bone development was somewhat more rapid than normal; skin conditions had improved, and muscle tone had increased. The children were stated to be in excellent physical condition. No differences were observed in growth, development, or health with any of the breads tested, but the B-vitamin reserves were somewhat better in those children who had eaten bread enriched to the whole-wheat levels. These results clearly demonstrated the nutritive efficiency of unusually large amounts of bread.

Cereal grains themselves are poor sources of calcium, but breakfast cereals and breads may serve as vehicles by which calcium is included in the diet. Two chemical additives commonly used by commercial bakers add significant amounts of utilizable calcium, namely: certain calcium salts, which are yeast foods or dough conditioners, and calcium propionate, which is a mold inhibitor. Most commercial breads now contain 4 per cent nonfat dry milk resulting in a further improvement of the calcium level as well as of the quality of the protein.

The nutritive contribution of bread is illustrated in Figure 46-3.

Kinds of bread. The Food and Drug Administration has established standards of identity for five kinds of bread: white, enriched, milk, raisin, and whole-wheat. Under these regulations specified levels of certain ingredients must be included for bread offered for interstate sale.[236] For numerous other breads on the market—potato, corn, wheat-and-soya, gluten, lysine-enriched and many others—no standards of identity have been developed. However, interstate trade requires that the ingredients of such breads be listed on the label in the order of the amounts used in the formula.

Enriched bread represents about 85 per cent of all white bread and rolls sold to the American public. The B vitamins and iron are included at levels to equal whole-wheat bread (see Fig. 46-3).

Whole-wheat flour is the only flour which may be used in bread labeled as "whole wheat," "graham," or "entire wheat" bread. This bread accounts for only a small proportion of bread sold in America today. Nutritively speaking, whole-wheat and enriched breads are so similar that one can be guided by taste preferences and cost of the loaf in making one's selection. On the other hand, many people buy breads labeled as "cracked wheat," "wheaten," "wheat," and "rye" in the mistaken belief that they are made with the whole grain. These breads, in fact, are made with white flour and varying proportions of cracked wheat, whole-wheat, or rye flours, as the case may be.

Numerous specialty breads are available in bakeries and supermarkets. For some of these, the advertising claims for superior nutritive qualities and for low-calorie benefits are misleading. For example, some breads are advertised as being made without sugar or shortening, the implication being that the caloric values are thereby considerably reduced. Often the caloric value of a thin slice of such bread is compared with the caloric value of a thicker slice of enriched bread. Actually, weight for weight, the caloric value of white, rye, whole-wheat, protein, and other specialty breads is so similar that there is no need to consider them separately.[237]

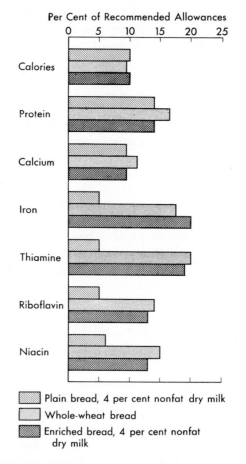

Per Cent of Recommended Allowances

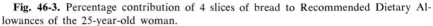

Fig. 46-3. Percentage contribution of 4 slices of bread to Recommended Dietary Allowances of the 25-year-old woman.

The use of soy flour, wheat germ, molasses, and other ingredients may increase the nutritive value of the loaf of bread, but how important that contribution is can be evaluated only in terms of the amounts used in the formula and in the amounts contributed to the daily intake.

Breakfast cereals. Whether hot or cold, enriched or whole-grain, from wheat, corn, rice, or oats, cereals are a mainstay of the breakfast (see p. 183). They may vary widely in mineral and vitamin content according to the grain used and the minerals and vitamins added, but when one chooses to eat a variety of cereals, one can be certain of high nutritive contributions.

Not only do breakfast cereals find wide usefulness as a main food for breakfast (see Fig. 46-4) but they may also be used in place of part of the

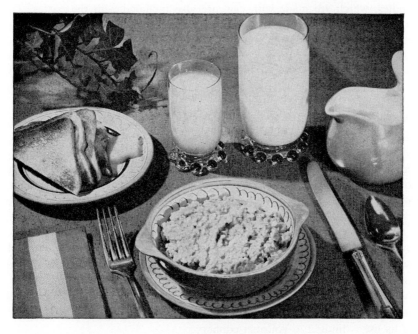

Fig. 46-4. A good breakfast supplies one-fourth to one-third of the day's nutrient needs. (*Courtesy, the Cereal Institute, Chicago, Illinois.*)

flour in quick breads and yeast breads, as an ingredient in many desserts, as extenders for main dishes such as meat loaf, and as crumb toppings for casserole dishes. Cereals may be served for lunch as well as for breakfast. Fried mush and Philadelphia scrapple are popular for lunch or even dinner.

While ready-to-serve cereals may be purchased in individual-serving-size packages, it is more economical to purchase the largest size package if the contents can be used in a reasonable length of time. During damp weather the crispness of the cereals may be restored by placing them in a shallow pan and heating them in the oven for a few minutes.

The uncooked oat and wheat cereals are usually more economical than ready-to-serve cereals. Almost all cereals are now of the quick-cooking variety and do not require long-cooking periods even when they are to be used for infant feeding. This is made possible through the use of a harmless salt such as disodium phosphate which is added during manufacture in order to bring about quicker gelatinization of the starch. Instead of using a salt, some quick-cooking cereals have been finely divided during manufacture to hasten the cooking process.

Pastes. A special kind of hard wheat flour—durum—is used in the manufacture of an almost endless variety of pastes, known as *pasta* to the Italian. Macaroni, spaghetti, and vermicelli will be most familiar to the reader. Noodles, which are made with egg, are also included with the pastes. These flour products are used in numerous dishes either as side dishes for the main meal or as a main dish when combined with cheese, meat, fish, or poultry.

Rice. About 95 per cent of the world's rice is grown in the Orient where it is the staple article of diet. Rice was first introduced into South Carolina in 1685 and has since become an important crop in Louisiana, Texas, Arkansas, and California.

White rice (polished) is preferred all over the world to the brown (unpolished) rice. Because it is a staple food for so many of the world's people, enrichment is a major goal in world nutrition. Rice may be enriched by coating the kernels with a mixture of the nutrients, in which case the rice should not be washed prior to cooking nor should an excessive amount of water be used so that the vitamins are dissolved out in water which is discarded. Another process has been developed whereby the rice is parboiled or steamed so that the thiamine is distributed throughout the kernel with only a slight loss taking place during washing and cooking. Precooked rice, now available in many markets, requires the addition of hot water and a short period of standing before it is ready to be served.

Wild rice is harvested in northern Minnesota and Wisconsin, but is not a true rice. It is prized for its flavor and texture, although it is so expensive that its use is limited to gourmet cookery.

Cookery of cereals and pastes. Cereals are cooked in order to soften or rupture the cellulose walls of the starch cells so as to render the starch more easily digested. The cooking of cereals also improves their flavor. Starch cells absorb water, expand, and become gelatinized on boiling.

The proportions of liquid to cereal which are indicated in recipes should be followed to obtain satisfactory results. The dry cereal should be added slowly to rapidly boiling salted water so that boiling does not stop. If very fine cereals are to be cooked, lumping can be avoided by mixing the cereal with a small amount of cold water before adding it to the boiling liquid. It is necessary to stir constantly while cooking over direct heat; however, quick-cooking cereals require cooking for only a few minutes. Well-cooked breakfast cereal is free from lumps, neither too thick nor too thin, and full-flavored.

Rice may be steamed, using just enough water for complete absorption by the grain, or it may be cooked in a large quantity of rapidly boiling water so that the kernels remain separate and distinct. Macaroni and spaghetti are also cooked in a large amount of boiling water, and then drained as soon as cooking is complete to avoid excessive pastiness.

Recipes for cereals may be found on page 678.

FLOUR MIXTURES

Classification of flour mixtures. *Dough* is a mixture of flour, liquid, and other ingredients, the proportion of liquid being just sufficient to allow kneading or rolling into a sheet. Yeast breads, baking-powder biscuits, piecrust, and rolled cookies are examples of doughs. *Batters* are semiliquid mixtures which can be poured or dropped from a spoon. They are classified as "pour" or "drop" batters. Popovers, griddle cakes, and waffles are examples of pour batters, while muffins, cakes, drop cookies, and drop biscuits are examples of drop batters.

Ingredients of batters and doughs. Flour, fats, sugar, eggs, liquid, leavening agents, and flavorings are ingredients used in varying proportions depending upon the product which is being prepared.

Fats. Butter, margarine, cream, hydrogenated fats, lard, and oils constitute the fats used in cooking and baking. All fats are the most concentrated sources of energy in the diet, but margarine, cream, and butter are the only fats which contain vitamin A. Fats deteriorate because of oxidation, hydrolysis of the fatty acids, and absorption of other flavors. They should be protected from light, air, and moisture by keeping them in a closed container in a cool place. Hydrogenated fats have better keeping qualities than lard or butter.

Fats are used in batters and doughs to separate the flour particles, thereby giving a more tender product, and to act as solvents for substances used in flavoring so that the flavoring agent is more effective. Lard and hydrogenated fats are suitable for batters and doughs and also find wide usefulness in frying, since the point at which decomposition occurs is at a relatively high temperature. Butter and margarine are preferred by many for fine cakes of bland flavor, but these fats are less suitable for frying because of their low smoking point.

Oils are used widely for frying and are used with success in recipes which specify melted fats—in muffins, for example. Recipes have been developed for chiffon cakes, pastries, and biscuits that use oil as the shortening; these products are of fine, light texture.

The choice of fat for cooking purposes may be dictated by certain requirements for therapeutic diets. Thus, oils high in polyunsaturated fatty acids and blended rather than hydrogenated margarines might be the only fats allowed. Some techniques have been described by Vail for their use in foods.[238]

Sugar. The tremendous variety of baked goods today would not be possible except for the abundance and low cost of sugar. Sugar from cane and from beets is of equal sweetening value, cane sugar comprising the primary source of sweets in America. It is purchased as granulated, powdered, confectioners', brown, and tablet sugar. Corn sugar (Cerelose, Dyno, glucose, or dextrose), corn sirup, molasses, honey, and maple sirup and sugar are other sweetenings of varying importance.

Sugar is used in batters and doughs to give sweetness to the product and thus modify the flavor, to provide crispness, to lessen the development of gluten, thus giving a more tender product, and to assist in browning. An excess of sugar may cause the product to spread and run over the sides of the pan. The presence of sugar helps to prevent the formation of tunnels in muffins and cakes.

Eggs function as a leavening agent and as a binder to hold the ingredients together. The yolk of egg increases the fineness of the texture and the tenderness of the finished product. Whenever egg whites are used, the following precautions should be observed: (1) the whites and yolks must be completely separated; (2) the whites should be whipped stiff but not dry. Only the number of eggs called for in the recipe should be used, since too many eggs increase the protein content to such an extent that the finished product will be dry and tough when baked.

Milk increases the nutritive value of the product and improves both flavor and texture. Water acts as a substitute for milk, but the texture of the finished product is less fine. The use of nonfat dry milk greatly enhances the nutritive value of baked products at low cost.

Leavening agents. The function of leavening agents is to raise the product and give it lightness and porosity. Leavening agents include carbon dioxide, air, and steam.

Steam is used as a leavening agent for batters such as popovers and cream puffs. In these mixtures the high temperatures used vaporize part of the moisture, and the resultant steam expands the product to give it lightness.

Air may be incorporated into egg whites, and its leavening properties are utilized for making angel food and sponge cakes, soufflés, and omelets. This method may be used in combination with the production of carbon dioxide as in the preparation of batters in which egg whites are beaten separately and folded in. Air is also beaten into sugar-fat mixtures during the process of creaming, and is of some value in improving texture.

Yeast is the oldest known agent in which carbon dioxide was used to leaven the product. It is a tiny plant cell which grows best at 75° to 95° F, with a temperature of 82° F being considered optimum. When temperatures exceed the upper limit, the yeast is destroyed. Cold, on the other hand, does not destroy the yeast but greatly retards its growth. Sugar, oxygen, and moisture are necessary for yeast growth. An enzyme in yeast converts sugar to yield carbon dioxide and alcohol. During baking the alcohol is driven off, while the carbon dioxide continues to raise the dough. Yeast gives a light product of excellent flavor and texture not duplicated by other leavening agents. One disadvantage of its use is the length of time required for leavening, but by doubling the quantity of yeast one can obtain breads in a much shorter period of time.

Both granular yeast and the moist compressed yeast cakes are sold in the retail markets. The keeping properties of granular yeast are much better than those of the moist yeast, and no refrigeration is required. However, it is important to hydrate the yeast before adding it to the flour mixtures.

Baking soda (sodium bicarbonate) is used with an acid such as sour milk or molasses to yield carbon dioxide, water, and a neutral salt. If soda is used in excess of the neutralizing power of the acid, the bitter flavor and yellow color of the sodium carbonate residue are noted in the product. Sour milk may vary greatly in the amount of acid present, and consequently in its neutralizing properties. In general, ½ teaspoon of soda is used for 1 cup of sour milk, and ¾ teaspoon of soda is required for 1 cup of molasses. Soda is mixed with the dry ingredients rather than with the sour milk or molasses, as formerly practiced, since the latter method results in considerable escape of carbon dioxide and loss of leavening power.

Baking powder consists of an acid salt, baking soda, and starch. Reaction takes place between the acid salt and the soda in the presence of moisture. Even a trace of moisture will promote the reaction, and therefore baking powders understandably may deteriorate in humid climates, with resultant baking failures unless precautions are taken for continuous storage in tight containers. There are three common types of baking powder:

1. Tartrate powders use cream of tartar and tartaric acid singly or in combination and are quick-acting; that is, reaction with the soda occurs immediately when moisture is added.

2. Phosphate powders employ calcium acid phosphate, and are also quick-acting.

3. Sodium aluminum sulfate phosphate (also known as "S.A.S.," "double-acting," or "combination type") contains monocalcium phosphate which reacts with soda as soon as moisture is introduced, and sodium aluminum sulfate which reacts with soda only in the presence of heat and moisture.

When quick-acting baking powders are used, mixing should be kept at a minimum after adding the baking powder. On the other hand, mixtures using the slow-acting aluminum salt may be beaten longer and may be allowed to stand for a short time before baking.

In general the following proportions of baking powder are used:

1½ to 2 teaspoons tartrate or phosphate (quick-acting) powder to 1 cup of flour

1 to 1½ teaspoons S.A.S. phosphate (double-acting) powder to 1 cup of flour.

Quick breads use the larger proportion and cakes the smaller proportion. Egg whites reduce somewhat the amount of baking powder needed.

Preparation of batters and doughs. The retail markets of today sell not only a variety of yeast breads, rolls, muffins, cakes, and pastries all ready to serve, but they also include an array of biscuit, muffin, popover, cookie, cake, and roll mixes as well as frozen foods ready to be baked. Excellent results are obtained when the few simple directions are exactly followed. The nurse is infrequently required to prepare quick breads, and scarcely ever is it necessary for her to bake cakes, pastries, and yeast breads. To do so would demand an unreasonable proportion of her time away from the patient. When occasion does arise to prepare these foods, the nurse should consult any standard cookbook which will present methods and variety far beyond the scope of this book. The recipes for quick breads in Chapter 54 illustrate the methods of mixing batters and doughs.

PROBLEMS AND REVIEW

1. *Problem*. Tabulate the protein, fat, carbohydrate, calories, thiamine, riboflavin, and niacin in 100 gm of each of the following: oatmeal; Puffed Wheat; unenriched and enriched farina; corn flakes; unenriched and enriched corn meal.

2. *Problem*. Calculate the number of servings of each of the above cereals one can purchase for 10 cents. Allow 20 gm of dry cereal for each serving.

3. *Problem*. Calculate the food value of one serving of oatmeal with ½ cup milk and 1 teaspoon sugar.

4. What contributions do cereals make to the nutritive value of the daily diet? To the variety in the diet?

5. Why is an adequate enrichment program so important?

6. Give three examples of (a) whole-grain cereals, (b) refined cereals, (c) enriched cereals.

7. State the principles for the cooking of cereals.

8. Why are the proteins of cereals of lower biologic value than protein from animal sources?

9. Enumerate the various leavening agents and give examples when each is used. What are the advantages and disadvantages of each?

10. Why is bread called the "staff of life"?

11. Differentiate between these kinds of bread: enriched, whole-wheat, wheaten, graham, rye, cracked wheat, entire wheat.

12. Should bread and cereal be eliminated from a reducing diet? Explain your answer.

13. What is the objection to prolonged stirring in the preparation of breads leavened with baking powder?

14. *Problem*. Calculate the food value for one of the muffin recipes. What is the value for one muffin?

15. *Problem*. Compare the nutritive value of a slice of whole-wheat bread, white bread, and enriched bread. How can you be sure that the loaf of bread you buy is enriched?

CHAPTER 47

White Sauces and Soups

WHITE SAUCES

Variations of sauces. White sauce is a basic sauce consisting of milk which has been thickened and which may be used as a foundation for cream soups, creamed and scalloped dishes, croquettes, and soufflés. White or cream sauces are a means of using milk in the daily diet, thereby improving the nutritive value. Moreover, they introduce variety in the menu. They may be varied by:

1. Using milk, cream, vegetable juices, or meat broths singly or in combination as the liquid
2. Using butter, margarine, oil, or meat drippings as the fat
3. Using flour, browned flour, cornstarch, or tapioca as the thickening
4. Adding finely chopped or puréed vegetables
5. Using commercial colorings, spices, and herbs of many kinds. When sugar, chocolate, caramel, or other flavorings are used, many simple desserts can be prepared.

Principles of cookery. Cream sauces must be of the proper thickness for the purpose for which they are intended, smooth, suitably seasoned, and sufficiently cooked to overcome the raw taste of starch. Careful measurement of ingredients is essential for a uniform product.

The thickening agent is blended with the fat to separate the starch granules. Liquid is added gradually to the starch paste, stirring to obtain a smooth mixture. The starch cells absorb liquid, and, when heated, thickening occurs. While stirring constantly, the sauce is cooked over low heat until thickened and until there is no taste of raw starch; or it may be placed in a double boiler over hot water to continue cooking. Variations and uses of white sauces are included in the recipe section, page 701.

SOUPS

Place in the diet. Soups have occupied a place on the menu for centuries. They have been served at the beginning of all formal dinners and at numerous other times as well. They have a double purpose in stimulating the appetite and in providing nourishment.

Clear soups are one of the ways of introducing liquids when only a clear-liquid diet is used. They are of negligible protein and caloric value, but they contribute sodium chloride, potassium, and small amounts of other minerals. Those prepared with meat stock are rich in extractives, full-flavored, and stimulating to the appetite. Moreover, they have a definite value as stimuli to the secretory cells of the stomach.

Some soups are rich, hearty, and highly nutritious, with chunks of meat, vegetables, and noodles, macaroni, rice, or barley. They may contain milk, thus adding to the variety of ways in which the daily quota of milk is met.

Terms used to describe soup. The following definitions will help the student to differentiate between the many soups available:

Stock is the liquid obtained from the long cooking of meat, poultry, or fish in water. It is seasoned with herbs, spices, and vegetables.

Brown stock is made from lean beef and bone. Part of the meat is browned before it is added to water.

White stock is made from veal or chicken. The meat is not browned.

Broth is the liquid resulting when meat or poultry is simmered in water.

Bouillon is prepared from brown stock, lightly seasoned, and clarified.

Consommé is made from two or more kinds of meat (beef, veal, and chicken). It is highly seasoned, clarified, and strained.

Vegetable soup may be made with or without meat stock. When it contains meat and a considerable proportion of vegetables, it provides satisfying bulk, some protein, and energy value, and may serve as the main dish of a meal.

Cream soup is a combination of white sauce and a purée of vegetables or fish, such as cream of pea, tomato, asparagus, carrot, celery, corn, spinach, bean, and oyster or clam bisque. The term "bisque" is applied to cream soups prepared from shellfish.

Chowders are unstrained soups made with milk, fish, shellfish, or vegetables such as potato, onion, and corn.

Gumbo is a mixture of chicken, oysters, crab, shrimp, tomatoes, okra, and seasonings.

Preparation of soups. Less tender cuts of meat or poultry are rich in extractives and, together with bone, provide the ideal combination for full-flavored meat stock. The meat or chicken should be cut in pieces to increase the surface and thus facilitate the extraction of purines. Long cooking at a simmering temperature is essential for maximum extraction of purines. Diced vegetables, salt, spices, and herbs are added during the last hour of the cooking period for best flavor.

In the preparation of cream soups it is customary to use 1 part of vegetable or fish purée to 1½ to 2 parts of thin cream sauce. Puréed vegetables such as are used for infant feeding may be used, or vegetables may be sieved after they have been cooked sufficiently to become soft. The heated purée should be added gradually to the hot sauce to prevent lumping and curdling. This is especially important in the preparation of cream of tomato or cream of asparagus soups, since the acid present in these vegetables is likely to produce curdling.

The nurse may need to prepare cream soups but is seldom required to use her time in the preparation of stock. There are many excellent canned, dehydrated, and frozen soups, both clear and creamed, which are a time-saving factor to the nurse who has many other duties. Bouillon cubes and various meat extracts, when properly diluted with water, are also good substitutes for home-prepared broths. Recipes for a variety of soups are given on page 701.

PROBLEM AND REVIEW

1. *Problem.* Calculate the carbohydrate, protein, fat, and caloric values for each of the four basic recipes for white sauce (see p. 701).

2. Give the progressive steps in the preparation of cream sauces. Give the reasons for each step.

3. Name six ways in which cream sauces may be used.

4. What is the value of soup in the diet?

5. Which type of soup furnishes the greatest amount of nourishment? What nutrients are present in appreciable amounts?

6. Give an example of each of four types of soup.

CHAPTER 48 /

Vegetables

Vegetables include the edible parts of a large number of plant foods. They are valued equally for the variety which they lend to the menu and the significant contributions they make to the vitamin-A, ascorbic acid, B-complex, and mineral levels of the daily diet.

Classification. It will be noted in the following botanic classification that practically every part of the plant is represented.

1. Flowers: broccoli, cauliflower, French artichokes, asparagus tips
2. Green leaves: Brussels sprouts, cabbage, chard, dandelion, endive, lettuce, mustard greens, parsley, spinach, turnip greens, water cress
3. Fruits: cucumbers, eggplant, green peppers, okra, pumpkin, squash, tomatoes
4. Stems: asparagus, celery, leeks
5. Roots: beets, carrots, kohlrabi, parsnips, rutabagas, salsify, sweet potatoes, turnips
6. Tubers: Jerusalem artichokes, Irish potatoes, tara, peanuts
7. Bulbs: mature onions, shallots
8. Seeds: fresh beans, corn, peas; dried legumes including beans, lentils, peas, soybeans
9. Fungi: mushrooms

Composition. The nutritive values of vegetables vary somewhat with the variety and the climatic conditions. More significant variations are brought about by the methods employed for handling from field to consumer, the storage in the home, and the preparation practices.

Water constitutes 75 to 96 per cent of the weight of fresh vegetables. Cucumbers, for example, contain 96 per cent water; raw potatoes are 78 per cent water. Legumes such as dry beans contain only 12 per cent water, but they absorb large amounts of water in cooking.

Energy. The caloric value of vegetables is, in general, low. Potatoes, Lima beans, sweet potatoes, and legumes in average serving portions provide 100 calories, more or less, while leafy vegetables such as spinach, lettuce, and cabbage yield about 20 calories per serving.

Protein. With the exception of legumes and peanuts, the protein of vege-

630

tables is of inferior quality and of low concentration, ranging from 1 to 2 per cent. The quality of protein in soybeans and peanuts is superior to that in other beans and dried peas. When legumes are served at the same meal with a small quantity of complete protein food such as meat, milk, and eggs, the proportion and quantity of amino acids are as satisfactory as if complete protein were the sole source.

Fat. Vegetables contain only traces of fat.

Carbohydrate. Starch, dextrins, sugars, and cellulose are found in vegetables. The leafy and stem vegetables contain the least carbohydrate, while the tubers, roots, and seeds are the richest in carbohydrate. A simplified classification of vegetables is now widely used in the calculation of measured diets (see Table 4, p. 769). Those vegetables classed as Group A contain so little carbohydrate that they are used as desired without calculating the carbohydrate, fat, or protein. Group B vegetables including carrots, beets, peas, winter squash, and others average 7 gm carbohydrate per ½ cup serving. Vegetables somewhat higher in carbohydrate content (potato, Lima beans, corn, etc.) are listed as bread exchanges (see list 4); they have been grouped as C vegetables in the lists for the sodium-restricted diet (see p. 512), but it will be noted that one unit of these vegetables equals one bread exchange.

Minerals. Turnip greens, mustard greens, collards, kale, and broccoli are excellent sources of calcium. The calcium of spinach, poke, dock, beet greens, chard, and lamb's-quarters is probably not nutritionally available because of the high oxalic acid content which results in an insoluble calcium salt.

The leafy vegetables are fair to good sources of iron. A ½ cup serving of cowpeas, kale, spinach, mustard greens, and turnip greens will supply 20 to 25 per cent of the adult's daily allowance for iron, while other vegetables supply smaller, but significant, amounts. With few exceptions, vegetables are low in sodium content and contribute varying amounts of potassium, phosphorus, magnesium, copper, and other mineral elements.

The mineral elements present in vegetables contribute to an alkaline end reaction in the body, and consequently vegetables aid in the maintenance of the acid-base balance of the body.

Vitamins. As good sources of carotene, the dark green leafy and the deep yellow vegetables like spinach, kale, turnip greens, carrots, and sweet potatoes are without equal (see Fig. 48-1). The carotene content is directly related to the depth of the green or yellow color.

Vegetables rank with fruits in meeting the dietary need for ascorbic acid. Especially important is the vitamin-C content of raw or canned tomatoes and tomato juice, raw cabbage, and other raw vegetables. Many cooked vegetables, when prepared under conditions as described below, likewise contribute importantly in this respect. Broccoli, mustard greens, dandelion greens, spinach, Brussels sprouts, kale, and many others are especially high in ascorbic acid. While potatoes and sweet potatoes do not contain such high concentrations of the vitamin, the amounts which may be eaten daily make them a source of great value.

Succulent vegetables contribute small amounts of thiamine, riboflavin, and niacin to the diet. Thiamine occurs more abundantly in the legumes and peanuts.

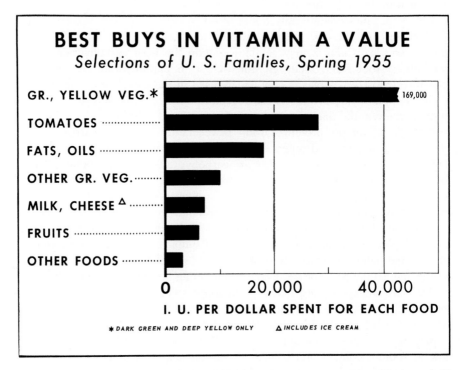

Fig. 48-1. Best buys in vitamin-A value according to data from the 1955 household survey. (*Courtesy, Agricultural Research Service, U.S. Department of Agriculture.*)

Digestibility. Properly cooked vegetables are digested with ease under normal conditions. The fiber of vegetables is highly desirable because of its capacity to hold water and stimulate peristalsis, thus aiding laxation. In young children and in some disturbances of the gastrointestinal tract such as peptic ulcer, this fiber may produce some mechanical irritation. In such situations, it is customary to allow only cooked vegetables in which the fiber has been considerably softened or to reduce even further the fiber content by pressing (puréeing) the cooked vegetable through a strainer.

A number of vegetables are classified as strongly flavored; these include broccoli, Brussels sprouts, dried beans, cabbage, cauliflower, cucumber, leeks, onions, peppers, radishes, and turnips. Individuals with cardiac disease, gallbladder disease, or gastrointestinal disturbances frequently experience distressing abdominal distention, flatulence, or belching following meals which have included these vegetables. It is customary to omit them in the planning of diets for such patients, but it should be emphasized that many persons can and do eat some or all of them without harm if the vegetables are not over-cooked. Consequently, restriction should not be employed when it is known the patient can tolerate the suspected foods.

Selection and care of fresh vegetables. Because of rapid transportation from distant points, fresh vegetables are now available throughout the year in most urban areas. The consumption of leafy vegetables has increased, but potatoes—valuable for a number of nutrients—are eaten in smaller amounts (see Fig. 48-2). Those that are grown abundantly in nearby areas are

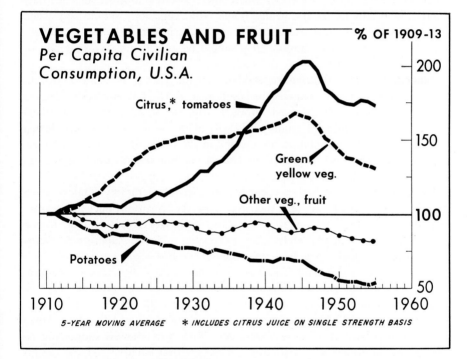

Fig. 48-2. Per capita consumption of vegetables and fruits in the United States. (*Courtesy, Agricultural Research Service, U.S. Department of Agriculture.*)

inexpensive, while others in limited supply are more expensive. The cost increases when highly perishable products must be shipped great distances, when the yield per acre of ground is small as compared with that for other foods, when harvesting and subsequent handling increase labor costs, and when adverse weather conditions have yielded a small crop. In consideration of economy, every effort should be made to purchase fresh vegetables at the peak of their season, and when feasible to produce some in a home garden. In rural areas a year-round supply may often be obtained at greatest economy by home canning or freezing during the height of the season.

Crisp, ripe, but not overmature vegetables that are firm in texture and free from blemishes, mold, and rot should be selected. As vegetables become too mature, the lignocellulose which is formed gives the characteristic stringy or woody texture which cannot be overcome by cookery. Wilted vegetables are lower in carotene and ascorbic acid content than fresh, crisp vegetables.

Vegetables should be used as soon as possible after their purchase. They deteriorate rapidly in palatability and nutritive value unless proper storage facilities are provided. Potatoes, carrots, beets, onions, and turnips may be stored in a cool, dark, dry room where there is circulation of air, but they deteriorate rapidly in the dry, heated home. Most vegetables should be washed to remove dirt, insects, worms, sprays, and bacteria before storing in the refrigerator. To avoid dehydration, they should be kept in the hydrator pan or in a plastic bag which retains the moisture.

Canned, frozen, and dried vegetables. A wide variety of canned, frozen, and dried vegetables is available in addition to those that are fresh. Canned vegetables approximate the fresh product from the standpoint of nutritional value, since in commercial canning it is possible to use vacuum closure. When vegetables other than tomatoes are canned in the home, it is necessary to use a pressure cooker since no other method of canning will assure safety from botulinus poisoning (see Chap. 21).

The consumption of frozen vegetables is expanding rapidly. Quick-frozen vegetables are usually more expensive than the fresh product in season. The nutritive values are equal to those of fresh vegetables; in fact, frozen vegetables packed immediately after harvesting may be superior to many fresh products which have been improperly handled.

Frozen vegetables are convenient because they involve little time in preparation and somewhat shorter cooking time. When they are brought into the home, they should be stored at 0° F in a freezer until they are to be used. When they are placed in the freezing compartment of a refrigerator, they should be used within a week. Vegetables which have thawed should not be refrozen because marked deterioration of quality thus occurs.

The sales for instant potatoes—mashed, scalloped, au gratin, and hashed brown—are rapidly increasing. Beans which have been precooked are also available. Dried beans and peas are available in considerable variety and might well occupy a more important place in the dietary than they do now.

Principles of cookery. The cooking of vegetables softens the cellulose and breaks the starch cells so that the carbohydrates are more accessible to the starch-splitting enzymes. The flavor and palatability of many vegetables are improved by cooking. Properly cooked vegetables should be tender yet firm and crisp, rather than hard and tough or soft and soggy. Some color change in green vegetables is unavoidable because heat decomposes the chlorophyll, but this can be kept to a minimum if overcooking is avoided.

The carotene of vegetables is not affected by cooking procedures. On the other hand, the manner of cookery can importantly influence the contribution which vegetables make to the dietary level of water-soluble minerals and water-soluble, heat-labile vitamins. Thiamine and ascorbic acid are extremely soluble in water, while riboflavin and niacin are much less so. Vitamin and mineral losses through solubility can be materially lessened by (1) keeping pieces as large as practical in order to avoid excessive surface exposure, (2) cooking with skins on whenever possible, (3) avoiding long soaking in water which is later discarded, (4) using a minimum quantity of water in cookery, and (5) saving water in which vegetables were cooked or canned for use in soups, sauces, or gravies.

Goodly amounts of vitamins and minerals are lost when peelings and skins are discarded, since vitamins and minerals occur in greatest concentration near the skin. Moreover, the exposure to air hastens oxidation, with the result that dicing in small pieces, chopping, grinding, and stirring during cookery greatly hastens destruction.

Some destruction of vitamins during cookery is unavoidable, but this can be kept at a minimum. The water in which vegetables are cooked should be rapidly boiling before vegetables are added and should be quickly brought to the boiling point again. This facilitates prompt destruction of enzymes which may oxidize the vitamins. Continuous boiling rather than simmering is most effective in giving a tender product in the shortest length of time. This does not mean that excessively high heat, with consequent rapid escape of steam and danger of scorching, is necessary. For most vegetables a tightly covered pot, using a minimum quantity of water, is desirable. Even such strongly flavored vegetables as cabbage may be cooked in this way.

The use of baking soda to retain color and shorten cooking time is destructive of water-soluble vitamins and also modifies flavor if used in excessive amounts. Recent studies indicate that alkali in properly controlled amounts may not be as harmful as formerly believed, and that the decreased loss of vitamins through the shortened cooking time may more than compensate for the destruction effected by the alkali itself. Further studies in this direction will no doubt clarify details of effective procedure.

Methods used in cooking vegetables. Boiling, steaming, and baking are the most commonly used methods of cooking vegetables.

1. *Boiling.* Many vegetables such as string beans, turnip and mustard greens, spinach, carrots, and green peas may be cooked in a covered vessel with a small amount of water to preserve flavor, reduce mineral loss, and keep oxidation at a minimum. Washed greens require no additional water.

2. *Steaming.* Spinach, chard, broccoli, and asparagus are especially adapted to this method. A closed vessel is used.

3. *Pressure cooker.* For preservation of flavor, color, and nutritive value the use of a pressure cooker is good. However, the cooking time must be carefully controlled, and the instructions of the manufacturer should be followed carefully since the cooking time is materially shortened and over-cooking can readily occur.

4. *Baking,* with or without removing the skin. This method retains the minerals which lie close to the skin, if the vegetables are not pared. Potatoes, eggplant, and squash are well suited to baking.

5. *Sautéing.* Eggplant, green or ripe tomatoes, and cucumbers are cooked to advantage with this method. The slices of vegetable are rolled in crumbs and browned in small amounts of fat. They should be drained to remove excess grease.

6. *Broiling.* Vegetables may be cooked under an open flame for a short time at high temperature. Tomatoes lend themselves well to broiling.

Vegetables may be served with butter and seasoned with salt, pepper, and herbs. They may be served with white sauce, hollandaise sauce, cheese sauce, sweet or sour sauces, or in cream. Details for the preparation and cookery of vegetables are given in Chapter 54.

PROBLEMS AND REVIEW

1. Give the approximate composition of vegetables. What are the chief reasons for including vegetables in the daily diet?

2. Give examples of vegetables in each botanic grouping.

3. What vegetables are outstanding sources of calcium; of iron; of ascorbic acid; of thiamine; of niacin; of provitamin A?

4. *Problem.* Outline the steps in the selection, storage, preparation, and cookery of (a) white potato, (b) spinach, and (c) cream of carrot soup.

5. *Problem.* List the vegetables in your own diet for 2 days. Calculate the calcium, iron, vitamin A, thiamine, and ascorbic acid content of these vegetables. Approximately what proportion of your daily allowance for each of these minerals and vitamins is provided by vegetables?

6. *Problem.* Illustrate how each of the several methods of cookery may be used for the preparation of carrots, cabbage, and tomatoes.

CHAPTER 49 /

Fruits

Fruits are the fleshy seed-bearing parts of plants. On a botanic basis nuts, cereal grains, and legumes are also fruits, but their composition and uses are so different that they are considered separately. The attractive appearance, delicate flavor, and pleasing odor of fruits make an appeal to the appetite second to that of no other food. Fruits contribute an ever-increasing proportion of the ascorbic acid content of the diet as they become more widely used by everyone. The consumption of citrus fruits has tripled in the last 50 years. On the other hand, the use of apples has been declining. Fruits are included with the Four Food Groups, the daily use of one citrus and one other fruit being recommended.

Composition. Fruits are much alike in their proximate composition but vary widely in their individual characteristics, flavor, color, odor, and palatability. As a group they are important for the vitamins, especially ascorbic acid, which they contain. Water is the chief constituent of fresh fruit, composing about 75 to 95 per cent of the total weight.

Energy. The caloric value of fruit is, generally speaking, low. An average serving of many fruits contains less than 50 calories, while others such as banana, a large apple, and some canned fruits will provide 100 calories or less.

Protein and fat. Fruits contain very little protein and are practically fat free. Avocados and olives, however, contain appreciable amounts of fat.

Carbohydrates. The carbohydrate content of fruit varies widely, from 5 per cent in rhubarb and cantaloupe to 32 per cent in native persimmons. The carbohydrate is in the form of sugars, particularly sucrose, fructose, and glucose, and starch, pectin, and cellulose. The kind of sugar present in fruit is determined by the degree of ripeness; that is, green fruits have more starch and less invert sugar than ripe fruits.

In the meal exchange lists (see Table 4, p. 770) unsweetened fruits are listed in the amounts which will provide 10 gm carbohydrate. Thus, it will be readily seen that a small amount of a relatively high-carbohydrate fruit will supply as much carbohydrate as a much larger measure of a low-carbohydrate fruit. This list serves for the substitution of one fruit for another in measured diets such as the low-calorie or diabetic diets.

The skins, seeds, and fibers are made up of cellulose, which is an unavailable carbohydrate. The texture of fruits is dependent on their fiber structure; thus one finds the variations between orange sections, crisp apples, somewhat fibrous pineapple, and smooth or grainy pears. Pectin is responsible for the ability of fruits to gel when cooked with sugar.

Minerals. Fruits supply a number of minerals although the concentration is usually low. Fresh or dried apricots, raisins, prunes, dates, figs, peaches, and berries are good sources of iron. Calcium is found in small amounts in citrus fruits, figs, and strawberries, but the contribution to the daily diet cannot be considered important. Fruits contain negligible amounts of sodium, but are rather rich in potassium.

Most fruits yield an alkaline ash upon metabolism and thus serve to neutralize the acid ash of foods such as eggs, cereals, and meats. It should be noted that the acid- or sour-tasting fruits also give an alkaline reaction in the body since the organic acids which account for the acid taste are oxidized in the body. Plums, prunes, rhubarb, and cranberries, however, give an acid reaction when metabolized because they contain benzoic acid, which cannot be utilized in the body.

Organic acids. Characteristic flavors in fruits are due to certain volatile compounds and to organic acids, the chief of which are:

1. Citric acid found in oranges, grapefruit, lemons, tangerines, strawberries, raspberries, and others;

2. Malic acid found in apples, peaches, apricots, plums, prunes, and cherries;

3. Tartaric acid found in grapes, cherries, and berries. These acids are metabolized in the body to yield energy, carbon dioxide, and water.

Vitamins. Fruits are especially prized for their ascorbic acid content (see Fig. 49-1), but some of them also contribute appreciable amounts of vitamin A. Citrus fruits are outstanding for their ascorbic acid content. Oranges are so rich in vitamin C that one medium-size orange will supply the amount needed daily by an adult. Frozen and canned juices compare favorably with fresh juices in their level of ascorbic acid and acceptability.

Fresh strawberries, cantaloupe, and honeydew melon are rich in ascorbic acid. Fresh pineapple, banana, apples, peaches, pears, and other berries also contain generous amounts of ascorbic acid, and are specially important if they are eaten often in relatively large amounts. Canned fruits and their juices are lower in their vitamin-C value; however, many juices today are being fortified with ascorbic acid. Unfortunately, the label information accompanying most products does not indicate the amount of ascorbic acid added.

Apricots, yellow peaches, prunes, and cantaloupe rank high as important sources of vitamin A. These fruits retain their vitamin-A content well during dehydration if they are subjected to the sulfuring process, and consequently, weight for weight, dried apricots contain four to five times as much vitamin A

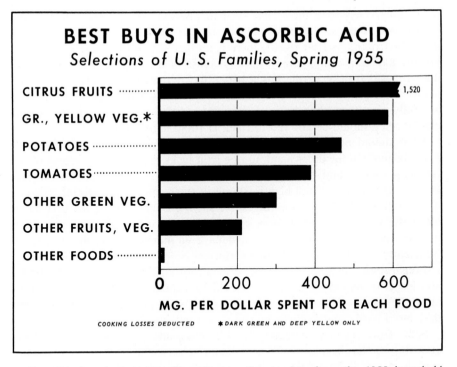

BEST BUYS IN ASCORBIC ACID
Selections of U. S. Families, Spring 1955

CITRUS FRUITS ·········· 1,520

GR., YELLOW VEG.*

POTATOES ·····················

TOMATOES·····················

OTHER GREEN VEG.

OTHER FRUITS, VEG.

OTHER FOODS ··············

0   200   400   600

MG. PER DOLLAR SPENT FOR EACH FOOD

COOKING LOSSES DEDUCTED   *DARK GREEN AND DEEP YELLOW ONLY

Fig. 49-1. Best buys in ascorbic acid according to data from the 1955 household survey. (*Courtesy, Agricultural Research Service, U.S. Department of Agriculture.*)

as fresh apricots. Deep yellow peaches contain much more vitamin A than pale varieties.

Digestibility. Fruits are readily digestible and consequently have a prominent place even in invalid dietaries. The cellulose of fruit, although indigestible, is important to health since it absorbs water and thus stimulates peristalsis and good elimination. Prunes, rhubarb, and figs are especially known for their laxative action. As a juice, fruits help to quench thirst and to supply needed fluids. They may be included in almost all therapeutic diets, either in raw or cooked form. When fiber content must be kept at a minimum, the only raw fruits permitted may be ripe bananas and strained citrus juices. Other fruits may be cooked and puréed for use in such diets as the bland diet.

Place in the diet. Fruits are highly useful because of their aesthetic value, their ability to stimulate the gastric secretion and appetite, their significant contributions of vitamins, especially ascorbic acid, and their functions as body regulators. They may be used as breakfast fruits, either raw or cooked, or as juices; as fruit cups at the beginning of luncheon or dinner; as salads, which lend color and flavor to any meal. Fruits for dessert, always high in favor, are used cooked or uncooked, in pies, cakes, whips, gelatins, water ices, and ice creams. They lend themselves well to low-sodium and low-calorie diets.

Selection and care. Fruits may be selected as fresh, canned, preserved, dried, or frozen. As fruit ripens, there is an increase in the sugar content and volatile flavoring compounds, with a decrease in the organic acid and starch. Tree-ripened fruit as a rule has a better flavor than fruits picked green and allowed to ripen in storage. Peaches and pears are usually picked before they are fully ripe since they bruise easily. If they are slightly green when purchased, they should be allowed to ripen at room temperature.

Fruit should not be overripe when used since fermentation may have already begun. On the other hand, unripe fruit lacks the flavor and aroma of the ripened product, and the sugar content will not have been fully developed. Bananas, for example, are high in starch in their green state. During ripening this starch is changed to more digestible sugars. Bananas have the best flavor when the skin shows speckles of brown (not bruised or decayed spots). A tinge of green at the stem end of a banana is an indication that the fruit is not sufficiently ripe for use in its raw form.

Preparation. All fruit should be washed thoroughly to remove dirt, sprays, and insect contamination. Berries should be kept in a refrigerator until they are to be used and should be washed just before they are to be served, since they mold easily and become mushy if washed in advance.

Some fruits, such as bananas, apples, pears, and peaches, darken quickly after the skin has been removed and should be served as soon as possible after cutting. A sprinkling of lemon juice will help to retard discoloration. Maximum flavor and ascorbic acid content are retained if fruits are not cut until just before they are to be used.

Citrus fruits retain practically all of the initial vitamin C even 24 hours or more after cutting and juice extraction, since the vitamin is stable in acid. A goodly amount of ascorbic acid is found in the pulp of the orange; hence, the eating of a whole orange with the white membrane around it, or the use of unstrained orange juice are desirable practices. (See also Figure 49-2.) If citrus juices are prepared in advance, they should be kept in a covered jar in the refrigerator.

Most fruits are more palatable if chilled before their service. However, bananas and pineapple should be kept at room temperature.

Fruits may be stewed or baked for variety. Cooking diminishes the acute flavors of fresh fruits, brings about a change in color, and softens the cellulose. A higher proportion of sugars is inverted during the cooking so that it is usually necessary to add some sugar to the final product. Fruits retain their shape better if sugar is added at the beginning of the stewing process, but the flavor in many cases is superior if the sugar is added at the end of the cooking period. Boiling brings about a rapid loss of volatile flavoring compounds, and fruit should therefore be simmered, rather than boiled, in a deep covered pan just long enough to give a tender product.

Prunes and raisins account for the greater part of dried-fruit consumption, although apricots, peaches, dates, figs, and apples are also available. A pound of dried fruit is equivalent to about 4 to 6 pounds of fresh fruit. Dried fruits are pasteurized and hydrated so that preliminary washing and soaking is not now necessary.

Fruits may be canned with or without the addition of sugar. Preserves and jellies owe their keeping qualities to the high concentration of sugar used and to the sterilization in the preserving process. Canned fruits may be chilled in the can before opening for table service. Water-packed fruits may be purchased in most supermarkets at moderate cost for those diets restricted in calories and carbohydrate. Some of these fruits include an artificial sweetening agent.

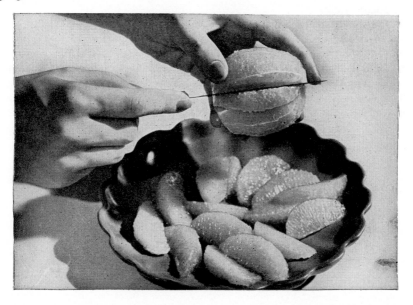

Fig. 49-2. Sectioning an orange. (*Courtesy, California Fruit Growers Exchange, Los Angeles, Calif.*)

Frozen fruits and juices are available in ever-increasing amounts and variety. They may be frozen with or without the addition of sugar. They should be kept in a freezer or the freezing compartment of a refrigerator until 3 or 4 hours before they are to be used. Frozen juice concentrates need not be thawed before reconstitution with water. Thawed fruit must never be refrozen, as marked deterioration of quality will take place. Frozen fruits may be kept in the freezing compartment of the refrigerator for about 1 week, and for several months in a freezer at 0° F.

Recipes for the use of fruits are given on pages 689–91 and for fruit beverages on pages 672–74.

PROBLEMS AND REVIEW

1. Give the approximate composition of fruits. On the basis of this composition what would you say was the chief nutritive importance of fruit in the diet?

2. Which fruits are most valuable for each of the following nutrients: iron, calcium, ascorbic acid, vitamin A?

3. Some individuals are allergic to certain fruits (Chap. 39). Which fruits are most frequent offenders in this respect?

4. List five ways in which fruits may be combined with other foods for variety.

5. When you select fresh fruits, what points would you especially note?

6. *Problem.* Calculate the carbohydrate, calcium, iron, vitamin-A, and ascorbic acid value of 200 gm of fresh orange juice.

7. *Problem.* Compare the caloric value of 100 gm of fresh apricots with 100 gm of dried apricots.

8. *Problem.* Calculate your own ascorbic acid intake for 2 days. What proportion of the total comes from fruits?

9. *Problem.* Calculate the amount (in grams) of each of the following fruits necessary to replace the carbohydrate of 100 gm of orange: cantaloupe, blueberries, grapefruit, strawberries, grapes, bananas, peaches.

10. *Problem.* Calculate the cost of 10 mg ascorbic acid from each of five fruits available in your market.

CHAPTER 50 /

Salads and Salad Dressings

Value of salads in the diet. Because of their rich mineral and vitamin value, salads have ceased being considered a luxury and have become an integral part of the meal. They are, moreover, one of the best ways of increasing the fiber content of the diet. A salad is a good source of protein when such materials as cheese, fish, eggs, or meat constitute the chief ingredients. When served with an oil dressing, it adds materially to the caloric value of the meal. Salads serve to balance the meal, and by their color, crisp texture, and variety of flavors enhance the attractiveness of food service.

Types of salads. According to the place they hold in menu planning, salads may be classified as appetizer, relish, main-course, main-course accompaniment, separate-course, and dessert salads. They may also be grouped according to their basic ingredients.

1. Certain vegetables such as radishes, celery, carrot sticks, and scallions may be used without dressing as relishes or may be included with other salads as a garnish or as an integral part of the salad.

2. Green salads are made of crisp, raw salad greens such as lettuce, romaine, chicory, escarole, endive, shredded cabbage, or water cress (see Fig. 50-1). They are appropriately used as the appetizer or first course at luncheon or dinner, or they may be served with the main course of a meal. A French dressing is usually served with such a salad.

3. Vegetable salads consist of raw or cooked vegetables such as potatoes, carrots, cucumbers, tomatoes, beets, asparagus, or green peppers, used singly or in combinations of two or three. Small, light vegetable salads are usually served with the main course of the meal or occasionally as a separate course, while a more substantial salad may be used together with meat or cheese for the main course; for example, potato salad with cold cuts of meat.

4. Fruit salads may consist of a single fruit or combinations of two or three of the following: oranges, grapefruit, pineapple, apple, grapes, melon, banana, pear, peach, prune, or others. They are used in place of a dessert or frequently when a light refreshment is desired. Some of them may be used with the main course of a meal. They may be served with variations of French dressing, mayonnaise, or a fruit-salad dressing.

643

5. Jellied salads are combinations of fruit or vegetable gelatins and pieces of fruit or vegetables, respectively. Depending upon the type, they are served with the main course of the meal or as a separate salad course.

6. Salads of frozen fruit or vegetables are popular desserts. Fruits or vegetables are folded into a mixture of whipped cream and mayonnaise or other salad dressing, placed in a mold or refrigerator tray, and frozen.

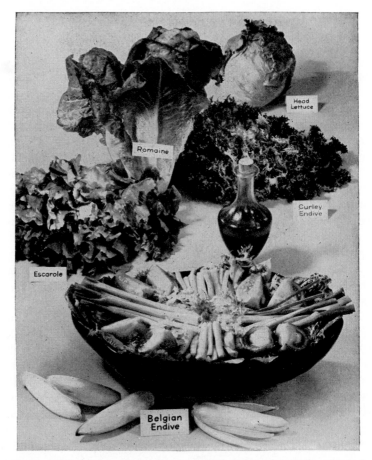

Fig. 50-1. A variety of salad greens provides interesting variations in texture and flavor. (*Courtesy, United Fresh Fruit and Vegetable Association.*)

7. Protein salads contain cooked meat, chicken, fish, eggs, soybeans, or cheese as the main ingredient. Salad greens and various vegetable combinations are used with the protein foods. These salads are used primarily as the main course of the meal where they substitute for the meat and vegetable which would otherwise be served.

Examples of each type of salad are to be found in the recipe section. (See p. 695.)

Essentials for a good salad. The success or failure of a salad is dependent on the observation of certain rules. The salad should be planned to complement the textures, flavors, and color of the rest of the meal. Appropriate combinations of food in the salad, together with a suitable dressing, are essential. Salad greens are proper and attractive bases for any kind of salad. Well-chosen garnishes also lend eye appeal. Simple, rather than elaborate, arrangements of food are to be desired, for too precise, exact arrangement suggests unnecessary handling of food. Meat and vegetables should be cut in uniform, attractive, small pieces, while most fruits may be cut in somewhat larger pieces.

No salad is successful unless it is fresh, cold, crisp, and dry. This necessitates thorough chilling of the salad plate or bowl and of the ingredients, as well as careful draining of foods packed in juices. Salads should be prepared just before serving; in some instances, however, the ingredients are marinated with dressing for an hour or so to develop the flavor. Certain fruits, such as bananas, peaches, apples, and pears, discolor readily. If they are cut with a silver, stainless-steel, or glass knife and are sprinkled with lemon juice or mixed with salad dressing immediately after cutting, such discoloration can be mainly avoided.

SALAD DRESSINGS

Salad dressing binds the ingredients of a salad together and gives the final touch in flavor and color as well as contributing calories. There are a number of dressings, but all fall under three main headings.

1. Mayonnaise, which is a mixture of egg, oil, acid, and seasoning, is so blended that a permanent or stable emulsion results.

2. French dressing is a combination of acid, oil, and seasoning blended to form a temporary emulsion.

3. Cooked dressing is a mixture thickened with egg or flour. It usually contains an appreciable amount of acid.

Oils used in salad dressings. Olive oil is preferred by some for salad dressings because of its fine flavor. It may be imported or domestic and may be obtained in three grades. Because olive oil is rather expensive, it represents only a small fraction of the total oils used in salad dressings.

Cottonseed, corn, soybean, and peanut oils are all used extensively in this country for the preparation of salad dressings. Peanut oil contains moderate amounts of linoleic acid, while the other oils are rich in this essential fatty acid. These oils are light in color, bland in flavor, and have better keeping qualities than olive oil.

Mineral oil should not be used because it interferes with the absorption of some minerals and the fat-soluble vitamins.

Salad oils are pure fats and must be stored in nonmetal air-tight containers. Light and air encourage rancidity.

Principles in preparation of salad dressings. Mayonnaise is a permanent emulsion of oil and acid with egg as an emulsifying agent. An emulsion is a dispersion of one liquid within another. To make it permanent, an emulsifying agent such as egg, starch, or gelatin must be used.

In the preparation of mayonnaise, egg is mixed with the seasonings and lemon juice or vinegar. Oil is added drop by drop, beating continuously to break up the oil in minute droplets to permit complete emulsification. It is important to use a narrow, deep bowl rather than a wide, shallow one so that the beater can be kept well under the surface of the mixture and so that beating can be thorough. Emulsification is more rapidly accomplished when all ingredients are at room temperature. As the volume of the mixture increases, the oil can be added more rapidly without danger of breaking the emulsion.

Mayonnaise may demulsify or curdle during its preparation as a result of too rapid addition of oil, too much oil, too much salt, or insufficient beating. Stirring or shaking the mayonnaise after it has been prepared may also break the emulsion. When this occurs, it is only necessary to begin again with another egg yolk and a little water and to add the curdled mixture very gradually until emulsion takes place; then proceed to use up the entire mixture which has curdled and the remaining oil, if any.

French dressing is a temporary emulsion of acid and oil; it is necessary to shake the mixture vigorously just before it is used. Sugar and seasonings not only affect the flavor of the dressing but are effective aids in forming the emulsion. French dressing is sometimes used to *marinate* cooked foods; that is, diced potatoes or other vegetables or meat may be mixed with the dressing and allowed to stand for a while to improve the flavor.

Cooked dressing is prepared in a double boiler according to the same principles used for the preparation of white sauce (Chap. 47).

PROBLEM AND REVIEW

1. Why are salads important parts of a menu?
2. Name the minerals and vitamins supplied by a citrus-fruit salad.
3. Give two illustrations for each type of salad. State what salad dressing you would use with each salad.
4. Outline the standards for a good salad.
5. State the essentials for salad making.
6. Why is an acid used in the preparation of mayonnaise?
7. What makes French dressing a temporary rather than a stable emulsion?

8. List variations for each of the following salad dressings: mayonnaise, French dressing, cooked dressing.

9. *Problem.* Calculate the protein, calories, calcium, iron, vitamin-A, ascorbic acid, thiamine, and riboflavin value of a salad made with green pepper stuffed with cream cheese.

CHAPTER 51 /

Desserts

In most countries the word "dessert" represents the final sweet at the end of the meal: pudding, pastry, or similar prepared dishes. In England the term "dessert" means the fruit, nuts, raisins, and wine served after the pudding when the table has been cleared.

Place of desserts in the diet. Desserts are important for their psychologic as well as their nutritive value. People have come to regard them as giving a satisfactory finish to a meal. They are attractive in color, they are delightful to the palate, and their sweetness gives satiety value to the meal. Of equal or even greater importance is the fact that desserts can incorporate foods supplying essential proteins, calories, minerals, and vitamins which might otherwise not be taken in optimum amounts. Light desserts may provide acceptable between-meal feedings for those who require additional nourishment.

Desserts may be misused in the diet, and then the disadvantages outweigh their advantages. Heavy desserts such as pies or rich puddings at the end of a substantial meal consisting of foods like roasts, potatoes, one or two vegetables, hot breads, and salads contribute excessively to the energy intake and may unduly prolong digestion. As a rule, rich desserts have no place in the diet of young children or of invalids. If desserts are eaten just before a meal, they may destroy the appetite for other essential foods. Likewise, a dessert and beverage (apple pie and coffee or milk) cannot be used to replace a meal. When the same desserts are used day after day, they, like other foods, become monotonous and lose their appeal.

Classification of desserts and their nutritive value. Desserts may be classed in several categories according to (1) the type of ingredients used; (2) nutritive value as high or low in calories, high or low in protein, high in vitamins, etc.; (3) whether they are light or heavy. The combination of ingredients makes it impossible to group desserts in rigid classes, and the student must understand that much overlapping occurs in the classification given below. According to ingredients and general procedures in preparation, desserts may be grouped as follows:

1. Fruits of all kinds are excellent for desserts. They may be served alone as fresh, stewed or baked, canned or preserved, or frozen, with or without

sugar. They are light desserts suitable at the end of a large meal. When prepared without sugar, they provide the final course for low-calorie or diabetic diets. They are fair to rich sources of minerals and ascorbic acid but provide little protein.

Fruits adapt themselves readily to use with egg white as in fruit whips or soufflés; in fruit puddings as apple tapioca; in frozen desserts as water ices, sherbets, and ice creams; and in fruit pies. In such combinations, of course, the caloric and satiety value may be greatly increased by the additional ingredients employed. Fruit whips provide light, airy desserts for a heavy meal, while pastries are suitable for lighter meals.

2. Gelatin desserts may be made with fruit juices and gelatin alone, or they may consist of jellies with added whole fruit or whipped jelly with whipped egg white or cream. Orange Bavarian cream and Spanish cream illustrate the latter type of gelatin dessert.

Gelatin is collagen which is extracted by boiling the connective tissue, cartilage, and bone of animals. Dry gelatin contains 86 per cent protein and 14 per cent water. The amount of gelatin used in a dessert will provide no more than about 2 gm protein. The protein of gelatin lacks some of the essential amino acids, but it is of good supplementary value when used with eggs or milk.

Plain gelatin desserts are relatively low in calories and protein, but the fruit or juices used in them may contribute significantly to the ascorbic acid level of the diet. When milk or cream is used, the caloric and protein values are greatly enhanced.

3. Milk desserts with or without egg are possible in almost endless variety as custards, Junkets, puddings, sherbets, mousses, ice cream. They are the most nutritious of all desserts since they make valuable contributions to the protein, calcium, phosphorus, vitamin-A, B-complex, and caloric levels of the diet. They are among the most readily digested foods.

Junket is a coagulated milk preparation that is made by adding the enzyme rennin to sweetened milk heated to a temperature not to exceed 100° F. The enzyme is destroyed by excess heat and is inactive in cold temperatures. Therefore, the successful preparation of rennet desserts depends upon the proper temperature of the milk.

Simple milk desserts lend themselves readily to most therapeutic diets. When saccharin is substituted for sugar, they may be used by diabetic patients, providing that the ingredients are considered in the total food allowances for the given meal.

4. Starchy desserts combine various cereals such as rice, tapioca, cornstarch, or bread with milk and, usually, eggs. Rice, tapioca, and bread puddings are examples of such desserts. They provide the nutrients of milk and eggs plus the carbohydrate of the cereal.

Cakes, cookies, and pastries are popular desserts which are high in carbohydrate and often high in fat. Fruit is frequently used in pastries, as for example in apple pie.

5. Frozen desserts include water ices, milk sherbets, mousses, and ice creams. Water ices are relatively low in calories, but the use of milk (fresh or evaporated) alone or of milk and cream raises the energy and protein values considerably.

Essentials for a good dessert. A successful dessert is one that completes the meal but does not dominate it. It must fit in with the particular meal; that is, a heavy meal requires a light dessert, while a light meal may require supplementary protein, calories, etc., which can be provided by a heavier dessert. A dessert must appeal to the appetite by reason of its attractive service, color, or flavor. It should be properly flavored and correct in both texture and temperature. A lumpy or pasty cornstarch pudding, a lukewarm piece of cantaloupe, a curdled custard, gummy tapioca pudding, or rubbery gelatin may destroy an individual's taste for that dessert forever. Variety in the selection of desserts is essential if interest in this part of the meal is to be maintained.

Preparation. By the time the student has reached the point of making desserts she should have acquired an appreciation of the principles of cookery for eggs, milk, cereals, and fruits. A review of these principles together with the careful following of instructions given in recipes will lead to the successful preparation of simple desserts.

Commercial preparations. Powders in great variety are available for gelatin dishes, cornstarch puddings, Junkets, tapioca puddings, ice cream, and sherbets which require only the addition of liquid. Mixes for piecrust, pie fillings, gingerbread, cookies, cakes, icings, cream puffs, meringues, and other desserts may be purchased at moderate cost. These products are time-saving, and if directions are carefully followed many interesting desserts can be prepared. Whipped cream, nuts, and fresh fruit add variety when properly employed.

Recipes for desserts are found in Chapter 54, page 681.

PROBLEM AND REVIEW

1. What are the important steps in the preparation of each of these simple desserts: soft custard, baked custard, Junket, chocolate pudding? What are the reasons for each of these steps?

2. What is gelatin? Name three ways of incorporating gelatin in the diet.

3. Outline the steps in the preparation of a fruit-juice gelatin and give the reasons for each step.

4. Desserts may be varied by the use of different sweetening and flavoring agents. Give a list of such flavoring agents and include an example of a dessert which employs each one you have mentioned.

5. List five desserts suitable for a soft diet.

6. *Problem.* Calculate the protein, carbohydrate, caloric, vitamin-A, thiamine, riboflavin, and ascorbic acid content of the recipe for baked custard and for orange jelly. In what ways could the caloric and protein content of the custard be increased?

CHAPTER 52 /

Cheese

Types. Cheese is a milk product representing the solids or curd of milk. The curd may be produced by the action of rennet or of lactic acid. As the milk casein coagulates and becomes semisolid, the whey separates out. The difference in varieties of cheese is due to the kind of milk used—cow (most common), goat, or sheep; the method used for curding the milk—rennet or lactic acid; the temperature and humidity for ripening; the amount of salt and seasonings used; the amount of moisure retained; and the type of bacteria or mold used for ripening.

Cheese is generally classified as hard, semihard, and soft. In hard cheeses the microorganisms are distributed through the cheese and act in a uniform manner all through the cheese, but in soft cheeses the organisms act only on the surface and gradually penetrate the mass. Soft cheeses consequently are made in small sizes. Over 400 varieties of cheese are known, those more widely used being listed here.

Soft
   Unripened: cottage, cream
   Bacteria ripened: Liederkranz, Limburger
   Mold ripened: Brie, Camembert
Semihard
   Bacteria ripened: brick, Muenster
   Mold ripened: blue, Gorgonzola, Roquefort
Hard
   Cheddar, Edam, Gouda, Gruyère, Parmesan, pineapple, Swiss

Process cheese consists of a blending of mild American cheese with other cheeses, followed by pasteurization. An emulsifying agent, such as disodium phosphate or sodium citrate, gives a smooth texture and keeps the fat from separating out. The process cheeses have a consistently uniform flavor and texture, and they keep well; they do not have the fine flavor of an aged Cheddar.

Of the hard cheeses, Cheddar—also known as American—cheese accounts for the bulk of the market. Cottage and cream cheese are increasing in popularity year by year.

651

Nutritive value. The composition of cheese depends upon the kind of milk used—whole or skim—and the amount of water present. A pound of hard cheese contains the casein and fat of 1 gallon of milk (see Fig. 52-1). Only a small amount of the lactalbumin of milk is retained. The proteins in cheese contain all the essential amino acids, and therefore are of high biologic value. During the process of ripening some of the protein becomes digested to

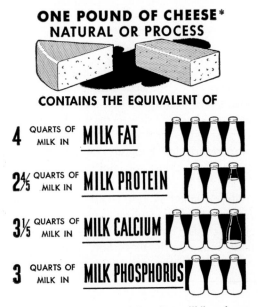

ONE POUND OF CHEESE*
NATURAL OR PROCESS

CONTAINS THE EQUIVALENT OF

4 QUARTS OF MILK IN **MILK FAT**

2⅘ QUARTS OF MILK IN **MILK PROTEIN**

3⅗ QUARTS OF MILK IN **MILK CALCIUM**

3 QUARTS OF MILK IN **MILK PHOSPHORUS**

* NOTE: Based on average composition of "market milk" and average composition of process and natural American Cheddar cheese. (*Courtesy, Kraft Foods Company, Consumer Service Department.*)

Fig. 52-1. Both cheese and milk are good food sources of Vitamins A and B₂.

soluble protein; that is, to proteoses, peptones, and even amino acids. Only a trace of the lactose present in milk remains in the cheese. Varying amounts of calcium, thiamine, and riboflavin are lost depending upon the method of preparation.

The average composition of hard cheese is: protein, 25 per cent; fat, 32 per cent; water, 37 per cent; calcium, 0.73 per cent, and phosphorus, 0.68 per cent. It ranks high as a source of vitamin A and riboflavin.

Soft cheeses vary widely in their composition. If made with skim milk, cottage cheese will contain as little as 1 per cent of fat; the protein content is about 19 per cent. Creamed cottage cheese is made by mixing the curd with cream or a cream-milk mixture; the fat content of the final product is about 4 per cent. Cottage cheese is considerably lower than Cheddar cheese in its calcium content since some of the calcium is lost in the whey with acid coagulation. While about 1¼ ounces of Cheddar cheese provide the calcium equivalent of 1 cup milk, almost 11 ounces of cottage cheese are needed for the same amount of calcium.

Cream cheese which is made from whole milk with cream added contains approximately 9 per cent protein and 37 per cent fat. It is therefore high in calories but is not a good substitute for cottage or hard cheese in terms of protein. Its calcium content is even less than that of cottage cheese.

Digestibility. Cheese is almost completely digested and leaves little residue in the intestine. It is probably digested with no more difficulty than a similar amount of meat. Cottage and cream cheese are common and useful foods for the invalid. Mild hard cheeses may be used in sauces for menu variety in many therapeutic diets.

Occasionally the volatile acids developed in well-ripened cheese may irritate the sensitive mucous membranes. In actual practice, the reputed indigestibility of cheese can usually be explained by the custom of serving cheese at the end of a substantial meal already more than sufficient. If used instead of dessert following an ordinary well-balanced meal in which the protein supply is not great, and especially if the cheese is well masticated, it should not cause discomfort.

Place in the diet. Cheese is gradually finding a more prominent place in the American diet. It supplements a meal otherwise low in protein or where protein is of poor quality; it is an economical substitute for meat, poultry, and fish; and its uses are so many and varied that it lends interest to every-day and company meals. Only a few of the many ways in which cheese may be used are suggested here.

1. Main dishes at luncheon or supper as a substitute for meat or fish, in the form of omelet, soufflé, fondue, Welsh rarebit, croquettes
2. In combination with macaroni, spaghetti, rice, noodles
3. As filling for sandwiches
4. As cheese sauce for vegetables such as broccoli, cauliflower, potatoes
5. As a hearty salad, such as peppers or tomatoes stuffed with cottage cheese; or fruit salad with cottage cheese
6. In salad dressings—Roquefort cheese with French dressing
7. Grated—on salads, soups (potato and onion), spaghetti, Melba toast
8. As a dessert at the end of dinner using a highly ripened cheese such as Roquefort, Camembert, Stilton, and crisp crackers; or pie with cheese; or fruit and cheese
9. Cheese dips for crackers, potato chips, pretzels

Recipes for cheese dishes may be found on page 679.

Selection and care. Cheddar, processed, and cottage cheese are economical while some imported cheeses which require exact and long ripening are costly. Cheddar cheese is specially useful in many cooked dishes. It is of good quality when it has a smooth, waxy texture, uniform color, and a nutty, slightly acid flavor. If it melts readily when it is held on the tongue, it is suitable for dishes requiring heat in their preparation. A cheese that has ripened for 6 months or longer is superior in cooking qualities to one which has had little ripening.

Cheese must be protected from disease-producing organisms since a number of gastrointestinal epidemics have been traced to cheese contaminated with streptococci and staphylococci. Unpasteurized cheese, particularly, may spoil and assume a strong unpleasing flavor because of mold or bacterial infiltration. Soft cheeses require constant refrigeration because they deteriorate rapidly. Cheese should be wrapped in wax paper, plastic, or foil, excluding as much air as possible, and kept in a cool place. If mold appears on hard cheese, it may be scraped away with little effect on the cheese. If Cheddar cheese becomes hardened before it is used, it may be grated for use in soups, cream sauces, etc.

Principles of cookery. Whenever cheese is used as an ingredient of cooked dishes, its protein nature should be remembered. Cheddar cheese softens and then melts at low temperatures. It toughens or becomes rubbery and stringy at 185° F or with overlong cooking. In the preparation of sauces a double boiler should be used, or the sauces may be cooked over low heat with continuous stirring. However, one should never attempt to melt cheese over direct heat. Dishes such as soufflés are set in a pan of hot water during baking to keep a uniform low temperature.

When cheese is to be served as an accompaniment to pie or with crackers, it should be allowed to come to room temperature before serving.

PROBLEMS AND REVIEW

1. *Problem.* Calculate the food value of the recipe for cheese soufflé.

2. *Problem.* Compare in table form the carbohydrate, protein, fat, caloric, calcium, vitamin-A, and riboflavin values of 100 gm of Cheddar, cottage, cream, Swiss, and Roquefort cheese.

3. *Problem.* About how much American cheese must be used in the diet to replace the protein and calcium of 1 cup (240 gm) of milk?

4. Visit your local market to see what cheeses are available. Classify them as to type.

5. List the factors which determine the flavor of cheese.

6. What reasons can you give for encouraging a more widespread use of cheese than it now enjoys?

7. Give various ways in which cheese may be used in the diet. Illustrate.

8. What precautions are necessary to avoid heavy cheese soufflé with a curdled appearance; stringy macaroni and cheese; grilled cheese sandwich with a rubbery texture?

CHAPTER 53 /

Meat, Poultry, and Fish

Meat is the name given to the flesh of such animals as beef, veal, mutton, lamb, and pork. As an inclusive term, it may also be applied to poultry and fish.

Place of meat in the diet. Since the days of the cave man and all through ancient and medieval history, meat has occupied a position of first importance in the diet. The pioneers of this country had an abundance of meat, and even as recently as 50 years ago the use of it three times a day was commonplace. Today meat is the most expensive item of the daily menu and accounts for a large proportion of the food budget. Even at lower income levels most families manage to have a fairly liberal allowance of meat.

Per capita consumption. On the basis of available food supplies, the per capita consumption each year of meat is about 160 pounds; [239] of poultry, 31 pounds; and of fish, 10 pounds.[240] About half of the meat consumed is beef, while pork accounts for almost two fifths. Thus, veal, lamb, and mutton together account for about 10 per cent of the meat consumed (see Fig. 53-1).

The use of variety meats depends to no small extent on family traditions and beliefs. The tongue, liver, brain, and heart of beef, lamb, veal, or pork, the sweetbreads or thymus gland of calves, and tripe of beef are all useful and highly nutritious meats.

Fish and poultry in the diet. Fish and shellfish are gradually gaining in popularity. However, some reasons for the more limited use of fish may be the idea held by some people that fish is inferior food because it is used on fast days instead of meat; that it is a food selected by the poor; that it has not always been available far away from the seacoast, lake, or river regions; and that it is so often poorly cooked and unpalatable. As a food, fish is equal in nutritive value to meat except that the caloric value is usually lower by reason of the lower fat concentration. The small amount of connective tissue in fish makes it especially suitable for diets of the sick. Some people are allergic to shellfish in particular, and this fact must be kept in mind.

Chicken and turkey have become increasingly popular during recent years.

Young chickens suitable for broiling or frying are available during the entire year, while turkeys of smaller size are being produced in greater numbers for year-round use by the average family.

Acceptability of meat and fish. Aside from its high nutritive value, meat is an important dietary item because the aromas and flavors given by meat extractives stimulate the appetite. Meat and fish have a high satiety value because the protein and fat content prolong the digestive period. The often heard comment "It doesn't seem like a meal without meat" attests to the importance of this food on a popular and psychologic basis.

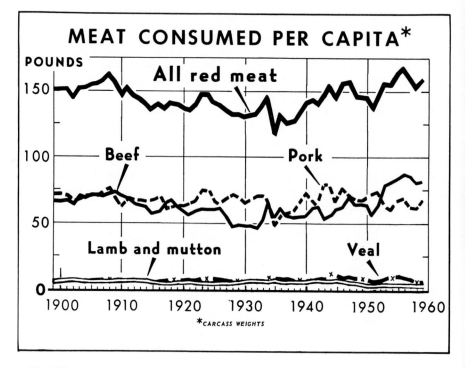

Fig. 53-1. Per capita consumption of meat. (*Courtesy, Agricultural Marketing Service, U.S. Department of Agriculture.*)

Meat alternates. It is wise to use organ meats and fish to an increasing extent, and to appreciate the role of cheese, eggs, legumes, and nuts as meat substitutes. Cheese and eggs are excellent sources of complete protein (Chaps. 45 and 52); legumes (Chap. 48) and nuts are high in protein concentration, but the protein is of lower biologic value. When supplemented with milk, these foods are inexpensive and excellent sources of protein. Peanuts and soybeans have a somewhat higher biologic value than other nuts and legumes.

The wide use of many kinds of meat, fish, and meat alternates is economically advisable and provides greater interest to menus.

Composition of flesh foods. Variations in the composition of meat, from one cut to another, and from one kind to another, are due largely to the proportion of lean and fat tissue. Considering the entire carcass, the proportion of fat is greater in older animals than in young animals; it is also higher in pork than in beef, and in lamb than in veal, and so on. Moreover, one cut of meat may be extremely lean, that from another part of the animal may be well marbled with fat—that is, tiny fat streaks are intertwined with the muscle fibers and inseparable from them, and that from still another part may be high in adipose tissue and low in muscle fiber.

Such considerations as the above do not necessarily modify the nutritive value of meat as consumed since (1) fat may be trimmed off and discarded before meat is cooked, (2) fat lost in drippings may not be used, and (3) surrounding fat on meat may be left as plate waste. Obviously, it is important to know the values for cooked meat as it is actually consumed. Leverton and Odell [241] have conducted extensive analyses of cooked meat and have suggested the following values as a guide in dietary planning:

	CALORIES	PROTEIN	FAT
	(per 100 gm cooked meat)		
		gm	gm
Extremely lean portion	200	32	8
Lean-plus-marble portions	255	28	16

The extremely lean portion would represent a selection of meat suitable for fat-restricted diets; it would contain no visible traces of fat. The lean-plus-marble portion represents meat as it is usually consumed.

Leverton and Odell found that no one kind of cooked lean meat or of lean-plus-marble meat was distinctly different from other kinds. Cooked pork was no higher in fat than similar portions of beef, veal, or lamb. For most dietary purposes, then, the four kinds of meat may be used interchangeably on a protein, fat, and caloric basis.

Minerals. The mineral content of meat is directly proportional to the protein content. Meat is an excellent source of iron; organ meats such as liver and heart contain much more iron than muscle meats. Meats are rich in phosphorus, sulfur, and potassium, moderately high in sodium, and quite low in their calcium content. Salt-water fish contains an appreciable amount of iodine.

Vitamins. Meats are good sources of the B-complex vitamins including thiamine, niacin, riboflavin, vitamin B_6, vitamin B_{12}, and others. Pork, liver, and other organ meats are excellent for their thiamine content; for the other vitamins the different kinds of meat are comparable.

Liver is an outstanding source of vitamin A; other organs such as the kidney contain some vitamin A. Otherwise, meats do not provide vitamin A, nor are they a source of ascorbic acid.

Extractives and purines. Various nonprotein nitrogenous substances, especially the purines, give to meat its characteristic flavor. They are readily extracted from meat with water, as in the preparation of broth. They have very little nutritive value.

Digestibility. Like other animal foods, meat is almost completely digested and absorbed, there being little if any residue in the intestinal tract. The rate of digestion is dependent upon the amount of fat eaten and the method of cooking. The less fat and connective tissue the meat contains, the more complete is its disintegration and the more rapid its passage from the stomach.

Selection of meat. Many factors should be considered in the choice of meat.

Safety as a food. Inspection of meat by the government is strictly enforced whenever interstate sale is concerned. The government seal of inspection, a small purple mark stamped on meat, indicates that the meat has been inspected for freedom from disease, and that it has been made ready for the market under sanitary conditions. As a rule, the period of hanging, the temperature of the cold room, and the internal temperature of the meat itself are all factors affecting the safety as well as the tenderness of meat. Soiled hands on the part of the butcher, dirty meat blocks and meat grinders, as well as dust and dirt coming in contact with openly exposed meat are among the factors militating against the safety of meat, since the bacterial count of such meat is likely to be too high for safety. (See also Chap. 21.)

Tenderness and texture. The tenderness of meat is dependent on the (1) muscular development, (2) part of the animal or cut of meat, (3) age, and (4) amount and kind of connective tissue. Meat cut from resting muscles is more tender than the cuts taken from muscles constantly energized (the flank, for example). The latter are rich in extractives and if properly prepared are both palatable and economical. The meat from cattle and poultry allowed to range is never as tender as that from animals which have been pen fed. The meat of old animals may be tough and stringy, while that of the young animal is tender. Mature animals as a rule show richer fat deposits than immature animals. The process of ripening brings about enzymatic action which accomplishes chemical and physical changes so that the fibers are more tender.

Cooking time. The cooking time required for meat is determined by the tenderness. As a rule, expensive tender cuts of meat require a short cooking time, while the less costly, tougher cuts demand a long, slow cooking period.

Economy. It is necessary to consider the cost of meat in terms of edible portions. The least expensive cuts of meat, when interpreted in terms of protein and other nutrients and the amount of fuel used in cookery, may sometimes be more costly in the end than more expensive cuts. The popular steaks, chops, and tender roasts as a rule are the more expensive cuts of meat. Poultry, because of its high proportion of bone, is usually more expensive than meat. Fish, on the other hand, is inexpensive, although shrimp and lobster are costly items.

The characteristics and cuts of meat, fish, and poultry are summarized below and in the tables on pages 663, 664, and 665. (See also Figures 53-2, 3, 4, and 5.)

BEEF CHART

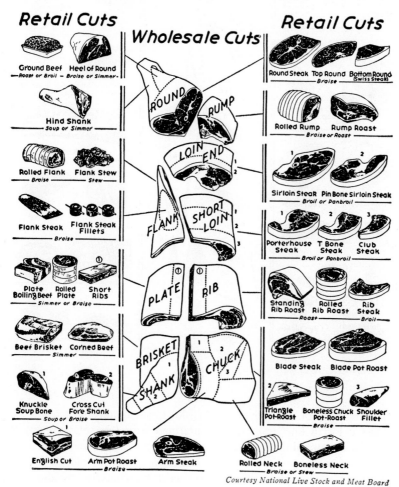

Courtesy National Live Stock and Meat Board

Fig. 53-2.

VEAL CHART

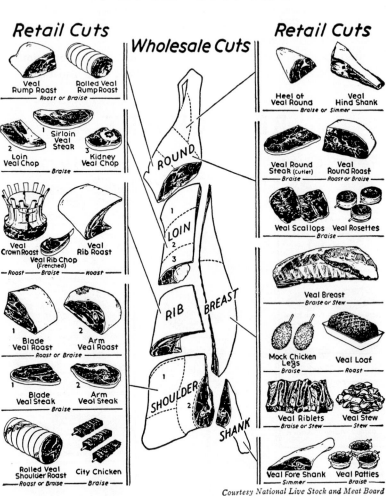

Courtesy National Live Stock and Meat Board

Fig. 53-3.

Beef is the flesh of cattle over 1 year old. Good quality beef has a bright, cherry red color; a fine grain texture marbled with fat; solid creamy-white layers of fat surrounding the muscle bundles; and porous red bones.

Choice *veal* is the flesh of a calf 6 weeks to 3 months old. It has a fine grain texture; grayish pink color; clear, hard fat sparsely distributed; and porous red bones.

LAMB CHART

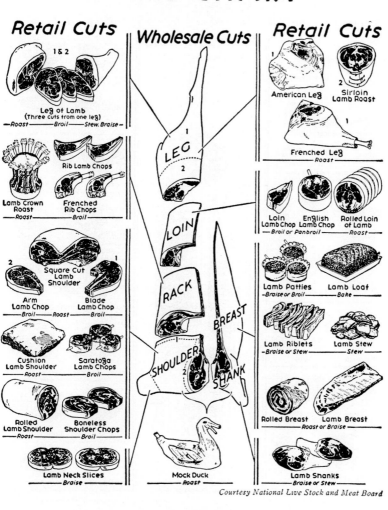

Courtesy National Live Stock and Meat Board

Fig. 53-4.

Lamb is the flesh of sheep 2 to 3 months old, but a well-fed animal may still be classed as lamb, rather than mutton, at 1 year. The flesh is firm and fine grained; pink in color; and the fat is firm, white, and flaky.

Pork includes the flesh of a suckling pig to a mature medium-size pig. Its flesh is fine and firm with a minute layer of fat coating the fibers; the color is grayish pink; the fat is smooth and white; and the bones are soft and tinged with red.

PORK CHART

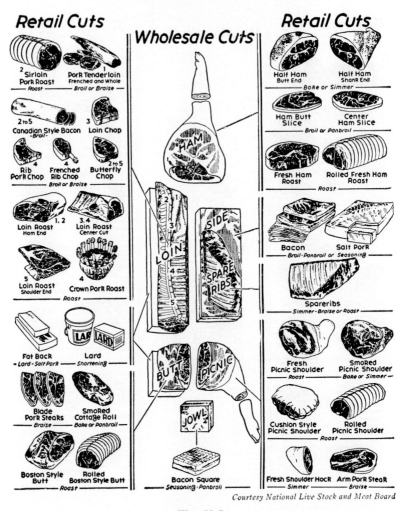

Courtesy National Live Stock and Meat Board

Fig. 53-5.

Care of meat, poultry, and fish. Meat or poultry should be unwrapped immediately after purchase and stored uncovered or lightly covered with a wax paper in the coldest part of the refrigerator. Because of its odor fish should be kept in a closed container until it is to be used. Since organ meats, ground meats, and fish spoil more rapidly than other meats, they should be used within 24 hours; or they should be stored in the freezing compartment of the refrigerator for use within a few days.

Meat, poultry, and fish may be purchased in the frozen state. If they are

METHODS OF COOKERY FOR VARIOUS CUTS OF MEAT

TYPE	DRY HEAT		MOIST HEAT	
	Broiling	Roasting	Braising	In Liquid
Beef	Steaks	Loaf	Brisket	(Large cuts and
	club	Rib	Plate	stews)
	hamburg	rolled	Pot roast	Brisket
	loin tip	standing	Shank	Corned beef
	porterhouse	Rump	Short ribs	Flank
	rib		Steaks	Heel of round
	sirloin		arm	Neck
	T-bone		blade	Plate
	tenderloin		flank	Shank
	top round		round	Short ribs
				Stew meat
Veal	Too lean for	Leg	Breast	Breast
	broiling	Loaf	Chops	Flank
		Loin	rib	Heel of round
		Rack	loin	Neck
		Shoulder, bone in	Cubes	Riblets
		or rolled	Steaks	Shank
				Shoulder
				Stew meat
Lamb	Chops	Leg	Breast	Breast
	loin	Loaf	Chops, shoul-	Flank
	rib	Shoulder, bone in	der	Neck
	shoulder	or rolled	Neck slices	Riblets
	sirloin		Shank	Shank
	Patties			Stew meat
	Steaks			
Pork	Bacon	Boston butt	Chops	Smoked:
	Canadian bacon	Loin	Hocks	ham
	Ham slice	Sirloin	Shoulder steaks	picnic ham
	Smoked shoulder	Spareribs	Spareribs	shank
	slice	Ham, fresh or smoked	Tenderloin	shoulder butt
	Fresh pork should	Picnic ham, fresh		
	not be broiled	or smoked		
		Ham loaf		
Variety	Brains		Brains	Brains
	Kidneys		Heart	Heart
	Liver, lamb or veal		Kidney	Kidney
	Sweetbreads		Liver	Sweetbreads
			Sweetbreads	Tongue

to be used within the week such frozen foods may be kept in the freezing compartment of the refrigerator, but for longer storage frozen meats must be kept at about 0° F or lower in a freezer. They must be tightly wrapped in good quality freezer paper, excluding all air, if they are to maintain good quality. Frozen meats should never be allowed to thaw and then be refrozen.

Cured and smoked hams and other cured meats also require refrigeration

KIND	CHARACTERISTICS AND TESTS FOR QUALITY	METHODS OF PREPARATION
Fish		Large fish may be baked; small fish broiled or fried
fatty	Colored flesh as a rule: mackerel, herring, sardines, eel, shad	
		Steaks and fillets from large fish broiled or sautéed
lean	White flesh usually: cod, haddock, black bass, bluefish, flounder, pickerel	
		Butter or fat should be added to lean fish if it is broiled
	Eyes: full and bright Gills: pink Flesh: firm and elastic; does not keep a dent when pressed with finger Odor: clean, fresh fish odor	Thaw frozen fish and prepare as fresh fish
Fish roe	Shad, sturgeon (caviar)	Fresh: broiled, baked
Shellfish	Fresh, frozen, canned	Short cooking for all shellfish to avoid toughening
mollusks	Soft unsegmented body	
oysters	Firm, plump; available September through April	Raw, fried, creamed, stew, scalloped
clams	Hard shell (quahaugs, round) available all year Little-neck (round) Soft shell (long) available May to October Select those with unbroken shells	Steamed, chowder, broiled Raw Boiled, steamed, chowder
scallops	Available September to March	Fried, fritters, chowders
crustaceans	Crustlike shell	
lobster	Select live, if not already boiled; active response to touch; available especially in summer	Broiled; boiled: à la Newburg, salads, cocktails, casserole dishes
lobster tails	Frozen	Boiling, broiling
shrimp	Available all year; fresh or frozen	Boiled: cocktails, fried, salads, curried, casserole dishes
crab	Hard shell—all year Soft shell—summer Grades in descending order of quality: claw, white, special lump, back fin	Salads, cocktails, scalloped, deviled, casserole dishes

SELECTION OF POULTRY

TESTS FOR QUALITY	KIND	WEIGHT pounds	METHODS OF PREPARATION
Breastbone: flexible; breast well-fleshed Wings: flexible; will spring back into place when pulled out Skin: dry, firm; age is indicated by hair on older chicken; pin feathers on young birds Fat: well-distributed and not abundant Legs: short and well-fleshed; not bony or long	Squab Cornish hen Broiler	¾–1 ¾–1 Small: ¾–1 Regular: 1–2	Squab and Cornish hens may be baked stuffed or unstuffed Broilers should be split down the back and cooked in a broiler or on a grill over live coals
	Fryer, whole or pieces	2–3	Fryers are disjointed and dipped in batter (chicken à la Maryland) or dipped in flour (southern fried chicken) and immersed in hot fat
	Roasting chicken Capon Duck Turkey Fowl	3–6 3–6 1½–4 5–20 3–6	Roast poultry is cooked whole, usually stuffed Fowl may be stewed for fricassee, salads, etc.

and should be kept in the package in which they are purchased. Canned hams also require refrigeration.

Leftover cooked meats should be stored in a covered dish in the refrigerator and should be used within 24 hours as a rule.

Principles of cookery. Meat is cooked in order to improve the flavor, increase digestibility, and destroy harmful bacteria. Cooking results in a change of color, loss of moisture, coagulation of protein, melting of the fat, and a change of collagen to gelatin (moist heat). Meat may be cooked by dry or moist heat.

There are two classes of proteins in meat, soluble and insoluble. The albumins and globulins of muscle fiber are soluble in dilute salt solution, while albumin is also soluble in water and in dilute acid solution. These proteins are coagulated by heat much below the boiling point; boiling water toughens albumin and hardens the globulin.

The proteins of connective tissue are insoluble and are of two kinds, collagen and elastin. Collagen is the chief constituent of white connective tissue which binds the muscle fibers to each other and to the bones. It is changed to gelatin when subjected to moist heat for a prolonged cooking time but is hardened by dry heat. The change from collagen to gelatin may be hastened by the use of acid; thus, tomato juice as in the preparation of Swiss steak, or vinegar, sometimes used in the marination of meat, helps to give a more tender product in a shorter cooking time.

Elastin, the main component of yellow connective tissue which is found in the ligaments, walls of the blood vessels, and between the muscle fibers, is not affected by moist heat but is hardened by dry heat.

The presence of fat in meat helps to retain moisture when it is subjected to dry heat. Very lean meats do not lend themselves well to cookery by dry heat. Meats such as liver and veal or lean fish should be brushed with butter or other fat if they are to be broiled to compensate for the absence of fat and to prevent dryness.

The length of cooking time is dependent upon the amount of connective tissue present and the toughness of the muscle fiber. The tender cuts of meat using dry heat require only a short cooking period, but tougher cuts of meat with much connective tissue require longer cookery. Fish contains such a small amount of connective tissue that the cooking time is very short. High temperatures give a tasteless, dry product. Fish is done when it "flakes" or separates on being touched with the point of a sharp knife.

Frozen meats may be cooked after thawing or without thawing if additional cooking time is allowed. Thawing requires a few hours at room temperature, depending upon the size and thickness of the cut, or about 24 hours if kept on a shelf in the refrigerator.

Cooking by dry heat. Oven or pan broiling, and baking in an oven or roasting over live coals or electrically heated wires are used for tender cuts of meat. A low temperature used throughout the cooking period results in less shrinkage, more juiciness, more attractive appearance, and greater tenderness. Searing is not only unnecessary, but it is undesirable.

Roasting. Large tender cuts of beef, veal, pork, lamb, or ground-meat loaves are roasted in an uncovered pan with a rack to permit circulation of heat around the meat. The fat side is placed up so that the meat bastes itself. No water is used. A temperature of 300° F is used for all meats except pork which requires a temperature of 350° F. Pork must be cooked so thoroughly that no tinge of pink remains in the meat itself or along the bone. Trichinella infestations are common in pork and may cause serious illness unless the parasite is destroyed by thorough cooking of the meat. A meat thermometer is an invaluable aid in determining when meat is cooked. The meat may be seasoned with salt and pepper at the beginning of the roasting or later, since salt penetrates only to a depth of about ½ inch.

Broiling is used for tender chops, steaks, meat patties, or fish. The meat is placed 2 or 3 inches away from the heat and is broiled until the top surface is browned. Here again, excessive heat is to be avoided, since the surface of thick pieces will become hardened and dry before the center is cooked, while thinner chops and steaks will be toughened throughout. Salt and pepper is added to the browned surface and the meat is turned; to add salt at the beginning would extract considerable amounts of juices and thus retard browning and detract from flavor. While fish, liver, and veal may be broiled, they lend themselves better to other methods of cookery. Broiling is not recommended for fresh pork.

In *pan broiling* the meat should be cooked without the addition of fat or water in a heavy uncovered pan. The meat is turned occasionally as it browns. Fat is poured off as it accumulates; otherwise the meat would be fried rather than broiled.

Cooking by moist heat. Less tender cuts of meat are cooked by braising, simmering, or stewing. Long cooking in the presence of moisture is necessary to soften the collagen and convert it to gelatin. Braising is also recommended for liver, and steaks and chops of pork and veal. The meat may be dredged with flour or coated with egg and crumbs, if desired. It is browned in fat, after which liquid is added together with salt, pepper, herbs, spices, and vegetables, depending upon the dish which is being prepared. The meat may be cut in small pieces to increase the surface area and to give a highly flavored broth. The flavor is further developed by long, slow cooking over a flame or in an oven.

Recipes for meats may be found in Chapter 54, pages 691–95.

Retention of vitamins in meat. Extensive research has been carried on to determine the effect of cooking meat by various methods. Braising and stewing resulted in greater losses of all the B vitamins than did broiling, roasting, and pan frying. This is explained in part by the solubility of these vitamins in water, and emphasizes the necessity for using liquids and drippings from meat cookery in either gravies, sauces, or soups. Losses were much higher in the instance of thiamine than they were for riboflavin and niacin. In the latter vitamins the losses could be explained almost entirely on the basis of extraction into the drippings.

When meats were roasted or broiled they retained 65 and 70 per cent of the thiamine, respectively; pan-fried meats still contained 90 per cent of the original thiamine. On the other hand, stewed meats retained only 25 per cent of the thiamine, while an additional 25 per cent was present in the liquid.

PROBLEM AND REVIEW

1. What foods are included in the general term "meat"?
2. Describe the composition of meat.
3. List the factors which determine the quality of meat.
4. What factors should be noted, especially when selecting poultry? Fish?
5. Why are not all so-called cheap cuts of meat necessarily economical?
6. How may meat be preserved?
7. Which is the more difficult to preserve, meat or fish?
8. Why is it important to cook pork thoroughly?

9. Name the cuts of meat you would select for preparing the following: Swiss steak, meat balls, filet mignon, beef stew.

10. *Problem.* Complete the following table:

	COST PER POUND	PROTEIN PER POUND AS PURCHASED, GRAMS	COST PER 100 GRAMS PROTEIN
Lamb chop		83	
Lamb neck		66	
Pork shoulder		59	
Pork loin chop		70	
Beef rib roast		69	
Beef round		88	
Frankfurter		65	
Frying chicken		69	

CHAPTER 54 /

Recipes

Beverages

Beverages may be reinforced for nutritive value in various ways or may be modified for therapeutic needs.

Calories. 1. Use light cream for part or all of the milk.

2. Add 1 to 2 small dips ice cream to milk beverages.

3. Substitute 2 to 3 teaspoons glucose for each teaspoon cane sugar, thus increasing the caloric value of the beverage.

Protein. 1. One to 3 tablespoons nonfat dry milk may be added to each glass of milk beverage.

2. Whole egg, egg white, or egg yolk may be used in fruit juices or in milk beverages.

Low Fat. For low-fat diets:

1. Use skim liquid or dry milk.

2. Use white of egg only.

3. Omit cream.

TEA

Tea is made by infusion; that is, it is never boiled. Bring freshly drawn cold water to the boiling point. Scald an earthenware or china pot. Allow 1 level teaspoon tea or 1 tea ball to each cup of boiling water. Put tea in pot, and pour boiling water over leaves. Cover closely, and allow to stand from 1 to 3 minutes according to the strength desired. Serve immediately with sugar, lemon, cream, or milk. Tea should never be reheated.

ICED TEA

Prepare hot tea using a double quantity of tea leaves. When steeped, pour over crushed ice. Garnish with a slice of lemon or a sprig of mint. Serve with lemon or cream, and sugar.

GENERAL INSTRUCTIONS FOR PREPARING COFFEE

1. Select grind of coffee suitable for type of coffee maker—coarse for boiling, medium for percolation, fine for drip, and very fine for vacuum methods.

2. Use freshly roasted and ground coffee. Keep coffee tightly covered and in a cool place.

3. Use pot of right size for amount of coffee to be made.

4. Measure 2 level tablespoons ground coffee for each measuring cup of water. Use freshly boiled water.

5. Serve beverage immediately after it has been brewed. Never reheat coffee.

6. Keep pot scrupulously clean. Rinse pot immediately after use. Wash with hot soapy water. Rinse with hot water.

BOILED COFFEE

2 tablespoons ground coffee	¼ cup cold water
2 teaspoons egg white	1 cup boiling water

Method. Mix coffee with egg white and half of cold water, place in pot, and pour freshly boiling water over coffee. Allow to simmer for 3 minutes. Remove from direct heat and add remaining cold water to settle grounds. Allow to steep from 5 to 7 minutes. Strain and serve in heated coffee pot.

PERCOLATED COFFEE

Place measured coffee in upper part of pot, water in lower section, and put over flame, or attach plug if electric percolator is used. When percolation begins, lower flame so that the process will continue slowly rather than violently for 5 to 10 minutes. The strength of the beverage depends upon the length of time it is allowed to percolate.

DRIP COFFEE

Put coffee basket over lower portion of pot and measure coffee into it. Measure freshly boiled, bubbling water and pour over the coffee. Cover and allow to filter through. Remove coffee basket, cover lower pot, and serve immediately.

VACUUM DRIP COFFEE

Place measured amount of water in bottom part of coffee maker. Put finely ground coffee in funnel, and place pot over low heat. When water has risen into funnel, allow to gurgle for ½ minute. Remove from heat, stir, and allow to stand in warm place. The vacuum formed in the bottom part of the pot will cause steeped beverage to flow down in a minute or so. Remove funnel and serve at once.

ICED COFFEE

Use 3 to 4 level tablespoons coffee for each cup of water. Prepare coffee by any of the methods described above. As soon as brewed, pour over crushed ice in a tall glass. Serve with cream and powdered sugar. It may also be served with 2 tablespoons vanilla ice cream in each glass.

COCOA

2 teaspoons cocoa	¼ cup water
1 to 2 teaspoons sugar	¾ cup milk

Method. Mix cocoa with sugar and water. Cook to a thick sirup over direct flame. Add milk and heat to the scalding point. Beat briskly with a Dover beater to avoid formation of scum. Serve with or without whipped cream.

Reinforcements. Protein: One to 2 tablespoons of dried milk may be mixed with the sugar and cocoa.

HOT CHOCOLATE

¼ square bitter chocolate	¼ cup boiling water
1 tablespoon sugar	¾ cup milk

Method. Melt the chocolate in top of double boiler over hot water; stir in the sugar and water gradually, and boil 1 minute over direct flame. Add milk, heat over hot water to scalding point, and beat briskly with egg beater until beverage is smooth. This may be served with whipped cream, or a marshmallow may be placed in cup before pouring the chocolate.

COCOA SIRUP (CHOCOLATE SAUCE) (about 1½ cups)

1 cup sugar	1½ cups boiling water
1 cup cocoa	½ teaspoon vanilla
⅛ teaspoon salt	

Method. Mix sugar, cocoa, and salt. Stir into boiling water and cook gently until of a creamy consistency. Cool, add vanilla, pour into jar, cover, and place in refrigerator.

Use 1 to 2 tablespoons of this sirup for each cup of milk beverage.

MILK SHAKE

¾ cup milk	¼ teaspoon vanilla
1 tablespoon sugar	1 egg white

Method. Combine the ingredients in a shaker and shake for a few minutes to blend them well. Pour over cracked ice.

Variations. Caramel, coffee, or maple flavorings may be used.

MILK PUNCH

½ cup milk	1 egg white
¼ cup cream	2 to 3 teaspoons sugar
1 tablespoon whisky, sherry,	Few grains nutmeg or cinnamon
or	
2 tablespoons strong coffee	

Method. Place the ingredients in shaker and shake a few minutes to mix them thoroughly. Pour over cracked ice; sprinkle cinnamon or nutmeg over top.

HIGH-PROTEIN MILK (basic recipe)

	For 1 quart	For 1 cup
Whole milk	3½ cups	¾ cup
Nonfat dry milk	1 cup	¼ cup

Method. Place milk in deep bowl. Sprinkle dried milk over it and beat with rotary beater until smooth. Allow to stand in a refrigerator for a few hours to permit foam to disappear. Serve ice cold.

Variations. 1. Add 1 tablespoon cocoa sirup to 1 glass of high-protein milk. Stir well.

2. Use skim milk for low-fat diets.

3. Add 2 tablespoons ice cream to each glass of high-protein milk.

CHOCOLATE MALTED MILK

3 tablespoons malted milk	1 tablespoon cocoa sirup
¾ cup milk	¼ teaspoon vanilla
2 teaspoons sugar	

Method. Mix malted milk with a little cold milk to make a smooth paste. Add remaining milk, sugar, cocoa sirup, and vanilla. Beat briskly with a rotary beater until smooth. Pour over crushed ice.

Variations. To add protein: Beat whole egg with sugar and chocolate sirup; add to malted-milk mixture.

To increase calories: Add ¼ cup cream and 1 tablespoon vanilla or chocolate ice cream to finished drink.

To serve hot: Heat milk to scalding point before adding it to malted milk paste.

EGGNOG

1 egg	Few grains salt
¾ cup milk	3 to 4 drops vanilla
1 to 2 teaspoons sugar	

Method. Beat egg well, and add milk, sugar, salt, and vanilla. Stir until sugar is dissolved. Strain to remove any shreds of unbeaten egg. Sprinkle with nutmeg, if desired.

Variations. One to 2 tablespoons cocoa sirup may be added to the eggnog for varied flavor. Malted-milk powder may also be used for variety.

High-protein eggnog: Beat 3 tablespoons nonfat dry milk into the prepared eggnog.

ORANGE OR GRAPEFRUIT JUICE

Method. Wash fruit and cut in half across sections. Extract juice with nonmetal hand squeezer or electric juicer. Remove any seeds. Do not strain except for low-fiber diets, since the pulp contains an important amount of ascorbic acid. Stir juice just before serving to keep the particles evenly suspended. Place glass in bowl of crushed ice, but do not add ice to the juice itself.

Frozen juices. Keep in freezer or freezing section of refrigerator until the can is opened. Add cold water according to the amounts stated on the can—usually 3 cans of water to each can of juice. Stir well until evenly suspended, and serve in 4-ounce glass.

Left over juices. Keep in a closed container in the refrigerator. Little loss of ascorbic acid and of flavor occurs within 24 to 48 hours.

KEY RULE FOR FRUITADES

KIND OF JUICE	AMOUNT tablespoons	SUGAR tablespoons	LEMON JUICE tablespoons	CRUSHED ICE	WATER OR OTHER LIQUID
Orange	6	1	1	⅓ glass	Fill 8-ounce glass to ½ in. from rim
Pineapple	6	1	1	⅓ glass	Fill 8-ounce glass to ½ in. from rim
Grape	6	none	1	⅓ glass	Fill 8-ounce glass to ½ in. from rim
Grapefruit	6	1	none	⅓ glass	Fill 8-ounce glass to ½ in. from rim
Lemon	2–3	1	—	⅓ glass	Fill 8-ounce glass to ½ in. from rim

Method. Mix fruit juices and sugar. Pour over crushed ice. Add water to fill glass and stir well.

HIGH-CARBOHYDRATE LEMONADE

1 cup glucose
1 cup boiling water

¼ cup lemon juice
Crushed ice

Method. Dissolve glucose in boiling water. Cool, and add lemon juice. Add sufficient crushed ice to make 2 glasses (200 ml each).

Each glass of lemonade will contain approximately 100 gm of carbohydrate.

FRUIT PUNCH

½ cup orange juice
2 tablespoons lemon juice
¼ cup pineapple juice

1 tablespoon sugar
Carbonated water, or plain water, to fill glass

Method. Mix the fruit juices and sugar; pour over ⅓ glass crushed ice. Add carbonated water to fill glass.

Peach, pear, raspberry, strawberry, or grape juice may be substituted for the pineapple juice.

CREAM, EGG, AND VICHY

1 egg white
⅓ cup whipping cream
2 teaspoons sugar

3 to 4 drops vanilla
Vichy to fill glass

Method. Whip egg white until stiff but not dry; whip cream and add sugar. Add vanilla, and fold in egg white. Pour over cracked ice and fill glass with Vichy.

FRUIT JUICE WITH EGG WHITE

⅓ cup orange juice
1 tablespoon lemon juice
1 tablespoon sugar

1 egg white
⅓ glass crushed ice

Method. Add sugar to fruit juices. Clip egg white with scissors or silver knife and fork and add to fruit juice. Strain through fine strainer or double thickness of cheese cloth. Pour carefully over crushed ice and add water to fill glass. Stir with a fork instead of a spoon to avoid foam.

Any fruit juice such as grape, grapefruit, or pineapple may be used in place of the orange juice. Omit sugar when sweet juices are used.

EGG AND ORANGE JUICE

1 egg
1 tablespoon sugar
⅓ cup orange juice

2 tablespoons lemon juice
⅓ glass crushed ice

Method. Beat egg, sugar, and juices together and pour over crushed ice. The yolk and white may be separated, if desired; mix yolk, sugar, and juices, fold in stiffly beaten egg white, and pour over crushed ice.

PINEAPPLE EGGNOG

1 egg
1 tablespoon sugar
⅓ cup pineapple juice

1 tablespoon lemon juice
⅓ cup whipping cream

Method. Beat egg yolk and sugar together; add fruit juices. Fold in the stiffly beaten egg white and then the whipped cream. Pour over crushed ice.

Quick Breads, Toast, and Sandwiches

Use enriched white flour unless other kinds of flour are specified. Assemble ingredients before starting the mixing process. Preheat oven for 10 minutes at the designated temperature. Grease pans before mixing is begun. Sift flour before measuring. Avoid overmixing, since muffins will be too compact and tunnels will appear throughout the muffin, while biscuits will not be light.

PLAIN MUFFINS (6 muffins)

1 cup flour
¼ teaspoon salt
1½ teaspoons baking powder
1–2 tablespoons sugar

½ cup milk
2 tablespoons melted fat or oil
½ egg

Method. Sift flour, measure, and sift again with salt, baking powder, and sugar. Beat whole egg and then divide into two equal parts. Mix milk, fat, and half egg. Pour into flour mixture, stirring quickly only until flour is moist (about 10 to 15 strokes). The batter need not be smooth and free of lumps. Fill paper muffin cups (or well-greased muffin tins) ⅔ full and bake from 15 to 20 minutes in a hot oven (425° F). When tins are very small, the temperature should be a little higher and the baking period shorter than that required for average-size muffins.

Variations. (1) Add ½ cup raisins or nuts to dry ingredients and proceed as above. If dates are used, cut in strips and add to milk which has been heated; allow to cool before adding egg. Then proceed as in original recipe. (2) *Whole-wheat muffins.* Use ½ cup unsifted whole-wheat flour and ⅜ cup (6 tablespoons) white flour and proceed as in original recipe.

CORN-MEAL MUFFINS

1 cup corn meal (not too fine)	1 egg
¼ cup flour	1 cup buttermilk
½ teaspoon baking soda	1 tablespoon melted fat or oil
1 teaspoon salt	

Method. Mix dry ingredients. Beat egg and buttermilk together just enough to mix, and stir into dry ingredients. Add fat, and stir quickly just to remove lumps. Pour into well-greased muffin tins or cornstick pans. Bake in a hot oven (425° F) for 25 to 30 minutes.

SPOON BREAD * (serves 3 to 4)

¾ cup corn meal	1 cup milk
1 teaspoon salt	2 eggs
3 tablespoons melted fat or oil	2 teaspoons baking powder
1 cup boiling water	

Method. Mix corn meal, salt, and butter; add boiling water, beating until smooth. Add milk, well-beaten eggs, and baking powder. When well mixed, turn into a greased baking dish or pan and bake in moderate oven (350° F) for 40 to 50 minutes.

BAKING-POWDER BISCUITS (8 to 12 biscuits)

1 cup sifted flour	2 tablespoons shortening
½ teaspoon salt	¼ to ⅓ cup milk
1½ teaspoons baking powder	

Method. Measure sifted flour into cup with a spoon, add salt and baking powder, and sift into mixing bowl. Mix in shortening with tips of fingers or cut in with two knives. Stir in milk to make a soft but not sticky dough. Knead gently on a lightly floured board for 20 to 30 seconds. Roll or pat to a thickness of ½ to ¾ inch; cut with a sharp knife into squares, strips, or triangles as desired. Place fairly close together on a lightly greased baking sheet and bake in a hot oven (425° F) 10 to 12 minutes, depending on thickness of biscuits.

Variations. (1) Use 2 tablespoons orange juice and ½ teaspoon grated orange

---

* Courtesy of Sally F. Hill, Editor, Home Department, *The Progressive Farmer.*

rind in place of the milk. (2) Add 2 tablespoons grated cheese to dry ingredients just before the milk is added.

CINNAMON PINWHEELS (12–16 rolls)

1 recipe baking-powder biscuit dough (above)	¼ cup white or brown sugar
	½ teaspoon cinnamon
2 tablespoons melted butter	Chopped nuts, if desired

Method. Prepare baking-powder biscuit dough as in preceding recipe. Mix sugar and cinnamon. Roll dough into a rectangle ¼ inch thick. Brush with melted butter, sprinkle evenly with sugar, cinnamon, and chopped nuts, if desired. Roll from long side of the rectangle, keeping roll firm but without crushing. Slice about ¾ inch thick, place cut side down about 1 inch apart in well-greased pan. Bake at 425° F for 10–15 minutes until light brown.

TOAST, DRY OR BUTTERED

Method. Use bread sliced ¼ to ½ inch thick. Cut into desired shapes before toasting. A toaster may be used, or the toast may be made in the broiling oven by placing the toast about 3 inches from the heat. Care must be taken to turn the bread before the surface becomes too dark. Well-made toast is golden brown on both sides, and should be slightly mellow in the center. Butter the toast as soon as it is made, if it is not to be served dry.

MELBA TOAST

Method. Cut bread in thin slices and place in a very slow oven, the temperature not to exceed 250° F. Dry out and allow to become yellow. The toast should be thoroughly crisp and brittle. Melba toast may be made in sufficient amounts to be served for several days. Crisp in oven before serving.

CINNAMON TOAST

1 slice bread	2 teaspoons granulated sugar
1 teaspoon butter	¼ teaspoon cinnamon

Method. Cut bread in slices from ¼ to ⅓ inch thick. Remove crusts, and cut into desired shapes. Toast one side in the broiling oven, turn over, butter lightly, and spread with a mixture of the cinnamon and sugar. Return to broiler, and allow to heat until mixture blends lightly with the bread.

CROUTONS

Method. Cut bread in slices ½ inch thick and then into ½-inch cubes. Place in pan in oven, at 300° F and allow to toast, stirring occasionally to brown cubes on all sides. Dot with a small amount of butter if desired. Return to oven, and stir to spread butter over all. Croutons are served with soup or in cream soups as a garnish.

MILK TOAST

1 slice bread	½ cup hot milk
1 teaspoon butter	Few grains salt

Method. Toast the bread on both sides, and butter it; place in a deep plate, and pour the hot milk over it. Season with salt. For a variation, sprinkle toast with sugar and cinnamon, as for cinnamon toast, before adding hot milk.

GENERAL METHOD FOR SANDWICHES

Use bread 24 hours old. White, whole-wheat, rye, Boston brown, or nut bread may be used. Cut slices ½ inch thick for main-dish sandwiches and more thinly for tea sandwiches. Fresh bread will cut more easily if chilled (tightly wrapped) in a refrigerator for several hours.

Soften butter by allowing to stand at room temperature for 10 to 15 minutes, or work with a wooden spoon until soft. Depending upon the kind of sandwich to be made, mustard, chopped chives, horse-radish, onion, or parsley may be creamed with the butter, if desired.

Use any sandwich filling between slices of buttered bread. Crisp shredded lettuce or water cress, thinly sliced tomato, and mayonnaise may be used singly or in combination together with the selected fillings. Cut off crusts after spreading sandwich, and cut in strips.

Open-faced sandwiches may be prepared with any soft spread and eaten with a fork.

Tea sandwiches are made with thinly sliced bread and are cut in small assorted shapes. They may be served open-face, using spreads such as cream cheese with a variety of flavor combinations, soft sharp cheese, fish, chopped chicken, or meat.

SUGGESTIONS FOR SANDWICH FILLINGS

Carrot, grated raw, mixed with mayonnaise and nuts; whole wheat bread
Chicken or turkey, thinly sliced, or chopped with celery, mayonnaise, salt, pepper
Cream cheese, plain, or with
  1. Marmalade or jelly
  2. Olives, chopped, stuffed or ripe
  3. Nut meats
  4. Chopped preserved ginger, almonds
  5. Chopped ham
Cheese, American or Swiss, with or without mustard, pickle
Cucumbers, sliced thinly, on brown bread
Eggs, hard cooked, and finely chopped and mixed with
  1. Anchovy paste
  2. Chopped celery, mayonnaise, salt, pepper
Fish: crab, lobster, salmon, shrimp, tuna
Jelly or marmalade
Meat: cold sliced beef, pork, ham, luncheon meats
Peanut butter
  1. With jelly or marmalade
  2. With bacon
Tomato, bacon

Cereals

GENERAL RULE FOR BREAKFAST CEREALS

TYPE OF CEREAL	AMOUNT OF CEREAL tablespoons	LIQUID cups	SALT teaspoons	TIME FOR COOKING minutes
Oatmeal	4	1	¼	Most cereals are now quick-cooking
Wheatena	4	1	¼	and require 3 to 15 minutes cook-
Corn meal	2½	1	¼	ing time. Read instructions on
Farina	3	1	¼	package for cooking time.

Method. Heat water to boiling point, add salt, and sprinkle in dry cereal, stirring until all the cereal has been added. Cook quick-cooking cereals over direct heat for the length of time specified on the package, stirring from time to time. Regular cereals may be cooked over direct heat if the heat is kept low, or they may be placed in a double boiler to continue cooking for the required length of time.

Variations. Nonfat dry milk may be used with the cereal to enhance flavor and nutritive value. Mix milk powder with cereal and add to the boiling water, allowing 2 to 4 tablespoons of dry milk for each cup of liquid. Dates or raisins may be added to cereal before serving.

GRUEL

½ cup well-cooked fine or strained   ⅓ to ½ cup milk
    cereal

Method. Mix hot strained cereal with hot milk and serve immediately. Sugar may be added if desired.

BOILED RICE

1 quart boiling water   ½ teaspoon salt
3 tablespoons rice

Method. Wash rice. Add salt to boiling water, and allow to boil briskly before adding the rice. Boil rice for about 20 to 30 minutes or until tender. Empty rice into a strainer. Pour hot water over rice until each grain is separate and distinct. Place strainer over a saucepan of hot water, taking care that the bottom does not touch the water. Cover loosely, allowing space for steam to pass through. Serve rice hot with butter, or as a breakfast cereal with milk, sugar, and cinnamon, as desired.

Variations. Rice may be combined with canned tomato sauce, or cheese sauce, page 701, covered with crumbs, and baked in a moderate oven for 15 to 20 minutes.

STEAMED RICE

3 tablespoons rice   ¼ teaspoon salt
1 cup boiling water

Method. Wash rice thoroughly. Boil water in top part of double boiler over direct flame. Add salt and rice, and boil for 2 to 3 minutes. Place in double boiler over hot water, cover, and cook until the rice has absorbed all the water. If not entirely tender when the water has been absorbed, add a little more boiling water and continue the cooking. Avoid adding too much water at a time or the rice grains will not stay separate. When rice is tender, lift top saucepan out of hot water and place for a few minutes over low flame to dry out.

MACARONI, SPAGHETTI, OR NOODLES

¼ cup broken macaroni
or
1 ounce spaghetti or noodles

1 quart or more boiling water
1 teaspoon salt

Method. Cook in boiling salted water for 9 to 12 minutes or until tender but not too soft. Drain and dress with sauce and seasonings.

To cook spaghetti without breaking into pieces, hold spaghetti in hand and dip ends into boiling water. As the spaghetti softens, continue to coil it under the boiling water.

Sauces. These cooked pastas may be dressed with canned tomato sauce, or cheese sauce, page 701. They may be turned into a casserole, covered with crumbs and grated cheese, and baked in a moderate oven for 15 to 20 minutes. (See recipe for Macaroni and Cheese, p. 680.)

Cheese

Select a sharp variety of cheese for full, rich flavor in cooked dishes. Always cook cheese dishes at a low temperature. Melt cheese over hot water in a double boiler; or broil 4 to 5 inches from direct heat until it begins to melt. To facilitate melting and preparation of uniform mixtures, the cheese may be grated or shredded, or ground through a food chopper. One cup of grated cheese equals approximately ¼ pound.

CHEESE SOUFFLÉ

1 tablespoon butter
1 tablespoon flour
⅛ teaspoon salt

⅓ cup milk
⅓ cup grated cheese
1 egg

Method. Melt butter in top of double boiler over water. Add flour and salt, and mix to a smooth paste. Add milk, stirring constantly until thick. Mix cheese with white sauce, and cook until melted. Remove from hot water, and stir in unbeaten yolk of egg. Beat egg white until stiff but not dry, and fold into mixture. Pour into buttered baking dish, and set in a pan of hot water. Bake for about 45 minutes in a moderate oven (350° F). Test by inserting tip of knife into center; if none adheres to knife, cooking is complete. Soufflé must be served immediately.

CHEESE FONDUE

⅓ cup milk
⅓ cup soft bread crumbs
⅓ cup American cheese cut into cubes

1 teaspoon butter
⅛ teaspoon salt
Pepper
1 egg

Method. Scald milk in top of double boiler; add bread crumbs, cheese, butter, and seasoning. Remove from stove, and add unbeaten egg yolk. Whip egg white stiff, and fold into the mixture. Pour into a buttered baking dish, set in a pan of hot water, and bake in a moderate oven (350° F) for 30 to 40 minutes or until firm in center. Serve hot.

CREAMY CHEESE ON TOAST

½ cup milk
1 tablespoon flour
⅓ cup grated cheese

⅛ teaspoon salt
Pepper
1 slice bread

Method. Scald milk in double boiler; mix flour with a little cold water and stir into the hot milk. Add grated cheese, salt, and pepper, and cook until mixture is of the consistency of medium-thick white sauce. Toast bread, butter, and cut into cubes. Pour cheese sauce over toast cubes.

MACARONI AND CHEESE

¼ cup uncooked macaroni
½ cup medium white sauce (p. 701)

¼ cup grated cheese
1 tablespoon bread crumbs

Method. Cook macaroni for about 10 minutes in boiling salted water. Drain. Prepare white sauce and add grated cheese, stirring until cheese is melted. Combine macaroni with cheese sauce. Put into buttered baking dish, sprinkle with bread crumbs, and bake in a slow oven (325° F) until brown—about 15 minutes.

RAREBIT

⅛ teaspoon mustard
¾ cup grated cheese

¼ cup medium white sauce (p. 701)

Method. Add mustard and grated cheese to white sauce. Cook over hot water until cheese is melted. Serve immediately on toast or crackers.

BAKED RICE AND CHEESE

½ cup medium white sauce
¼ cup grated cheese

½ cup cooked rice

Method. Prepare white sauce as directed on page 701. Add grated cheese, and stir until cheese is melted. Combine with rice, and turn into buttered baking dish. Bake for 15 minutes in a moderately slow oven (325° F).

For other cheese recipes see Cheese Omelet, page 688; Cheese Sauce, page 701; Roquefort Dressing, page 701; Cottage Cheese Salad, page 699.

Desserts and Dessert Sauces

EGG AND MILK DESSERTS

SOFT CUSTARD (about 1¼ cups)

1 cup milk	Few grains salt
1 egg or 2 egg yolks	¼ teaspoon vanilla
1½ tablespoons sugar	

Method. Scald milk in top of double boiler. Beat egg, sugar, and salt together. Pour milk gradually over the egg mixture. Return to double boiler and cook over hot (not boiling) water, stirring constantly, until custard forms a coating on the spoon. Water in the lower part of the double boiler should not touch the upper pan because the custard will curdle if the egg is cooked at too high a temperature. Cool custard quickly by setting in a pan of cool water, stirring once in a while. Add vanilla and chill. Serve as dessert with whipped cream garnish, or as a sauce for fruit whips, stewed fruit, berries, or cake.

For diabetic diets. Substitute 1 saccharin or Sucaryl tablet for sugar in the above recipe. Protein 14 gm; fat 15 gm; carbohydrate 12 gm.

FLOATING ISLAND

1 egg white	3 to 4 drops vanilla
Few grains salt	Soft custard (see above)
2 tablespoons powdered sugar	

Method. Whip egg white until stiff but not dry. Fold in salt, sugar, and vanilla. Pour chilled custard into serving dishes, and garnish with meringue. The meringue may be browned slightly in an oven, if desired.

BAKED CUSTARD

¾ cup milk	Few grains salt
1 egg	¼ teaspoon vanilla
1½ tablespoons sugar	Few grains nutmeg

Method. Scald milk. Beat egg, sugar, and salt together slightly. Stir in milk and vanilla, strain, and pour into custard cups. Sprinkle top lightly with nutmeg. Place cups in a deep baking pan, and surround with hot water to about half the depth of the cup. Bake in a moderate oven (350° F) until a knife blade inserted just off the center of the custard comes out clean—about 25 to 30 minutes. Care must be taken not to allow the water to boil because the egg proteins will separate, making a watery, unpalatable, and unattractive mixture. Serve either hot or cold, with or without whipped cream. If chilled before serving, custard may be turned out of cup into a fruit saucer or sherbet glass.

PINEAPPLE OMELET

1 egg	¼ cup crushed pineapple
2 tablespoons lemon juice	2 tablespoons sugar

Method. Beat egg yolk; add 1 tablespoon of the lemon juice, 1 tablespoon of the pineapple, and 1 tablespoon of the sugar. Beat white of egg until stiff but not dry, and fold into the yolk mixture. Butter a smooth frying pan and heat. Pour omelet into hot pan, and cook on top of stove until bottom of omelet is brown. Place in oven, and bake until mixture will not adhere to the finger tips. During the baking process, heat all remaining ingredients in small saucepan, and, when ready to serve, pour over omelet.

JUNKET

1 tablespoon cold water	1 teaspoon sugar
½ rennin tablet	Few drops vanilla
⅔ cup milk	

Method. Crush rennin tablet and dissolve in water. Heat milk to 100° F. If milk thermometer is not available, test heated milk by allowing a drop of it to fall on inner side of wrist; if it is of the proper temperature, it will feel neither hot nor cold. Add sugar and vanilla. Stir dissolved rennin into milk, stirring for a few seconds only. Pour into molds promptly, and leave undisturbed until firm. Then place in refrigerator until needed.

Sweetened Junket powders in a variety of flavors are now available commercially. Package directions should be followed exactly.

For diabetic diets. Substitute 1 saccharin tablet (¼ grain) for the sugar. Protein 5; fat 6; carbohydrate 8.

STARCHY DESSERTS

BLANCMANGE (2–3 servings)

1 cup milk	2 tablespoons sugar
1½ tablespoons cornstarch	⅛ teaspoon salt
1 egg	½ teaspoon vanilla

Method. Scald ¾ cup milk in top of double boiler. Blend cornstarch and rest of milk until smooth, and add to the hot milk. Cook over hot water for 10 to 15 minutes, stirring constantly until thickening begins. Beat egg yolk slightly with sugar and salt. Add cooked mixture to egg gradually, return to double boiler, and cook for 1 minute. Add vanilla, and fold in stiffly beaten egg white. Pour into molds and chill. Unmold and serve with whipped cream, fruit sauce, fresh fruit, or chocolate or butterscotch sauce.

Variations. (1) For chocolate blancmange, add ½ square chocolate to milk before scalding; (2) ½ cup puréed banana and 1 teaspoon lemon juice may be added to pudding just before mixing with the egg yolk; (3) add 2 tablespoons coconut to plain or chocolate blancmange.

TAPIOCA CREAM (serves 2)

1 egg
3 tablespoons sugar
Few grains salt

1 tablespoon tapioca
1 cup milk
¼ teaspoon vanilla

Method. Beat egg white until foamy. Add 1½ tablespoons sugar gradually while beating with a rotary beater until mixture will stand in soft peaks. Set aside.

Mix egg yolk with remaining sugar and salt in top of double boiler. Add tapioca and milk. Cook over hot water, stirring frequently, until tapioca is transparent and mixture is slightly thick.

Pour hot mixture over the egg white, stirring constantly until blended. Add vanilla. Chill, and serve plain, with fruit, or with whipped cream.

Variation. For chocolate tapioca cream, add ½ square grated chocolate to milk mixture when cooking is started.

BAKED RICE PUDDING (serves 2)

1½ tablespoons rice
2 cups milk
2 tablespoons sugar

¼ teaspoon salt
¼ teaspoon nutmeg or cinnamon

Method. Wash rice thoroughly in cold water; add milk and other ingredients. Place in a buttered pan and bake in a slow oven for 2 hours, stirring from time to time as a scum forms on top of the milk.

Variations. (1) Raisins may be added to this pudding during the last half hour of baking. (2) This pudding may be cooked in a double boiler for 2 to 3 hours if it is not practical to bake it in the oven.

BREAD PUDDING (serves 2)

1 slice toast
1 cup milk
1 egg
1 tablespoon sugar

¼ teaspoon vanilla
Few grains nutmeg
Few grains salt

Method. Remove crusts from toast. Butter, and cut in cubes. Place in baking dish. Scald milk, and add to slightly beaten egg mixed with salt, sugar, and vanilla. Pour over diced toast. Sprinkle with nutmeg. Set dish in pan of hot water, and bake in moderate oven (350° F) for about 30 minutes or until knife comes out clean when inserted into center of custard.

Serve hot with fruit sauce or cold with whipped cream.

APPLE BETTY

1 slice toasted bread
½ cup thinly sliced apple
3 tablespoons brown sugar

¼ teaspoon cinnamon
1½ teaspoons butter

Method. Cover bottom of a small greased baking dish with small pieces of toasted bread, arrange half of apple slices over bread, sprinkle with half of sugar, and add a little cinnamon. Dot layer with butter and top with another layer of toast, apple, sugar, cinnamon and butter. Bake for about 20 minutes in a moderate oven. Serve hot with hard sauce or cream.

Variations. (1) Cover apple Betty before baking with ½ cup of soft custard (p. 681). Set in a pan of hot water and bake at 350° F. (2) Any fruit may be used instead of apples.

GELATIN DESSERTS

Preparation of gelatin. Use granulated or flaked gelatin which is unflavored and unsweetened. Allow 1 level tablespoon of gelatin to 1 pint of liquid. Soak gelatin for 5 minutes in a small quantity of the cold liquid in order to swell the granules. Heat the remaining liquid and dissolve the gelatin in it.

To mold jelly. Large or individual molds may be used. Pour mixture into molds and set in cold place to congeal—about 2 hours for small molds and 4 hours for large molds. When jelly is congealed, set mold in a pan of luke-warm water for ½–1 minute. Loosen the jelly by inserting the point of a knife around the edge. Invert mold over center of dish. When foods such as fruit are added, the jelly must first be allowed to thicken in order that foods will not settle to the bottom of the mold. Fresh pineapple cannot be added to jelly because an enzyme in the fruit splits the gelatin so that congealing will not take place; stewed or canned pineapple may be used.

For diabetic diets. Jelly recipes may be used for diabetic diets if 1 saccharin tablet is substituted for the sugar in the recipe. The fruit or fruit juice used is subtracted from the allowance of a given meal.

LEMON JELLY (serves 2)

1½ teaspoons granulated gelatin	¼ cup sugar
2 tablespoons cold water	¼ cup lemon juice
¼ cup boiling water	½ cup cold water

Method. Soak gelatin for 5 minutes in cold water, add boiling water, and stir until dissolved. Add sugar, lemon juice, and cold water. Strain into molds, and place in refrigerator to congeal. Serve with plain or whipped cream, or custard sauce.

ORANGE JELLY (serves 2)

1½ teaspoons granulated gelatin	2 drops orange extract *or*
2 tablespoons cold water	½ teaspoon grated orange rind
¼ cup boiling water	½ cup orange juice
3 tablespoons sugar	2 tablespoons lemon juice

Method. Proceed as directed for lemon jelly.

SNOW PUDDING (serves 2)

Lemon jelly	1 egg white

Method. Prepare lemon jelly (above) and place the bowl in a pan of cracked ice. When the mixture begins to stiffen, fold in well-beaten white of egg, beating it in with a rotary beater until the mixture is stiff. Pour the mixture into a mold or individual glasses, and set in refrigerator to congeal. Unmold, and serve with soft custard.

Orange or grape-juice jelly may be used in place of the lemon jelly.

ORANGE CHARLOTTE (serves 2)

½ cup orange jelly   ¼ cup cream, whipped

Method. Prepare orange jelly (p. 684), and pour it into a bowl surrounded with cracked ice. When it begins to stiffen, whip well, and fold in the stiffly beaten cream. Pour into molds or ice-cream glasses, and set in refrigerator to congeal.

Variations. (1) One stiffly beaten egg white may be substituted for the whipped cream. (2) The molds may be lined with sections of orange before putting the charlotte into them.

SPANISH CREAM (serves 2 to 3)

½ tablespoon granulated gelatin	2 tablespoons sugar
2 tablespoons cold milk	Few grains salt
⅔ cup scalded milk	¼ teaspoon vanilla
1 egg	

Method. Soak gelatin for 5 minutes in cold milk and dissolve in scalded milk. Beat egg yolk slightly, and add sugar and salt. Stir milk mixture into egg, and cook in double boiler until slightly thickened. Remove top of double boiler from stove and place in cold water until the mixture is of the consistency of unbeaten egg white. Add vanilla. Beat egg white until stiff, with rotary beater, and fold into custard. Pour into individual molds and chill. Serve with whipped cream, if desired.

FRUIT WHIPS

GENERAL RULE FOR FRUIT WHIPS

¼ cup fruit pulp	1 egg white
2 tablespoons powdered sugar	Few grains salt
2 tablespoons lemon juice	

Method. Cook apple, apricots, or prunes in a small amount of water until tender. Press through sieve, and measure ¼ cup for each serving. Add sugar and lemon juice. Whip egg white until stiff but not dry, and fold into the fruit pulp. Serve with a soft custard sauce or with cream.

Fresh fruit such as strawberries or peaches can be mashed and sieved. Lemon juice is not necessary for fresh-fruit whips.

For diabetic diet. Substitute 1 saccharin tablet for the powdered sugar. Use fruit pulp from the diet allowance. One egg white will add 3 gm protein to the value of the fruit used.

SWEET SAUCES

BUTTERSCOTCH SAUCE (about 1¼ cups)

¾ cup brown sugar   ⅛ teaspoon salt
½ cup light corn sirup   ½ cup coffee cream
¼ cup water   ½ teaspoon vanilla
3 tablespoons butter

Method. Mix sugar, corn sirup, water, butter, and salt in saucepan. Cook over low heat until a very thick sirup. Remove from the stove, cool, add cream and vanilla. Stir well, and serve cold as a sauce for ice cream or over cup cakes. Sauce may be served hot by reheating in a double boiler.

LEMON SAUCE (1 cup)

½ cup sugar   1½ to 2 tablespoons lemon juice
1 tablespoon cornstarch   Grated rind of lemon
1 cup boiling water   1 tablespoon butter

Method. Mix sugar and cornstarch, stir in the boiling water gradually, and cook 8 to 10 minutes, stirring continuously. Then add the lemon juice, grated rind, and butter. Serve sauce hot on puddings or cupcakes.

WINE OR FRUIT SAUCE (about ½ cup)

1 egg   ½ cup orange juice and 1 tablespoon
½ cup powdered sugar   lemon juice
1 wineglass sherry wine or whisky *or*   1 teaspoon hot milk

Method. Beat yolk and white of egg separately. Add sugar to yolk and beat until creamy. Add wine or fruit juice, fold in egg white, and add the hot milk last. Serve at once.

CHOCOLATE SAUCE

Use recipe for Cocoa Sirup, page 671.

Eggs

Only the freshest eggs should be used for the invalid dietary, since a single egg of poor quality may result in the patient's continued refusal to eat them. They should be cooked at a low temperature, since their proteins are easily toughened, and should be served immediately after being prepared.

POACHED EGG

1 egg   1 teaspoon salt
1 pint water

Method. Fill a small saucepan with water to a depth of 2½ inches, and add salt. Allow water to come to the boiling point. Break egg carefully into a saucer, and slip it gently into the hot water; cover, and allow to stand for 5 to 7 minutes until white becomes opaque and of jelly-like consistency, and a thin white film forms over the yolk. Never allow water to boil after inserting egg. Remove egg with a perforated spoon and serve on buttered toast.

Variation. Egg may be served on hot toast with cheese sauce, page 701.

CODDLED EGG

1 egg   Boiling water to cover egg

Method. Put water into small saucepan, and heat to boiling point. Place egg in water, and remove pan from flame. Allow to stand covered for 5 to 7 minutes. If very soft egg is desired, allow to remain in water for 3 to 5 minutes. Serve immediately.

HARD-COOKED EGG

1 egg   Water to cover egg

Method. Wash egg, drop in saucepan of cold water, and bring slowly to boil. Lower the flame so that water is kept at simmering temperature, and allow to cook for 20 minutes. Plunge into cold water to avoid discoloration of the yolk. Remove shell when entirely cold. The method used for coddled eggs (above) may be used by allowing the egg to remain in the water for about 40 minutes.

SCRAMBLED EGGS

2 eggs $\frac{1}{4}$ teaspoon salt
2 tablespoons milk, cream, or tomato   1 teaspoon butter
    juice

Method. Beat eggs slightly, add liquid and salt. Heat butter slowly in frying pan, and pour eggs into hot pan. Cook over low flame, and stir with spatula until creamy—about 3 minutes. Serve at once.

A double boiler may be used instead of the frying pan to ensure cooking at a low temperature.

CREAMY EGG ON TOAST

$\frac{1}{4}$ cup milk $\frac{1}{8}$ teaspoon salt
1 teaspoon butter   1 slice buttered toast
1 egg

Method. Heat milk with butter in double boiler to scalding temperature, stir in the beaten egg, and cook until mixture is of a creamy consistency. Season and serve on buttered toast.

PUFFY OMELET

1 egg   1 tablespoon water, milk, or tomato
$\frac{1}{8}$ teaspoon salt   juice
Few grains pepper   1 teaspoon butter

Method. Separate yolk from white; beat yolk with liquid, salt, and pepper. Whip white until stiff but not dry, and fold into yolk mixture. Pour into a hot, lightly buttered pan, and cook slowly on top of stove, lifting edge of omelet to determine when it has become brown. As soon as brown, place pan in moderate oven and cook until the mixture will not adhere to the finger—about 5 minutes. Place on warm plate, making a crease down middle of omelet, fold, and garnish with parsley. Jelly or chopped asparagus may also be used for a garnish.

Variations. (1) Add slice of crisply cooked and finely chopped bacon to top of omelet while baking. (2) One tablespoon of grated cheese may be added to egg yolk before folding in the egg white, or may be sprinkled over omelet during the cooking process. (3) When tomato juice is used, a tomato sauce may be poured over omelet at serving time.

FRENCH OMELET

2 eggs	2 tablespoons water or milk
¼ teaspoon salt	2 teaspoons butter
Few grains pepper	

Method. Beat eggs slightly; add salt, pepper, and liquid. Melt fat in small frying pan and grease the bottom and sides well. Pour in the egg mixture and cook slowly, pricking the mixture with a fork during the cooking to allow the uncooked portions on top to reach the pan. Avoid scrambling. When the entire mixture reaches a creamy consistency and is light brown on the bottom, fold and turn onto hot plate. A very smooth pan is necessary for making omelets.

BAKED EGGS (SHIRRED EGGS)

1 egg	Pepper
1 tablespoon cream	Grated cheese, if desired
Salt	2 teaspoons bread crumbs

Method. Butter individual baking dish. Break egg into it. Add cream and season with salt and pepper. Sprinkle with grated cheese and bread crumbs. Set in pan of hot water and bake in a moderate oven (350° F) until the white is set—about 20 minutes. Sprinkle with paprika before serving.

EGG À LA GOLDENROD

1 tablespoon butter	½ cup milk
1 tablespoon flour	1 hard-cooked egg
¼ teaspoon salt	1 slice toast

Method. Make white sauce with butter, flour, salt, and milk. Separate white of the hard-cooked egg from yolk, chop white, and add to white sauce. Pour over the toast. Press the yolk through a strainer, covering the top of the toast. Garnish with parsley.

Variation: White and yolk may be chopped and added to the white sauce, and served as creamed eggs.

For other important egg dishes, see Beverages, pages 669–74; Custards, page 681; and Stuffed-egg Salad, page 699.

Fruits

All fruits should be washed before they are served. It is preferable to chill fruit (except bananas and pineapple) before cutting in order to minimize the chilling time after preparation and thus avoid discoloration and loss of nutrients. Canned fruit may be chilled in the can before opening. Frozen fruits should be allowed to thaw at room temperature before serving. This requires 3 to 4 hours if the fruit remains in the carton in which it was packed. Thawed fruits must never be refrozen.

BERRIES

Method. Remove undesirable berries and leaves. Place in sieve and wash berries under gently running water. Drain thoroughly. Strawberries and other berries may be served with caps removed and sugar added just before serving. Specimen strawberries are sometimes offered with caps on, arranged on green leaves around a mound of powdered sugar, as a first course at luncheon. These large berries are eaten from the stem, which is held with the fingers.

FRUIT CUP

Method. A variety of fresh or canned fruit or a combination of both may be used for fruit cup. Sprinkle lemon juice on any raw fruits which discolor readily, such as banana, apple, peach, and pear. Chill fruit, cut in attractive pieces, and mix. A tablespoon of fruit juice, sweet cider, or wine may be added. Powdered sugar may be used for very tart fruits if desired. Garnish with a sprig of mint or fruit ice, if available.

The following are suggested combinations for fruit cup:

1. Orange sections—4; grapefruit sections—2; fresh pineapple—$\frac{1}{3}$ cup
2. Equal parts of fresh or canned pineapple, sweet cherries, sliced banana
3. Equal parts of peaches, pears, pineapple
4. Equal parts of oranges, diced apples, canned peaches, Tokay grapes
5. Equal parts of orange sections and sliced banana with grated coconut

CANTALOUPE

Method. Chill melon thoroughly. Cut melon in half or sections, depending on size, and remove seeds. A potato-ball cutter may be used to cut fruit into balls, which are served on a mound of crushed ice.

Honeydew and Persian melons are served in the same way. A slice of lemon or lime may be served with honeydew.

GRAPEFRUIT OR ORANGE HALVES

Method. Select medium-size, thin-skinned grapefruit or large navel orange. Wash fruit and cut along line midway between stem and bud ends. Run sharp, pointed knife around each section, separating the pulp from the skin and inner membrane. Remove center and seeds and serve without sugar unless additional sweetening is desired. Grapefruit, like oranges, may also be served in sections.

BROILED GRAPEFRUIT

½ grapefruit   1 tablespoon sherry (optional)
1 tablespoon sugar   1 cherry

Method. Prepare grapefruit as described above. Sprinkle with sugar and place under broiler with moderate flame. When grapefruit is hot and beginning to brown at the edges, place on serving plate. Pour sherry over the fruit, garnish with a cherry, and serve immediately.

ORANGE OR GRAPEFRUIT SECTIONS

Method. Wash fruit and pare as you would an apple, using a sawing motion with the knife. Remove the white inner skin with the peel. Using a sharp, pointed knife, separate the sections from the dividing membrane without breaking sections. (See Fig. 49-2, p. 641.)

APPLESAUCE

2 tart apples   1 to 2 tablespoons sugar

Method. Wash and pare apples. Cut into quarters and remove core. Add just enough water to keep the apple from scorching, cover, and cook slowly until apple mashes readily with a spoon—about 10 to 15 minutes. Add the sugar and beat well. The apple need not be peeled if the sauce is to be strained.

For serving at breakfast, no spices are added. Nutmeg, cinnamon, or lemon juice may be used for applesauce which is to be served as a dessert.

BAKED APPLE

1 apple   ¼ cup water
2 tablespoons sugar   Dash of nutmeg
1 teaspoon butter

Method. Wash and core the apple, leaving the blossom end intact. Place in small pan or baking dish, and fill cavity in apple with the sugar and butter. Add water, and bake in moderately hot oven (375° F) for about ½ hour or until fruit can be readily pierced with a toothpick. This may be a breakfast dish or a simple dessert. It may be served warm or cold, with or without cream.

STEWED PEAR

2 pears   1 slice lemon
½ cup water   1 small piece stick cinnamon or a few
¼ cup sugar   cloves

Method. Wash fruit and pare. Cut in half and remove core. Bring sugar and water to a boil, add the slice of lemon, cinnamon, and pear halves. Cover and cook gently until tender. If spices are omitted, the pears may be served when cold with 1 tablespoon crème de menthe.

STEWED DRIED FRUIT

4 to 6 prunes   Sugar to taste
   or
4 to 6 apricot halves
   or
3 peach halves

Method. Cover fruit with cold water, bring to a boil, and simmer gently for 25 to 30 minutes. Add sugar to taste, stir until dissolved, and cool the fruit. Prunes usually do not require additional sugar, but a slice of lemon may be cooked with them. Let fruit stand overnight in refrigerator before serving, if possible.

Stewed fruit may be served alone or with whipped cream. It provides a welcome variation when served on breakfast cereal.

Meat, Poultry, and Fish

Only recipes for quickly cooked meats which require little preparation time are presented here, since the nurse will rarely be expected to prepare other cuts. For the preparation of meats requiring longer cooking such as roasts and stews, any standard cookbook may be consulted.

OVEN-BROILED STEAK, CHOPS, OR HAMBURG PATTIES

Method. Heat broiling oven for 5 to 10 minutes, and grease the broiler rack. Wipe meat (except hamburg) with a damp cloth, and place on rack about 3 inches below the flame. Cook until brown on one side, season with salt and pepper, and turn. Continue to cook until done. The table on page 692 gives approximate broiling time for various cuts of meat. Lift meat to a hot plate, place 1 teaspoon butter on it, dust the surface with salt and pepper, and serve hot. Parsley may be used as a garnish.

For hamburg patties, shape ground meat in large or small cakes with as little handling as possible. Ground meat dries quickly, and overcooking should be avoided.

OVEN-BROILED HAM SLICE

Method. Preheat broiling oven for 5 to 10 minutes. Wipe meat and place on rack about 3 inches below the flame. Broil on one side, turn, and partially cook the other side. Spread with brown sugar, if desired, and continue broiling until the sugar melts. Do not add salt.

PAN-BROILED STEAK, CHOPS, HAM SLICE, OR HAMBURG

Method. Pan broiling is done on the top of the stove in a heavy frying pan. Without greasing the pan, place the meat in the pan, with or without preheating. Cook slowly until done, turning occasionally. Pour off the fat as it accumulates. Season with butter, salt (except ham), and pepper. Garnish with parsley and serve immediately.

If pork chops are being cooked, the pan should be covered after the chops have browned and cooking continued over very low heat until the chops are well done—25 to 30 minutes for 1-inch chops.

TIME TABLE FOR COOKING STEAKS AND CHOPS

KIND OF MEAT	COOKING TIME minutes
Steak, 1½ inches thick	8–15
Lamb chops, 1 inch	10–15
Lamb chops, 1½ inches	15–20
Ham, ¼ inch	8–12
Ham, ½ inch	15–20
Hamburg	6–12

VEAL CUTLET

1 egg yolk
1 tablespoon water
¼ pound veal cutlet

3 tablespoons bread crumbs
1 tablespoon fat

Method. Mix egg yolk with water; dip cutlet first in egg and then in bread crumbs. Sauté in slightly greased frying pan. Add ½ cup hot water, broth, or tomatoes, cover, and simmer about 30 minutes or until tender. Serve plain or with thickened sauce.

VEGETABLES AND MEAT EN CASSEROLE

½ cup diced cooked meat
½ cup mixed vegetables

Gravy

Method. Carrots, potatoes, onions, celery, and turnips are suitable for the vegetable mixture. Place meat and vegetables in a deep baking dish; season with salt and pepper. Cover with gravy and bake in a moderately slow oven (325° F) for ½ hour or more.

BROILED LIVER

1 slice veal or lamb liver, ½ inch
    thick

1 teaspoon butter
Salt and pepper

Method. Remove membrane and veins from liver, and wipe with a damp cloth. Preheat broiler for 5 to 10 minutes and grease the broiler rack. Dot liver with butter or cover with a strip of bacon. Broil under direct flame for about 5 to 8 minutes or until tender. Liver will be toughened if it is overcooked.

SAUTÉED LIVER

1 slice liver ½ inch thick
Flour

Salt and pepper

Method. Remove outer membrane and veins from liver and wipe with a damp cloth. Dredge with flour and cook in a well-greased pan for 6 to 7 minutes, turning frequently. Liver may be served with strips of bacon or with sautéed onions.

Calves' liver is very tender, but beef, lamb, or pig liver is equally nutritious and much less expensive.

BACON

Method. Arrange bacon in a cold frying pan and cook over a moderate flame until edges begin to curl. If the bacon has just been removed from the refrigerator, the strips may be separated as the bacon cooks. Turn each slice separately, and remove before fat of bacon looks dry. Pour off the fat as it accumulates. Place in pan lined with absorbent paper to drain. Properly cooked bacon is crisp and readily broken with a fork; if underdone, it will be tough and have to be cut with a knife.

SWISS STEAK (serves 6)

1½ pounds round steak	2 tablespoons fat
Flour	1 cup stewed tomatoes
Salt and pepper	

Method. Pound as much flour as possible into the meat, season, and brown in hot fat. Add tomatoes; cover, and cook slowly until done—about 45 minutes to 1 hour. Serve with sauce in which it was cooked. Garnish with parsley.

MEAT BALLS (serves 3)

½ cup bread or cracker crumbs	1 egg
¼ teaspoon salt	½ pound ground lean beef
Pepper to season	4 slices bacon
⅛ teaspoon nutmeg	1½ cups tomato juice

Method. Mix ¼ cup of bread crumbs, salt, pepper, nutmeg, and slightly beaten egg with meat. Form in balls the size of a walnut, and roll in remaining crumbs. Line pan with bacon, place balls on top, and pour tomato juice over all. Bake in moderate oven (350° F) from 20 to 30 minutes. Serve on hot platter garnished with parsley.

POULTRY

Ready-to-cook (eviscerated) poultry. Remove any pin feathers. Singe, if necessary. Remove bits of lung and kidney remaining in the cavity. Cut out oil sac if it has not been removed. Clean giblets and wash chicken and giblets.

Dressed (not drawn) poultry. To draw poultry, cut head off at shoulders; loosen craw at base of neck and remove. Cut off oil sac and vent above tail, and slit under the tail to remove the viscera, including the lungs. Hold under running water and wash well. Clean and wash the giblets.

BROILED CHICKEN

½ broiler (¾ to 1 pound)   1–2 tablespoons oil
Salt and pepper   Parsley for garnish

Method. Wash chicken. Brush generously on all sides with oil or melted fat. Season with salt and pepper. Place skin side down on broiler 5 to 7 inches from heat. Regulate heat so that chicken just begins to brown in 10 minutes. Turn and brush with fat two or three times during cooking. Continue to cook until done —about 35 to 50 minutes. Chicken is done when meat in thickest part of drumstick cuts easily and has no tinge of pink. Serve on hot platter, garnished with parsley, tomato slices, or toast points.

STEWED CHICKEN

1 stewing chicken, cut in pieces   2 stalks celery, diced
1 sliced onion   1 bay leaf
1 carrot, sliced   Salt and pepper

Method. Add onion, carrot, celery, and bay leaf to about 1 quart water and bring to a boil. Drop pieces of washed chicken in water, and simmer for about 1 hour. Add seasonings and cook for about 1 hour or until tender. If chicken is to be used for salad or is to be creamed, allow it to cool in the broth before removing.

Fricassee chicken. Melt 4 tablespoons butter or chicken fat. Add 4 tablespoons flour and stir until well blended. Add 2 cups hot chicken stock gradually, bring to a boil, and season as needed with salt and pepper; 1 cup of milk, or milk and cream, may be substituted for 1 cup of chicken stock. Place pieces of chicken in gravy, and reheat before serving.

CREAMED CHICKEN

⅓ cup diced chicken   ½ cup medium white sauce (p. 701)
⅓ cup sliced mushrooms, cooked or   1 slice toast
   canned

Method. Mix chicken and mushrooms with hot white sauce; serve on one slice of toast. Garnish with parsley.

Variations. Creamed chicken may also be served in the center of a macaroni ring or ring of boiled rice, in croustades, pastry shells, or on waffles. Cold meat of turkey, fish, crab, lobster, or shrimp may be prepared by the same rule.

FRIED CHICKEN

2–3 pounds chicken   Salt and pepper
Flour   Fat for frying

Method 1. Have chicken cut in attractive pieces. Wash chicken, and wipe with a damp cloth. Roll chicken in flour to which salt and pepper have been added. Heat ½ inch of fat in a skillet. Add pieces of chicken, turning as necessary with a pair of tongs until brown—about 15 to 20 minutes. Cover and cook slowly until tender—15 to 30 minutes. Uncover during last 5 to 10 minutes of cooking to recrisp the skin.

Method 2. Roll washed chicken in flour, and season with salt and pepper. Drop pieces into deep hot fat (375° F) and fry until golden brown. Remove chicken and drain on unglazed paper.

OVEN-BROILED FISH

Method. Wipe fish with a cloth after washing thoroughly. Dot with butter, season with salt and pepper, and place skin side down on a greased broiler rack. Cook for 8 to 12 minutes or until fish is brown and flakes when touched with a pointed knife. Serve with parsley butter sauce or tartar sauce.

PAN-BROILED FISH

Method. Wash fish, and wipe with a cloth. Melt 1 tablespoon butter or fat in a frying pan. Dip fish in flour, season with salt and pepper, and sauté until brown on both sides.

CREAMED FISH

$\frac{1}{3}$ cup cooked or canned fish	$\frac{1}{2}$ cup medium white sauce (p. 701)
$\frac{1}{2}$ hard-cooked egg	1 slice buttered toast

Method. Flake the fish into small pieces, and add with chopped egg white to the cream sauce; pour over the toast. Press the egg yolk through sieve over the fish, and garnish with parsley or strips of pimento.

Salads and Salad Dressings

GENERAL RULES FOR PREPARATION OF SALADS

Prepare salads only a short time before serving in order to present the best appearance, texture, and flavor, and to conserve vitamin values.

All greens such as lettuce, water cress, romaine, chicory, endive, and escarole should be washed thoroughly in cold water and drained as much as possible. They are then placed in wax paper, aluminum foil, a plastic bag, or damp cloth, and chilled for 1 hour or more before use.

To prepare leaves of head lettuce, remove core of head with a sharp knife. Wash under cold running water to loosen leaves, and remove leaves carefully from the head. If the lettuce is not to be used immediately, the head should be drained thoroughly before storage, since excess moisture encourages discoloration of the leaves.

Chill all ingredients thoroughly before making the salad. Salad plates or bowls must also be cold.

Add salad dressings to salad at time of serving, except where ingredients are marinated with dressing to develop the flavor.

Season salads to taste; avoid flatness of flavor or excessive seasoning.

Drain fruits and vegetables well before combining with other salad ingredients. They should be cut in attractive pieces easily taken with a fork. Green pepper, pimento, and raw carrots used as a garnish should be finely shredded. Because many cut fruits discolor on standing, a stainless steel, silver, or glass knife should be used for cutting. Sprinkling fruits with a little acid such as lemon juice, or mixing immediately with salad dressing, when possible, also helps to retard discoloration.

Precise architectural arrangements of food on salad greens should be avoided. The "candle" salad and "wheel" arrangements, for example, are not in good taste.

VEGETABLE SALADS

Vegetable salads may be served as the first course of a meal, as a relish, as an accompaniment to the main course, or as a separate course following the main course.

RELISHES

Relishes are more appetizing when completely chilled and crisp. They should be prepared an hour or so before serving and kept in the refrigerator. Because of the loss of water-soluble minerals and vitamins, prolonged standing in water should be avoided.

Radishes. Wash carefully. Remove tips and leaves, retaining enough of stem for attractive appearance. To make radish roses, cut strips to resemble petals from the tip end toward the stem, being careful not to break off the cut portion. Keep in ice water until serving time.

Celery. Wash carefully. Serve hearts whole, or in individual stalks. To prepare celery curls, cut each stalk lengthwise in about five strips, and immerse in ice water until serving time.

Carrots. Wash and scrape. Cut thin strips, and chill thoroughly. Thin strips will curl if put immediately into ice water.

Cucumber. Wash and chill. Cucumbers may be peeled or not, as desired. Slice thinly. If serrated edges are desired, pull silver fork lengthwise along peeled cucumber to make parallel grooves; then slice.

MIXED GREEN SALAD

Method. Use a combination of well-dried, crisp, and thoroughly chilled greens such as lettuce, romaine, chicory, escarole, endive, tender spinach, dandelion greens, or water cress. Finely sliced radishes, cucumbers, carrots, or tomatoes, flowerets of cauliflower, or fine slivers of ham, tongue, cheese, chicken, or bacon are sometimes used with the greens.

Tear greens into small pieces before putting into wooden bowl. Pour over French dressing, and toss lightly with two forks until greens are well coated with dressing. Serve immediately.

Greens are sometimes mixed at the table, or may be served to the patient in a bowl with a separate pitcher of French dressing.

SHREDDED CARROT AND CABBAGE SALAD

¼ cup shredded cabbage	French dressing
¼ cup shredded carrots	Salad greens

Method. Marinate cabbage and carrots with French dressing, and serve on salad greens.

STUFFED TOMATO

1 medium tomato	1 tablespoon diced celery
⅛ teaspoon salt	1 tablespoon chopped green pepper
1 tablespoon diced cucumber	2 teaspoons mayonnaise

Method. Remove skin from tomato by turning over flame until skin blisters. Cut slice from top and remove pulp, sprinkle inside with salt, and allow to drain. Fill cavity with mixture of cucumber, celery, green pepper, tomato pulp, and 1 teaspoon of the mayonnaise. Place on lettuce and garnish with thinly sliced rings of pepper and mayonnaise.

TOMATO JELLY

1½ teaspoons granulated gelatin	3 cloves
2 tablespoons cold water	1 tablespoon minced parsley
1 cup canned tomatoes or tomato juice	½ teaspoon salt
2 tablespoons diced celery	1 bay leaf
	1 tablespoon mild vinegar

Method. Soak gelatin in cold water. Simmer remaining ingredients gently for 20 minutes; press through a sieve, and measure. Add water to make 1 cup liquid, and bring to a boil. Pour over the soaked gelatin and stir until gelatin is dissolved. Pour into molds, and chill until set.

Variation. One or more of the following may be added when the jelly begins to thicken: finely chopped or sliced celery, green pepper, olives, carrots, or flaked fish.

POTATO SALAD

½ cup cold, boiled, diced potato	1 tablespoon cooked dressing or mayonnaise
2 tablespoons diced celery	
1 tablespoon diced cucumber	Lettuce
1 tablespoon French dressing	Radishes, parsley, or hard-cooked egg

Method. Marinate potato, celery, and cucumber with French dressing. Before serving, mix with cooked dressing and place on lettuce. Garnish with radishes, parsley, or hard-cooked egg.

COLESLAW (serves 4)

1 slice bacon	1 tablespoon chopped onion
1 tablespoon vinegar	¼ cup cooked dressing
2 cups shredded cabbage	Salt and pepper
½ cup diced celery	

Method. Cut bacon into small pieces and cook until crisp enough to crumble, taking care not to allow any pieces to burn. Add vinegar to bacon. Pour over cabbage, celery, and onion and mix lightly. Add salad dressing or mayonnaise.

Variation. This may be made into a hearty salad by the addition of a hard-cooked egg.

FRUIT SALADS

Fruit salads may be served as an accompaniment to the main course of a lunch or dinner or as a dessert. When they are used at the end of a meal, they are frequently combined with nuts, whipped cream, or marshmallows. They are sometimes frozen in the freezing tray of a refrigerator.

ORANGE AND GRAPEFRUIT SALAD

4 sections orange	Lettuce or water cress
3 sections grapefruit	French dressing

Method. Section fruit according to the method described on page 690. Arrange alternate sections of orange and grapefruit on salad greens, and serve with French dressing.

WALDORF SALAD

1 apple	2 teaspoons mayonnaise
2 tablespoons English walnuts	Lettuce
2 tablespoons diced celery	

Method. Select firm, tart apples. Pare, core, and cut apple into ½-inch cubes. Break the walnuts into pieces. Mix the ingredients together, and add mayonnaise. Place upon lettuce leaves or other salad greens.

COMBINATION FRUIT SALAD

1 slice canned pineapple	Lettuce
2 sections grapefruit	Mayonnaise
6 white grapes or cherries	1 orange cut in sections

Method. Dice pineapple, add shredded grapefruit, and grapes or cherries. Mix with mayonnaise. Arrange small inner leaves of lettuce on a salad plate. Pile mixture in center of lettuce. Arrange orange sections about the fruit mixture.

Variations. Jellied: Line mold with orange sections, and then fill with other ingredients. Pour over all a gelatin mixture of 1 teaspoon gelatin soaked in 1 tablespoon cold fruit juice and dissolved in ¼ cup boiling fruit juice. Pineapple juice from canned fruit may be used. Chill and serve, when jellied, with mayonnaise.

SALADS WITH PROTEIN FOODS

Salads which contain a protein food such as eggs, cheese, fish, or meat, may be used as the main course for luncheon or dinner. The protein is usually combined with a vegetable or fruit to give taste appeal.

STUFFED-EGG SALAD

1 hard-cooked egg	Lettuce leaves
1 teaspoon anchovy paste	Mayonnaise
Green pepper	

Method. Cut egg lengthwise. Mash yolk through sieve, and add anchovy paste and a little mayonnaise. Return yolk paste to the white, and arrange on slices of green pepper. Place on lettuce, and serve with mayonnaise or any preferred salad dressing.

Anchovy paste may be omitted and the yolk mixed with cream and mayonnaise, and seasoned to taste.

CHICKEN SALAD

$\frac{1}{3}$ cup diced chicken	2 tablespoons chopped almonds
$\frac{1}{3}$ cup diced celery	$1\frac{1}{2}$ tablespoons mayonnaise
1 tablespoon French dressing	Lettuce
1 tablespoon chopped olives	

Method. Marinate chicken and celery with French dressing for 1 hour or more in refrigerator. Add olives, nuts, and mayonnaise. Season to taste and serve on lettuce.

COTTAGE-CHEESE SALAD

$\frac{1}{3}$ cup cottage cheese	French dressing
1 teaspoon minced green pepper	Paprika
Salad greens	

Method. Mix cottage cheese with minced green pepper and serve on lettuce or other salad greens with French dressing. Garnish with paprika.

Variations. The above cottage-cheese mixture may be served with:

(1) Sliced pineapple, halves of pear or peach, as stuffing for prunes or apricots, or to accompany any fruit salad

(2) Sliced tomato, or whole tomato stuffed with the mixture

FISH SALAD

$\frac{1}{3}$ cup shrimp, flaked salmon, tuna, crabmeat, or lobster	1 tablespoon mayonnaise
	Lettuce
$\frac{1}{3}$ cup diced celery	$\frac{1}{2}$ hard-cooked egg
1 tablespoon French dressing	$\frac{1}{2}$ tomato

Method. Mix fish, celery, and French dressing. Chill for 1 hour, and mix with mayonnaise. Serve on lettuce and garnish with slices of hard-cooked egg and wedges of tomato.

Variation. A whole tomato from which the pulp has been removed may be stuffed with the above mixture.

SALAD DRESSINGS

These may be stored in a refrigerator for future use, and therefore quantities larger than individual portions may be prepared. Dressings to which other foods have been added, as in Russian or Thousand Island dressing, should be mixed just before use.

COOKED DRESSING (about 1½ cups)

2 tablespoons flour	¾ cup hot water or milk
1 tablespoon sugar	¼ cup mild vinegar
1 teaspoon salt	1 egg
½ teaspoon dry mustard	2 tablespoons butter or other fat
⅛ teaspoon red pepper	

Method. Mix flour, sugar, and seasonings and slowly add liquid. Cook until thickened, stirring constantly. Add vinegar, and blend well. Pour mixture over slightly beaten egg, and cook for 1 to 2 minutes longer. Add butter, and cool before using.

FRENCH DRESSING (about 1¼ cups)

½ teaspoon salt	1 to 2 teaspoons powdered sugar
½ teaspoon paprika	¼ to ⅓ cup lemon juice or vinegar
⅛ teaspoon red pepper	1 cup salad oil

Method. Add dry ingredients to oil and lemon juice in jar. Cover closely, and shake briskly until emulsified, or place in a deep bowl, and beat well with a rotary beater. If the dressing is not to be used at once, shake well before serving.

Variations. (1) Add 1½ teaspoons onion juice and 2½ teaspoons Worcestershire sauce to 1 cup French dressing. (2) Add 1 finely chopped pimento, ½ green pepper, and 1 green onion.

MAYONNAISE (about 1½ cups)

1 egg yolk, or 1 whole egg	1½ tablespoons lemon juice or vinegar
¼ teaspoon dry mustard	1 cup salad oil
½ teaspoon salt	

Method. Mix dry ingredients with egg. Add lemon juice, and stir well. With a rotary beater, beat in oil a few drops at a time until the mixture begins to thicken; then add in gradually larger quantities. Beat until stiff. If whole egg is used, increase salad oil to 1½ cups.

The emulsion may break because of too rapid addition of oil or incontinuous beating. If this occurs, beat an egg yolk in a clean bowl, and add the broken emulsion drop by drop until completely added; then continue to add the remainder of the oil.

Variations. (1) Add ½ cup Roquefort cheese to 1 cup of mayonnaise. (2) Mix equal quantities of whipped cream and mayonnaise.

Sauces and Soups

PROPORTIONS FOR WHITE SAUCES (1 cup)

CONSISTENCY	MILK cups	FAT tablespoons	FLOUR tablespoons	SALT teaspoons	USES
Very thin	½	½	½	½	Cream soups made with starchy vegetables such as peas, Lima beans, corn
Thin	1	1	1	½	Cream soups made with nonstarchy vegetables
Medium	1	2	2	½	Cream soups, creamed vegetables, creamed meats or fish
Thick	1	3	3	½	Croquettes, soufflés

Method. Melt the fat in top of double boiler, and mix in the salt and flour to make a smooth paste. Add liquid gradually to the flour mixture, and continue stirring until thickened sufficiently. Cover, and cook for 10 to 15 minutes, stirring from time to time.

The sauce may also be made in this way: Melt fat in saucepan over direct heat. Add flour, and stir until smooth. Add liquid gradually, stir constantly, and cook over low heat until sauce comes to a boil.

VARIATIONS FOR WHITE SAUCE

Thickening agents may be varied if the following relationships are observed:
  2 tablespoons browned flour equal 1 tablespoon raw flour. In order to brown flour, melt fat over direct heat, and add flour. Stir until brown over low heat.
  ⅔ tablespoon cornstarch equals 1 tablespoon raw flour.
  1 teaspoon tapioca equals 1 tablespoon raw flour.
  1 egg yolk equals 1 tablespoon raw flour.
Liquid may be varied by using cream, vegetable juices, or meat broths for part or all of the milk.
Flavorings may be varied by adding minced parsley, grated carrot, minced pimento, minced onion or chives, herbs, or spices such as mace, nutmeg, paprika, curry powder.

CHEESE SAUCE (1 cup)

¼ to ½ cup (1–2 ounces) grated   1 cup thin white sauce
    American cheese

Method. Heat white sauce over hot water, stir in grated cheese, and continue to stir until cheese is melted and completely incorporated.

MOCK HOLLANDAISE SAUCE

½ cup medium white sauce   1 tablespoon butter
1 egg yolk   1 tablespoon lemon juice

Method. Make white sauce in double boiler. Beat egg yolk slightly. Mix some of white sauce with egg yolk, and stir into the remainder of the white sauce. Add the butter and lemon juice; stir well and remove from heat.

This sauce is less likely to separate than a true hollandaise sauce, and is therefore recommended for the inexperienced cook.

SOUPS

Service of soups. All soups should be served in a heated cup or cream soup dish and covered when possible to retain maximum heat until eaten. Croutons (p. 676) may be placed in the soup at serving time, or Melba toast or crackers may be served on a separate plate.

BROTH WITH EGG

1 egg   ⅔ cup hot broth

Method. Beat egg slightly. Add broth gradually to the egg, stirring continuously in order to avoid overcooking the egg. Serve immediately.

TOMATO BOUILLON

½ cup tomato juice   Salt and pepper
⅔ cup broth

Method. Mix the ingredients and bring to the boiling point. Serve in a heated container.

GENERAL METHOD FOR CREAM SOUPS

PREPARATION OF VEGETABLES

Allow ½ cup purée per serving of soup. This will require ¾ to 1 cup, or more, of cooked vegetable because of loss on the sieve. To prepare fresh vegetables: carrots should be scraped and diced; potatoes pared and diced; celery or asparagus cut into 1-inch pieces; onions chopped; cauliflower broken into small flowerets; and spinach washed through several waters to remove all grit. Cook vegetables in about ½ cup boiling salted water until very tender. Press through a sieve. A blender may be used to reduce the vegetable to a smooth consistency, but if the soup is to be used on a diet in which fiber is restricted it may still be necessary to strain through a sieve.

Canned green peas, Lima beans, carrots, corn, and asparagus may be used for the purée. If they are not very soft, they should be cooked in their own juice before sieving them.

Purées for infant feeding may also be used in cream soups.

PREPARATION OF SOUP

2 teaspoons fat

2 teaspoons flour

½ teaspoon salt

¾ cup milk

½ cup vegetable purée (asparagus, carrot, green bean, Lima bean, corn, celery, pea, or spinach)

Method. Melt fat in top of double boiler and mix in the salt and flour to make a smooth paste. Add milk gradually to the flour mixture and continue stirring until thickened. Cook over hot water for 5 to 10 minutes. Heat vegetable purée and add gradually to the white sauce. Add a little milk if it seems too thick. Serve piping hot in covered soup dish.

Cream soups may be garnished with paprika, whipped cream, grated cheese, or minced parsley, chives, celery leaves, or green peppers.

CREAM OF TOMATO SOUP

¾ cup tomato juice

1 thin slice onion

2 whole cloves

¾ cup thin white sauce (p. 701)

Method. Simmer tomato juice with small slice onion and cloves for 5 minutes. Strain. Prepare white sauce and add hot tomato juice gradually while continuing to stir. If slight curdling should occur, beat vigorously with a rotary beater.

One-eighth teaspoon baking soda may be added to the tomatoes before mixing with the white sauce to minimize curdling; this practice, however, will reduce the ascorbic acid content.

Serve soup immediately in a hot covered soup dish. Chopped parsley, chives, or whipped cream may be used for a garnish.

CREAM OF POTATO SOUP

½ cup diced potatoes

2 to 3 slices onion

½ cup thin white sauce

1 sprig parsley or caraway seeds

Method. Boil potatoes and sliced onion together in about ½ cup water. When potatoes and onion are soft, rub through sieve with water in which they were cooked. Heat white sauce in double boiler, and add puréed potato mixture. Beat well; garnish with minced parsley or caraway seeds.

OYSTER STEW

1 cup milk

⅓ cup oysters

1 tablespoon butter

Salt and pepper

Sprig parsley

Method. Strain liquid from oysters to remove any sand and particles of shell. Cook oysters in their own liquid slowly until edges curl—about 3 to 5 minutes.

Heat milk with butter in top of double boiler, add oysters to milk, and season. Garnish with chopped parsley and serve.

Vegetables

PREPARATION AND COOKING OF FRESH VEGETABLES

Select only fresh, crisp, ripe but not overmature vegetables. Use vegetables as soon as possible after purchase to retain maximum vitamin content. Plan preliminary preparation as follows:

Spinach and other greens. Cut off roots and remove bad parts. Wash under running water or in several changes of water to remove all sand. Lukewarm water with a little salt added may be used for the first washings to help remove the sand, but the vegetables must not be allowed to soak.

Peas, beans, corn. Remove shells or husks just before these vegetables are to be cooked.

Broccoli, cabbage, cauliflower, Brussels sprouts. To remove any insects, cauliflower, broccoli, and Brussels sprouts may be soaked for a few minutes in salty water. Remove outer leaves just before use. Cook cauliflower whole or in flowerets. Quarter cabbage or shred. Remove base of sprouts. Peel off hard outer covering of stems of broccoli. Cut thick broccoli stems in half.

Root vegetables. Scrub with brush before peeling or scraping. Beets are usually cooked without peeling since there is less loss of color. Potatoes and sweet potatoes may also be cooked without removing the skin.

COOKING TIME FOR FRESH VEGETABLES

	COOKING TIME minutes		COOKING TIME minutes
Artichokes	20–40	Corn on the cob	8–12
Asparagus, butts	15–25	Dandelion	10–20
tips	5–10	Eggplant	10–20
Beans, Lima	20–30	Kale	20–30
string	15–30	Kohlrabi	20–40
Beet greens	10–20	Okra	20–40
Beets		Onions	25–30
old	1–2 hours	Parsnips	30–40
young	30–45	Peas	10–20
Broccoli	20–25	Potatoes, Irish	20–30
Brussels sprouts	10–20	sweet	20–30
Cabbage		Rutabagas	20–60
quartered	20–30	Spinach and other greens	5–15
shredded	8–12	Squash, Hubbard	20–30
Cauliflower, flowerets	10–15	summer	5–15
whole	20–30	Tomatoes	5–10
Celery	20–30	Turnips, white	20–30

Boiling vegetables. Use a saucepan with a tightly fitting cover. Add vegetables to boiling water, using about ½ inch water in the pan. No water is needed for greens since the water clinging from the washing is adequate. Cover pan and bring to the boiling point as rapidly as possible. Boil gently until just tender. The addition of 1 teaspoon sugar improves the flavor of mature vegetables which have lost their sweetness.

The table on page 704 gives approximate cooking time, but the time will vary depending upon the degree of maturity and the size of the pieces.

FROZEN VEGETABLES

For method of cookery, read carefully the directions which accompany vegetables. Preliminary thawing is not necessary except in the case of corn on the cob. Drop frozen vegetable into rapidly boiling salted water, and bring quickly to the boiling point. Cover, and cook until tender. The length of time for cooking is less than that for fresh vegetables.

CANNED VEGETABLES

Drain liquor from vegetables, and reduce volume by boiling. Then add vegetables, season to taste, and heat thoroughly. Liquor may be used in sauces, gravies, or soups if not boiled down and used with the vegetables.

SERVICE OF VEGETABLES

Vegetables may be served in a variety of ways: (1) *Buttered:* Add 1 to 2 teaspoons butter with a dash of salt and pepper to ½ cup diced and cooked vegetables. Minced parsley with potatoes or carrots, a dash of nutmeg with green beans, lemon juice with spinach, minced green pepper and pimento with corn, mint leaves with peas suggest a few of many possibilities for enhancing flavor and interest of vegetables. (2) *With cream:* Add 1 tablespoon hot cream to ½ cup of hot buttered vegetables. (3) *With sauces* of blending or contrasting flavor: (a) pour ¼ cup hot white sauce (medium) over ½ cup cooked vegetable; (b) cheese sauce (p. 701) is especially suitable for cabbage, cauliflower, asparagus; (c) hollandaise sauce (p. 702) lends a piquant flavor to asparagus, broccoli. (4) *Escalloped:* Mix ½ cup cooked vegetables with ¼ to ½ cup medium white sauce (p. 701). Place in a buttered baking dish, and cover with bread or cracker crumbs. Dot with butter, and bake in oven until crumbs are brown.

HARVARD BEETS

1 tablespoon butter	⅛ teaspoon salt
½ tablespoon flour	¼ cup mild vinegar
¼ cup sugar	½ cup sliced beets

Method. Melt butter in top part of double boiler. Add flour, sugar, and salt, and stir in vinegar gradually. Cook for 10 to 15 minutes, and add sliced beets. Allow to stand in warm place until sauce takes on a rich red color before serving.

GLAZED SWEET POTATOES OR CARROTS

2 small sweet potatoes	3 tablespoons sugar, white or brown
or	1 tablespoon butter
4 carrots	1 teaspoon water

Method. Wash sweet potatoes or carrots. If carrots are used scrape off the skin before boiling; sweet potatoes are peeled after boiling. Boil in small amount of boiling salted water until tender; drain. Peel potato, and cut in half lengthwise. Put sugar, butter, and water in skillet and cook over slow heat until blended. Reheat potatoes or carrots in this mixture until they become glazed and slightly brown.

Variation. Carrots or potatoes may be placed in a buttered baking dish with the sugar and butter, and cooked in a slow oven for about 20 minutes.

BAKED POTATO

1 medium-size potato	1 teaspoon butter

Method. Scrub potato with a brush; dry and slightly grease the surface. Place in a moderately hot oven (425° F) and bake about 45 to 50 minutes. The potato should feel tender under pressure. When done, make an incision of 1 inch in the skin and gently press the potato so that excess moisture can escape. Put butter in the cut and serve immediately.

BAKED STUFFED POTATO

1 potato	Salt and pepper
1 teaspoon butter	2 teaspoons grated cheese
1 tablespoon cream or milk	Paprika

Method. Bake potato as directed above. Cut thin slice from side of potato, and remove pulp from casing. Mash, and mix with butter and hot cream. Season with salt and pepper, and beat until creamy. Return to potato shell and sprinkle with cheese and paprika. Place in hot oven and cook until cheese is melted and browned.

MASHED POTATO

1 cooked medium-sized potato	1 tablespoon hot milk or cream
1 teaspoon butter	Salt and pepper

Method. Mash potato until free of lumps, add butter, hot cream, and salt and pepper to taste. Beat until creamy.

BAKED SQUASH

Squash (acorn or Hubbard)	1 teaspoon butter
Salt; pepper	1 teaspoon brown sugar

Method. Wash squash. Without cutting bake for about 30 minutes at 400° F. Cut squash in serving size pieces, remove seeds, and season with salt, pepper, butter, and brown sugar. Put pieces on a shallow pan, and continue baking for 20 to 30 minutes until very tender.

A medium acorn squash will serve two persons, while a Hubbard squash, depending upon size, will provide 6 or more servings.

BROILED TOMATO

1 teaspoon butter	Salt and pepper
1 tablespoon fine bread crumbs	1 tomato

Method. Melt butter, brown bread crumbs, and season with salt and pepper. Wash tomato, remove core end, and cut in half. Dust with salt and pepper, and sprinkle bread crumbs on each half. Place on greased broiler rack about 3 inches below direct flame. Broil for about 10 minutes or until tender.

WHOLE TOMATO STUFFED WITH RICE

1 medium-size tomato	1 teaspoon butter
2 tablespoons rice	Salt and pepper

Method. Remove the center from the tomato, dust the inside with salt and a very little pepper, and set aside. Boil the rice for about 20 minutes, drain, and add the tomato pulp, butter, salt, and pepper. Fill the center with rice. Set the tomato in a lightly buttered pan, and bake in a moderate oven 20 minutes.

Sodium-restricted Recipes

Adaptation of recipes for sodium-restricted diets. Almost all recipes in this text and from standard cookbooks may be adapted to sodium-restricted diets by making certain very simple changes. The following important modifications apply:

1. Omit salt in any recipe.
2. Substitute low-sodium leavening agent whenever baking powder or baking soda are specified.
   - *a.* Potassium bicarbonate instead of sodium bicarbonate, using the quantity specified in the recipe
   - *b.* Sodium-free baking powder instead of regular baking powder. Most drug stores and many food stores which sell dietetic foods can supply one of several brands. If not available in the community, the druggist can prepare a baking powder using the following formula:

potassium bicarbonate	39.8 gm
cornstarch	28.0 gm
tartaric acid	7.5 gm
potassium bi-tartrate	56.1 gm

     Use 1½ teaspoons sodium-free baking powder for each teaspoon regular baking powder.
3. Use unsalted fats: sweet butter, unsalted margarine, lard, hydrogenated vegetable fats, vegetable oils.

4. Substitute low-sodium ingredients for salted ingredients:

> low-sodium (dietetic) tomato juice or canned vegetables for salted canned vegetables and juice
>
> low-sodium (dietetic) bouillon cubes for regular bouillon cubes
>
> low-sodium (dietetic) cheese for regular cheese; unsalted cottage cheese
>
> plain gelatin for sweetened gelatin powders

5. Count any of the following ingredients as part of the day's food allowance since they are naturally high in sodium: milk, whole eggs, meat, fish, and poultry. For example, the recipe for blancmange (p. 682) makes 2 to 3 servings. From the day's food allowance one would subtract ½ cup milk and ½ egg. On the other hand, the amount of egg and of milk represented in one plain muffin (see below) would be so small that no allowance need be made except in severely restricted diets.

Low-sodium milk may be substituted for regular milk whenever diets are severely restricted (usually below 500 mg sodium). Unless calories or protein are restricted in the diet, the low-sodium milk need not be subtracted from the day's allowance.

Egg yolks are much lower in sodium content than are egg whites. In many recipes an egg yolk (or two) may be used satisfactorily instead of one whole egg: for example, puddings, custard, mayonnaise, brownies.

6. Omit recipes which include bacon, ham, more than one egg white.

The following illustrates the adaptation of a recipe:

PLAIN MUFFINS (recipe, p. 674)

(6 muffins)

1 cup flour	1 tablespoon sugar
Omit salt	½ cup milk
2¼ teaspoons sodium-free baking powder	2 tablespoons unsalted fat
	½ egg

Follow directions for preparation on page 674.

Seasonings for low-sodium diets. Since ancient times, herbs and spices have been used as medicines, perfumes, and for seasoning food. Many people today do not realize the intriguing flavors which can be given to foods by using them judiciously. Observation of the following simple rules in herb and spice cookery will yield satisfying results:

1. Begin experimenting with herbs and spices sparingly until you learn what they can do for food. Their effect can be subtle and illusive, but if used with a heavy hand they can be overwhelming.

2. Herbs and spices contain volatile flavors which are lost if they are kept too long. Buy them in small quantities and keep them tightly covered at all times.

3. Start with about ¼ teaspoon dried herbs in a dish for four people. When using fresh herbs, use about three to four times this quantity.

4. Cutting, crushing, or mincing fresh herbs brings out the volatile oils and true flavors.

5. For foods which are not to be cooked, such as vegetable juices, add herbs well in advance—even overnight—of serving time. The herbs may be tied in a cheesecloth bag and removed from the juice just before serving.

6. For a quickly cooked dish, or for a salad, moisten the herbs first with a little milk, unsalted butter, lemon juice, or oil and add to the prepared dish; allow a salad to stand for about ½ hour before serving.

7. For dishes cooked a long time (soups and stews), add herbs during the last hour of cookery.

Herb, spice, and flavoring shelf. A complete list of flavoring aids is included on page 516. Until one is accustomed to using herbs and spices in cookery, one may wish to try a few at the time. The following might be used as a "starter shelf."

HERBS	SPICES	FLAVORING EXTRACTS
Basil	Cinnamon	Almond
Bay leaf	Cloves	Lemon
Chives	Curry	Maple
Marjoram	Ginger	Orange
Mint	Mustard, dry	Peppermint
Parsley	Nutmeg	Vanilla
Rosemary	Paprika	
Sage	Pepper	
Savory		
Thyme		

Suggestions for using herbs, spices, and garnishes in cookery. The suggestions presented here are useful for enhancing the flavor of foods for the family fare, but lend special interest to the sodium-restricted diet. Herb butters may be used to brush meats before broiling or to season cooked vegetables. To prepare herb butter:

Cream ½ cup unsalted butter. Blend in 3 tablespoons lemon juice and 2 tablespoons minced fresh herbs or 1 teaspoon dried herbs. This mixture may be kept in the refrigerator for a few days, or may be frozen.

Meat, Poultry, Fish, Eggs

Beef: bay leaf, lemon juice, marjoram, dry mustard, mushrooms, nutmeg, onion, green pepper, pepper, sage, thyme; currant or grape jelly

Chicken or turkey: basil, bay leaf, lemon juice, marjoram, onion, pepper, rosemary, sage, sesame seeds, thyme; cranberry sauce

Lamb: curry, garlic, mint, onion, oregano, parsley, rosemary, thyme; mint jelly, broiled pineapple

Pork: garlic, lemon juice, marjoram, sage; applesauce, spiced apples, cranberries

Veal: bay leaf, curry, dill seed, ginger, marjoram, oregano, summer savory; currant jelly; broiled apricots or peaches

Fish: bay leaf, curry, dill, garlic, lemon juice, mushrooms, mustard, onion, paprika, pepper

Eggs: basil, chives, curry, mustard, parsley, green pepper, rosemary, diced tomato

Vegetables. Add a dash of sugar while cooking vegetables to bring out flavor.

Asparagus: lemon juice, caraway; unsalted chopped nuts

Green beans: dill, lemon, marjoram, nutmeg, onion, rosemary; slivered almonds

Broccoli: lemon juice, oregano, tarragon

Corn: chives, parsley, green pepper, pimento, tomato

Peas: mint, mushroom, onion, parsley, green pepper

Potatoes: chives, mace, onion, parsley, green pepper

Squash: basil, ginger, mace, onion, oregano

Sweet potatoes: cinnamon, nutmeg; brown sugar

Tomatoes: basil, marjoram, oregano, parsley, sage

LOW-SODIUM BREAD

1 cup lukewarm water	2 tablespoons soft fat, unsalted
3 tablespoons sugar	2¾ to 3 cups sifted flour
½ cake compressed yeast	

Method. Mix water and sugar in large bowl. Crumble yeast into mixture. Add fat and about half of the flour. Mix well. Add flour and stir to a soft dough. Turn out dough on a floured board, cover, and let stand for about 5 minutes. Knead dough until it is smooth and elastic. Place in a greased bowl large enough to permit the dough to double in bulk. Cover, keep in a warm place, and let rise until doubled in bulk—about 1–1½ hours. Knead again, and shape into a loaf. Place in a greased one-loaf pan, 9 x 5 x 3 inches. Let rise again and bake at 400° F for 30 to 35 minutes.

CINNAMON ROLLS

Dough for low-sodium bread	Cinnamon
Soft unsalted butter	Unsalted nuts, chopped
Brown sugar	

Method. Prepare dough as for low-sodium bread above. After first rising, roll out dough into a rectangle to about ¼ inch. Spread with soft butter, sprinkle generously with brown sugar, cinnamon, and chopped nuts. Roll tightly, and slice in pieces 1 inch thick. Place cut side down on greased pan. Let rise until double in bulk. Bake in oven at 400° F for 15 to 20 minutes—light golden brown.

WAFFLES

1 cup scalded milk, regular or low-sodium	1 package compressed yeast
¼ cup soft fat	1 egg
1 tablespoon sugar	3 cups sifted flour
1½ cups water	

Method. Mix milk, fat, and sugar. Add water, cooling the mixture to lukewarm temperature. Crumble yeast and mix well with milk mixture. Add slightly beaten egg. Stir in flour and mix until well blended. Allow batter to stand for 15–30 minutes until bubbles begin to form on surface. Bake on heated waffle iron.

If a freezer is available, the baked waffles may be frozen, kept wrapped in freezer paper, and reheated by placing the waffle in a toaster.

POPOVERS (6 large popovers)

2 eggs	1 cup sifted flour
1 cup milk, regular or low-sodium	1 teaspoon melted fat or oil

Method. Combine all ingredients in a mixing bowl and beat with a rotary beater until smooth. Butter (unsalted) custard cups well, and fill each about ⅔ with batter. Place cups on a baking sheet and bake at 425° F until golden brown—about 35 minutes. Serve immediately.

One popover made with regular milk: 45 mg sodium.

MEAT LOAF

½ pound ground beef	⅛ teaspoon poultry seasoning
¼ pound ground pork	½ cup milk, warm
¼ pound ground veal	2 slices unsalted bread
2 tablespoons minced onion	1 egg
⅛ teaspoon pepper	¼ cup dry bread crumbs, unsalted
⅛ teaspoon sage	½ cup tomatoes, unsalted
⅛ teaspoon dry mustard	

Method. Combine meat, onion, and seasonings and mix well. Soak bread in milk and add egg. Combine the meat and bread-milk mixtures, and shape into a loaf. Roll in dry bread crumbs, and place in loaf pan. Cover with tomatoes and bake at 350° F for about 1 hour. Baste with liquid in pan at 15-minute intervals.

PIECRUST (double crust)

2 cups flour	4–5 tablespoons cold water
⅔ cup soft shortening, unsalted	

Method. Cut shortening into sifted flour with two knives or a pastry blender until the crumbs are the size of small peas. Add water, a tablespoon at the time, mixing in with a fork. Use just enough water to hold the ingredients together; the dough should not be sticky. Turn out on a lightly floured board. Divide dough in half and roll each piece into a circle to fit an 8-inch pie tin.

APPLE PIE

6–8 tart apples	½ teaspoon nutmeg
¾ cup sugar	1 tablespoon unsalted butter

Method. Pare apples, quarter them, and take out the core. Slice thinly and mix with sugar and nutmeg. Line piepan with one crust. Pile apples into crust. Place slits with a knife in the top crust so that steam can escape. Carefully place top crust over pie so that it fits evenly. Turn edges of top crust under the lower crust, and build up a fluted edge with a fork or with thumb and forefinger. Bake at 400° F for about 50 minutes—until crust is light brown and apples are cooked.

NORWEGIAN BUTTER COOKIES (about 3 dozen)

¾ cup unsalted butter	1 teaspoon grated orange rind
½ cup sugar	2 cups sifted flour
2 hard-cooked egg yolks	

Method. Cream butter until light and fluffy, adding a little sugar at the time. Press egg yolks through sieve and blend with butter-sugar mixture. Stir in orange rind and sifted flour. Chill dough in the refrigerator. Break off small pieces of dough and roll to thickness of a pencil and about 5 inches long. Bring ends together and overlap as in a pretzel. Place on ungreased baking sheet, and bake for about 10 minutes at 375° F until set but not brown.

BROWNIES

2 squares unsweetened chocolate	¾ cup sifted flour
⅓ cup unsalted fat	½ teaspoon sodium-free baking powder
1 cup sugar	
2 egg yolks	½ cup chopped nuts

Method. Melt chocolate and fat over hot water. Beat in sugar and egg yolks. Add flour, baking powder, and nuts; stir until blended. Spread in greased pan, 8 inches square. Bake at 350° F for about 30 minutes until top has dull crust. Cool slightly, and cut into squares.

RECIPE INDEX

713

APPENDIX /

TABLE I /

EXPLANATION

The uses of a food table have been described in Chapter 3. Each food table should be carefully studied to determine what information it provides, and how it can be best used. Table 1 which follows is reproduced from the publication of the Institute of Home Economics in 1960 *Nutritive Value of Foods*. The explanation provided in the bulletin for this table is reproduced here in part: *

Foods listed. Foods are grouped under the following main headings: Milk; eggs; meat, poultry, and fish; dry beans and peas, nuts; vegetables; fruits; grain products; fats; sugars; and miscellaneous items.

Most of the foods listed are in ready-to-eat form. Some are basic products widely used in food preparation, such as flour, fat, and cornmeal.

Weight in grams is shown for an approximate measure of each food as it is described; if inedible parts are included in the description, both measure and weight include these parts.

The approximate measure shown for each food is in cups, ounces, pounds, a piece of a certain size, or some other well-known unit. The measure shown can be calculated readily to larger or smaller amounts by multiplying or dividing. However, because the measures are approximate (some are rounded for convenient use), calculated nutritive values for very large quantities of some food items may be less representative than those for smaller quantities.

The cup measure refers to the standard measuring cup of 8 fluid ounces or $\frac{1}{2}$ liquid pint. The ounce refers to $\frac{1}{16}$ of a pound avoirdupois, unless fluid ounce is indicated. The weight of a fluid ounce varies according to the food measured.

Food values. Values are shown for protein; fat; fatty acids; total carbohydrate; two minerals—calcium and iron; and five vitamins—vitamin A, thiamine, riboflavin, niacin, and ascorbic acid (vitamin C). Calories are shown also, in the column headed "Food energy." . . .

Water content is also shown in the table because the percentage of moisture present is needed for identification and comparison of many food items.

Nutritive values are shown for only the parts of food customarily eaten—corn without the cob, meat without bone, potatoes without the skin, American-type grapes without seeds and skin, European-type grapes without seeds. If additional parts are eaten—the skin of the potato, for example—amounts of some nutrients obtained will be somewhat greater than those shown.

For many of the prepared items, values have been calculated from the in-

* Institute of Home Economics, Agricultural Research Service: *Nutritive Value of Foods.* Home and Garden Bull. 72, U.S. Department of Agriculture, Washington, D.C., 1960.

718

gredients in typical recipes. Examples of such items are: Biscuits, corn muffins, oyster stew, macaroni and cheese, and custard and a number of other dessert-type items.

For vegetables and for toast, the values are shown for the food without any fat added, either during preparation or at the table.

For meat, the values are for the meat as cooked and drained and without drippings. For many cuts, values are shown for the meat both with and without the fat that can be trimmed off in the kitchen or on the plate.

TABLE 1.—NUTRITIVE VALUES OF

[Dashes show that no basis could be found for imputing a value although there was some

ITEM NO.	FOOD, approximate measure, and weight (in grams)			WATER	FOOD ENERGY	PROTEIN	FAT (total lipid)
			gm	per cent	calories	gm	gm
	Milk, cream, cheese; related products						
	Milk, cow's						
1	fluid, whole	1 cup	244..	87	165	9	10
2	fluid, nonfat (skim)	1 cup	246..	90	90	9	Trace
3	buttermilk, cultured, from skim milk	1 cup	246..	90	90	9	Trace
4	evaporated, unsweetened, undiluted	1 cup	252..	74	345	18	20
5	condensed, sweetened, un-diluted	1 cup	306..	26	985	25	25
6	dry, whole	1 cup	103..	2	515	27	28
7	dry, nonfat	1 cup	80...	3	290	29	1
8	Milk, goat's: fluid, whole ..	1 cup	244..	88	165	8	10
	Cream						
9	half-and-half (milk and cream)	1 cup	242..	80	330	8	29
10		1 tablespoon .	15...	80	20	Trace	2
11	light, table or coffee	1 cup	240..	71	525	7	52
12		1 tablespoon .	15...	71	35	Trace	3
	whipping, unwhipped (volume about double when whipped)						
13	medium	1 cup	239..	61	745	6	78
14		1 tablespoon .	15...	61	45	Trace	5
15	heavy	1 cup	238..	56	860	5	93
16		1 tablespoon .	15...	56	55	Trace	6
	Cheese						
17	blue mold (Roquefort type)	1 ounce	28...	40	105	6	9
	Cheddar or American						
18	ungrated	1-inch cube .	17...	36	70	4	6
19	grated	1 cup	112..	36	455	28	37
20		1 tablespoon .	7....	36	30	2	2
21	Cheddar, process	1 ounce	28...	39	105	7	9
22	cheese foods, Cheddar ...	1 ounce	28...	43	95	6	7
	cottage cheese, from skim milk						
23	creamed	1 cup	225..	78	240	30	11
24		1 ounce	28...	78	30	4	1
25	uncreamed	1 cup	225..	79	195	38	1
26		1 ounce	28...	79	25	5	Trace
27	cream cheese	1 ounce	28...	51	105	2	11
28		1 tablespoon .	15...	51	55	1	6
29	Swiss	1 ounce	28...	39	105	7	8
	Milk beverages						
30	cocoa	1 cup	242..	79	235	9	11

THE EDIBLE PART OF FOODS *

reason to believe that a measurable amount of the constituent might be present]

SATU-RATED (total)	UNSATURATED OLEIC	LINO-LEIC	CARBO-HY-DRATE	CAL-CIUM	IRON	VITA-MIN-A VALUE	THIA-MINE	RIBO-FLA-VIN	NIA-CIN	ASCOR-BIC ACID	ITEM NO.
gm	gm	gm	gm	mg	mg	I.U.	mg	mg	mg	mg	
6	3	Trace	12	285	0.1	390	0.08	0.42	0.2	2	1
—	—	—	13	298	.1	10	.10	.44	.2	2	2
—	—	—	13	298	.1	10	.10	.44	.2	2	3
11	7	1	24	635	.3	820	.10	.84	.5	3	4
14	8	1	170	829	.3	1,020	.24	1.21	.5	3	5
15	9	1	39	968	.5	1,160	.30	1.50	.7	6	6
—	—	—	42	1,040	.5	20	.28	1.44	.7	6	7
6	2	Trace	11	315	.2	390	.10	.27	.7	2	8
16	10	1	11	259	.1	1,190	.07	.39	.1	2	9
1	1	Trace	1	16	0	70	0	.02	0	Trace	10
29	17	2	10	238	.1	2,140	.07	.35	.1	Trace	11
2	1	Trace	1	15	0	130	0	.02	0	Trace	12
43	26	2	8	196	.1	3,200	.06	.29	.1	Trace	13
3	2	Trace	1	12	0	200	0	.02	0	Trace	14
51	31	3	7	164	0	3,800	.05	.24	.1	Trace	15
3	2	Trace	Trace	10	0	240	0	.02	0	Trace	16
5	3	Trace	Trace	122	.2	350	.01	.17	.1	0	17
3	2	Trace	Trace	133	.2	230	Trace	.08	Trace	0	18
20	12	1	2	874	1.2	1,510	.03	.53	.1	0	19
1	1	Trace	Trace	55	.1	90	.02	.03	Trace	0	20
5	3	Trace	Trace	214	.2	350	Trace	.12	Trace	0	21
4	2	Trace	2	163	.2	300	.01	.17	Trace	0	22
6	4	Trace	6	207	0.9	430	.07	.66	.2	0	23
1	Trace	Trace	1	25	.1	50	.01	.08	Trace	0	24
Trace	Trace	Trace	6	202	.9	20	.07	.64	.2	0	25
—	—	—	1	26	.1	Trace	.01	.08	Trace	0	26
6	4	Trace	1	18	.1	440	Trace	.07	Trace	0	27
3	2	Trace	Trace	9	Trace	230	Trace	.04	Trace	0	28
4	3	Trace	1	271	.3	320	.01	.06	Trace	0	29
6	4	Trace	26	286	.9	390	.09	.45	.4	2	30

* Institute of Home Economics, Agricultural Research Service: *Nutritive Value of Foods*. Home and Garden Bull. 72, U.S. Department of Agriculture, Washington, D.C., 1960.

TABLE 1.—NUTRITIVE VALUES OF THE

ITEM NO.	FOOD, approximate measure, and weight (in grams)			WATER	FOOD EN- ERGY	PRO- TEIN	FAT (total lipid)
			gm	per cent	calo- ries	gm	gm
	Milk beverages (*Continued*)						
31	chocolate-flavored milk drink	1 cup	250..	83	190	8	6
32	malted milk	1 cup	270..	78	280	13	12
	Milk desserts						
33	cornstarch pudding, plain (blanc mange)	1 cup	248..	76	275	9	10
34	custard, baked	1 cup	248..	77	285	13	14
	ice cream, plain, factory packed						
35	slice or cut brick, ⅛ of quart brick	1 slice or cut brick	71...	62	145	3	9
36	container	3½ fluid ounces	62...	62	130	2	8
37	container	8 fluid ounces	142..	62	295	6	18
38	ice milk	1 cup	187..	67	285	9	10
39	Yoghurt, from partially skimmed milk	1 cup	246..	89	120	8	4
	Eggs						
	Eggs, large, 24 ounces per dozen raw						
40	whole, without shell ...	1 egg	50...	74	80	6	6
41	white of egg	1 white	33...	88	15	4	Trace
42	yolk of egg	1 yolk	17...	51	60	3	5
	cooked						
43	boiled, shell removed ..	2 eggs	100..	74	160	13	12
44	scrambled, with milk and fat	1 egg	64...	72	110	7	8
	Meat, poultry, fish, shellfish; related products						
45	Bacon, broiled or fried crisp	2 slices	16...	8	95	5	8
	Beef, trimmed to retail basis,* cooked cuts braised, simmered, or pot-roasted						
46	lean and fat	3 ounces	85...	53	245	23	16
47	lean only	2.5 ounces ..	72...	62	140	22	5
	hamburger, broiled						
48	market ground	3 ounces	85...	54	245	21	17
49	ground lean	3 ounces	85...	60	185	23	10
	roast, oven-cooked, no liquid added relatively fat, such as rib						
50	lean and fat	3 ounces	85...	38	390	16	36
51	lean only	1.8 ounces ..	51...	57	120	14	7

* Outer layer of fat on the cut was removed to within approximately ½ inch of the lean. Deposits of fat within the cut were not removed.

EDIBLE PART OF FOODS—Continued

	FATTY ACIDS		CARBO-HY-DRATE	CAL-CIUM	IRON	VITA-MIN-A VALUE	THIA-MINE	RIBO-FLA-VIN	NIA-CIN	ASCOR-BIC ACID	ITEM NO.
SATU-RATED (total)	UNSATURATED										
	OLEIC	LINO-LEIC									
gm	gm	gm	gm	mg	mg	I.U.	mg	mg	mg	mg	
3	2	Trace	27	270	0.4	210	0.09	0.41	0.2	2	*31*
7	4	Trace	32	364	.8	670	.17	.56	—	2	*32*
6	3	Trace	39	290	.1	390	.07	.40	.1	2	*33*
6	5	1	28	278	1.0	870	.10	.47	.2	1	*34*
5	3	Trace	15	87	.1	370	.03	.13	.1	1	*35*
4	3	Trace	13	76	.1	320	.03	.12	.1	1	*36*
10	6	1	29	175	.1	740	.06	.27	.1	1	*37*
6	3	Trace	42	292	.2	390	.09	.41	.2	2	*38*
2	1	Trace	13	295	.1	170	.09	.43	.2	2	*39*
2	3	Trace	Trace	27	1.1	590	.05	.15	Trace	0	*40*
—	—	—	Trace	3	Trace	0	Trace	.09	Trace	0	*41*
2	2	Trace	Trace	24	.9	580	.04	.07	Trace	0	*42*
4	5	1	1	54	2.3	1,180	.09	.28	.1	0	*43*
3	4	1	1	51	1.1	690	.05	.18	Trace	0	*44*
3	4	1	1	2	.5	0	.08	.05	.8	—	*45*
8	7	Trace	0	10	2.9	30	.04	.18	3.5	—	*46*
2	2	Trace	0	10	2.7	10	.04	.16	3.3	—	*47*
8	7	Trace	0	9	2.7	30	.07	.02	4.6	—	*48*
5	4	Trace	0	10	3.0	20	.08	.20	5.1	—	*49*
17	16	1	0	7	2.1	70	.04	.13	3.0	—	*50*
3	3	Trace	0	6	1.8	10	.04	.11	2.6	—	*51*

TABLE 1.—NUTRITIVE VALUES OF THE

ITEM NO.	FOOD, approximate measure, and weight (in grams)		gm	WATER per cent	FOOD EN-ERGY calo-ries	PRO-TEIN gm	FAT (total lipid) gm
	roast, oven-cooked (*Continued*)						
	relatively lean, such as round						
52	lean and fat	3 ounces	85...	56	220	23	14
53	lean only	2.5 ounces ..	71...	63	130	21	4
	steak, broiled						
	relatively fat, such as sirloin						
54	lean and fat	3 ounces	85...	44	330	20	27
55	lean only	2 ounces	56...	59	115	18	4
	relatively lean, such as round						
56	lean and fat	3 ounces	85...	55	220	24	13
57	lean only	2.4 ounces ..	69...	61	130	22	4
	Beef, canned						
58	corned beef	3 ounces	85...	59	180	22	10
59	corned beef hash	3 ounces	85...	70	120	12	5
60	Beef, dried or chipped	2 ounces	57...	48	115	19	4
61	Beef and vegetable stew	1 cup	235..	82	185	15	10
62	Beef potpie: individual pie, 4¼-in. diam., weight before baking about 8 ounces	1 pie, baked ..	227..	63	460	18	28
	Chicken, cooked						
63	flesh and skin, broiled	3 ounces with-out bone	85...	61	185	23	9
	breast, fried, ½ breast						
64	with bone	3.3 ounces ..	94...	52	215	24	12
65	flesh and skin only	2.8 ounces ..	79...	52	215	24	12
	leg, fried (thigh and drumstick)						
66	with bone	4.3 ounces ..	121..	52	245	27	15
67	flesh and skin only	3.1 ounces ..	89...	52	245	27	15
68	Chicken, canned, boneless ..	3 ounces	85...	62	170	25	7
	Chicken potpie. *See* Poultry potpie.						
	Chile con carne, canned						
69	with beans	1 cup	250..	72	335	19	15
70	without beans	1 cup	255..	67	510	26	38
71	Heart, beef, trimmed of fat, braised	3 ounces	85...	61	160	26	5
	Lamb, trimmed to retail basis,* cooked						
72	chop, thick, with bone, broiled	1 chop, 4.8 ounces	137..	47	405	25	33
73	lean and fat	4 ounces	112..	47	405	25	33
74	lean only	2.6 ounces ..	74...	62	140	21	6
	leg, roasted						
75	lean and fat	3 ounces	85...	54	235	22	16
76	lean only	2.5 ounces ..	71...	62	130	20	5
	shoulder, roasted						
77	lean and fat	3 ounces	85...	50	285	18	23
78	lean only	2.3 ounces ..	64...	61	130	17	6

* Outer layer of fat on the cut was removed to within approximately ½ inch of the lean. Deposits of fat within the cut were not removed.

EDIBLE PART OF FOODS—Continued

SATU-RATED (total)	UNSATURATED		CARBO-HY-DRATE	CAL-CIUM	IRON	VITA-MIN-A VALUE	THIA-MINE	RIBO-FLA-VIN	NIA-CIN	ASCOR-BIC ACID	ITEM NO.
	OLEIC	LINO-LEIC									
gm	gm	gm	gm	mg	mg	I.U.	mg	mg	mg	mg	
7	6	Trace	0	10	3.0	30	0.06	0.18	4.2	—	52
2	2	Trace	0	9	2.7	10	.05	.16	3.8	—	53
13	12	1	0	8	2.5	50	.05	.16	4.0	—	54
2	2	Trace	0	7	2.2	10	.05	.14	3.6	—	55
6	6	Trace	0	11	3.0	20	.07	.19	4.8	—	56
2	2	Trace	0	9	2.6	10	.06	.16	4.2	—	57
5	4	Trace	0	17	3.7	20	.01	.20	2.9	—	58
2	2	Trace	6	22	1.1	10	.02	.11	2.4	—	59
2	2	Trace	0	11	2.9	—	.04	.18	2.2	—	60
5	4	Trace	15	31	2.8	2,530	.13	.18	4.4	14	61
10	15	1	32	20	2.5	2,830	.07	.14	3.0	Trace	62
3	4	2	0	10	1.4	260	.04	.15	7.1	—	63
3	6	2	—	10	1.1	60	.03	.06	9.4	—	64
3	6	2	—	10	1.1	60	.03	.06	9.4	—	65
4	7	2	—	13	1.8	220	.05	.18	4.7	—	66
4	7	2	—	13	1.8	220	.05	.18	4.7	—	67
2	3	1	0	12	1.5	160	.03	.14	5.4	—	68
7	7	Trace	30	98	4.2	150	.08	.20	3.5	—	69
18	17	1	15	97	3.6	380	.05	.31	5.6	—	70
2	2	Trace	1	14	5.9	30	.23	1.05	6.8	3	71
18	12	1	0	10	3.1	—	.14	.25	4.5	—	72
18	12	1	0	10	3.1	—	.14	.25	5.6	—	73
3	2	Trace	0	9	2.5	—	.11	.20	4.5	—	74
9	6	Trace	0	9	2.8	—	.13	.23	4.7	—	75
3	2	Trace	0	9	2.6	—	.12	.21	4.4	—	76
13	8	1	0	8	2.4	—	.11	.20	4.0	—	77
3	2	Trace	0	8	2.2	—	.10	.18	3.7	—	78

TABLE 1.—NUTRITIVE VALUES OF THE

ITEM NO.	FOOD, approximate measure, and weight (in grams)		gm	WATER per cent	FOOD EN- ERGY calo- ries	PRO- TEIN gm	FAT (total lipid) gm
79	Liver, beef, fried	2 ounces	57...	57	120	13	4
	Pork, cured, cooked						
80	ham, smoked, lean and fat luncheon meat	3 ounces	85...	48	290	18	24
81	cooked ham, sliced	2 ounces	57...	48	170	13	13
82	canned, spiced or un- spiced	2 ounces	57...	55	165	8	14
	Pork, fresh, trimmed to retail basis,* cooked						
83	chop, thick, with bone ...	1 chop, 3.5 ounces	98...	42	260	16	21
84	lean and fat	2.3 ounces ..	66...	42	260	16	21
85	lean only	1.7 ounces ..	48...	53	130	15	7
	roast, oven-cooked, no liq- uid added						
86	lean and fat	3 ounces	85...	46	310	21	24
87	lean only	2.4 ounces ..	68...	55	175	20	10
	cuts simmered						
88	lean and fat	3 ounces	85...	46	320	20	26
89	lean only	2.2 ounces ..	63...	60	135	18	6
90	Poultry potpie (chicken or turkey): individual pie, 4¼-inch-diameter, about 8 ounces	1 pie	227..	60	485	17	28
	Sausage						
91	bologna, slice 4.1 by 0.1 inch	8 slices	227..	56	690	27	62
92	frankfurter, cooked	1 frankfurter	51...	58	155	6	14
93	pork, bulk, canned	4 ounces	113..	55	340	18	29
94	Tongue, beef, simmered	3 ounces	85...	61	205	18	14
	Turkey potpie. *See* Poultry potpie.						
	Veal, cooked						
95	cutlet, broiled	3 ounces with- out bone	85...	60	185	23	9
96	roast, medium fat, medium done: lean and fat	3 ounces	85...	55	305	23	14
	Fish and shellfish						
97	bluefish, baked or broiled .	3 ounces	85...	68	135	22	4
	clams						
98	raw, meat only	3 ounces	85...	80	70	11	1
99	canned, solids and liquid	3 ounces	85...	87	45	7	1
100	crabmeat, canned or cooked	3 ounces	85...	77	90	14	2

* Outer layer of fat on the cut was removed to within approximately ½ inch of the lean. Deposits of fat within the cut were not removed.

EDIBLE PART OF FOODS—Continued

	FATTY ACIDS		CARBO-HY-DRATE	CAL-CIUM	IRON	VITA-MIN-A VALUE	THIA-MINE	RIBO-FLA-VIN	NIA-CIN	ASCOR-BIC ACID	ITEM NO.
SATU-RATED (total)	UNSATURATED										
	OLEIC	LINO-LEIC									
gm	gm	gm	gm	mg	mg	I.U.	mg	mg	mg	mg	
2	2	Trace	6	5	4.4	30,330	0.15	2.25	8.4	18	79
9	10	2	1	8	2.2	0	.39	.15	3.1	—	80
5	5	1	0	5	1.5	0	.57	.15	2.9	—	81
5	6	1	1	5	1.2	0	.18	.12	1.6	—	82
8	9	2	0	8	2.2	0	.63	.18	3.8	—	83
8	9	2	0	8	2.2	0	.63	.18	3.8	—	84
3	3	1	0	7	1.9	0	.54	.16	3.3	—	85
9	10	2	0	9	2.7	0	.78	.22	4.7	—	86
4	4	1	0	9	2.6	0	.73	.21	4.4	—	87
9	11	2	0	8	2.5	0	.46	.21	4.1	—	88
2	3	1	0	8	2.3	0	.42	.19	3.7	—	89
8	15	3	39	41	1.6	1,860	.07	.14	3.2	Trace	90
26	27	3	2	16	4.1	—	.36	.49	6.0	—	91
6	6	1	1	3	.8	—	.08	.10	1.3	—	92
10	12	3	0	10	2.6	0	.23	.27	3.4	—	93
7	6	Trace	Trace	7	2.5	—	.04	.26	3.1	—	94
4	4	Trace	0	9	2.7	—	.06	.21	4.6	—	95
7	6	Trace	0	10	2.9	—	.11	.26	6.6	—	96
—	—	—	0	25	.6	40	.09	.08	1.6	—	97
—	—	—	3	82	6.0	90	.08	.15	1.4	—	98
—	—	—	2	74	5.4	70	.04	.08	.9	—	99
—	—	—	1	38	.8	—	.04	.05	2.1	—	100

TABLE 1.—NUTRITIVE VALUES OF THE

ITEM NO.	FOOD, approximate measure, and weight (in grams)			WATER	FOOD EN- ERGY	PRO- TEIN	FAT (total lipid)
			gm	per cent	calo- ries	gm	gm
	Fish and shellfish (*Continued*)						
101	fishsticks, breaded, cooked, frozen; stick, 3.8 by 1.0 by 0.5 inch	10 sticks or 8-ounce package	227	66	400	38	20
102	haddock, fried	3 ounces	85	67	135	16	5
	mackerel						
103	broiled, Atlantic	3 ounces	85	62	200	19	13
104	canned, Pacific, solids and liquid	3 ounces	85	66	155	18	9
105	ocean perch, breaded (egg and breadcrumbs), fried	3 ounces	85	59	195	16	11
106	oysters, meat only: raw, 13–19 medium selects	1 cup	240	85	160	20	4
107	oyster stew, 1 part oysters to 3 parts milk by vol- ume, 3–4 oysters	1 cup	230	84	200	11	12
108	salmon, pink, canned	3 ounces	85	70	120	17	5
109	sardines, Atlantic type, canned in oil, drained solids	3 ounces	85	57	180	22	9
110	shad, baked	3 ounces	85	64	170	20	10
111	shrimp, canned, meat only	3 ounces	85	66	110	23	1
112	swordfish, broiled with but- ter or margarine	3 ounces	85	65	150	24	5
113	tuna, canned in oil, drained solids	3 ounces	85	60	170	25	7
	Mature dry beans and peas, nuts, peanuts; related products						
114	Almonds, shelled	1 cup	142	5	850	26	77
	Beans, dry common varieties, such as Great Northern, navy, and others, canned						
115	red	1 cup	256	76	230	15	1
	white, with tomato or molasses						
116	with pork	1 cup	261	69	330	16	7
117	without pork	1 cup	261	69	315	16	1
118	Lima, cooked	1 cup	192	64	260	16	1
119	Brazil nuts, broken pieces	1 cup	140	5	905	20	92
120	Cashew nuts, roasted	1 cup	135	5	770	25	65
	Coconut						
121	fresh, shredded	1 cup	97	50	330	3	31
122	dried, shredded, sweetened	1 cup	62	3	345	2	24

EDIBLE PART OF FOODS—Continued

SATU-RATED (total) gm	UNSATURATED OLEIC gm	LINO-LEIC gm	CARBO-HY-DRATE gm	CAL-CIUM mg	IRON mg	VITA-MIN-A VALUE I.U.	THIA-MINE mg	RIBO-FLA-VIN mg	NIA-CIN mg	ASCOR-BIC ACID mg	ITEM NO.
5	4	10	15	25	0.9	—	0.09	0.16	3.6	—	101
1	3	Trace	6	15	.5	50	.03	.08	2.2	—	102
—	—	—	0	5	1.0	450	.13	.23	6.5	—	103
—	—	—	0	221	1.9	20	.02	.28	7.4	—	104
—	—	—	6	14	1.3	50	.09	.10	1.7	—	105
—	—	—	8	226	13.2	740	.30	.39	6.6	—	106
—	—	—	11	269	3.3	640	.12	.40	1.7	—	107
1	1	—	0	159*	.7	60	.03	.16	6.8	—	108
2	2	4	1	367	2.5	190	.02	.18	4.6	—	109
—	—	—	0	20	.5	20	.11	.22	7.3	—	110
—	—	—	—	98	2.6	50	.01	.03	1.9	—	111
—	—	—	0	23	1.1	1,750	.03	.04	9.3	—	112
2	1	4	0	7	1.2	70	.04	.10	10.9	—	113
6	52	15	28	332	6.7	0	.34	1.31	5.0	Trace	114
—	—	—	42	74	4.6	0	.13	.13	1.5	Trace	115
3	3	1	54	172	4.4	140	.13	.10	1.3	5	116
—	—	—	60	183	5.2	140	.13	.10	1.3	5	117
—	—	—	48	56	5.6	Trace	.26	.12	1.3	Trace	118
18	44	24	15	260	4.8	Trace	1.21	—	—	—	119
11	46	5	35	51	5.1	—	.49	.46	1.9	—	120
27	2	—	13	15	1.7	0	.06	.03	.5	4	121
21	2	—	33	13	1.6	0	.04	.02	.4	0	122

* If bones are discarded, calcium content is much lower. Bones equal about 2 per cent by weight of total contents of can.

TABLE 1.—NUTRITIVE VALUES OF THE

ITEM NO.	FOOD, approximate measure, and weight (in grams)		gm	WATER per cent	FOOD EN-ERGY calo-ries	PRO-TEIN gm	FAT (total lipid) gm
123	Cowpeas or blackeye peas, dry, cooked	1 cup	248..	80	190	13	1
	Peanuts, roasted, shelled						
124	halves	1 cup	144..	2	840	39	71
125	chopped	1 tablespoon .	9....	2	50	2	4
126	Peanut butter	1 tablespoon .	16...	2	90	4	8
127	Peas, split, dry, cooked	1 cup	250..	70	290	20	1
	Pecans						
128	halves	1 cup	108..	3	740	10	77
129	chopped	1 tablespoon .	7.5 ..	3	50	1	5
	Walnuts, shelled						
130	black or native, chopped .	1 cup	126..	3	790	26	75
	English or Persian						
131	halves	1 cup	100..	4	650	15	64
132	chopped	1 tablespoon .	8....	4	50	1	5
	Vegetables and vegetable products						
	Asparagus						
133	cooked, cut spears	1 cup	175..	92	35	4	Trace
	canned spears, medium						
134	green	6 spears	96...	92	20	2	Trace
135	bleached	6 spears	96...	92	20	2	Trace
	Beans						
136	Lima, immature, cooked .	1 cup	160..	75	150	8	1
	snap, green						
	cooked						
137	in small amount of water, short time	1 cup	125..	92	25	2	Trace
138	in large amount of water, long time	1 cup	125..	92	25	2	Trace
	canned						
139	solids and liquid	1 cup	239..	94	45	2	Trace
140	strained or chopped .	1 ounce	28...	93	5	Trace	Trace
	Bean sprouts. *See* Sprouts.						
141	Beets, cooked, diced	1 cup	165..	88	70	2	Trace
142	Broccoli spears, cooked	1 cup	150..	90	45	5	Trace
143	Brussels sprouts, cooked ...	1 cup	130..	85	60	6	1
	Cabbage						
	raw						
144	finely shredded	1 cup	100..	92	25	1	Trace
145	coleslaw	1 cup	120..	84	100	2	7
	cooked						
146	in small amount of water, short time	1 cup	170..	92	40	2	Trace
147	in large amount of water, long time	1 cup	170..	92	40	2	Trace

EDIBLE PART OF FOODS—Continued

FATTY ACIDS			CARBO-HY-DRATE	CAL-CIUM	IRON	VITA-MIN-A VALUE	THIA-MINE	RIBO-FLA-VIN	NIA-CIN	ASCOR-BIC ACID	ITEM NO.
SATU-RATED (total)	UNSATURATED										
	OLEIC	LINO-LEIC									
gm	gm	gm	gm	mg	mg	I.U.	mg	mg	mg	mg	
—	—	—	34	42	3.2	20	0.41	0.11	1.1	Trace	*123*
16	31	21	28	104	3.2	0	.47	.19	24.6	0	*124*
1	2	1	2	6	.2	0	.03	.01	1.5	0	*125*
2	4	2	3	12	.4	0	.02	.02	2.8	0	*126*
—	—	—	52	28	4.2	120	.36	.22	2.2	Trace	*127*
5	49	15	16	79	2.6	140	.93	.14	1.0	2	*128*
Trace	3	1	1	5	.2	10	.06	.01	.1	Trace	*129*
4	26	36	19	Trace	7.6	380	.28	.14	.9	—	*130*
4	10	40	16	99	3.1	30	.33	.13	.9	3	*131*
Trace	1	3	1	8	.2	Trace	.03	.01	.1	Trace	*132*
—	—	—	6	33	1.8	1,820	.23	.30	2.1	40	*133*
—	—	—	3	18	1.8	770	.06	.08	.9	17	*134*
—	—	—	4	15	1.0	70	.05	.07	.8	17	*135*
—	—	—	29	46	2.7	460	.22	.14	1.8	24	*136*
—	—	—	6	45	.9	830	.09	.12	.6	18	*137*
—	—	—	6	45	.9	830	.06	.11	.5	12	*138*
—	—	—	10	65	3.3	990	.08	.10	.7	9	*139*
—	—	—	1	10	.3	120	.01	.02	.1	1	*140*
—	—	—	16	35	1.2	30	.03	.07	.5	11	*141*
—	—	—	8	195	2.0	5,100	.10	.22	1.2	111	*142*
—	—	—	12	44	1.7	520	.05	.16	.6	61	*143*
—	—	—	5	46	.5	80	.06	.05	.3	50	*144*
1	1	4	9	47	.5	80	.06	.05	.3	50	*145*
—	—	—	9	78	.8	150	.08	.08	.5	53	*146*
—	—	—	9	78	.8	150	.05	.05	.3	32	*147*

TABLE 1.—NUTRITIVE VALUES OF THE

ITEM NO.	FOOD, approximate measure, and weight (in grams)		gm	WATER per cent	FOOD EN-ERGY calo-ries	PRO-TEIN gm	FAT (total lipid) gm
	Cabbage, celery or Chinese						
148	raw, leaves and stem, 1-inch pieces	1 cup	100..	95	15	1	Trace
149	cooked	1 cup	190..	95	25	2	1
	Carrots raw						
150	whole, 5½ by 1 inch (25 thin strips)	1 carrot	50...	88	20	1	Trace
151	grated	1 cup	110..	88	45	1	Trace
152	cooked, diced	1 cup	145..	92	45	1	1
153	canned, strained or chopped	1 ounce	28...	92	5	Trace	0
154	Cauliflower, cooked, flower-buds	1 cup	120..	92	30	3	Trace
	Celery, raw						
155	stalk, large outer, 8 by about 1½ inches at root end	1 stalk	40...	94	5	1	Trace
156	pieces, diced	1 cup	100..	94	20	1	Trace
157	Collards, cooked	1 cup	190..	87	75	7	1
	Corn, sweet						
158	cooked, ear 5 by 1¾ inches	1 ear	140..	76	65	2	1
159	canned, solids and liquid .	1 cup	256..	80	170	5	1
160	Cowpeas, cooked, immature seeds	1 cup	160..	75	150	11	1
	Cucumbers, 10-ounce; 7½ by about 2 inches						
161	raw, pared	1 cucumber .	207..	96	25	1	Trace
162	raw, pared, center slice ⅛-inch thick	6 slices	50...	96	5	Trace	Trace
163	Dandelion greens, cooked ..	1 cup	180..	86	80	5	1
164	Endive, curly (including esca-role)	2 ounces	57...	93	10	1	Trace
165	Kale, cooked	1 cup	110..	87	45	4	1
	Lettuce, headed, raw						
166	head, looseleaf, 4-inch-di-ameter	1 head	220..	95	30	3	Trace
167	head, compact, 4¾-inch-diameter, 1 pound	1 head	454..	95	70	5	1
168	leaves	2 large or 4 small	50...	95	5	1	Trace
169	Mushrooms, canned, solids and liquid	1 cup	244..	93	30	3	Trace
170	Mustard greens, cooked	1 cup	140..	92	30	3	Trace
171	Okra, cooked, pod 3 by ⅝ inch	8 pods	85...	90	30	2	Trace

EDIBLE PART OF FOODS—Continued

SATU-RATED (total)	UNSATURATED		CARBO-HY-DRATE	CAL-CIUM	IRON	VITA-MIN-A VALUE	THIA-MINE	RIBO-FLA-VIN	NIA-CIN	ASCOR-BIC ACID	ITEM NO.
	OLEIC	LINO-LEIC									
gm	gm	gm	gm	mg	mg	I.U.	mg	mg	mg	mg	
—	—	—	2	43	0.9	260	0.03	0.04	0.4	31	*148*
—	—	—	5	82	1.7	490	.04	.06	.6	42	*149*
—	—	—	5	20	.4	6,000	.03	.03	.3	3	*150*
—	—	—	10	43	.9	13,200	.06	.06	.7	7	*151*
—	—	—	9	38	.9	18,130	.07	.07	.7	6	*152*
—	—	—	2	7	.2	3,400	.01	.01	.1	1	*153*
—	—	—	6	26	1.3	110	.07	.10	.6	34	*154*
—	—	—	1	20	.2	0	.02	.02	.2	3	*155*
—	—	—	4	50	.5	0	.05	.04	.4	7	*156*
—	—	—	14	473	3.0	14,500	.15	.46	3.2	84	*157*
—	—	—	16	4	.5	300*	.09	.08	1.1	6	*158*
—	—	—	41	10	1.3	520*	.07	.13	2.4	14	*159*
—	—	—	25	59	4.0	620	.46	.13	1.3	32	*160*
—	—	—	6	21	.6	0	.07	.09	.4	18	*161*
—	—	—	1	5	.2	0	.02	.02	.1	4	*162*
—	—	—	16	337	5.6	27,310	.23	.22	1.3	29	*163*
—	—	—	2	45	1.0	1,700	.04	.07	.2	6	*164*
—	—	—	8	248	2.4	9,220	.08	.25	1.9	56	*165*
—	—	—	6	48	1.1	1,200	.10	.18	.4	17	*166*
—	—	—	13	100	2.3	2,470	.20	.38	.9	35	*167*
—	—	—	1	11	.2	270	.02	.04	.1	4	*168*
—	—	—	9	17	2.0	0	.04	.60	4.8	—	*169*
—	—	—	6	308	4.1	10,050	.08	.25	1.0	63	*170*
—	—	—	6	70	.6	630	.05	.05	.7	17	*171*

* Vitamin A value is based on yellow corn; white corn contains only a trace.

TABLE 1.—NUTRITIVE VALUES OF THE

ITEM NO.	FOOD, approximate measure, and weight (in grams)		gm	WATER per cent	FOOD EN-ERGY calo-ries	PRO-TEIN gm	FAT (total lipid) gm
	Onions						
	mature						
172	raw, onion 2½-inch-di-ameter	1 onion	110	88	50	2	Trace
173	cooked	1 cup	210	90	80	2	Trace
174	young green, small, without tops	6 onions	50	88	25	Trace	Trace
175	Parsley, raw, chopped	1 tablespoon	3.5	84	1	Trace	Trace
176	Parsnips, cooked	1 cup	155	84	95	2	1
	Peas, green						
177	cooked	1 cup	160	82	110	8	1
178	canned, solids and liquid	1 cup	249	82	170	8	1
179	canned, strained	1 ounce	28	86	10	1	Trace
180	Peppers, hot, red, without seeds, dried; ground chili powder	1 tablespoon	15	13	50	2	1
	Peppers, sweet						
	raw, medium, about 6 per pound						
181	green pod without stem and seeds	1 pod	62	93	15	1	Trace
182	red pod without stem and seeds	1 pod	60	91	20	1	Trace
183	canned, pimientos, medium	1 pod	38	92	10	Trace	Trace
	Potatoes, medium, about 3 per pound						
184	baked, peeled after baking	1 potato	99	75	90	3	Trace
	boiled						
185	peeled after boiling	1 potato	136	80	105	3	Trace
186	peeled before boiling	1 potato	122	80	90	3	Trace
	French-fried, piece 2 by ½ by ½ inch						
187	cooked in deep fat, ready to eat	10 pieces	57	45	155	2	7
188	frozen, ready to heat for serving	10 pieces	57	64	95	2	4
	mashed						
189	milk added	1 cup	195	80	145	4	1
190	milk and butter added	1 cup	195	76	230	4	12
191	Potato chips, medium, 2-inch-diameter	10 chips	20	3	110	1	7
192	Pumpkin, canned	1 cup	228	90	75	2	1
193	Radishes, raw, small, without tops	4 radishes	40	94	10	Trace	Trace
194	Sauerkraut, canned, drained solids	1 cup	150	91	30	2	Trace
	Spinach						
195	cooked	1 cup	180	91	45	6	1
196	canned, drained solids	1 cup	180	91	45	6	1

EDIBLE PART OF FOODS—Continued

SATU-RATED (total) gm	UNSATURATED OLEIC gm	UNSATURATED LINO-LEIC gm	CARBO-HY-DRATE gm	CAL-CIUM mg	IRON mg	VITA-MIN-A VALUE I.U.	THIA-MINE mg	RIBO-FLA-VIN mg	NIA-CIN mg	ASCOR-BIC ACID mg	ITEM NO.
—	—	—	11	35	0.6	60	0.04	0.04	0.2	10	*172*
—	—	—	18	67	1.0	110	.04	.06	.4	13	*173*
—	—	—	5	68	.4	30	.02	.02	.1	12	*174*
—	—	—	Trace	7	.2	290	Trace	.01	.1	7	*175*
—	—	—	22	88	1.1	0	.09	.16	.3	19	*176*
—	—	—	19	35	3.0	1,150	.40	.22	3.7	24	*177*
—	—	—	32	62	4.5	1,350	.28	.15	2.6	21	*178*
—	—	—	2	5	.3	160	.03	.02	.3	2	*179*
—	—	—	9	20	1.2	11,520	.03	.20	1.6	2	*180*
—	—	—	3	6	.4	260	.05	.05	.3	79	*181*
—	—	—	4	8	.4	2,670	.05	.05	.3	122	*182*
—	—	—	2	3	.6	870	.01	.02	.1	36	*183*
—	—	—	21	9	.7	Trace	.10	.04	1.7	20	*184*
—	—	—	23	10	.8	Trace	.13	.05	2.0	22	*185*
—	—	—	21	9	.7	Trace	.11	.04	1.4	20	*186*
2	1	4	20	9	.7	Trace	.06	.04	1.8	8	*187*
1	1	2	15	4	.8	Trace	.08	.01	1.2	10	*188*
—	—	—	30	47	1.0	50	.17	.11	.2	17	*189*
7	4	Trace	28	45	1.0	470	.16	.10	1.6	16	*190*
2	2	4	10	6	.4	Trace	.04	.02	.6	2	*191*
—	—	—	18	46	1.6	7,750	.04	.14	1.2	—	*192*
—	—	—	2	15	.4	10	.01	.01	.1	10	*193*
—	—	—	7	54	.8	60	.05	.10	.2	24	*194*
—	—	—	6	223*	3.6	21,200	.14	.36	1.1	54	*195*
—	—	—	6	223*	3.6	13,740	.04	.21	.7	26	*196*

* Calcium may not be usable because of presence of oxalic acid.

TABLE 1.—NUTRITIVE VALUES OF THE

ITEM NO.	FOOD, approximate measure, and weight (in grams)		gm	WATER per cent	FOOD EN-ERGY calo-ries	PRO-TEIN gm	FAT (total lipid) gm
	Spinach (*Continued*)						
197	canned, strained and creamed	1 ounce	28...	90	10	1	Trace
	Sprouts, raw						
198	mung bean	1 cup	90...	92	20	3	Trace
199	soybean	1 cup	107..	86	50	7	1
	Squash						
	cooked						
200	summer, diced	1 cup	210..	95	35	1	Trace
201	winter, baked, mashed .	1 cup	205..	86	95	4	1
202	canned, winter, strained or chopped	1 ounce	28...	92	10	Trace	Trace
	Sweetpotatoes						
	cooked, medium, 5 by 2 inches, weight raw about 6 ounces						
203	baked, peeled after bak-ing	1 sweetpotato	110..	64	155	2	1
204	boiled, peeled after boil-ing	1 sweetpotato	147..	71	170	2	1
205	candied, 3½ by 2¼ inches	1 sweetpotato	175..	60	295	2	6
206	canned, vacuum or solid pack	1 cup	218..	72	235	4	Trace
	Tomatoes						
207	raw, medium, 2 by 2½ inches, about 3 per pound	1 tomato ...	150..	94	30	2	Trace
208	canned or cooked	1 cup	242..	94	45	2	Trace
209	Tomato juice, canned	1 cup	242..	94	50	2	Trace
210	Tomato catsup	1 tablespoon .	17...	70	15	Trace	Trace
211	Turnips, cooked, diced	1 cup	155..	92	40	1	Trace
	Turnip greens						
	cooked						
212	in small amount of wa-ter, short time	1 cup	145..	90	45	4	1
213	in large amount of wa-ter, long time	1 cup	145..	90	45	4	1
214	canned, solids and liquid .	1 cup	232..	94	40	3	1
	Fruits and fruit products						
215	Apples, raw, medium, 2½-inch-diameter, about 3 per pound	1 apple	150..	85	70	Trace	Trace
216	Apple brown Betty	1 cup	230..	64	350	4	8
217	Applejuice, fresh or canned .	1 cup	249..	86	125	Trace	0
	Applesauce, canned						
218	sweetened	1 cup	254..	80	185	Trace	Trace
219	unsweetened	1 cup	239..	88	100	Trace	Trace

EDIBLE PART OF FOODS—Continued

SATU-RATED (total) gm	UNSATURATED OLEIC gm	LINO-LEIC gm	CARBO-HY-DRATE gm	CAL-CIUM mg	IRON mg	VITA-MIN-A VALUE I.U.	THIA-MINE mg	RIBO-FLA-VIN mg	NIA-CIN mg	ASCOR-BIC ACID mg	ITEM NO.
—	—	—	2	19*	0.3	750	0.01	0.03	0.1	1	*197*
—	—	—	4	26	.7	10	.06	.08	.5	14	*198*
—	—	—	6	51	1.1	190	.24	.21	.9	14	*199*
—	—	—	8	32	.8	550	.08	.15	1.3	23	*200*
—	—	—	23	49	1.6	12,690	.10	.31	1.2	14	*201*
—	—	—	2	7	.1	510	.01	.01	.1	1	*202*
—	—	—	36	44	1.0	8,970	.10	.07	.7	24	*203*
—	—	—	39	47	1.0	11,610	.13	.09	.9	25	*204*
2	3	1	60	65	1.6	11,030	.10	.08	.8	17	*205*
—	—	—	54	54	1.7	17,110	.12	.09	1.1	30	*206*
—	—	—	6	16	.9	1,640	.08	.06	.8	35	*207*
—	—	—	9	27	1.5	2,540	.14	.08	1.7	40	*208*
—	—	—	10	17	1.0	2,540	.12	.07	1.8	38	*209*
—	—	—	4	2	.1	320	.02	.01	.4	2	*210*
—	—	—	9	62	.8	Trace	.06	.09	.6	28	*211*
—	—	—	8	376	3.5	15,370	.09	.59	1.0	87	*212*
—	—	—	8	376	3.5	15,370	.07	.52	.9	65	*213*
—	—	—	7	232	3.7	10,210	.03	.21	1.3	45	*214*
—	—	—	18	8	.4	50	.04	.02	.1	3	*215*
4	3	Trace	69	41	1.4	270	.13	.10	.9	Trace	*216*
—	—	—	34	15	1.2	90	.05	.07	Trace	2	*217*
—	—	—	50	10	1.0	80	.05	.03	.1	3	*218*
—	—	—	26	10	1.0	70	.05	.02	.1	3	*219*

* Calcium may not be usable because of presence of oxalic acid.

TABLE 1.—NUTRITIVE VALUES OF THE

ITEM NO.	FOOD, approximate measure, and weight (in grams)			WATER	FOOD EN- ERGY	PRO- TEIN	FAT (total lipid)
			gm	per cent	calo- ries	gm	gm
	Apricots						
220	raw, about 12 per pound .	3 apricots ...	114..	85	55	1	Trace
	canned in heavy sirup						
221	halves and sirup	1 cup	259..	77	220	2	Trace
222	halves, medium, and sirup	4 halves; 2 tablespoons sirup	122..	77	105	1	Trace
	dried						
223	uncooked, 40 halves, small	1 cup	150..	25	390	8	1
224	cooked, unsweetened, fruit and liquid	1 cup	285..	76	240	5	1
225	Apricots and applesauce, canned (strained or chopped)	1 ounce	28...	80	20	Trace	Trace
226	Apricot nectar	1 cup	250..	85	140	1	Trace
	Avocados, raw						
	California varieties, mainly Fuerte						
227	10-ounce avocado, about 3⅛ by 4¼ inches, peeled, pitted	½ avocado ..	108..	74	185	2	18
228	½-inch cubes	1 cup	152..	74	260	3	26
	Florida varieties						
229	13-ounce avocado, about 4 by 3 inches, peeled, pitted	½ avocado ..	123..	78	160	2	14
230	½-inch cubes	1 cup	152..	78	195	2	17
231	Bananas, raw, 6 by 1½ inches, about 3 per pound	1 banana ...	150..	76	85	1	Trace
232	Blackberries, raw	1 cup	144..	85	85	2	1
233	Blueberries, raw	1 cup	140..	83	85	1	1
234	Cantaloupes, raw, medium, 5-inch-diameter, about 1⅔ pounds	½ melon	385..	94	40	1	Trace
	Cherries						
235	raw, sour, sweet, hybrid ..	1 cup	114..	83	65	1	1
236	canned, red, sour, pitted ..	1 cup	247..	88	105	2	1
237	Cranberry juice cocktail, canned	1 cup	250..	85	140	Trace	Trace
238	Cranberry sauce, sweetened, canned or cooked	1 cup	277..	48	550	Trace	1
239	Dates, "fresh" and dried, pitted, cut	1 cup	178..	20	505	4	1
	Figs						
240	raw, small, 1½-inch-diam- eter, about 12 per pound	3 figs	114..	78	90	2	Trace
241	dried, large, 2 by 1 inch ..	1 fig	21...	23	60	1	Trace

EDIBLE PART OF FOODS—Continued

SATU-RATED (total)	UNSATURATED		CARBO-HY-DRATE	CAL-CIUM	IRON	VITA-MIN-A VALUE	THIA-MINE	RIBO-FLA-VIN	NIA-CIN	ASCOR-BIC ACID	ITEM NO.
	OLEIC	LINO-LEIC									
gm	gm	gm	gm	mg	mg	I.U.	mg	mg	mg	mg	
—	—	—	14	18	0.5	2,890	0.03	0.04	0.7	10	*220*
—	—	—	57	28	.8	4,520	.05	.06	.9	10	*221*
—	—	—	27	13	.4	2,130	.02	.03	.4	5	*222*
—	—	—	100	100	8.2	16,390	.02	.24	4.9	19	*223*
—	—	—	62	63	5.1	10,130	.01	.13	2.8	8	*224*
—	—	—	5	3	.2	440	.01	.01	.1	Trace	*225*
—	—	—	36	22	.5	2,380	.02	.02	.5	7	*226*
4	8	2	6	11	.6	310	.12	.21	1.7	15	*227*
5	12	3	9	15	.9	430	.16	.30	2.4	2	*228*
3	6	2	11	12	.7	350	.13	.24	2.0	17	*229*
3	8	2	13	15	.9	430	.16	.30	2.4	21	*230*
—	—	—	23	8	.7	190	.05	.06	.7	10	*231*
—	—	—	19	46	1.3	290	.05	.06	.5	30	*232*
—	—	—	21	21	1.4	140	.04	.08	.6	20	*233*
—	—	—	9	33	.8	6,590*	.09	.07	1.0	63	*234*
—	—	—	15	19	.4	650	.05	.06	.4	9	*235*
—	—	—	26	37	.7	1,680	.07	.06	.4	13	*236*
—	—	—	36	10	.5	20	.02	.02	.1	5	*237*
—	—	—	142	22	.8	80	.06	.06	.3	5	*238*
—	—	—	134	105	5.7	100	.16	.17	3.9	0	*239*
—	—	—	22	62	.7	90	.06	.06	.6	2	*240*
—	—	—	15	40	.7	20	.02	.02	.1	0	*241*

* Vitamin A value is based on deeply colored yellow varieties.

TABLE 1.—NUTRITIVE VALUES OF THE

ITEM NO.	FOOD, approximate measure, and weight (in grams)		gm	WATER per cent	FOOD EN-ERGY calo-ries	PRO-TEIN gm	FAT (total lipid) gm
242	Fruit cocktail, canned in heavy sirup, solids and liquid	1 cup	256..	80	195	1	1
	Grapefruit raw, medium, 4¼-inch-diameter, size 64						
243	white	½ grapefruit .	285..	89	50	1	Trace
244	pink or red	½ grapefruit .	285..	89	55	1	Trace
245	raw sections, white	1 cup	194..	89	75	1	Trace
	canned						
246	sirup pack, solids and liquid	1 cup	249..	81	170	1	Trace
247	water pack, solids and liquid	1 cup	240..	91	70	1	Trace
	Grapefruit juice						
248	fresh	1 cup	246..	90	95	1	Trace
	canned						
249	unsweetened	1 cup	247..	89	100	1	Trace
250	sweetened	1 cup	250..	86	130	1	Trace
	frozen, concentrate, unsweetened						
251	undiluted, can, 6 fluid ounces	1 can	207..	62	300	4	1
252	water added	1 cup	247..	89	100	1	Trace
	frozen, concentrate, sweetened						
253	undiluted, can, 6 fluid ounces	1 can	211..	57	350	3	1
254	water added	1 cup	249..	88	115	1	Trace
	dehydrated						
255	crystals, can, net weight 4 ounces	1 can	114..	1	430	5	1
256	water added	1 cup	247..	90	100	1	Trace
	Grapes, raw						
257	American type (slip skin), such as Concord, Delaware, Niagara, and Scuppernong	1 cup	153..	82	70	1	1
258	European type (adherent skin), such as Malaga, Muscat, Sultanina (Thompson Seedless), and Flame Tokay	1 cup	160..	81	100	1	Trace
259	Grape juice, bottled	1 cup	254..	83	165	1	Trace
260	Lemons, raw, medium, 2⅕-inch-diameter, size 150	1 lemon	106..	90	20	1	Trace
	Lemon juice						
261	fresh	1 cup	246..	91	60	1	Trace
262		1 tablespoon .	15...	91	5	Trace	Trace
263	canned, unsweetened	1 cup	245..	92	60	1	Trace

EDIBLE PART OF FOODS—Continued

SATU-RATED (total)	UNSATURATED		CARBO-HY-DRATE	CAL-CIUM	IRON	VITA-MIN-A VALUE	THIA-MINE	RIBO-FLA-VIN	NIA-CIN	ASCOR-BIC ACID	ITEM NO.
	FATTY ACIDS										
	OLEIC	LINO-LEIC									
gm	gm	gm	gm	mg	mg	I.U.	mg	mg	mg	mg	
—	—	—	50	23	1.0	360	0.04	0.03	1.1	5	242
—	—	—	14	21	.5	10	.05	.02	.2	50	243
—	—	—	14	21	.5	590	.05	.02	.2	48	244
—	—	—	20	31	.8	20	.07	.03	.3	72	245
—	—	—	44	32	.7	20	.07	.04	.5	75	246
—	—	—	18	31	.7	20	.07	.04	.5	72	247
—	—	—	23	22	.5	20	.09	.04	.4	92	248
—	—	—	24	20	1.0	20	.07	.04	.4	84	249
—	—	—	32	20	1.0	20	.07	.04	.4	78	250
—	—	—	72	70	.8	60	.29	.12	1.4	286	251
—	—	—	24	25	.2	20	.10	.04	.5	96	252
—	—	—	85	59	.6	50	.24	.11	1.2	245	253
—	—	—	28	20	.2	20	.08	.03	.4	82	254
—	—	—	103	99	1.1	90	.41	.18	2.0	399	255
—	—	—	24	22	.2	20	.10	.05	.5	92	256
—	—	—	16	13	.4	100	.05	.03	.3	4	257
—	—	—	26	18	.6	150	.08	.04	.4	7	258
—	—	—	42	28	.8	—	.10	.05	.6	Trace	259
—	—	—	6	18	.4	10	.03	.01	.1	38	260
—	—	—	20	17	.5	40	.08	.03	.2	113	261
—	—	—	1	1	Trace	Trace	Trace	Trace	Trace	7	262
—	—	—	19	17	.5	40	.07	.03	.2	102	263

TABLE 1.—NUTRITIVE VALUES OF THE

ITEM NO.	FOOD, approximate measure, and weight (in grams)		gm	WATER per cent	FOOD ENERGY calories	PROTEIN gm	FAT (total lipid) gm
	Lemonade concentrate, frozen, sweetened						
264	undiluted, can, 6 fluid ounces	1 can	220..	48	430	Trace	Trace
265	water added	1 cup	248..	88	110	Trace	Trace
	Lime juice						
266	fresh	1 cup	246..	90	65	1	Trace
267	canned	1 cup	246..	90	65	1	Trace
	Limeade concentrate, frozen, sweetened						
268	undiluted, can, 6 fluid ounces	1 can	218..	50	405	Trace	Trace
269	water added	1 cup	248..	89	105	Trace	Trace
	Oranges, raw						
270	Navel, California (winter), size 88, 2⅖-inch-diameter	1 orange	180..	85	60	2	Trace
271	other varieties, 3-inch-diameter	1 orange	210..	86	70	1	Trace
	Orange juice fresh						
272	California, Valencia, summer	1 cup	249..	88	120	2	1
	Florida varieties						
273	early and midseason .	1 cup	247..	90	100	1	Trace
274	late season, Valencia .	1 cup	248..	88	110	1	Trace
275	canned, unsweetened	1 cup	249..	87	120	2	Trace
	frozen concentrate						
276	undiluted, can, 6 fluid ounces	1 can	210..	58	330	5	Trace
277	water added	1 cup	248..	88	110	2	Trace
	dehydrated						
278	crystals, can, net weight 4 ounces	1 can	113..	1	430	6	2
279	water added	1 cup	248..	88	115	1	Trace
	Orange and grapefruit juice frozen concentrate						
280	undiluted, can, 6 fluid ounces	1 can	209..	59	330	4	1
281	water added	1 cup	248..	88	110	1	Trace
282	Papayas, raw, ½-inch cubes .	1 cup	182..	89	70	1	Trace
	Peaches raw						
283	whole, medium, 2-inch-diameter, about 4 per pound	1 peach	114..	89	35	1	Trace
284	sliced	1 cup	168..	89	65	1	Trace

EDIBLE PART OF FOODS—Continued

SATU-RATED (total) gm	OLEIC gm	LINO-LEIC gm	CARBO-HY-DRATE gm	CAL-CIUM mg	IRON mg	VITA-MIN-A VALUE I.U.	THIA-MINE mg	RIBO-FLA-VIN mg	NIA-CIN mg	ASCOR-BIC ACID mg	ITEM NO.
—	—	—	112	9	0.4	40	0.05	0.06	0.7	66	*264*
—	—	—	28	2	.1	10	.01	.01	.2	17	*265*
—	—	—	22	22	.5	30	.05	.03	.3	80	*266*
—	—	—	22	22	.5	30	.05	.03	.3	52	*267*
—	—	—	108	11	.7	Trace	.02	.02	.2	262	*268*
—	—	—	27	2	.2	Trace	.01	Trace	Trace	6	*269*
—	—	—	16	49	.5	240	.12	.05	.5	75	*270*
—	—	—	18	63	.3	290	.12	.03	.4	66	*271*
—	—	—	26	27	.7	500	.22	.06	.9	122	*272*
—	—	—	23	25	.5	490	.22	.06	.9	127	*273*
—	—	—	26	25	.5	500	.22	.06	.9	92	*274*
—	—	—	28	25	1.0	500	.17	.05	.6	100	*275*
—	—	—	80	69	.8	1,490	.63	.10	2.4	332	*276*
—	—	—	27	22	.2	500	.21	.03	.8	112	*277*
—	—	—	100	95	1.9	1,900	.76	.24	3.3	406	*278*
—	—	—	27	25	.5	500	.20	.06	.9	108	*279*
—	—	—	78	61	.8	790	.47	.06	2.3	301	*280*
—	—	—	26	20	.2	270	.16	.02	.8	102	*281*
—	—	—	18	36	.5	3,190	.07	.08	.5	102	*282*
—	—	—	10	9	.5	1,320*	.02	.05	1.0	7	*283*
—	—	—	16	15	.8	2,230*	.03	.08	1.6	12	*284*

* Vitamin A value of yellow-fleshed varieties; the value is negligible in white-fleshed varieties.

TABLE 1.—NUTRITIVE VALUES OF THE

ITEM NO.	FOOD, approximate measure, and weight (in grams)			WATER	FOOD EN-ERGY	PRO-TEIN	FAT (total lipid)
			gm	per cent	calo-ries	gm	gm
	Peaches (*Continued*)						
	canned, yellow-fleshed, solids and liquid						
	sirup pack, heavy						
285	halves or slices	1 cup	257..	79	200	1	Trace
286	halves, medium, and sirup	2 halves and 2 table-spoons sirup	117..	79	90	Trace	Trace
287	water pack	1 cup	245..	91	75	1	Trace
288	strained	1 ounce	28...	82	20	Trace	Trace
	dried						
289	uncooked	1 cup	160..	25	420	5	1
290	cooked, unsweetened, 10–12 halves and 6 table-spoons liquid	1 cup	270..	77	220	3	1
	frozen						
291	carton, 12 ounces	1 carton	340..	79	265	1	Trace
292	can, 16 ounces	1 can	454..	79	355	2	Trace
293	Peach nectar, canned	1 cup	250..	87	115	Trace	Trace
	Pears						
294	raw, 3 by 2½-inch-diame-ter	1 pear	182..	83	100	1	1
	canned, solids and liquid						
	sirup pack, heavy						
295	halves or slices	1 cup	255..	80	195	1	1
296	halves, medium, and sirup	2 halves and 2 table-spoons sirup	117..	80	90	Trace	Trace
297	water pack	1 cup	243..	91	80	Trace	Trace
298	strained	1 ounce	28...	84	15	Trace	Trace
299	Pear nectar, canned	1 cup	250..	86	130	1	Trace
300	Persimmons, Japanese or Kaki, raw, seedless, 2½-inch-diameter	1 persimmon .	125..	79	75	1	Trace
	Pineapple						
301	raw, diced	1 cup	140..	85	75	1	Trace
	canned, sirup pack, solids and liquid						
302	crushed	1 cup	260..	78	205	1	Trace
303	sliced, slices and juice..	2 small or 1 large and 2 tablespoons juice	122..	78	95	Trace	Trace
304	Pineapple juice, canned	1 cup	249..	86	120	1	Trace
	Plums, all except prunes						
305	raw, 2-inch-diameter, about 2 ounces	1 plum	60...	86	30	Trace	Trace

EDIBLE PART OF FOODS—Continued

SATU-RATED (total) gm	UNSATURATED OLEIC gm	LINO-LEIC gm	CARBO-HY-DRATE gm	CAL-CIUM mg	IRON mg	VITA-MIN-A VALUE I.U.	THIA-MINE mg	RIBO-FLA-VIN mg	NIA-CIN mg	ASCOR-BIC ACID mg	ITEM NO.
—	—	—	52	10	0.8	1,100	0.02	0.06	1.4	7	285
—	—	—	24	5	.4	500	.01	.03	.7	3	286
—	—	—	20	10	.7	1,100	.02	.06	1.4	7	287
—	—	—	5	2	.2	150	Trace	.01	.2	Trace	288
—	—	—	109	77	9.6	6,240	.02	.31	8.5	28	289
—	—	—	58	41	5.1	3,300	.01	.15	4.2	6	290
—	—	—	69	20	1.4	1,770	.04	.10	1.8	99*	291
—	—	—	92	27	1.8	2,360	.05	.14	2.4	132*	292
—	—	—	31	10	.5	1,070	.02	.05	1.0	1	293
—	—	—	25	13	.5	30	.04	.07	.2	7	294
—	—	—	50	13	.5	Trace	.03	.05	.3	4	295
—	—	—	23	6	.2	Trace	.01	.02	.2	2	296
—	—	—	20	12	.5	Trace	.02	.05	.3	4	297
—	—	—	4	3	.1	Trace	Trace	.01	.1	Trace	298
—	—	—	33	8	.2	10	.01	.05	Trace	1	299
—	—	—	20	6	.4	2,740	.03	.02	.1	11	300
—	—	—	19	22	.4	180	.12	.04	.3	33	301
—	—	—	55	75	1.6	210	.20	.04	.4	23	302
—	—	—	26	35	.7	100	.09	.02	.2	11	303
—	—	—	32	37	1.2	200	.13	.04	.4	22	304
—	—	—	7	10	.3	200	.04	.02	.3	3	305

* Content of frozen peaches with added ascorbic acid; when not added the content is 14 milligrams per 12-ounce carton and 18 milligrams per 16-ounce can.

TABLE 1.—NUTRITIVE VALUES OF THE

ITEM NO.	FOOD, approximate measure, and weight (in grams)		gm	WATER per cent	FOOD EN-ERGY calo-ries	PRO-TEIN gm	FAT (total lipid) gm
	Plums (*Continued*)						
	canned, sirup pack (Italian prunes)						
306	plums and juice	1 cup	256	79	185	1	Trace
307	plums (without pits) and juice	3 plums and 2 tablespoons juice	122	79	90	Trace	Trace
	Prunes, dried						
	medium, 50–60 per pound						
308	uncooked	4 prunes	32	24	70	1	Trace
309	cooked, unsweetened, 17–18 prunes and ⅓ cup liquid	1 cup	270	65	305	3	1
310	canned, strained	1 ounce	28	73	25	Trace	Trace
311	Prune juice, canned	1 cup	240	80	170	1	Trace
312	Raisins, dried	1 cup	160	18	460	4	Trace
	Raspberries, red						
313	raw	1 cup	123	84	70	1	1
314	frozen, 10-ounce carton	1 carton	284	74	280	2	1
315	Rhubarb, cooked, sugar added	1 cup	272	63	385	1	Trace
	Strawberries						
316	raw, capped	1 cup	149	90	55	1	1
317	frozen, 10-ounce carton	1 carton	284	72	300	2	1
318	frozen, 16-ounce can	1 can	454	72	485	3	2
319	Tangerines, raw, medium, 2½-inch-diameter, about 4 per pound	1 tangerine	114	87	40	1	Trace
	Tangerine juice						
320	canned, unsweetened	1 cup	248	89	105	1	Trace
	frozen concentrate						
321	undiluted, can, 6 fluid ounces	1 can	210	58	340	4	1
322	water added	1 cup	248	88	115	1	Trace
323	Watermelon, raw, wedge, 4 by 8 inches (¹⁄₁₆ of 10- by 16-inch melon, about 2 pounds with rind)	1 wedge	925	92	120	2	1
	Grain products						
324	Barley, pearled, light, un-cooked	1 cup	203	11	710	17	2
325	Biscuits, baking powder, with enriched flour, 2½-inch-di-ameter	1 biscuit	38	28	130	3	4
326	Bran flakes (40 per cent bran) with added thiamine	1 ounce	28	4	85	3	1

EDIBLE PART OF FOODS—Continued

SATU-RATED (total) gm	FATTY ACIDS UNSATURATED OLEIC gm	LINO-LEIC gm	CARBO-HY-DRATE gm	CAL-CIUM mg	IRON mg	VITA-MIN-A VALUE I.U.	THIA-MINE mg	RIBO-FLA-VIN mg	NIA-CIN mg	ASCOR-BIC ACID mg	ITEM NO.
—	—	—	50	20	2.7	560	0.07	0.06	0.9	3	*306*
—	—	—	25	10	1.3	280	.03	.03	.5	1	*307*
—	—	—	19	14	1.0	430	.02	.05	.4	1	*308*
—	—	—	81	60	4.5	1,850	.08	.19	1.8	3	*309*
—	—	—	7	8	.4	170	.01	.01	.2	1	*310*
—	—	—	45	34	9.8	—	.01	.03	1.1	4	*311*
—	—	—	124	99	5.6	30	.18	.13	.9	2	*312*
—	—	—	17	27	1.1	160	.03	.09	.9	31	*313*
—	—	—	70	79	1.7	220	.03	.12	.5	45	*314*
—	—	—	98	112*	1.1	70	.02	—	.2	17	*315*
—	—	—	13	31	1.5	90	.04	.10	.9	87	*316*
—	—	—	75	62	1.7	120	.05	.14	.5	116	*317*
—	—	—	121	100	2.7	190	.08	.23	.8	186	*318*
—	—	—	10	34	.3	360	.05	.01	.1	26	*319*
—	—	—	25	45	.5	1,050	.14	.04	.3	56	*320*
—	—	—	80	130	1.5	3,070	.43	.12	.9	202	*321*
—	—	—	27	45	.5	1,020	.14	.04	.3	67	*322*
—	—	—	29	30	.9	2,530	.20	.22	.7	26	*323*
Trace	1	1	160	32	4.1	0	.25	.17	6.3	0	*324*
1	2	Trace	18	61	.7	Trace	.09	.09	.7	Trace	*325*
—	—	—	22	17	1.1	0	.13	.07	2.5	0	*326*

* Calcium may not be usable because of presence of oxalic acid.

TABLE 1.—NUTRITIVE VALUES OF THE

ITEM NO.	FOOD, approximate measure, and weight (in grams)			WATER	FOOD EN-ERGY	PRO-TEIN	FAT (total lipid)
			gm	per cent	calo-ries	gm	gm
	Breads						
327	Boston brown bread, made with degermed cornmeal, slice, 3 by ¾ inch	1 slice	48...	45	100	3	1
	cracked-wheat bread						
328	loaf, 1-pound, 20 slices	1 loaf	454..	35	1,190	39	10
329	slice	1 slice	23...	35	60	2	1
	French or Vienna bread						
330	enriched, 1-pound loaf	1 loaf	454..	31	1,315	41	14
331	unenriched, 1-pound loaf	1 loaf	454..	31	1,315	41	14
	Italian bread						
332	enriched, 1-pound loaf	1 loaf	454..	32	1,250	41	4
333	unenriched, 1-pound loaf	1 loaf	454..	32	1,250	41	4
	raisin bread						
334	loaf, 1-pound, 20 slices	1 loaf	454..	35	1,190	30	13
335	slice	1 slice	23...	35	60	2	1
	rye bread						
	American, light (⅓ rye, ⅔ wheat)						
336	loaf, 1-pound, 20 slices	1 loaf	454..	36	1,100	41	5
337	slice	1 slice	23...	36	55	2	Trace
338	pumpernickel, dark, loaf, 1 pound	1 loaf	454..	34	1,115	41	5
	white bread, enriched *						
	1 to 2 per cent nonfat dry milk						
339	loaf, 1-pound, 20 slices	1 loaf	454..	36	1,225	39	15
340	slice	1 slice	23...	36	60	2	1
	3 to 4 per cent nonfat dry milk						
341	loaf, 1-pound	1 loaf	454..	36	1,225	39	15
342	slice, 20 per loaf ..	1 slice	23...	36	60	2	1
343	slice, toasted	1 slice	20...	24	60	2	1
344	slice, 26 per loaf ..	1 slice	17...	36	45	1	1
	5 to 6 per cent nonfat dry milk						
345	loaf, 1-pound, 20 slices	1 loaf	454..	35	1,245	41	17
346	slice	1 slice	23...	35	65	2	1
	white bread, unenriched *						
	1 to 2 per cent nonfat dry milk						
347	loaf, 1-pound, 20 slices	1 loaf	454..	36	1,225	39	15
348	slice	1 slice	23...	36	60	2	1
	3 to 4 per cent nonfat dry milk						
349	loaf, 1-pound	1 loaf	454..	36	1,225	39	15
350	slice, 20 per loaf ..	1 slice	23...	36	60	2	1
351	slice, toasted ...	1 slice	20...	24	60	2	1
352	slice, 26 per loaf ..	1 slice	17...	36	45	1	1
	5 to 6 per cent nonfat dry milk						
353	loaf, 1-pound, 20 slices	1 loaf	454..	35	1,245	41	17
354	slice	1 slice	23...	35	65	2	1

* When the amount of nonfat dry milk in commercial white bread is unknown, use values for bread with 3 to 4 per cent nonfat dry milk.

EDIBLE PART OF FOODS—Continued

SATU-RATED (total) gm	UNSATURATED OLEIC gm	LINO-LEIC gm	CARBO-HY-DRATE gm	CAL-CIUM mg	IRON mg	VITA-MIN-A VALUE I.U.	THIA-MINE mg	RIBO-FLA-VIN mg	NIA-CIN mg	ASCOR-BIC ACID mg	ITEM NO.
—	—	—	22	43	0.9	0	0.05	0.03	0.6	0	*327*
2	5	2	236	399	5.0	Trace	.53	.42	5.8	Trace	*328*
—	—	—	12	20	.3	Trace	.03	.02	.3	Trace	*329*
3	8	2	251	195	10.0	Trace	1.26	.98	11.3	Trace	*330*
3	8	2	251	195	3.2	Trace	.39	.39	3.6	Trace	*331*
1	1	2	256	77	10.0	0	1.31	.93	11.7	0	*332*
1	1	2	256	77	3.2	0	.39	.27	3.6	0	*333*
3	8	2	243	322	5.9	Trace	.24	.42	3.0	Trace	*334*
—	—	—	12	16	.3	Trace	.01	.02	.2	Trace	*335*
1	2	2	236	340	7.3	0	.81	.33	6.4	0	*336*
—	—	—	12	17	.4	0	.04	.02	.3	0	*337*
1	2	2	241	381	10.9	0	1.05	.63	5.4	0	*338*
3	9	2	229	318	10.9	Trace	1.13	.77	10.4	Trace	*339*
—	—	—	12	16	.6	Trace	.06	.04	.5	Trace	*340*
3	9	2	229	381	11.3	Trace	1.13	.95	10.8	Trace	*341*
—	—	—	12	19	.6	Trace	.06	.05	.6	Trace	*342*
—	—	—	12	19	.6	Trace	.05	.05	.6	Trace	*343*
—	—	—	9	14	.4	Trace	.04	.04	.4	Trace	*344*
4	10	2	228	435	11.3	Trace	1.22	.91	11.0	Trace	*345*
—	—	—	12	22	.6	Trace	.06	.05	.6	Trace	*346*
3	9	2	229	318	3.2	Trace	.40	.36	5.6	Trace	*347*
—	—	—	12	16	.2	Trace	.02	.02	.3	Trace	*348*
3	9	2	229	381	3.2	Trace	.31	.39	5.0	Trace	*349*
—	—	—	12	19	.2	Trace	.02	.02	.3	Trace	*350*
—	—	—	12	19	.2	Trace	.01	.02	.3	Trace	*351*
—	—	—	9	14	.1	Trace	.01	.01	.2	Trace	*352*
4	10	2	228	435	3.2	Trace	.32	.59	4.1	Trace	*353*
—	—	—	12	22	.2	Trace	.02	.03	.2	Trace	*354*

TABLE 1.—NUTRITIVE VALUES OF THE

ITEM NO.	FOOD, approximate measure, and weight (in grams)		gm	WATER per cent	FOOD EN-ERGY calo-ries	PRO-TEIN gm	FAT (total lipid) gm
	Breads (*Continued*)						
	whole-wheat, graham, entire-wheat bread						
355	loaf, 1-pound, 20 slices	1 loaf	454..	36	1,105	48	14
356	slice	1 slice	23...	36	55	2	1
357	toast	1 slice	19...	24	55	2	1
358	Breadcrumbs, dry, grated ...	1 cup	88...	6	345	11	4
	Cakes						
359	angel food cake; sector, 2-inch (1/12 of 8-inch-diameter cake)	1 sector	40...	32	110	3	Trace
360	chocolate cake, fudge icing; sector, 2-inch (1/16 of 10-inch-diameter layer cake)	1 sector	120..	24	420	5	14
361	fruitcake, dark; piece, 2 by 2 by ½ inch	1 piece	30...	23	105	2	4
362	gingerbread; piece, 2 by 2 by 2 inches	1 piece	55...	30	180	2	7
	plain cake and cupcakes, without icing						
363	piece, 3 by 2 by 1½ inches	1 piece	55...	27	180	4	5
364	cupcake, 2¾-inch-diameter	1 cupcake ...	40...	27	130	3	3
	plain cake and cupcakes, with icing						
365	sector, 2-inch (1/16 of 10-inch layer cake)	1 sector	100..	25	320	5	6
366	cupcake, 2¾-inch-diameter	1 cupcake ...	50...	25	160	3	3
367	pound cake; slice, 2¾ by 3 by ⅝ inch	1 slice	30...	19	130	2	7
368	sponge cake; sector, 2-inch (1/12 of 8-inch-diameter cake)	1 sector	40...	32	115	3	2
	Cookies						
369	plain and assorted, 3-inch-diameter	1 cooky	25...	5	110	2	3
370	fig bars, small	1 fig bar	16...	14	55	1	1
371	Corn-cereal mixture (mainly degermed cornmeal), puffed, with added thiamine, niacin, and iron	1 ounce	28...	3	115	2	1
	Corn flakes, with added thiamine, niacin, and iron						
372	plain	1 ounce	28...	4	110	2	Trace
373	presweetened	1 ounce	28...	3	110	1	Trace

* If the fat used in the recipe is butter or fortified margarine, the vitamin-A value for chocolate cake with fudge icing will be 520 I.U. per 2-inch sector, item 360; 120 I.U. for fruitcake, item 361; for plain cake without icing, 200 I.U. per piece, item 363; 150 I.U.

EDIBLE PART OF FOODS—Continued

FATTY ACIDS			CARBO-HY-DRATE	CAL-CIUM	IRON	VITA-MIN-A VALUE	THIA-MINE	RIBO-FLA-VIN	NIA-CIN	ASCOR-BIC ACID	ITEM NO.
SATU-RATED (total)	UNSATURATED										
	OLEIC	LINO-LEIC									
gm	gm	gm	gm	mg	mg	I.U.	mg	mg	mg	mg	
3	7	4	216	449	10.4	Trace	1.17	1.03	12.9	Trace	355
—	—	—	11	23	.5	Trace	.06	.05	.7	Trace	356
—	—	—	11	23	.5	Trace	.05	.05	.7	Trace	357
1	2	1	65	107	3.2	Trace	.19	.26	3.1	Trace	358
—	—	—	23	2	.1	0	Trace	.05	.1	Trace	359
5	7	1	70	118	.5	140*	.03	.10	.3	Trace	360
1	2	Trace	17	29	.8	50*	.04	.04	.3	Trace	361
2	4	Trace	28	63	1.4	50	.02	.05	.6	Trace	362
1	3	Trace	31	85	.2	70*	.02	.05	.2	Trace	363
1	2	Trace	23	62	.2	50*	.01	.03	.1	Trace	364
2	3	Trace	62	117	.4	90*	.02	.07	.2	Trace	365
1	1	Trace	31	58	.2	50*	.01	.04	.1	Trace	366
2	4	1	15	16	.5	100*	.04	.05	.3	Trace	367
1	1	Trace	22	11	.6	210*	.02	.06	.1	Trace	368
1	2	Trace	19	6	.2	0	.01	.01	.1	0	369
—	—	—	12	11	.2	0	Trace	.01	.1	0	370
—	—	—	23	6	1.2	—	.15	.04	.6	0	371
—	—	—	24	3	.5	—	.12	.03	.6	0	372
—	—	—	26	3	.4	—	.12	.01	.5	0	373

per cupcake, item 364; for plain cake with icing, 280 I.U. per 2-inch sector, item 365; 140 I.U. per cupcake, item 366; and 300 I.U. for pound cake, item 367.

TABLE 1.—NUTRITIVE VALUES OF THE

ITEM NO.	FOOD, approximate measure, and weight (in grams)			WATER	FOOD ENERGY	PROTEIN	FAT (total lipid)
			gm	per cent	calories	gm	gm
	Corn grits, white, degermed, cooked						
374	enriched	1 cup	242..	87	120	3	Trace
375	unenriched	1 cup	242..	87	120	3	Trace
	Cornmeal, white or yellow, dry						
376	whole ground	1 cup	118..	12	420	11	5
377	degermed, enriched	1 cup	145..	12	525	11	2
378	Corn muffins, made with enriched, degermed cornmeal; muffin, 2¾-inch-diameter	1 muffin	48...	30	155	4	5
379	Corn, puffed, presweetened, with added thiamine, riboflavin, niacin, and iron	1 ounce	28...	3	110	1	Trace
380	Corn and soy shreds, with added thiamine and niacin	1 ounce	28...	4	100	5	Trace
	Crackers						
381	graham	4 small or 2 medium	14...	6	55	1	1
382	saltines, 2 inches square ..	2 crackers ...	8....	5	35	1	1
	soda, plain						
383	cracker, 2½ inches square	2 crackers ...	11...	6	45	1	1
384	oyster crackers	10 crackers ..	10...	6	45	1	1
385	Cracker meal	1 tablespoon .	10...	6	45	1	1
386	Doughnuts, cake type	1 doughnut ..	32...	19	135	2	7
387	Farina, cooked; enriched to minimum levels for required nutrients and for the optional nutrient, calcium	1 cup	238..	89	105	3	Trace
	Macaroni, cooked						
	enriched						
388	cooked 8–10 minutes (undergoes additional cooking in a food mixture)	1 cup	130..	64	190	6	1
389	cooked until tender	1 cup	140..	72	155	5	1
	unenriched						
390	cooked 8–10 minutes (undergoes additional cooking in a food mixture)	1 cup	130..	64	190	6	1
391	cooked until tender	1 cup	140..	72	155	5	1
392	Macaroni, enriched, and cheese, baked	1 cup	220..	58	475	18	25

EDIBLE PART OF FOODS—Continued

FATTY ACIDS			CARBO-HY-DRATE	CAL-CIUM	IRON	VITA-MIN-A VALUE	THIA-MINE	RIBO-FLA-VIN	NIA-CIN	ASCOR-BIC ACID	ITEM NO.
SATU-RATED (total)	UNSATURATED										
	OLEIC	LINO-LEIC									
gm	gm	gm	gm	mg	mg	I.U.	mg	mg	mg	mg	
—	—	—	27	2	0.7	Trace	0.11	0.08	1.0	0	374
—	—	—	27	2	.2	Trace	.04	.01	.4	0	375
1	2	2	87	12	2.8	600*	.45	.13	2.4	0	376
Trace	1	1	114	9	4.2†	430*	.64†	.38†	5.1†	0	377
2	2	Trace	22	79	.9	170‡	.10	.15	.8	Trace	378
—	—	—	26	3	.5	—	.12	.05	.6	0	379
—	—	—	21	24	1.2	—	.19	.04	.6	0	380
—	—	—	10	3	.3	0	.04	.02	.2	0	381
—	—	—	6	2	.1	0	Trace	Trace	.1	0	382
—	—	—	8	2	.1	0	.01	.01	.1	0	383
—	—	—	7	2	.1	0	.01	Trace	.1	0	384
—	—	—	7	2	.1	0	.01	Trace	.1	0	385
2	2	3	17	23	.4	40	.05	.04	.4	0	386
—	—	—	22	31	.8	0	.11	.07	1.0	0	387
—	—	—	39	14	1.4	0	.23	.14	1.9	0	388
—	—	—	32	11	1.3	0	.19	.11	1.5	0	389
—	—	—	39	14	.6	0	.02	.02	.5	0	390
—	—	—	32	11	.6	0	.02	.02	.4	0	391
14	8	1	44	394	2.0	970	.22	.46	1.9	Trace	392

* Vitamin A value based on yellow cornmeal; white cornmeal contains only a trace.
† Iron, thiamine, riboflavin, and niacin are based on minimal level of enrichment specified in standards of identity promulgated under the Federal Food, Drug, and Cosmetic Act.
‡ Based on recipe using white cornmeal; if yellow cornmeal is used the vitamin-A value is 240 I.U.

TABLE 1.—NUTRITIVE VALUES OF THE

ITEM NO.	FOOD, approximate measure, and weight (in grams)			WATER	FOOD EN-ERGY	PRO-TEIN	FAT (total lipid)
			gm	per cent	calo-ries	gm	gm
393	Muffins, with enriched white flour; muffin, 2¾-inch-di-ameter	1 muffin	48	39	135	4	5
	Noodles (egg noodles), cooked						
394	enriched	1 cup	160	70	200	7	2
395	unenriched	1 cup	160	70	200	7	2
396	Oat-cereal mixture, mainly oats, with added B vitamins and minerals	1 ounce	28	3	115	4	2
397	Oatmeal or rolled oats, regular or quick-cooking, cooked	1 cup	236	85	150	5	3
	Pancakes (griddlecakes), 4-inch-diameter						
398	wheat, enriched flour (home recipe)	1 cake	27	53	60	2	2
399	buckwheat (buckwheat pan-cake mix)	1 cake	27	62	45	2	2
	Piecrust, plain, baked enriched flour						
400	lower crust, 9-inch shell	1 crust	135	10	655	10	36
401	double crust, 9-inch pie	1 double crust	270	10	1,315	20	73
	unenriched flour						
402	lower crust, 9-inch shell	1 crust	135	10	655	10	36
403	double crust, 9-inch pie	1 double crust	270	10	1,315	20	73
	Pies; sector, 4-inch, ¹⁄₇ of 9-inch-diameter pie						
404	apple	1 sector	135	48	330	3	13
405	cherry	1 sector	135	46	340	3	13
406	custard	1 sector	130	58	265	7	11
407	lemon meringue	1 sector	120	47	300	4	12
408	mince	1 sector	135	43	340	3	9
409	pumpkin	1 sector	130	59	265	5	12
410	Pizza (cheese), 5½-inch sec-tor, ⅛ of 14-inch-diameter pie	1 sector	75	47	180	8	6
411	Popcorn, popped	1 cup	14	4	55	2	1
412	Pretzels, small stick	5 sticks	5	8	20	Trace	Trace
	Rice, cooked						
413	parboiled	1 cup	176	72	205	4	Trace
414	white	1 cup	168	71	200	4	Trace
415	Rice, puffed, with added thi-amine, niacin, and iron	1 cup	14	5	55	1	Trace
416	Rice flakes, with added thia-mine and niacin	1 cup	30	5	115	2	Trace
	Rolls						
	plain, pan; 12 per 16 ounces						
417	enriched	1 roll	38	31	115	3	2

EDIBLE PART OF FOODS—Continued

FATTY ACIDS			CARBO-HY-DRATE	CAL-CIUM	IRON	VITA-MIN-A VALUE	THIA-MINE	RIBO-FLA-VIN	NIA-CIN	ASCOR-BIC ACID	ITEM NO.
SATU-RATED (total)	UNSATURATED										
	OLEIC	LINO-LEIC									
gm	gm	gm	gm	mg	mg	I.U.	mg	mg	mg	mg	
1	3	Trace	19	74	0.7	60	0.08	0.11	0.7	Trace	393
1	1	Trace	37	16	1.4	60	.23	.14	1.8	0	394
1	1	Trace	37	16	1.0	60	.04	.03	.7	0	395
Trace	1	1	21	45	1.2	0	.22	.04	.5	0	396
1	1	1	26	21	1.7	0	.22	.05	.4	0	397
Trace	1	Trace	8	34	.3	30	.05	.06	.3	Trace	398
1	1	Trace	6	67	.3	30	.04	.04	.2	Trace	399
8	24	3	72	15	2.7	0	.29	.23	3.0	0	400
17	47	5	143	30	5.4	0	.58	.47	5.9	0	401
8	24	3	72	15	.7	0	.05	.03	.7	0	402
17	47	5	143	30	1.4	0	.09	.06	1.4	0	403
4	7	1	53	9	.5	220	.04	.02	.3	1	404
4	7	1	55	14	.5	520	.04	.02	.3	2	405
4	6	1	34	162	1.6	290	.07	.21	.4	0	406
4	6	1	45	24	.6	210	.04	.10	.2	1	407
2	6	1	62	22	3.0	10	.09	.05	.5	1	408
5	6	1	34	70	1.0	2,480	.04	.15	.4	0	409
3	3	Trace	23	157	.7	570	.03	.09	.8	8	410
—	—	—	11	2	.4	0	.05	.02	.3	0	411
—	—	—	4	1	0	0	Trace	Trace	Trace	0	412
—	—	—	45	14	.5	0	.10	.02	1.9	0	413
—	—	—	44	13	.5	0	.02	.01	.7	0	414
—	—	—	12	2	.3	—	.06	.01	.6	0	415
—	—	—	26	9	.5	—	.11	.01	1.7	0	416
1	1	Trace	20	28	.7	Trace	.11	.07	.8	Trace	417

TABLE 1.—NUTRITIVE VALUES OF THE

ITEM NO.	FOOD, approximate measure, and weight (in grams)			WATER	FOOD EN-ERGY	PRO-TEIN	FAT (total lipid)
			gm	per cent	calo-ries	gm	gm
	Rolls (*Continued*)						
418	unenriched	1 roll	38...	31	115	3	2
419	hard, round; 12 per 22 ounces	1 roll	52...	25	160	5	2
420	sweet, pan; 12 per 18 ounces	1 roll	43...	31	135	4	4
421	Rye wafers, 1⅞ by 3½ inches	2 wafers	13...	6	45	2	Trace
	Spaghetti, cooked until tender						
422	enriched	1 cup	140..	72	155	5	1
423	unenriched	1 cup	140..	72	155	5	1
424	Spaghetti with meat sauce	1 cup	250..	76	285	13	10
425	Spaghetti in tomato sauce with cheese	1 cup	250..	80	210	6	5
426	Waffles, with enriched flour, ½ by 4½ by 5½ inches	1 waffle	75...	34	240	8	9
	Wheat, puffed						
427	with added thiamine, nia-cin, and iron	1 ounce	28...	4	100	4	Trace
428	with added thiamine and niacin; presweetened	1 ounce	28...	3	105	1	Trace
429	Wheat, rolled; cooked	1 cup	236..	80	175	5	1
430	Wheat, shredded, plain (long, round, or bite-size)	1 ounce	28...	6	100	3	1
431	Wheat and malted barley ce-real, with added thiamine, niacin, and iron	1 ounce	28...	3	105	3	Trace
432	Wheat flakes, with added thiamine, niacin, and iron	1 ounce	28...	4	100	3	Trace
	Wheat flours						
433	whole-wheat, from hard wheats, stirred	1 cup	120..	12	400	16	2
	all-purpose or family flour						
434	enriched, sifted	1 cup	110..	12	400	12	1
435	unenriched, sifted	1 cup	110..	12	400	12	1
	self-rising						
436	enriched	1 cup	110..	12	385	10	1
437	unenriched	1 cup	110..	12	385	10	1
438	Wheat germ, stirred	1 cup	68...	11	245	17	7
	Fats, oils						
	Butter, 4 sticks per pound						
439	sticks, 2	1 cup	224..	16	1,605	1	181
440	stick, ⅛	1 tablespoon	14...	16	100	Trace	11
441	pat or square (64 per pound)	1 pat	7....	16	50	Trace	6

EDIBLE PART OF FOODS—Continued

SATU-RATED (total)	UNSATURATED OLEIC	LINO-LEIC	CARBO-HY-DRATE	CAL-CIUM	IRON	VITA-MIN-A VALUE	THIA-MINE	RIBO-FLA-VIN	NIA-CIN	ASCOR-BIC ACID	ITEM NO.
gm	gm	gm	gm	mg	mg	I.U.	mg	mg	mg	mg	
1	1	Trace	20	28	0.3	Trace	0.02	0.03	0.3	Trace	*418*
1	1	Trace	31	24	.4	Trace	.03	.05	.4	Trace	*419*
1	2	Trace	21	37	.3	30	.03	.06	.4	0	*420*
—	—	—	10	6	.6	0	.04	.03	.2	0	*421*
—	—	—	32	11	1.3	0	.19	.11	1.5	0	*422*
—	—	—	32	11	.6	0	.02	.02	.4	0	*423*
3	3	3	35	25	2.0	690	.07	.10	2.1	13	*424*
2	1	2	36	45	1.0	830	.07	.08	1.0	15	*425*
3	5	1	30	124	1.4	310	.14	.21	1.1	Trace	*426*
—	—	—	22	8	1.2	0	.16	.06	2.2	0	*427*
—	—	—	26	4	.5	0	.12	.01	1.4	0	*428*
—	—	—	40	19	1.7	0	.17	.06	2.1	0	*429*
—	—	—	23	13	1.0	0	.06	.03	1.3	0	*430*
—	—	—	24	13	1.0	0	.13	.05	1.5	0	*431*
—	—	—	23	13	1.2	0	.16	.05	1.8	0	*432*
Trace	1	1	85	49	4.0	0	.66	.14	5.2	0	*433*
—	—	—	84	18	3.2*	0	.48*	.29*	3.8*	0	*434*
—	—	—	84	18	.9	0	.07	.05	1.0	0	*435*
—	—	—	81	299	3.2*	0	.48*	.29*	3.8*	0	*436*
—	—	—	81	299	1.1	0	.08	.05	1.3	0	*437*
1	2	3	34	57	5.5	0	1.39	.54	3.1	0	*438*
100	60	5	1	45	Trace	7,400†	—	—	—	0	*439*
6	4	Trace	Trace	3	Trace	460†	—	—	—	0	*440*
3	2	0	Trace	1	Trace	230†	—	—	—	0	*441*

* Iron, thiamine, riboflavin, and niacin are based on the minimal level of enrichment specified in the standards of identity promulgated under the Federal Food, Drug, and Cosmetic Act.

† Year-round average.

TABLE 1.—NUTRITIVE VALUES OF THE

ITEM NO.	FOOD, approximate measure, and weight (in grams)			WATER	FOOD EN- ERGY	PRO- TEIN	FAT (total lipid)
			gm	per cent	calo- ries	gm	gm
	Fats, cooking						
442	lard	1 cup	220..	0	1,985	0	220
443		1 tablespoon .	14...	0	135	0	14
444	vegetable fats	1 cup	200..	0	1,770	0	200
445		1 tablespoon .	12.5 .	0	110	0	12
	Margarine, 4 sticks per pound						
446	sticks, 2	1 cup	224..	16	1,615	1	181
447	stick, ⅛	1 tablespoon .	14...	16	100	Trace	11
448	pat or square (64 per pound)	1 pat	7....	16	50	Trace	6
	Oils, salad or cooking						
449	corn	1 tablespoon .	14...	0	125	0	14
450	cottonseed	1 tablespoon .	14...	0	125	0	14
451	olive	1 tablespoon .	14...	0	125	0	14
452	soybean	1 tablespoon .	14...	0	125	0	14
	Salad dressings						
453	blue cheese	1 tablespoon .	16...	28	90	1	10
454	commercial, plain; mayon- naise type	1 tablespoon .	15...	48	60	Trace	6
455	French	1 tablespoon .	15...	42	60	Trace	6
456	home cooked, boiled	1 tablespoon .	17...	68	30	1	2
457	mayonnaise	1 tablespoon .	15...	14	110	Trace	12
458	Thousand Island	1 tablespoon .	15...	38	75	Trace	8
	Sugars, sweets						
	Candy						
459	caramels	1 ounce	28...	7	120	1	3
460	chocolate, sweetened, milk	1 ounce	28...	1	145	2	9
461	fudge, plain	1 ounce	28...	5	115	Trace	3
462	hard candy	1 ounce	28...	1	110	0	0
463	marshmallow	1 ounce	28...	15	90	1	0
464	Chocolate sirup	1 tablespoon .	20...	39	40	Trace	Trace
465	Honey, strained or extracted	1 tablespoon .	21...	20	60	Trace	0
466	Jams, marmalades, preserves	1 tablespoon .	20...	28	55	Trace	Trace
467	Jellies	1 tablespoon .	20...	34	50	0	0
	Molasses, cane						
468	light (first extraction)	1 tablespoon .	20...	24	50	—	—
469	blackstrap (third extrac- tion)	1 tablespoon .	20...	24	45	—	—
470	Sirup, table blends	1 tablespoon .	20...	25	55	0	0
	Sugar						
471	granulated, cane or beet	1 cup	200..	Trace	770	0	0
472		1 tablespoon .	12...	Trace	50	0	0
473	lump, 1⅛ by ⅝ by ⅛ inch	1 lump	7....	Trace	25	0	0

EDIBLE PART OF FOODS—Continued

SATURATED (total) gm	UNSATURATED OLEIC gm	UNSATURATED LINOLEIC gm	CARBOHYDRATE gm	CALCIUM mg	IRON mg	VITAMIN-A VALUE I.U.	THIAMINE mg	RIBOFLAVIN mg	NIACIN mg	ASCORBIC ACID mg	ITEM NO.
84	101	22	0	0	0	0	0	0	0	0	442
5	6	1	0	0	0	0	0	0	0	0	443
46	130	14	0	0	0	0	0	0	0	0	444
3	8	1	0	0	0	0	0	0	0	0	445
47	103	16	1	45	Trace	7,400*	—	—	—	0	446
3	6	1	Trace	3	Trace	460*	—	—	—	0	447
1	3	1	Trace	1	Trace	230*	—	—	—	0	448
1	4	7	0	0	0	—	0	0	0	0	449
3	3	7	0	0	0	—	0	0	0	0	450
2	11	1	0	0	0	—	0	0	0	0	451
2	3	7	0	0	0	—	0	0	0	0	452
2	2	5	1	11	Trace	30	Trace	.02	Trace	Trace	453
1	1	3	2	2	Trace	30	Trace	Trace	Trace	0	454
1	1	3	2	3	.1	0	0	0	0	0	455
1	1	Trace	3	15	.1	80	.01	.03	Trace	Trace	456
2	3	6	Trace	2	.1	40	Trace	Trace	Trace	0	457
1	2	4	1	2	.1	60	Trace	Trace	Trace	2	458
2	1	Trace	22	36	.7	50	.01	.04	Trace	Trace	459
5	3	Trace	16	61	.3	40	.03	.11	.2	0	460
2	1	Trace	23	14	.1	60	Trace	.02	Trace	Trace	461
—	—	—	28	0	0	0	0	0	0	0	462
—	—	—	23	0	0	0	0	0	0	0	463
—	—	—	11	3	.3	—	—	—	—	—	464
—	—	—	17	1	.2	0	Trace	.01	Trace	1	465
—	—	—	14	2	.1	Trace	Trace	Trace	Trace	1	466
—	—	—	13	2	.1	Trace	Trace	Trace	Trace	1	467
—	—	—	13	33	.9	—	.01	.01	Trace	—	468
—	—	—	11	116	2.3	—	.02	.04	.3	—	469
—	—	—	15	9	.8	0	0	Trace	Trace	0	470
—	—	—	199	—	—	0	0	0	0	0	471
—	—	—	12	—	—	0	0	0	0	0	472
—	—	—	7	—	—	0	0	0	0	0	473

* Based on the average vitamin A content of fortified margarine. Federal specifications for fortified margarine require a minimum of 15,000 I.U. of vitamin A per pound.

TABLE 1—NUTRITIVE VALUES OF THE

ITEM NO.	FOOD, approximate measure, and weight (in grams)		gm	WATER per cent	FOOD EN- ERGY calo- ries	PRO- TEIN gm	FAT (total lipid) gm
	Sugar (*Continued*)						
474	powdered, stirred before measuring	1 cup	128..	Trace	495	0	0
475		1 tablespoon .	8....	Trace	30	0	0
476	brown, firm-packed	1 cup	220..	3	815	0	0
477		1 tablespoon .	14...	3	50	0	0
	Miscellaneous items						
478	Beer (average 4 per cent alcohol)	1 cup	240..	90	†	1	Trace
	Beverages, carbonated						
479	ginger ale	1 cup	230..	91	80	—	—
480	Kola type	1 cup	230..	88	105	—	—
481	Bouillon cube, ⅝ inch	1 cube	4....	5	2	Trace	Trace
	Chili powder. *See* Vegetables, Peppers.						
482	Chili sauce (mainly tomatoes)	1 tablespoon .	17...	69	15	Trace	Trace
	Chocolate						
483	bitter or unsweetened	1 ounce	28...	2	145	2	15
484	sweetened	1 ounce	28...	1	135	1	8
	Cider. *See* Fruit, Applejuice.						
	Gelatin, dry						
485	plain	1 tablespoon .	10...	13	35	9	Trace
486	dessert powder, 3-ounce package	½ cup	85...	2	325	8	Trace
	Gelatin dessert, ready-to-eat						
487	plain	1 cup	239..	83	155	4	Trace
488	with fruit	1 cup	241..	81	170	3	Trace
	Olives, pickled						
489	green	12 Extra Large or 7 Jumbo	66...	78	65	1	7
490	ripe: Mission; other varieties, such as Ascolano, Manzanillo, and Sevillano	12 Extra Large or 7 Jumbo	66...	76	85	1	9
	Pickles, cucumber						
491	dill, large, 4 by 1¾ inches	1 pickle	135..	93	15	1	Trace
492	sweet, 2¾ by ¾ inch	1 pickle	20...	70	20	Trace	Trace
	Popcorn. *See* Grain products.						
493	Sherbet, factory packed	1 cup	193..	68	235	3	Trace
	Soups, canned; ready-to-serve						
494	bean	1 cup	250..	82	190	8	5
495	beef	1 cup	250..	92	100	6	4

† The value excluding energy derived from alcohol is 48 calories. If the energy from alcohol is considered available, the value is 114 calories.

EDIBLE PART OF FOODS—Continued

FATTY ACIDS			CARBO-HY-DRATE	CAL-CIUM	IRON	VITA-MIN-A VALUE	THIA-MINE	RIBO-FLA-VIN	NIA-CIN	ASCOR-BIC ACID	ITEM NO.
SATU-RATED (total)	UNSATURATED										
	OLEIC	LINO-LEIC									
gm	gm	gm	gm	mg	mg	I.U.	mg	mg	mg	mg	
—	—	—	127	—	—	0	0	0	0	0	474
—	—	—	8	—	—	0	0	0	0	0	475
—	—	—	210	167*	5.7	0	0	0	0	0	476
—	—	—	13	10*	.4	0	0	0	0	0	477
—	—	—	11	10	Trace	0	Trace	.06	.4	0	478
—	—	—	21	—	—	—	—	—	—	—	479
—	—	—	28	—	—	—	—	—	—	—	480
—	—	—	0	—	—	—	—	.07	1.0	0	481
—	—	—	4	2	.1	320	.02	.01	.4	2	482
8	6	Trace	8	28	1.2	20	.01	.06	.3	0	483
5	3	Trace	18	18	.8	10	.01	.04	.2	0	484
—	—	—	0	0	0	0	0	0	0	0	485
—	—	—	76	0	0	0	0	0	0	0	486
—	—	—	36	0	0	0	0	0	0	0	487
—	—	—	42	14	.7	270	.07	.05	.5	7	488
1	5	Trace	1	48	.9	170	Trace	—	—	—	489
1	7	1	2	45	.9	40	Trace	Trace	—	—	490
—	—	—	3	34	1.6	420	Trace	.09	.1	8	491
—	—	—	5	3	.3	20	0	Trace	Trace	1	492
—	—	—	58	96	.1	0	.03	.15	.1	0	493
2	2	Trace	30	95	2.8	—	.10	.10	.8	—	494
2	2	Trace	11	15	.5	—	—	—	—	—	495

* Calcium value is based on dark brown sugar; value is lower for light brown sugar.

TABLE 1—NUTRITIVE VALUES OF THE

ITEM NO.	FOOD, approximate measure, and weight (in grams)		gm	WATER per cent	FOOD EN- ERGY calo- ries	PRO- TEIN gm	FAT (total lipid) gm
	Soups, canned (*Continued*)						
496	bouillon, broth, consomme	1 cup	240	95	10	2	—
497	chicken	1 cup	250	94	75	4	2
498	clam chowder	1 cup	255	91	85	5	2
499	cream soup (asparagus, celery, mushroom)	1 cup	255	85	200	7	12
500	noodle, rice, barley	1 cup	250	90	115	6	4
501	pea	1 cup	245	86	140	6	2
502	tomato	1 cup	245	91	90	2	2
503	vegetable	1 cup	250	92	80	4	2
504	Starch, pure, including arrowroot, corn, etc.	1 cup	128	12	465	1	Trace
505		1 tablespoon	8	12	30	Trace	Trace
506	Tapioca, quick-cooking granulated, dry; stirred before measuring	1 cup	152	13	545	1	Trace
507		1 tablespoon	10	13	35	Trace	Trace
508	Vinegar	1 tablespoon	15	—	2	0	—
509	White sauce, medium	1 cup	265	73	430	10	33
	Yeast bakers'						
510	compressed	1 ounce	28	71	25	3	Trace
511	dry active	1 ounce	28	5	80	10	Trace
512	brewers', dry	1 tablespoon	8	5	25	3	Trace
	Yoghurt. *See* Milk, cream, cheese; related products.						

EDIBLE PART OF FOODS—Continued

SATU-RATED (total)	UNSATURATED		CARBO-HY-DRATE	CAL-CIUM	IRON	VITA-MIN-A VALUE	THIA-MINE	RIBO-FLA-VIN	NIA-CIN	ASCOR-BIC ACID	ITEM NO.
	OLEIC	LINO-LEIC									
gm	gm	gm	gm	mg	mg	I.U.	mg	mg	mg	mg	
—	—	—	0	2	1.0	0	0	0.05	0.6	0	496
1	1	Trace	10	20	.5	—	.02	.12	1.5	—	497
Trace	Trace	1	12	36	3.6	—	—	—	—	—	498
7	4	Trace	18	217	.5	200	.05	.20	.1	0	499
1	2	1	13	82	.2	30	.02	.05	.7	0	500
1	1	Trace	25	32	1.5	440	.17	.07	1.2	5	501
1	Trace	1	18	24	1.0	1,230	.02	.10	.7	10	502
1	1	Trace	14	32	.8	—	.05	.08	1.0	8	503
—	—	—	111	0	0	0	0	0	0	0	504
—	—	—	7	0	0	0	0	0	0	0	505
—	—	—	131	18	1.5	0	0	0	0	0	506
—	—	—	8	1	.1	0	0	0	0	0	507
—	—	—	1	1	.1	—	—	—	—	—	508
18	11	1	23	305	.3	1,350	.07	.42	.3	1	509
—	—	—	3	4	1.4	Trace	.20	.47	3.2	Trace	510
—	—	—	11	12	4.6	Trace	.66	1.53	10.4	Trace	511
—	—	—	3	17	1.4	Trace	1.25	.34	3.0	Trace	512

TABLE 2—FOOD COMPOSITION TABLE FOR SHORT METHOD OF DIETARY ANALYSIS (2nd revision) *

FOOD *	APPROXIMATE MEASURE	WEIGHT gm	CALO-RIES	PRO-TEIN gm	FAT gm	CAR-BOHY-DRATE gm	CAL-CIUM gm	PHOS-PHO-RUS gm	IRON mg	VITA-MIN A I.U.	ASCOR-BIC ACID mg	THIA-MINE mg	RIBO-FLA-VIN mg	NIA-CIN mg
Cereal products refined	1 slice bread (30 gm); ½ cup cooked cereal and cereal products (20 gm dry); ½–1 cup prep. cereal (20 gm); 3 soda crackers (20 gm); 1½ cups popcorn (20 gm); 1 griddle cake (4-in. diameter)		80	2.5	1	15	.01	.02	.2	—	—	.02	.02	.3
whole grain and enriched	1 slice bread (30 gm); ½ cup cooked cereal (20 gm dry); ½–1 cup prepared cereal (20 gm); 2 Graham crackers (20 gm)		80	2.5	1	15	.02	.03	.6	—	—	.07	.04	.6
Dairy products butter	1 teaspoon	5	35	—	4	—	—	—	—	165	—	—	—	—
cheese, cheddar type	1 cu. in.	30	125	7.5	10	1	.22	.15	.3	420	—	.01	.13	—
cheese, cottage, skim	½ cup	100	95	19.5	1	2	.10	.19	.3	20	—	.02	.31	.1
cream, light	⅛ cup (for heavy cream add ½ serving butter)	30	60	1.0	6	1	.03	.02	—	250	—	.01	.04	—
custard	½ cup	130	150	7.0	7	15	.15	.16	.6	440	—	.06	.26	.1
egg	1 medium	50	80	6.5	6	—	.03	.10	1.4	570	—	.05	.14	.1
ice cream	½ cup	80	165	3.0	10	16	.10	.08	.1	420	1	.03	.15	.1
milk buttermilk, skim	1 cup	240	85	8.5	—	12	.30	.23	.2	—	2	.10	.43	.2
whole	1 cup	240	165	8.5	9	12	.28	.22	.2	385	2	.10	.41	.2

Food	Measure													
Desserts														
cake, plain, chocolate	1 piece cake 2½ x 2½ x 2½ (75 gm), for iced add 1 serving sweets; 1 waffle, 6-in. diameter (60 gm); 2½ dough-nuts, cake type (add 1 serving fat)		250	5.0	8	40	.09	.10	.4	140	—	.02	.06	.2
cookies, plain	2 medium	40	175	2.5	5	30	.01	.03	.4	100	—	.02	.02	.2
pie crust	1/6 shell, single crust	25	110	1.5	6	12	—	.01	.4	—	—	.05	.04	.5
puddings, cream fillings	½ cup	140	150	4.5	5	22	.14	.13	.1	225	—	.04	.22	.1
Fats	2 slices bacon (20 gm raw); 1 tablespoon fat (12 gm); 1 tablespoon mayonnaise (15 gm); 1 cu. in. salt pork (15 gm); 2 tablespoons French dressing (30 gm)		105	1.5	11	—	—	.01	.2	15	—	.03	.02	.4
Fish														
cod, haddock, cooked	1 medium serving	75	55	13.5	—	—	.01	.15	.4	—	1	.04	.06	1.6
halibut, herring, tuna, white-fish, cooked	1 medium serving tuna (60 gm); others (75 gm)	60	115	17.0	5	—	.01	.19	.8	60	—	.04	.06	6.0
salmon, canned	1 medium serving	75	125	15.0	7	—	.11	.23	.8	135	—	.02	.12	5.6
Fruits														
banana	1 small	100	90	1.0	—	22	.01	.03	.6	430	10	.04	.05	.7
cantaloupe	½ melon, 4½-in. diameter	150	30	1.0	—	7	.02	.02	.6	5130	50	.07	.06	.8
citrus	1 medium orange; ½ medium grapefruit; ½ cup juice; 1 medium large lemon	100	45	.5	—	11	.03	.02	.4	115	45	.06	.02	.2
yellow—fresh, canned, dried	1 medium peach (100 gm); 1 medium fresh (100 gm); 2 to 3 apricots, 3 plums; dried (30 gm); for sweetened, canned, dried, or fresh, add ½ serving sweets	100	70	.5	—	17	.01	.03	.6	910	6	.01	.03	1.0

* Leichsenring, J. M., and Wilson, E. D.: "Food Composition Table for Short Method of Dietary Analysis (2nd Revision)," *J. Am. Dietet. A.* **27**:387–88, 1951.

The nutritive value of food mixtures such as macaroni and cheese, Spanish rice, chow mein, creamed vegetables, soups, and so on should be computed on the basis of the kind and approximate amount of the foods in the combination.

TABLE 2 (*Continued*)

FOOD	APPROXIMATE MEASURE	WEIGHT gm	CALORIES	PROTEIN gm	FAT gm	CARBOHYDRATE gm	CALCIUM gm	PHOSPHORUS gm	IRON mg	VITAMIN A I.U.	ASCORBIC ACID mg	THIAMINE mg	RIBOFLAVIN mg	NIACIN mg
Fruits (*Continued*)														
other—dried	3 to 4 dates; 1½ to 2 small figs; dried apple; ¼ cup raisins	30	80	.5	—	20	.03	.03	.9	15	—	.04	.03	.3
other—fresh and canned	½ cup	100	55	.5	—	13	.01	.01	.4	95	4	.04	.03	.2
Gravy, white sauce	¼ cup	65	105	2.5	8	6	.07	.06	.2	225	—	.04	.11	.2
Legumes														
beans, peas	½ cup cooked; dried (30 gm)		100	6.5	—	18	.05	.13	2.0	10	1	.19	.07	.7
soybeans	½ cup cooked; dried (30 gm)		105	10.5	5	4	.07	.18	2.4	35	—	.32	.09	.7
Meat														
beef, lamb, veal, cooked	1 medium serving	75	240	19.0	18	—	.01	.15	2.3	—	—	.07	.17	3.7
fowl, cooked	1 medium serving	75	150	15.0	10	—	.01	.16	1.7	—	—	.04	.08	5.2
liver, cooked	1 small serving	60	125	14.0	5	6	.01	.29	4.7	32,100	19	.16	2.38	8.9
luncheon meats, cooked	2 slices sausage, minced ham, dried beef, luncheon roll (30 gm); ½ frankfurter		85	6.0	7	—	.01	.05	.9	—	—	.08	.08	.8
pork, ham, cooked	1 medium serving	75	280	18.0	23	—	.01	.16	2.2	—	—	.47	.17	3.5
Nuts	1 tablespoon peanut butter; 8 to 15 walnut halves; 16 peanuts; 12 to 15 almonds; 12 pecan halves	15	90	4.0	7	3	.01	.06	.3	—	—	.04	.02	2.3
Sweets														
candy, sugar, sirup	1 tablespoon sugar, jelly, jam, sirup, honey; 1 serving plain Jello, plain candy (fondant or mints, 14 gm); 6-oz. bottle soft drink		55	—	—	14	—	—	—	—	—	—	—	
candy bar	1 2-oz. chocolate-coated bar	20	290	4.0	15	34	.06	.09	1.1	65	—	.04	.17	1.1
Molasses; sorghum	1 tablespoon		50	—	—	13	.04	.01	1.8	—	—	.02	.03	.6

Vegetables—														
cabbage— cooked and sauerkraut	⅔ cup	100	25	1.5	—	5	.05	.05	.5	90	30†	.05	.05	.3
cabbage, raw; cauliflower, cooked	1 cup cabbage (50 gm); ⅔ cup cauliflower (70 gm)		15	1.0	—	3	.02	.03	.5	50	22	.04	.04	.2
corn; parsnips, cooked	½ cup corn; 1 large parsnip	100	85	2.0	1	19	.03	.07	.6	195	10‡	.07‡	.09‡	.6†
green and yellow asparagus, cooked	⅔ cup	100	20	2.0	—	3	.02	.05	1.0	1040	18‡	.13‡	.17‡	1.2
broccoli, cooked	⅔ cup	100	30	3.0	—	5	.13	.08	1.3	3400	74	.07	.15	.8
carrots, cooked	⅔ cup	100	30	.5	—	7	.03	.03	.6	12,500	4‡	.05‡	.05‡	.4‡
green beans, cooked	½ cup	100	25	1.5	—	5	.04	.02	.7	660	14‡	.07‡	.10‡	.5‡
leafy green, cooked	⅔ cup spinach, turnip, kale, other greens	100	30	2.5	—	5	.20§	.05	2.7	10,400	33‡	.08‡	.21‡	.6‡
peas, fresh, cooked, canned	½ cup	100	70	4.0	—	13	.02	.09	1.8	630	15‡	.25‡	.14‡	2.3‡
sweet potato, cooked	½ large (100 gm); for fried add 1 to 2 servings fat; for French fried (50 gm) add 1 to 2 servings fat	100	140	2.0	1	31	.03	.05	.8	8605	22‡	.10‡	.06‡	.7†
potato, cooked	1 small (100 gm); for fried add 1 to 2 servings fat	85	85	2.0	—	19	.01	.06	.7	20	14‡	.09‡	.03	1.0
tomato, fresh, canned, or juice	½ cup; 1 small tomato (100 gm); for 2½ tablespoons catsup (50 gm), add ½ serving sweets		20	1.0	—	4	.01	.02	.5	1035	18	.09‡	.03	.8
other, cooked	½ cup beets, eggplant, onions, etc.	100	40	1.0	—	9	.03	.05	.6	80	8	.03	.04	.3
other, commonly served raw	2 pieces celery; 8 slices cucumber; ⅛ head lettuce	50	10	.5	—	2	.02	.02	.2	105	4	.02	.03	.2

† For sauerkraut, reduce by one-half.
‡ For canned, reduce by one-half.
§ Calcium may be unavailable in chard, spinach, and beet greens.

TABLE 3—COMPOSITION OF SOME ALCOHOLIC BEVERAGES

BEVERAGE	APPROXIMATE MEASURE	ml	ENERGY calories *	ALCOHOL (per cent by weight)	CARBOHYDRATE per cent
Ale, American	1 glass	250	155	6	5
Beer	1 glass	250	110	4	4
Brandy	1 cordial glass	20	65	45	
Creme de Menthe	1 cordial glass	20	75	36	30
Gin	1 jigger	45	126	40	
Rum	1 jigger	45	140	44	
Whisky	1 jigger	45	132	42	
Wine					
Champagne, dry	1 champagne glass	135	105	10	2
Champagne, sweet	1 champagne glass	135	161	10	13
California, red	1 claret glass	120	95	10	3
white	1 claret glass	120	89	9	3
port	1 sherry glass	30	50	15	14
sherry	1 sherry glass	30	38	15	6

* Alcohol yields 7 calories per gram. The percentages of alcohol vary widely in different brands.

TABLE 4—FOOD EXCHANGE LISTS FOR CALCULATING DIETS *

Foods are divided into six groups, according to their composition:

FOOD EXCHANGE	QUANTITY FOR ONE EXCHANGE Measure	Weight gm	CARBO-HYDRATE gm	PROTEIN gm	FAT gm	CALORIES
Milk	8 ounces	240	12	8	10	170
Vegetables—A	as desired	—	—	—	—	—
Vegetables—B	½ cup	100	7	2	—	36
Fruit	varies	—	10	—	—	40
Bread	varies	—	15	2	—	68
Meat	1 ounce	30	—	7	5	73
Fat	1 teaspoon	5	—	—	—	45

* Caso, E. K.: "Calculation of Diabetic Diets," *J. Am. Dietet. A.*, **26**:575, 1950.

TABLE 4—FOOD EXCHANGE LISTS (*Continued*)

List 1—Milk Exchanges

Per exchange: carbohydrate, 12 gm; protein, 8 gm; fat, 10 gm

	MEASURE	WEIGHT gm
Milk, whole (plain or homogenized)	1 cup (8 ounces)	240
Milk, skim, liquid *	1 cup	240
Milk, evaporated	½ cup	120
Milk, powdered whole	3–5 tablespoons †	35
Milk, nonfat dry *	3–5 tablespoons †	35
Buttermilk (from whole milk)	1 cup	240
Buttermilk (from skim milk) *	1 cup	240

* Since these forms of milk contain no fat, two fat exchanges may be added to the diet when they are used; or one exchange of these forms of milk may be calculated as carbohydrate, 12; protein, 8; and fat, 0.

† The amount of milk powder to use depends upon the brand used; read package direction for the equivalent for 1 cup liquid milk.

List 2—Vegetable Exchanges

GROUP A VEGETABLES—negligible carbohydrate, protein, and fat if 1 cup (200 gm) or less is used. Count each additional cup as one exchange of Group B vegetable.

Asparagus	Eggplant	Lettuce
Beans, string, young	Greens * beet greens	Mushrooms Okra
Broccoli *	chard, Swiss	Pepper *
Brussels sprouts	collard	Radish
Cabbage	dandelion	Sauerkraut
Cauliflower	kale	Squash, summer
Celery	mustard	Tomatoes *
Chicory *	spinach	Watercress *
Cucumbers	turnip greens	
Escarole *		

GROUP B VEGETABLES—per exchange: carbohydrate, 7 gm; protein, 2 gm; fat, negligible. One exchange = ½ cup = 100 gm.

Beets	Peas, green	Squash, winter *
Carrots *	Pumpkin *	Turnip
Onion	Rutabaga	

* These vegetables have high vitamin-A value. At least one serving should be included in the diet each day.

TABLE 4—FOOD EXCHANGE LISTS (*Continued*)

List 3—Fruit Exchanges

Per exchange: carbohydrate, 10 gm; protein, and fat, negligible

Fruits may be used fresh, cooked, canned or frozen, unsweetened

	MEASURE	WEIGHT gm
Apple	1 small, 2-in. diameter	80
Applesauce	½ cup	100
Apricots, dried	4 halves	20
Apricots, fresh	2 medium	100
Banana	½ small	50
Blackberries	1 cup	150
Blueberries	⅔ cup	100
Cantaloupe *	¼, 6-inch diameter	200
Cherries	10 large	75
Dates	2	15
Figs, dried	1 small	15
Figs, fresh	2 large	50
Grapefruit *	½ small	125
Grapefruit juice *	½ cup	100
Grape juice	¼ cup	60
Grapes	12	75
Honeydew melon *	⅛, 7-inch diameter	150
Mango	½ small	70
Nectarines	1 medium	80
Orange *	1 small	100
Orange juice *	½ cup	100
Papaya	⅓ medium	100
Peach	1 medium	100
Pear	1 small	100
Pineapple	½ cup cubed	80
Pineapple juice	⅓ cup	80
Plums	2 medium	100
Prunes, dried	2 medium	25
Raisins	2 tablespoons	15
Raspberries	1 cup	150
Strawberries *	1 cup	150
Tangerine	1 large	100
Watermelon	1 cup diced	175

* These fruits are rich sources of ascorbic acid. At least one exchange should be included in the diet each day.

TABLE 4—FOOD EXCHANGE LISTS (*Continued*)

List 4—Bread Exchanges

Per exchange: carbohydrate, 15 gm; protein, 2 gm; fat, negligible

	MEASURE	WEIGHT gm
Bread	1 slice	25
biscuit, roll (2 inch diameter)	1	30
muffin	1 medium	35
cornbread	1½-inch cube	35
Cereal, cooked	½ cup	100
Cereal, dry	¾ cup	20
Crackers, graham	2	20
oyster	20 (½ cup)	20
saltines (2 inches square)	5	20
soda (2½ inches square)	3	20
round, thin (1½ inch diameter)	6–8	20
Flour	2½ tablespoons	30
Grits	½ cup cooked	100
Ice cream, vanilla (omit two fat exchanges)	⅛ quart	70
Macaroni	½ cup cooked	100
Matzoth	½ (6½ inch square)	20
Noodles	½ cup cooked	100
Rice	½ cup cooked	100
Spaghetti	½ cup cooked	100
Sponge cake, no icing	1½-inch cube	25
Vegetables		
beans, baked; no pork	¼ cup	50
beans and peas, dried (includes kidney, Lima, navy beans, black-eyed, split, and cowpeas, etc.)	½ cup cooked	100
beans, Lima, fresh	½ cup	100
corn, popped	1 cup	20
corn, fresh	⅓ cup or ½ small ear	80
parsnips	⅔ cup	125
potatoes, white	1 small (2-inch diameter)	100
potatoes, white, mashed	½ cup	100
potatoes, sweet or yam	¼ cup	50

TABLE 4—FOOD EXCHANGE LISTS (*Continued*)

List 5—Meat Exchanges

Per exchange: carbohydrate, negligible; protein, 7 gm; fat, 5 gm
Measures and weights are for cooked meat

	MEASURE	WEIGHT gm
Meat, fish, and poultry (medium fat) (beef, lamb, pork, veal, liver, chicken, turkey, etc.)	1 ounce	30
cold cuts (bologna, liver sausage, luncheon loaf, boiled ham, salami, etc.)	1 slice, ⅛ inch thick	45
frankfurt	1	50
cod, haddock, halibut, herring, etc.	1 ounce	30
crab, lobster, salmon, tuna	¼ cup	30
clams, oysters, shrimp	5 small	45
sardines	3 medium	30
Cheese, Cheddar	1 ounce	30
cottage	¼ cup	45
Egg	1	50
Peanut butter *	2 tablespoons	30

* Limit to one exchange daily or adjust for carbohydrate. Deduct 5 gm carbohydrate for each additional exchange.

List 6—Fat Exchanges

Per exchange: fat, 5 gm; protein and carbohydrate, negligible

	MEASURE	WEIGHT gm
Butter or margarine	1 teaspoon	5
Bacon, crisp	1 slice	10
Cream, light, 20 per cent	2 tablespoons	30
Cream, heavy, 35–40 per cent	1 tablespoon	15
Cream cheese	1 tablespoon	15
French dressing	1 tablespoon	15
Mayonnaise	1 teaspoon	5
Nuts	6 small	10
Oil or cooking fat	1 teaspoon	5
Olives	5 small	50
Avocado	⅛, 4-inch diameter	25

TABLE 4—FOOD EXCHANGE LISTS (*Concluded*)

Foods Allowed As Desired

Protein, fat, and carbohydrate negligible

Coffee	Gelatin, unsweetened	Vinegar
Tea	Rennet tablets	Cranberries, unsweetened
Clear broth	Cyclamate, sodium or	Lemon
Bouillon	calcium	Mustard, dry
(fat free)	Saccharin	Pickle, dill, unsweetened
Herbs (see list p. 516)	Spices (see list p. 516)	Rhubarb, unsweetened

TABLE 5—BEST ESTIMATES OF SODIUM CONTENT OF FOODS *

FOOD	SODIUM mg/100 gm	FOOD	SODIUM mg/100 gm
Almonds, unsalted	3	Beans, snap, green and yellow	
Apples, raw	1	wax, frozen	2
cider	1	Beans, snap, green and yellow	
sauce, canned	2 †	wax, canned without salt	2 †
Apricots, raw	1	Beef, lean, raw	70
unpeeled, canned	4 †	heart, raw	85
dried	10 ‡	kidney, raw	200 ‡
Asparagus, raw	3	liver, raw	130 ‡
canned without salt	4 †	tongue, raw, unsmoked	80
Avocado, raw	3	Beets, raw	60 ‡
Bacon, raw, cured	700 † ‡	canned without salt	40 ‡
fried crisp	2400 † ‡	Beet greens, raw	130
Baking powder, ordinary		Beverages	
(av.)	9000 ‡	beer	7 ‡
low-sodium	35	soft drinks (cola drinks,	
Bananas	1	fruit soda, ginger ale,	
Barley, pearled	3	root beer, etc.)	7 ‡
Beans, dry (Navy, pea, etc.)	1	wine (average)	7 ‡
Beans, Lima, raw	1	Blackberries, raw	1
Lima, frozen	variable †	canned	1 †
Lima, canned without		Blueberries, raw	1
added salt	2 †	canned	1 †
Beans, snap, green and yellow		Brazil nuts	2
wax, raw	1	Bread, rye	600 † ‡

* Low-Sodium Diet Committee of Food and Nutrition Board: *Sodium Restricted Diets,* National Research Council, Washington, 1954.

† The estimated sodium values may be altered by various factors such as: (1) a high-sodium packing water in the case of canned foods, (2) quality separation by means of brine in the case of canned and frozen peas, Lima beans, etc., (3) lye peeling (canned peaches, citrus fruits, apricots, tomatoes), (4) variation in the amounts of sodium chloride or sodium-containing compounds added during manufacture (bread, cookies, cheese, meats, etc.).

‡ Variation is to be expected in the estimated sodium content of most foods listed. The sodium content of foods marked "‡" is reported as especially variable, and the estimated values must be taken as approximations.

The figures for canned foods also apply to the glass-packed product.

Many foods are especially prepared for use in low-sodium diets, and their sodium content should be stated on the label.

TABLE 5—BEST ESTIMATES OF SODIUM CONTENT OF FOODS (*Continued*)

FOOD	SODIUM mg/100 gm	FOOD	SODIUM mg/100 gm
Bread (*Continued*)		Swiss, domestic	700 †
rye, unsalted	30 † ‡	Cherries, raw	2
Bread, white, enriched	600 † ‡	frozen	2
white, unsalted	30 † ‡	canned	2 †
Bread, whole-wheat	600 † ‡	Chestnuts	7
whole-wheat, unsalted	30 † ‡	Chicken	75 ‡
Broccoli, raw	15	Chocolate, bitter	10
frozen	15	Cocoa, Dutch process	60 †
Brussels sprouts, raw	12	plain, Hershey	5
frozen	12	Coconut, raw	30
Butter, salted	1000 † ‡	dried, shredded	20
unsalted, or sweet	10 † ‡	Coffee, roasted, dry	2
Buttermilk, cultured	130	Corn, dry, white	1
Cabbage, raw	15	dry, yellow	1
Candy	variable †	sweet, raw	1
Cantaloupe	13	sweet, canned without salt	2 †
Carrots, raw	50	Corn meal	2
canned without salt	35 †	Crackers	variable †
Cashew nuts	13	graham	710
Cauliflower, raw	20	Ry-Krisp	1500
frozen	20	soda	1100
Celery	100	matzoth	variable †
Cereals, dry		matzoth, unsalted, plain	1
All-Bran	1400	Cranberries	1
corn flakes	660	sauce, canned	1 †
Cream of Wheat, plain	2	Cream	40
Cream of Wheat, quick-		Cucumber, raw	5 ‡
cooking, enriched	90	Currants, raw	2
Farina, unsalted	2	dried	20
Grape-Nuts	660	Dates	1
Instant Ralston	1	Duck	85
Maltex	4	Eggs, whole	130
Muffets	4	whites only	150
Pabena	640	yolks only	85
Pablum	620	Eggplant	2
Pettijohn's	2	Figs, raw	2
rice flakes	720	canned	2 †
rice, puffed	1	dried	34
rolled oats	2	Filberts	1
wheat, cracked	1	Fish and Shellfish	
wheat germ, malt-flavored,		bluefish, raw, unsalted	68
Zing	9	catfish, raw, unsalted	60
wheat flakes	1300	codfish, raw, unsalted	65
wheat flakes, unsalted	2	crab, boiled	370
wheat, puffed	4	flounder, raw, unsalted	68
wheat, shredded	2	haddock, raw, unsalted	125
Wheatena	2	halibut, raw, unsalted	56
Chard, raw	100 ‡	herring, raw, unsalted	100
Cheese, Cheddar	700 †	lobster, boiled	250 ‡
cottage	290 †	oysters, raw	variable
cottage, unsalted (curd)	20 †	rockfish, raw, unsalted	45
cream, Philadelphia	250 †	salmon, raw, unsalted	50
process	1500 †		

TABLE 5—BEST ESTIMATES OF SODIUM CONTENT OF FOODS (*Continued*)

FOOD	SODIUM mg/100 gm	FOOD	SODIUM mg/100 gm
Fish and Shellfish, salmon (*Cont.*)		Olives, pickled	2000 †
canned without salt	60 †	Onions	10 ‡
canned	540 †	Oranges	1
sardines, canned	550 † ‡	Orange juice, canned	1
shrimp, raw	140	Parsley, raw	30
tuna, canned	800 †	Parsnips, raw	8
canned without salt	50 †	Peaches, raw	1
Flour; bleached, enriched; whole-		frozen	3
wheat; rye; buckwheat, etc.	2	canned	2 †
Flour, self-rising	1500 †	Peanuts, roasted, unsalted	3
Fruit cocktail, canned	5 †	Peanut butter, prepared without	
Gelatin, plain	30 ‡	added sodium	5 †
dessert, flavored	330 ‡	Pears, raw	2
flavored, without added sodium	10 ‡	canned	2 †
Goose, raw	85 ‡	Peas, raw	2
Grapes	2	frozen	variable †
Grapefruit	1	canned without added salt	2 †
canned	2 †	dried	20 ‡
Grapefruit juice, canned	2 †	Pecans, raw	1
Ham, cured	1100 †	Peppers, green, raw	1
Hominy, canned	250 †	Pineapple, raw	1
Honey	7	frozen	1
Ice cream	90	canned	1 †
Kale	80 ‡	Pineapple juice, canned	1 †
Lamb, lean, raw	90	Plums, raw	1
Lemons, pulp and juice	1	canned	1 †
Lettuce, head	15 ‡	Pork, lean, raw	55
Liver, beef, raw	130 ‡	Potatoes, white, raw	3
chicken, raw	85	Prunes, raw	1
goose, raw	140	canned	3 †
pork, raw	80	dried	6
turkey, raw	50	Prune juice	2
Macaroni, plain	5 ‡	Pumpkin, raw	1
Margarine, salted	1100 †	Rabbit	40
unsalted	10 †	Radish	15 ‡
Mayonnaise, without added		Raisins	25
sodium	25 †	Raspberries, raw	1
Milk, fresh, whole or skim	50	canned	2 †
evaporated, canned	100	Rhubarb, raw	2
skim, dried	525	frozen	2
malted, dry	440	Rice, dry, polished	2
Lesofac (modified low-sodium		Sauerkraut, canned	650 †
milk powder)	13	Shortening (Crisco, Spry,	
Lonalac (modified low-sodium		lard, etc.)	negligible
milk powder)	15	Sirup, corn (Karo)	68
Molasses	40 ‡	maple	14
Mushrooms, raw	5	sorghum	20 ‡
canned without salt	3 †	table blends	60 ‡
Noodles, egg	10	Soybeans, dry	4
Nuts, all, unsalted (average)	4	Spaghetti, plain	5 ‡
Oils (corn, cottonseed, codliver,		Spices and herbs (all spices, with	
olive, peanut, etc.)	negligible	the exceptions of celery seed	
Okra, raw	1	and flakes, and parsley flakes	

TABLE 5—BEST ESTIMATES OF SODIUM CONTENT OF FOODS (*Concluded*)

FOOD	SODIUM mg/100 gm	FOOD	SODIUM mg/100 gm
Spices and herbs (*Continued*)		Tea, blend, dry	4
may be used in low-sodium		Tomatoes, raw	3
diets)		canned without added salt	3 †
Spinach, raw	85 ‡	Tomato juice, canned	230 †
canned without salt	60 † ‡	canned without added salt	5 †
frozen	80 ‡	Turkey, raw	65 ‡
Squash, raw, all types	1	Turnips, white	40 ‡
Starch, corn	4	yellow	5
Strawberries, raw	1	Turnip greens	10
Strawberries, frozen, sweetened	2	Veal, raw	100 ‡
canned	1 †	Vinegar	1
Sugar, white	negligible	Walnuts	2
light brown	25 ‡	Watermelon	1
Sweet potato, raw	5 ‡	Yeast, baker's	3
Tangerines	1	cultured, dry	variable
Tapioca, dry	4		

TABLE 6—POTASSIUM CONTENT OF FOODS *

FOOD	POTASSIUM mg/100 gm	FOOD	POTASSIUM mg/100 gm
Breads, Cereals, and Flours		Crackers	
Barley, pearled	160	graham	330
Bread		pretzel	130
Boston brown	360	Ry-Krisp	600
white, enriched	180	soda	120
whole-wheat	230	Flour	
Cereals		bleached, enriched	82
All-bran	1200	gluten	24
Corn Flakes	160	rye, dark	860
farina	85	whole-wheat	290
Grape-Nuts	230	Macaroni	160
Maltex	250	Matzoth, Passover	140
oats, rolled	340	Rice	
Pettijohn's	380	brown	150
Puffed Rice	100	polished	130
Puffed Wheat	340	Tapioca	19
rice flakes	180		
Shredded Wheat	330	*Dairy Products*	
wheat flakes	320	Butter	23
wheat germ	780	Casein, acid-wash	2
wheat meal	370	low-ash commercial	39
Corn meal, enriched,		Cheese, American Swiss	100
degerminated	120	Cheddar	92
Cornstarch	4	cottage	72

* Values are those reported by C. E. Bills, et al.: "Sodium and Potassium in Foods and Waters. Determination by the Flame Photometer," *J. Am. Dietet. A.*, **25:**304, 1949. In a few instances averages of two or more varieties have been listed.

Values are given for raw foods except as otherwise noted.

TABLE 6—POTASSIUM CONTENT OF FOODS (*Continued*)

FOOD	POTASSIUM mg/100 gm	FOOD	POTASSIUM mg/100 gm
Cheese (*Continued*)		Grape juice	120
cream, Philadelphia	74	Grapefruit	200
process	80	frozen	60
whey, Velveeta	270	Grapefruit juice	150
Cream, whipping	56	Nectarine	320
Egg, white	100	Oranges	170
whole	100	Orange juice	190
yolk	100	Peaches	160
Ice cream	90	canned	31
Milk, buttermilk	140	dried	1100
cow's, condensed	340	frozen	120
evaporated	270	Pears	100
skim	150	canned	52
whole, dry	1100	Pineapple	210
liquid	140	canned	120
human	51	frozen	38
low-sodium (Lonalac)	1300	Pineapple juice	140
malted	720	Plums	170
		canned	110
Fats and Oils		Prunes, fresh	210
		dried	600
Bacon, fried crisp	390	Prune juice	260
Lard	0.2	Raisins	725
Mayonnaise	25	Raspberries, black	190
Oleomargarine	58	red	130
Peanut oil	0.1	Rhubarb	70
Shortening, vegetable	0	Strawberries	180
		Tangerines	110
Fruits and Fruit Juices		Tangerine juice, canned	170
		Watermelon	110
Apples	80		
juice	100	*Meat, Poultry, Fish*	
Apricots	440		
canned	65	Beef	360
dried	1700	corned	60
Avocado	340	dried	200
Banana	420	Brain, pig	340
Blackberry	150	Catfish	330
Blueberry	89	Caviar, salmon	180
Cantaloupe	230	Chicken, breast	320
Cherries, dark	260	leg	250
canned	77	Cod	360
Cherries, light, canned	55	dried	160
Cranberry	65	frozen	400
sauce	17	Crab, canned	110
Currants	160	Duck, breast	360
dried	730	leg	210
Date, semidry	790	Goose	420
Fig	190	Halibut	540
canned	105	Ham	340
dried	780	Hash, corned beef, canned	200
Fruit cocktail, canned	160	Heart, beef	160
Grapes, Concord	84	Kidney, beef	310
Tokay	160		

TABLE 6—POTASSIUM CONTENT OF FOODS (*Continued*)

FOOD	POTASSIUM mg/100 gm	FOOD	POTASSIUM mg/100 gm
Lamb, chop, lean	340	Beans, dry, navy	1300
leg, lean	380	baked, navy	210
Liver, calf	380	green, snap	300
pig	350	canned	120
Lobster, boiled	180	frozen	110
Oyster	110	Lima	680
Pancreas, pig	240	canned	210
Pork, lean	260	frozen	580
salt	27	Beets	350
Salmon	410	canned	120
canned	300	Beet greens	570
Sardines, herring in oil	560	Broccoli	400
pilchards, in tomato sauce	320	frozen	250
Sausage, bologna	230	Brussels sprouts	450
frankfurter	230	frozen	300
pork	140	Cabbage	230
Scallops, frozen	420	Carrots	410
Shrimp	220	canned	110
Thymus, beef	360	Cauliflower	400
Tongue, beef	260	frozen	290
Tuna, canned	240	Celery	300
Turkey, breast	320	Chard, small leaves	380
leg	310	large leaves	720
Veal, lean	330	Cowpeas	560
		Cucumber	230
Nuts		Dandelion greens	430
		Eggplant	190
Almond	690	Endive	400
Brazil nut	670	Kale	410
Chestnut	410	Lentils, dry	1200
Coconut, dry	770	Lettuce, head	140
Filbert	560	Mushrooms	520
Peanut butter	820	canned	150
Peanuts	740	Mustard greens	450
Pecan	420	Onions	55
Walnuts, English	450	Peas	370
		canned	96
Sugars and Sweets		dried, split	880
		frozen	160
Candy, gum drop	18	Peppers	170
milk chocolate	420	Potatoes, white	410
sweet chocolate	230	Pumpkin	480
Honey	10	canned	240
Jam, grape	78	Radish	260
Maple sirup	130	Rutabaga	260
Marmalade, orange	19	Sauerkraut	140
Molasses, cane	1500	Soybeans, dry	1900
Sorghum sirup	600	Squash, summer	175
Sugar, light brown	230	winter	240
white	0.5	Sweet potato	530
		canned	200
Vegetables		Tomatoes	230
		canned	130
Asparagus	240		
canned	130		

TABLE 6—POTASSIUM CONTENT OF FOODS (*Concluded*)

FOOD	SODIUM mg/100 gm	FOOD	SODIUM mg/100 gm
Tomato juice	230	plain	22
Turnip, white	230	Ginger ale	0.6
Turnip greens	440	Pepsi-cola	3
		Root beer	0.5
Miscellaneous		Soup, beef, canned, diluted	
Bouillon cubes	100	for use	100
Brandy	4	Tea, dry	1800
Cider	100	Whisky	1
Coca-Cola	52	Wine	80
Cocoa, plain, Hershey	1400	Yeast, compressed	360
Coffee, regular, dry	1600	brewers' dry	1700
Gelatin, dessert, flavored	210		

TABLE 7—CHOLESTEROL CONTENT OF FOODS *

FOOD	mg per 100 gm	FOOD	mg per 100 gm
Dairy Products		Meat and poultry	
butter	280	*Muscle*	
casein, raw	65	beef round, medium fat	125
cheese		lean	95
American	160	chicken, dark	60
American, processed	155	light	90
Limburger, processed	135	duck	70
Monterey Jack	190	lamb	70
pimento cream, processed	140	pigeon	110
Swiss, processed	145	pork	60
ice cream	65	pork, spareribs	105
milk		rabbit, laboratory	50
skim, dry	4	wild	80
skim, liquid	0.4	veal	65–140
whole	11	*Organ*	
Egg, whole, dried	2140	brain, beef	2235
Egg, whole, fresh	495	heart, beef	145
Egg, whole, frozen	560	rabbit	200
Egg white	0	kidney, beef	405
Egg yolk, dried	2810–3900	liver, beef	260
Egg yolk, fresh	2000	calf	360
Egg yolk, frozen	1330	lamb	610
Fish and seafood		pork	420
cod	50	lung, beef	370
crab †	145	thymus, beef (sweet-	
frog	40	bread)	235–280
mackerel ‡	80	tripe	150
oysters, eastern †	230	Primex †	150
oysters, California †	280–470	Yeast, brewers' †	680
salmon	60		
sardines ‡	70		
shrimp	150		
tuna ‡	65		
turtle	65		

* Compiled chiefly from data by R. Okey: "Cholesterol Content of Food," *J. Am. Dietet. A.,* **21:**341, 1945.

Also: B. Nataf, et al.: "The Cholesterol Content of Cows' Milk," *J. Nutrition,* **36:**495, 1948; and

Geiger, E.: Queries and Minor Notes, *J.A.M.A.,* **139:**194, 1949.

† Total digitonin precipitable sterol. These foods are known to contain sterols other than cholesterol.

‡ Recomputed by authors of this text to approximate raw-food basis from dry-weight figures given by Geiger, cited above.

TABLE 8—AVERAGE WEIGHT FOR HEIGHT TABLE *

(For boys from birth to school age)

HEIGHT (INCHES)	AGE (MONTHS)											
	1	3	6	9	12	18	24	30	36	48	60	72
20	8											
21	9	10										
22	10	11										
23	11	12	13									
24	12	13	14									
25	13	14	15	16								
26		15	17	17	18							
27		16	18	18	19							
28			19	19	20	20						
29			20	21	21	21						
30			22	22	22	22	22					
31				23	23	23	23	24				
32				24	24	24	25	25				
33					26	26	26	26	26			
34						27	27	27	27			
35						29	29	29	29	29		
36							30	31	31	31		
37							32	32	32	32	32	
38								33	33	33	34	
39								35	35	35	35	
40									36	36	36	36
41										38	38	38
42										39	39	39
43										41	41	41
44											43	43
45											45	45
46												48
47												50
48												52
49												55

* Used by the courtesy of the American Child Health Association. Prepared by Robert M. Woodbury.

TABLE 9—AVERAGE WEIGHT FOR HEIGHT TABLE *

(For boys from 5 to 19 years)

HEIGHT (inches)	AGE (YEARS)														
	5	6	7	8	9	10	11	12	13	14	15	16	17	18	19
38	34	34													
39	35	35													
40	36	36													
41	38	38	38												
42	39	39	39	39											
43	41	41	41	41											
44	44	44	44	44											
45	46	46	46	46	46										
46	47	48	48	48	48										
47	49	50	50	50	50	50									
48		52	53	53	53	53									
49		55	55	55	55	55	55								
50		57	58	58	58	58	58	58							
51			61	61	61	61	61	61							
52			63	64	64	64	64	64	64						
53			66	67	67	67	67	68	68						
54				70	70	70	70	71	71	72					
55				72	72	73	73	74	74	74					
56				75	76	77	77	77	78	78	80				
57					79	80	81	81	82	83	83				
58					83	84	84	85	85	86	87				
59						87	88	89	89	90	90	90			
60						91	92	92	93	94	95	96			
61							95	96	97	99	100	103	106		
62							100	101	102	103	104	107	111	116	
63							105	106	107	108	110	113	118	123	127
64								109	111	113	115	117	121	126	130
65								114	117	118	120	122	127	131	134
66									119	122	125	128	132	136	139
67									124	128	130	134	136	139	142
68										134	134	137	141	143	147
69										137	139	143	146	149	152
70										143	144	145	148	151	155
71										148	150	151	152	154	159
72											153	155	156	158	163
73											157	160	162	164	167
74											160	164	168	170	171

* Used by the courtesy of the American Child Health Association. Prepared by Bird T. Baldwin and Thomas D. Wood.

TABLE 10—AVERAGE WEIGHT FOR HEIGHT TABLE *

(For girls from birth to school age)

HEIGHT (INCHES)	AGE (MONTHS)											
	1	3	6	9	12	18	24	30	36	48	60	72
20	8											
21	9	10										
22	10	11										
23	11	12	13									
24	12	13	14	14								
25	13	14	15	15								
26		15	16	17	17							
27		16	17	18	18							
28			19	19	19	19						
29			19	20	20	20						
30			21	21	21	21	21					
31				22	22	23	23	23				
32					23	24	24	24	25			
33						25	25	25	26			
34						26	26	26	27			
35						29	29	29	29	29		
36							30	30	30	30	31	
37							31	31	31	31	32	
38								33	33	33	33	
39								34	34	34	34	34
40									35	36	36	36
41										37	37	37
42										39	39	39
43										40	41	41
44											42	42
45												45
46												47
47												50
48												52

* Used by the courtesy of the American Child Health Association. Prepared by Robert M. Woodbury.

TABLE 11—AVERAGE WEIGHT FOR HEIGHT TABLE *

(For girls from 5 to 18 years)

HEIGHT (INCHES)	AGE (YEARS)													
	5	6	7	8	9	10	11	12	13	14	15	16	17	18
38	33	33												
39	34	34												
40	36	36	36											
41	37	37	37											
42	39	39	39											
43	41	41	41	41										
44	42	42	42	42										
45	45	45	45	45	45									
46	47	47	47	48	48									
47	49	50	50	50	50	50								
48		52	52	52	52	53	53							
49		54	54	55	55	56	56							
50		56	56	57	58	59	61	62						
51			59	60	61	61	63	65						
52			63	64	64	64	65	67						
53			66	67	67	68	68	69	71					
54				69	70	70	71	71	73					
55				72	74	74	74	75	77	78				
56					76	78	78	79	81	83				
57					80	82	82	82	84	88	92			
58					84	86	86	86	88	93	96	101		
59						87	90	90	92	96	100	103	104	
60						91	95	95	97	101	105	108	109	111
61							99	100	101	105	108	112	113	116
62							104	105	106	109	113	115	117	118
63								110	110	112	116	117	119	120
64								114	115	117	119	120	122	123
65								118	120	121	122	123	125	126
66									124	124	125	128	129	130
67									128	130	131	133	133	135
68									131	133	135	136	138	138
69										135	137	138	140	142
70										136	138	140	142	144
71										138	140	142	144	145

* Used by the courtesy of the American Child Health Association. Prepared by Bird T. Baldwin and Thomas D. Wood.

TABLE 12—DESIRABLE WEIGHTS FOR MEN OF AGES 25 AND OVER *

Weight in Pounds According to Frame (In Indoor Clothing)

HEIGHT (with shoes on) 1-inch heels Feet Inches	SMALL FRAME	MEDIUM FRAME	LARGE FRAME
5 2	112–120	118–129	126–141
5 3	115–123	121–133	129–144
5 4	118–126	124–136	132–148
5 5	121–129	127–139	135–152
5 6	124–133	130–143	138–156
5 7	128–137	134–147	142–161
5 8	132–141	138–152	147–166
5 9	136–145	142–156	151–170
5 10	140–150	146–160	155–174
5 11	144–154	150–165	159–179
6 0	148–158	154–170	164–184
6 1	152–162	158–175	168–189
6 2	156–167	162–180	173–194
6 3	160–171	167–185	178–199
6 4	164–175	172–190	182–204

TABLE 13—DESIRABLE WEIGHTS FOR WOMEN OF AGES 25 AND OVER *, †

Weight in Pounds According to Frame (In Indoor Clothing)

HEIGHT (with shoes on) 2-inch heels Feet Inches	SMALL FRAME	MEDIUM FRAME	LARGE FRAME
4 10	92– 98	96–107	104–119
4 11	94–101	98–110	106–122
5 0	96–104	101–113	109–125
5 1	99–107	104–116	112–128
5 2	102–110	107–119	115–131
5 3	105–113	110–122	118–134
5 4	108–116	113–126	121–138
5 5	111–119	116–130	125–142
5 6	114–123	120–135	129–146
5 7	118–127	124–139	133–150
5 8	122–131	128–143	137–154
5 9	126–135	132–147	141–158
5 10	130–140	136–151	145–163
5 11	134–144	140–155	149–168
6 0	138–148	144–159	153–173

* Metropolitan Life Insurance Company, New York.
† For girls between 18 and 25, subtract 1 pound for each year under 25.

TABLE 14—NORMAL CONSTITUENTS OF THE BLOOD IN THE ADULT

Physical measurements		
specific gravity		1.025–1.029
viscosity (water as unity)		4.5
bleeding time (capillary)	min	1–3
prothrombin time (plasma) (Quick)	sec	10–20
sedimentation rate (Wintrobe method)		
men	mm in 1 hr	0–9
women	mm in 1 hr	0–20
Hematologic studies		
cell volume	per cent	39–50
red blood cells	million per cu mm	4.25–5.25
white blood cells	per cu mm	5000–9000
lymphocytes	per cent	25–30
neutrophils	per cent	60–65
monocytes	per cent	4–8
eosinophils	per cent	0.5–4
basophils	per cent	0–1.5
platelets	per cu mm	125,000–300,000
Proteins		
total protein (serum)	gm per 100 ml	6.5–7.5
albumin (serum)	gm per 100 ml	4.5–5.5
globulin (serum)	gm per 100 ml	1.5–2.5
albumin: globulin ratio		1.8–2.5
fibrinogen (plasma)	gm per 100 ml	0.2–0.5
hemoglobin		
males	gm per 100 ml	14–17
females	gm per 100 ml	13–16
Nitrogen constituents		
nonprotein N (serum)	mg per 100 ml	20–36
(whole blood)	mg per 100 ml	25–40
urea (whole blood)	mg per 100 ml	18–38
urea N (whole blood)	mg per 100 ml	8–18
creatinine (whole blood)	mg per 100 ml	1–2
uric acid (whole blood)	mg per 100 ml	2.5–5.0
amino acid N (whole blood)	mg per 100 ml	3–6
Blood gases		
CO_2 content (serum)	volumes per cent	55–75
	mM per liter	(24.5–33.5)
CO_2 content (whole blood)	volumes per cent	40–60
	mM per liter	(18.0–27.0)
oxygen capacity (whole blood)		
males	volumes per cent	18.7–22.7
females	volumes per cent	17.0–21.0
oxygen saturation		
arterial blood	per cent	94–96
venous blood	per cent	60–85
Carbohydrates and lipids		
glucose (whole blood)	mg per 100 ml	70–90
ketones—as acetone (whole blood)	mg per 100 ml	1.5–2
fats (total lipids) (serum)	mg per 100 ml	570–820
cholesterol (serum)	mg per 100 ml	100–230
bilirubin (serum)	mg per 100 ml	0.1–0.25
icteric index (serum)	units	4–6
Acid-base constituents		
base, total fixed (serum)	m.eq. per liter	142–150

TABLE 14—NORMAL CONSTITUENTS OF THE BLOOD (*Concluded*)

Acid-base constituents (Continued)

sodium (serum)	mg per 100 ml	320–335
	m.eq. per liter	(139–146)
potassium (serum)	mg per 100 ml	16–22
	m.eq. per liter	(4.1–5.6)
calcium (serum)	mg per 100 ml	9.0–11.5
	m.eq. per liter	(4.5–5.8)
magnesium (serum)	mg per 100 ml	1.0–3.0
	m.eq. per liter	(1.0–2.5)
phosphorus, inorganic (serum)	mg per 100 ml	3.0–5.0
	m.eq. per liter	(1.0–1.6)
chlorides, expressed as Cl (serum)	mg per 100 ml	352–383
	m.eq. per liter	(99–108)
as NaCl (serum)	mg per 100 ml	580–630
	m.eq. per liter	(99–108)
sulfates, inorganic as SO_4 (serum)	mg per 100 ml	2.5–5.0
	m.eq. per liter	(0.5–1.0)
lactic acid (venous blood)	mg per 100 ml	10–20
	m.eq. per liter	(1.1–2.2)
serum protein base binding power	m.eq. per liter	(15.5–18.0)
base bicarbonate HCO_3 (serum)	m.eq. per liter	(19–30)
pH (blood or plasma at 38° C)		7.3–7.45

Miscellaneous

phosphatase (serum)	Bodansky units per 100 ml	5
iron (whole blood)	mg per 100 ml	46–55
ascorbic acid (whole blood)	mg per 100 ml	0.75–1.50
carotene (serum)	mcg per 100 ml	75–125

ml = milliliters
mg = milligrams   gm = grams
mcg = micrograms   cu mm = cubic millimeters
m.eq. = milli-equivalents

$$\text{m.eq. per liter} = \frac{\text{mg per liter}}{\text{equivalent weight}}$$

$$\text{equivalent weight} = \frac{\text{atomic weight}}{\text{valence of element}}$$

$$\text{mM (millimoles) per liter} = \frac{\text{mg per liter}}{\text{molecular weight}}$$

volumes per cent = mM per liter $\times$ 2.24

TABLE 15—NORMAL CONSTITUENTS OF THE URINE OF THE ADULT

Specific gravity		1.010–1.025
Reaction	pH	5.5–8.0
Volume	ml per 24 hr	800–1600

	gm per 24 hr
Total solids	55–70
Nitrogenous constituents	
total nitrogen	10–17
ammonia	0.5–1.0
amino acid N	0.4–1
creatine	none
creatinine	1–1.5
protein	none
purine bases	0.016–0.060
urea	20–35
uric acid	0.5–0.7
Acetone bodies	0.003–0.015
Bile	none
Calcium	0.2–0.4
Chloride (as NaCl)	10–15
Glucose	none
Indican	0–0.030
Iron	0.001–0.005
Magnesium (as MgO)	0.15–0.30
Phosphate, total (as phosphoric acid)	2.5–3.5
Potassium (as K_2O)	2.0–3.0
Sodium (as Na_2O)	4.0–5.0
Sulfates, total (as sulfuric acid)	1.5–3.0

TABLE 16—MEASURES AND WEIGHTS

3 teaspoons = 1 tablespoon		4 quarts = 1 gallon	
16 tablespoons = 1 cup		2 gallons = 1 peck	
2 cups = 1 pint		4 pecks = 1 bushel	
2 pints = 1 quart		16 ounces = 1 pound	

The following relationships are approximately correct for water and milk.

1 gram = 1 milliliter
1 teaspoon = 5 ml = 5 gm
1 tablespoon = 15 ml = 15 gm = ½ oz
2 tablespoons = 30 ml = 30 gm = 1 oz = ⅛ cup
16 tablespoons = 240 ml = 240 gm = 8 oz = 1 cup
1 kilogram = 2.2 pounds
28.35 grams = 1 ounce (approximate measure is 30 grams)
1 pound = 453.6 gm = approximately 2 cups
To convert ounces to grams, multiply the ounces by 30 (or 28.35)
To convert grams to ounces, divide the grams by 30 (or 28.35)
To convert pounds to kilograms, divide the pounds by 2.2
To convert kilograms to pounds, multiply the kilograms by 2.2

All foods do not weigh or measure alike. The following list shows the weight and measure of some of the most commonly used ones:

2 tablespoons butter	= 1 oz	2 cups rice	= 1 lb
2 cups butter	= 1 lb	2⅔ cups oatmeal	= 1 lb
2 cups granulated sugar	= 1 lb	4¾ cups rolled oats	= 1 lb
2½ cups powdered sugar	= 1 lb	4 tablespoons fat	= 2 oz
4 cups sifted flour	= 1 lb	2 tablespoons sugar	= 1 oz
1 pint milk or water	= 1 lb	4 tablespoons sifted flour	= 1 oz
8 medium-size eggs	= 1 lb	4 tablespoons powdered coffee	= 1 oz
10 eggs (without shells)	= 1 lb		

ABBREVIATIONS

METRIC	HOUSEHOLD	
Kilogram—kg	Teaspoon—tsp or t	Gallon—gal
Liter—l	Tablespoon—tbsp or T	Ounce—oz
Gram—gm	Cup—c	Pound—lb
Milligram—mg	Pint—pt	Peck—pk
Milliliter—ml	Quart—qt	Bushel—bu

TABLE 17—MINIMUM DAILY REQUIREMENTS OF SPECIFIC NUTRIENTS *

	INFANTS	CHIL-DREN years 1–5 in-clusive	CHIL-DREN years 6–11 in-clusive	CHIL-DREN 12 years and over	ADULTS	PREG-NANCY OR LACTA-TION
Calcium, gm	—	0.75	0.75	0.75	0.75	1.50
Phosphorus, gm	—	0.75	0.75	0.75	0.75	1.50
Iron, mg	—	7.5	10.0	10.0	10.0	15.0
Iodine, mg	—	0.1	0.1	0.1	0.1	0.1
Vitamin A, U.S.P. units	1500	3000	3000	4000	4000	
Thiamine, mg	0.25	0.50	0.75	1.00	1.00	
Riboflavin, mg	0.5			2.0	2.0	
Ascorbic acid, mg	10	20	20	30	30	
Vitamin D, U.S.P. units	400	400	400	400	400	

* Food and Drug Administration, Department of Health, Education and Welfare, published under section 403 (j), *Federal Register*, Nov. 22, 1941.

Cited References

1. Agricultural Research Service: *Food Consumption and Dietary Levels of Households in the United States,* ARS 62–6, U.S. Department of Agriculture, Washington, D.C., 1957.
2. Food and Nutrition Board: *Recommended Dietary Allowances—Revised 1958,* Pub. 589, National Academy of Sciences—National Research Council, Washington, D.C., 1958.
3. Clark, F.: "Dietary Levels of Families in the United States," *J. Am. Dietet. A.,* **34:** 378, 1958.
4. Hundley, J. M.: "Malnutrition—A Global Problem," *Federation Proc.,* **18** (No. 2, Part II): 76, 1959.
5. Lusk, G.: *Nutrition.* Paul B. Hoeber, Inc., New York, 1933.
6. McCay, C. M.: "Seven Centuries of Scientific Nutrition," *J. Am. Dietet. A.,* **15:**648, 1939.
7. McCay, C. M., and Todhunter, E. N.: "A Century of Progress in Nutrition," *J. Am. Dietet. A.,* **24:**737, 1948.
8. Rorer, S. T.: "Early Dietetics," *J. Am. Dietet. A.,* **10:**289, 1934.
9. Gilson, H. E.: "Some Historical Notes on the Development of Diet Therapy," *J. Am. Dietet. A.,* **23:**761, 1947.
10. Barber, M. I.: *History of the American Dietetic Association.* J. B. Lippincott Company, Philadelphia, 1959.
11. Pett, L. B.: "Limitations in the Use of Dietary Standards. Differences in American, British, and Canadian Standards," *J. Am. Dietet. A.,* **27:**28, 1951.
12. McHenry, E. W.: *Basic Nutrition.* J. B. Lippincott Company, 1957, p. 227.
13. Food and Agriculture Organization: *Calorie Requirements.* FAO Nutritional Studies, No. 15, Rome, 1957.
14. Food and Agriculture Organization: *Protein Requirements.* FAO Nutritional Studies, No. 16, Rome, 1957.
15. Maynard, L. A.: "Effect of Fertilizers on the Nutritional Value of Foods," *J.A.M.A.,* **161:**1478, 1956.
16. Vickery, H. B.: "The Origin of the Word Protein," *Yale J. Biol. Med.,* **22:**387, 1949.
17. Rose, W. C., et al.: "Further Experiments on the Role of Amino Acids in Human Nutrition," *J. Biol. Chem.,* **148:**457, 1943.
18. Scrimshaw, N. S.: "Progress in Solving World Nutrition Problems," *J. Am. Dietet. A.,* **35:**441, 1959.
19. Elvehjem, C. A.: "Amino Acid Balance in Nutrition," *J. Am. Dietet. A.,* **32:**305, 1956.
20. Staff Report: "Rose Reports Human Amino Acid Requirements," *Chem. Eng. News,* **27:**1364, 1949.
21. Rose, W. C., et al.: "The Amino Acid Requirements of Man. XV. The Valine Requirements; Summary and Final Observations," *J. Biol. Chem.,* **217:**987, 1955.
22. Leverton, R. M., et al.: "The Quantitative Amino Acid Requirements of Young Women," *J. Nutrition,* **58:**59, 83, 219, 341, 355, 1956.

23. Holt, L. E., and Snyderman, S. E.: "The Amino Acid Requirements of Children," in *Some Aspects of Amino Acid Supplementation,* W. H. Cole, ed., Rutgers University Press, Rutgers, 1956, p. 60.

24. Sherman, H. C.: *Chemistry of Food and Nutrition,* 8th ed. The Macmillan Company, New York, 1952.

25. Orr, M. L., and Watt, B. K.: *Amino Acid Content of Foods.* Home Economics Research Report No. 4, U.S. Department of Agriculture, Washington, D.C., 1957.

26. Youmans, J. B.: "The Clinical Detection of Protein Deficiency," *J.A.M.A.,* **128:**439, 1945.

27. Cowgill, G. R., and Anderson, W. E.: "Laxative Effects of Wheat Bran and 'Washed Bran' in Healthy Men. A Comparative Study," *J.A.M.A.,* **98:**1866, 1932.

28. Hardinge, M. G., et al.: "Nutritional Studies of Vegetarians. III. Dietary Levels of Fiber," *Am. J. Clin. Nutrition,* **6:**523, 1958.

29. Agricultural Research Service: *Dietary Levels of Households in the United States,* Household Food Consumption Survey 1955, Report No. 6, U.S. Department of Agriculture, Washington, D.C., 1957, p. 24.

30. Gortner, W. A., ed.: *The Role of Dietary Fat in Human Health,* Pub. 575, Food and Nutrition Board, National Academy of Sciences—National Research Council, Washington, D.C., 1958.

31. Hansen, A. E.: "Essential Fatty Acids in Infant Feeding," *J. Am. Dietet. A.,* **34:**239, 1958.

32. Keys, A., et al.: "Diet and Serum Cholesterol in Man. Lack of Effect of Dietary Cholesterol," *J. Nutrition,* **59:**39, 1956.

33. Committee on Calorie Conversion Factors and Food Composition Tables: *Energy-Yielding Components of Food and Computation of Calorie Values.* Food and Agriculture Organization of the United Nations, Washington, D.C., 1947.

34. Taylor, C. M., and MacLeod, G.: *Rose's Laboratory Handbook of Dietetics,* 5th ed. The Macmillan Company, New York, 1949, p. 73.

35. Passmore, R., and Durnin, J. V. G. A.: "Human Energy Expenditure," *Physiol. Rev.,* **34:**801, 1955.

36. Swift, R. W., et al.: "The Effect of High Versus Low Protein Equicaloric Diets on the Heat Production of Human Subjects," *J. Nutrition,* **65:**89, 1958.

37. Johnston, F. A.: "Calcium Retained by Young Women before and after Adding Spinach to the Diet," *J. Am. Dietet. A.,* **28:**933, 1952.

38. Hegsted, D. M., et al.: "A Study of the Minimum Calcium Requirements of Adult Men," *J. Nutrition,* **46:**181, 1952.

39. Wenger, J., et al.: "The Milk-Alkali Syndrome. Hypercalcemia, Alkalosis, and Temporary Renal Insufficiency during Milk-Antacid Therapy for Peptic Ulcer," *Am. J. Med.,* **24:**161, 1958.

40. Review: "Utilization of Phytin," *Nutrition Rev.,* **6:**202, 1948.

41. Moore, C. V., and Dubach, R.: "Metabolism and Requirements of Iron in the Human," *J.A.M.A.,* **162:**197, 1956.

42. Gubler, C. J.: "Absorption and Metabolism of Iron," *Science,* **123:**87, 1956.

43. Marine, D., and Kimball, O. P.: "Prevention of Goiter in Man," *J.A.M.A.,* **77:**1068, 1921.

44. Astwood, E. B.: "Iodine in Nutrition," *Borden's Review,* **16:**53, 1955.

45. Scrimshaw, N. S.: "Endemic Goiter," *Nutrition Rev.,* **15:**161, 1957.

46. Nelson, W. E.: *Textbook of Pediatrics,* 7th ed. W. B. Saunders Company, 1959, p. 1170.

47. Greer, M. A.: "Goitrogenic Substances in Food," *Am. J. Clin. Nutrition,* **5:**440, 1957.

48. Srinivasan, V., et al.: "Studies on Goitrogenic Agents in Food. I. Goitrogenic Action of Groundnut," *J. Nutrition,* **61:**87, 1957.

49. Review: "Present Knowledge of Fluorine in Nutrition," *Nutrition Rev.,* **5:**322, 1947.

50. Council on Foods and Nutrition: "The Use of Aluminum Cooking Utensils in the Preparation of Foods," *J.A.M.A.,* **146:**477, 1951.

51. Toomey, J. A., and Morissette, R. A.: "Hypervitaminosis A," *Am. J. Dis. Child.,* **73:**473, 1947.

52. Review: "Present Knowledge of Vitamin D in Nutrition," *Nutrition Rev.,* **5:**35, 1947.
53. Council of Foods and Nutrition: "Vitamin Preparations as Dietary Supplements and as Therapeutic Agents," *J.A.M.A.,* **169:**41, 1959.
54. Boyd, J. D.: "Nutrition as It Affects Tooth Decay," *J. Am. Dietet. A.,* **18:**211, 1942.
55. Review: "Osteomalacia Due to Increased Resistance to Vitamin D," *Nutrition Rev.,* **6:**79, 1948.
56. Horwitt, M. K., et al.: "Effects of Limited Tocopherol Intake in Man with Relationships to Erythrocyte Hemolysis and Lipid Oxidations," *Am. J. Clin. Nutrition,* **4:**408, 1956.
57. Hove, E. L., and Harris, P. L.: "Interrelation Between alpha-Tocopherol and Protein Metabolism," *J. Nutrition,* **34:**571, 1947.
58. Harris, P. L., et al.: "Covitamin Studies. VI. Effect of Tocopherol Supplementation on the Output of Vitamin A, Carotene and Fat by Dairy Cows," *J. Nutrition,* **33:**411, 1947.
59. Harris, P. L., et al.: "Vitamin E Content of Foods," *J. Nutrition,* **40:**367, 1950.
60. Williams, R. R.: "The World Beriberi Problem Today," *J. Clin. Nutrition,* **1:**513, 1953.
61. Horwitt, M. K.: "Niacin-Tryptophan Requirements of Man," *J. Am. Dietet. A.,* **34:**914, 1958.
62. Coursin, D. B.: "Convulsive Seizures in Infants with Pyridoxine-Deficient Diet," *J.A.M.A.,* **154:**406, 1954.
63. Glusman, M.: "The Syndrome of 'Burning Feet' (Nutritional Melalgia) as a Manifestation of Nutritional Deficiency," *Am. J. Med.,* **13:**211, 1947.
64. Sydenstricker, V. P.: " 'Egg White Injury' in Man and Its Cure with a Biotin Concentrate," *J.A.M.A.,* **118:**1199, 1942.
65. Magnus-Levy, A., quoted in L. G. Rowntree: "The Water Balance of the Body," *Physiol. Rev.,* **2:**116, 1922.
66. *Breakfast Source Book,* Cereal Institute, Chicago, 1959.
67. Stefferud, A., ed.: *Food, the Yearbook of Agriculture, 1959,* U.S. Department of Agriculture, Washington, D.C., 1959, p. 577.
68. Anliker, J., and Mayer, J.: "The Regulation of Food Intake. Some Experiments Relating Behavioral, Metabolic, and Morphologic Aspects," *Am. J. Clin. Nutrition,* **5:**148, 1957.
69. Montagu, M. F. A.: "Nature, Nurture, and Nutrition," *Am. J. Clin. Nutrition,* **5:**237, 1957.
70. Lee, D.: "Cultural Factors in Dietary Choice," *Am. J. Clin. Nutrition,* **5:**166, 1957.
71. Hacker, D. B., and Miller, E. D.: "Food Patterns of the Southwest," *Am. J. Clin. Nutrition,* **7:**224, 1959.
72. Kaufman, M.: "Adapting Therapeutic Diets to Jewish Food Customs," *Am. J. Clin. Nutrition,* **5:**676, 1957.
73. Torres, R. M.: "Dietary Patterns of the Puerto Rican People," *Am. J. Clin. Nutrition,* **7:**349, 1959.
74. Ramirez, M. E.: "Problems of Nutrition in Mexico," *J. Am. Dietet. A.,* **22:**293, 1946.
75. Cantoni, M.: "Adapting Therapeutic Diets to the Eating Patterns of Italian-Americans," *Am. J. Clin. Nutrition,* **6:**548, 1958.
76. Hepner, R.: "Maternal Nutrition and the Fetus," *J.A.M.A.,* **168:**1774, 1958.
77. Macy, I. G.: "Metabolic and Biochemical Changes in Normal Pregnancy," *J.A.M.A.,* **168:**2265, 1958.
78. Tompkins, W. T., and Wiehl, D. G.: "Nutritional Deficiencies as a Causal Factor in Toxemia and Premature Labor," *Am. J. Obst. & Gynec.,* **62:**898, 1951.
79. Stearns, G.: "Nutritional State of the Mother Prior to Conception," *J.A.M.A.,* **168:**1655, 1958.
80. Warkany, J.: "Production of Congenital Malformations by Dietary Measures (Experiments in Mammals)," *J.A M.A.,* **168:**2020, 1958.
81. Burke, B. S., et al.: "Nutrition Studies During Pregnancy," *Am. J. Obst. & Gynec.,* **46:**38, 1943.

82. McGanity, W. J., et al.: "Vanderbilt Cooperative Study of Maternal and Infant Nutrition. XII. Effect of Reproductive Cycle on Nutritional Status and Requirements," *J.A.M.A.,* **168:**2138, 1958.
83. Review: "The Vitamin Composition of Human Milk," *Nutrition Rev.,* **4:**134, 1946.
84. Rice, F. E.: "Lysine in Milk Proteins in Relation to Infant Needs," *J. Am. Dietet. A.,* **33:**1141, 1957.
85. Wiese, H. F., et al.: "Essential Fatty Acids in Infant Nutrition. I. Linoleic Acid Requirement in Terms of Serum Di-, Tri- and Tetraenoic Acid Levels," *J. Nutrition,* **66:**345, 1958.
86. Stearns, G.: "Infants and Toddlers," in *Food: The Yearbook of Agriculture 1959,* U.S. Department of Agriculture, Washington, D.C., 1959, p. 289.
87. Levine, S. Z.: "Protein Nutrition in Pediatrics," *J.A.M.A.,* **128:**283, 1945.
88. Spock, B.: "Avoiding Behavior Problems," *J. Pediat.,* **27:**363, 1945.
89. Morgan, A. F., ed.: *Nutritional Status, U.S.A.,* Bull. 769, California Agricultural Experiment Station, Berkeley, 1959.
90. Eppright, E. S., et al.: "Very Heavy and Obese School Children in Iowa," *J. Home Econ.,* **48:**168, 1956.
91. Johnson, M. L., et al.: "Relative Importance of Inactivity and Overeating in the Energy Balance of Obese High School Girls," *Am. J. Clin. Nutrition,* **4:**37, 1956.
92. Johnston, J. A.: "Nutritional Problems of Adolescence," *J.A.M.A.,* **137:**1587, 1948.
93. Macy, I. G., and Hunscher, H. A.: "Calories—A Limiting Factor in the Growth of Children," *J. Nutrition,* **45:**189, 1951.
94. Stearns, G.: "Human Requirement of Calcium, Phosphorus and Magnesium," in *Handbook of Nutrition,* The Blakiston Company, Philadelphia, 1951, Chap. 4.
95. Ohlson, M. A., and Stearns, G.: "Calcium Intake of Children and Adults," *Federation Proc.,* **18:**1076, 1959.
96. Beal, V. A.: "Nutritional Intake of Children. II. Calcium, Phosphorus and Iron," *J. Nutrition,* **53:**499, 1954.
97. Lowenberg, M. E.: "Food Preferences of Young Children," *J. Am. Dietet. A.,* **24:**430, 1948.
98. Young, C. M.: "Educating Adolescents and Adults in Proper Diet," Nutrition Symposium of the Melamine Council and Columbia University, New York, 1960.
99. Sandstrom, M. M.: "School Lunches," in *Food: Yearbook of Agriculture 1959,* U.S. Department of Agriculture, Washington, D.C., p. 697.
100. Martin, E. A.: *Robert's Nutrition Work with Children.* University of Chicago Press, Chicago, 1954.
101. Roberts, P. H., et al.: "Nutritional Status of Older Women—Nitrogen, Calcium, Phosphorus Retentions of Nine Women," *J. Am. Dietet. A.,* **24:**292, 1948.
102. Hollifield, G., and Parson, W.: "Overweight in the Aged," *Am. J. Clin. Nutrition,* **7:**127, 1959.
103. Tuohy, E. L.: "Feeding the Aged," *J.A.M.A.,* **121:**42, 1943.
104. Whedon, G. D.: "Effects of High Calcium Intakes on Bones, Blood and Soft Tissue; Relationship of Calcium Intake to Balance in Osteoporosis," *Federation Proc.,* **18:**1112, 1959.
105. "Canned Death," *Time,* Aug. 17, 1959, p. 89.
106. Libdeck, W. L., et al.: "Acute Sodium Fluoride Poisoning," *J.A.M.A.,* **121:**826, 1943.
107. Somers, I. I., and Reed, J. M.: "Promising Developments in Food Preservation," *J. Am. Dietet. A.,* **35:**230, 1959.
108. Welch, H.: "Problem of Antibiotics in Foods," *J.A.M.A.,* **170:**2093, 1959.
109. Food Protection Committee: *The Use of Chemical Additives in Food Processing,* Pub. 398, National Research Council, Washington, D.C., 1956.
110. Black, L. C., and Lewis, M. N.: "Effect on Bacterial Growth of Various Methods of Cooling Cooked Foods," *J. Am. Dietet. A.,* **24:**399, 1948.
111. Hundley, J. M.: "The Under-fed," Nutrition Symposium, Melamine Council, New York, February, 1960.
112. Bosley, B.: "Nutrition in the Indian Health Program," *J. Am. Dietet. A.,* **35:**305, 1959.

113. Janssen, W. F.: "Food Quackery—A Law Enforcement Problem," *J. Am. Dietet. A.,* **36:**110, 1960.
114. Williams, R. R.: "Can We Eradicate the Classical Deficiency Diseases," *J. Am. Dietet. A.,* **36:**31, 1960.
115. *Statements and Decisions of the Council on Foods and Nutrition.* American Medical Association, Chicago, 1957, p. 45.
116. Moore, H. B.: "Psychologic Facts and Dietary Fancies," *J. Am. Dietet. A.,* **28:**789, 1952.
117. Babcock, C. G.: "Problems in Sustaining the Nutritional Care of Patients," *J. Am. Dietet. A.,* **28:**222, 1952.
118. Young, C. M.: "Teaching the Patient Means Reaching the Patient," *J. Am. Dietet. A., 33:*52, 1957.
119. Young, C. M.: "The Interview Itself," *J. Am. Dietet. A.,* **35:**677, 1959.
120. Hildreth, H. M.: "Hunger and Eating," *J. Am. Dietet. A.,* **31:**561, 1955.
121. Caso, E.: "Calculation of Diabetic Diets," *J. Am. Dietet. A.,* **26:**575, 1950.
122. Elman, R.: "Protein Deficiency in Surgical Patients and Its Correction," *J. Am. Dietet. A.,* **18:**141, 1942.
123. Keys, A.: "Human Starvation and Its Consequences," *J. Am. Dietet. A.,* **22:**582, 1946.
124. Benditt, E. P., et al.: "The Dynamics of Protein Metabolism. II. The Relationship between the Level of Protein Intake and the Rate of Protein Utilization by Protein-depleted Men and Rats," *J. Lab. & Clin. Med.,* **33:**269, 1948.
125. Mayer, J.: "An Experimentalist's Approach to the Problem of Obesity," *J. Am. Dietet. A.,* **31:**230, 1955.
126. Young, C. M., et al.: "The Problem of the Obese Patient," *J. Am. Dietet. A.,* **31:**1111, 1955.
127. Mayer, J., and Stare, F. J.: "Exercise and Weight Control. Frequent Misconceptions," *J. Am. Dietet. A.,* **29:**340, 1953.
128. Herrick Memorial Hospital Project: "The Group Approach to Weight Reduction":
    (a) Simmons, W. D.: "I. A Review of the Project," *J. Am. Dietet. A.,* **30:**437, 1954.
    (b) Suczek, R. F.: "II. Psychologic Aspects of Obesity and Group Weight Reduction," *J. Am. Dietet. A.,* **30:**442, 1954.
    (c) Walsh, H. E.: "III. As the Nutritionist Sees It," *J. Am. Dietet. A.,* **30:**447, 1954.
129. Bowser, L., et al.: "Methods of Reducing. Group Therapy vs Individual Clinic Interview," *J. Am. Dietet. A.,* **29:**1193, 1953.
130. Cederquist, D. C., et al.: "Weight Reduction on Low Fat and Low Carbohydrate Diets. I. Clinical Results and Energy Metabolism," *J. Am. Dietet. A.,* **28:**113, 1952.
131. Brewer, W. D., et al.: "Weight Reduction on Low Fat and Low Carbohydrate Diets. II. Utilization of Nitrogen and Calcium," *J. Am. Dietet. A.,* **28:**213, 1952.
132. Young, C.: "Weight Reduction Using a Moderate Fat Diet. Clinical Responses and Energy Metabolism," *J. Am. Dietet. A.,* **28:**410, 1952.
133. Young C.: "Weight Reduction Using a Moderate Fat Diet. Biochemical Responses," *J. Am. Dietet. A.,* **28:**529, 1952.
134. Pennington, A. W.: "An Alternate Approach to the Problem of Obesity," *J. Clin. Nutrition,* **1:**100, 1953.
135. Wilcox, E. B., and Galloway, L. S.: "Children with and without Rheumatic Fever. II. Food Habits," *J. Am. Dietet. A.,* **30:**453, 1954.
136. Getz, H. R.: "Problems in Feeding the Tuberculosis Patient," *J. Am. Dietet. A.,* **30:**17, 1954.
137. Brewer, W. D., et al.: "Calcium and Phosphorus Metabolism of Women with Active Tuberculosis," *J. Am. Dietet. A.,* **30:**21, 1954.
138. Wilson, N. L., et al.: "Nutrition in Tuberculosis," *J. Am. Dietet. A.,* **33:**243, 1957.
139. Crandon, J. H.: "Nutrition in Surgical Patients," *J.A.M.A.,* **158:**264, 1955.
140. Hayes, M. A.: "Postoperative Diet Therapy," *J. Am. Dietet. A.,* **35:**17, 1959.
141. Krehl, W. A.: "Tube Feeding," *J.A.M.A.,* **169:**1153, 1959.
142. Barron, J.: "Preparation of Natural Foods for Tube Feeding," *Henry Ford Hosp. Med. Bull.,* **4:**18 (March) 1956.

143. Zollinger, R. M., and Ellison, E. H.: "Nutrition after Gastric Operations," *J.A.M.A.,* **154:**811, 1954.
144. Lewis, M. N., et al.: "Nutrition following Gastric Resection. I. The Immediate Postoperative Period," *J. Am. Dietet. A.,* **34:**1195, 1958.
145. Levenson, S. M., et al.: "Oral Fat Emulsions in the Feeding of Patients with Severe Burns," *Bull. New York Acad. Sc.,* **56:**37, 1952.
146. Pollack, H., and Halpern, S. L.: *Therapeutic Nutrition,* Food and Nutrition Board, National Research Council, Washington, D.C., 1952, pp. 47–51.
147. Kirsner, J. B.: "Current Status of Therapy in Peptic Ulcer," *J.A.M.A.,* **166:**1727, 1958.
148. Stare, F. J., and Thorn, G. W.: "Protein Nutrition in Problems of Medical Interest," *J.A.M.A.,* **127:**1120, 1945.
149. Sippy, B. W.: "Gastric and Duodenal Ulcers: Medical Cure by an Efficient Removal of Gastric Juice Erosion," *J.A.M.A.,* **64:**1625, 1915.
150. Wolf, S.: "A Critical Appraisal of the Dietary Management of Peptic Ulcer and Ulcerative Colitis," *J. Clin. Nutrition,* **2:**1, 1954.
151. Schneider, M. A., et al.: "The Effect of Spice Ingestion upon the Stomach," *Am. J. Gastroenterology,* **26:**722, 1956.
152. Shull, H. J.: "Diet in the Management of Peptic Ulcer," *J.A.M.A.,* **170:**124, 1959.
153. Meulengracht, E.: "Treatment of Hematemesis and Melena with Food," *Lancet,* **2:**1220, 1935.
154. Schiff, L.: "The Meulengracht Diet in the Treatment of Bleeding Peptic Ulcer," *J. Am. Dietet. A.,* **18:**298, 1942.
155. Andresen, A. F. R.: "Results of Treatment of Massive Gastric Hemorrhage," *Am. J. Digest. Dis.,* **6:**641, 1939.
156. Alvarez, W. C.: "How to Avoid Flare-ups of Peptic Ulcer," *J.A.M.A.,* **125:**903, 1944.
157. Kantor, J. L.: *Synopsis of Digestive Diseases.* The C. V. Mosby Company, St. Louis, 1937.
158. Hosoi, K., et al.: "Intestinal Absorption. A Search for a Low Residue Diet," *Arch. Int. Med.,* **41:**112, 1928.
159. Kirsner, J. B., and Palmer, W. L.: "The Irritable Colon," *Gastroenterology,* **34:**491, 1958.
160. Machella, T. E.: "Medical Aspects of Pancreatitis," *J.A.M.A.,* **169:**1571, 1959.
161. Review: "Cortisone and ACTH in Nontropical Sprue," *Nutrition Rev.,* **10:**169, 1952.
162. Mike, E. M.: "Practical Dietary Management of Patients with the Celiac Syndrome," *Am. J. Clin. Nutrition,* **35:**1184, 1959.
163. Berger, F. M.: "Diet in Infectious Hepatitis," *J. Am. Dietet. A.,* **22:**210, 1946.
164. Hoagland, C. L., et al.: "An Analysis of the Effect of Fat in the Diet on Recovery in Infectious Hepatitis," *Am. J. Pub. Health,* **36:**1287, 1946.
165. Davidson, C. S.: "Cirrhosis of the Liver Treated with Prolonged Sodium Restriction. Improvement in Nutrition, Hepatic Function, and Portal Hypertension," *J.A.M.A.,* **159:**1257, 1955.
166. Hundley, J. M.: "Diabetes—Overweight: U.S. Problems," *J. Am. Dietet. A.,* **32:**417, 1956.
167. Daughaday, W. H.: "Dietary Treatment of Adults with Diabetes Mellitus," *J.A.M.A.,* **167:**859, 1958.
168. Cohen, A. S.: "Current Concepts in Diabetes Mellitus," *J. Am. Dietet. A.,* **32:**102, 1956.
169. "ADA Meal Plans No. 1 through 9," The American Dietetic Association, Chicago, 1956.
170. Sobel, G. W., and Levine, R.: "Sulfonylureas in Diabetes Mellitus," *J. Am. Dietet. A.,* **34:**1072, 1958.
171. Conn, J. W.: "The Dietary Management of Spontaneous Hypoglycemia," *J. Am. Dietet. A.,* **23:**108, 1947.
172. Beeuwkes, A. M.: "The Dietary Treatment of Functional Hyperinsulinism," *J. Am. Dietet. A.,* **18:**731, 1942.

173. Conn, J. W.: "The Advantage of a High Protein Diet in the Treatment of Spontaneous Hypoglycemia," *J. Clin. Investigation,* **15:**673, 1936.

174. Puppel, I. D.: "Some Metabolic Factors in the Treatment of Hyperthyroidism," *Ann. Int. Med.,* **48:**1300, 1958.

175. Harkavy, J.: "Allergic Factors in Gout," *J.A.M.A.,* **139:**75, 1949.

176. Robinson, W. D.: "Nutrition and Joint Disease," *J.A.M.A.,* **166:**253, 1958.

177. Bartels, E. C.: "Gout—Now Amenable to Control," *Ann. Int. Med.,* **42:**1, 1955.

178. Brozek, J.: "Psychologic Effects of Thiamine Restriction and Deprivation in Normal Young Men," *Am. J. Clin. Nutrition,* **5:**109, 1957.

179. Jolliffe, N., et al.: "The Experimental Production of Vitamin B₁ Deficiency in Normal Subjects," *Am. J. Med. Sc.,* **198:**198, 1939.

180. Williams, R. D., et al.: "Observations on Induced Thiamine Deficiency in Man," *Arch. Int. Med.,* **66:**785, 1940.

181. Hussar, A. E., and Sturdevant, J. E.: "An Advisory Committee Considers Dietetic Problems in a Psychiatric Hospital," *J. Am. Dietet. A.,* **32:**1188, 1956.

182. Peterman, M. G.: "Epilepsy in Childhood; Newer Methods of Diagnosis and Treatment," *J.A.M.A.,* **138:**1012, 1948.

183. Hughes, J. G., and Jabbour, J. T.: "The Treatment of the Epileptic Child," *J. Pediat.,* **53:**66, 1958.

184. Fay, T.: "Symposium on Epilepsy: Therapeutic Effects of Dehydration," *Internat. Clin.,* **3:**78, 1930.

185. Keys, A.: "Diet and the Epidemiology of Coronary Heart Disease," *J.A.M.A.,* **164:**1912, 1957.

186. White, P. L.: "Dietary Fads in Heart Disease," *Illinois Med. J.,* **116:**308, 1959.

187. Brozek, J., et al.: "Drastic Food Restriction. Effect on Cardiovascular Dynamics in Normotensive and Hypertensive Conditions," *J.A.M.A.,* **137:**1569, 1948.

188. Newburgh, L. H., and Reimer, A.: "The Rationale and Administration of Low-Sodium Diets," *J. Am. Dietet. A.,* **23:**1047, 1947.

189. Council on Foods: "Low Sodium Milk," *J.A.M.A.,* **163:**739, 1957.

190. Kempner, W.: "Rice Diet in the Treatment of Hypertension and Vascular Diseases," *North Carolina M.J.,* **5:**125, 225, 1944; **6:**61, 117, 1945.

191. Smith, H. W.: *Lectures on the Kidney,* University Extension Division, University of Kansas, Lawrence, Kan., 1943.

192. Zimmerman, H. J.: "Nutritional Aspects of Acute Glomerulonephritis," *Am. J. Clin. Nutrition,* **4:**482, 1956.

193. Danowski, T. S.: "Low-Sodium Diets. Physiological Adaptation and Clinical Usefulness," *J.A.M.A.,* **168:**1886, 1958.

194. Borst, J. C. G.: "Protein Katabolism in Uraemia. Effects of Protein-Free Diets, Infections and Blood Transfusions," *Lancet,* **1:**824, 1948.

195. McDonald, D. F.: "Medical Management of Recurrent Urinary Calculi," *New York J. Med.,* **59:**4212, 1959.

196. Kushner, D. S.: "Calcium and the Kidney," *Am. J. Clin. Nutrition,* **4:**561, 1956.

197. Castle, W. B.: "Observations on the Etiologic Relationship of Achylia Gastrica to Pernicious Anemia," *Am. J. Med. Sc.,* **178:**748, 1929.

198. Frenchman, R., and Johnston, F. A.: "Relation of Menstrual Losses to Iron Requirement," *J. Am. Dietet. A.,* **25:**217, 1949.

199. Whipple, G. H.: "Experimental Anemias, Diet Factors and Related Pathologic Changes of Human Anemias," *J.A.M.A.,* **91:**863, 1928.

200. Moore, C. V.: "The Importance of Nutritional Factors in the Pathogenesis of Iron Deficiency Anemia," *Am. J. Clin. Nutrition,* **3:**3, 1955.

201. Murphy, W. P., and Minot, G. R.: "A Special Diet for Patients with Pernicious Anemia," *Boston M. & S.J.,* **195:**410, 1926.

202. Rabinovitch, R. D., and Fischoff, J.: "Feeding Children to Meet Their Emotional Needs," *J. Am. Dietet. A.,* **28:**614, 1952.

203. Lee, H. J., and Squier, T. L.: "Recognition of Food Allergy," *J.A.M.A.,* **142:**318, 1950.

204. Leibowitz, H., et al.: "Importance of Foods in Patients as Determined by Skin Testing and Intentional Feeding," *J.A.M.A.,* **144:**990, 1950.

205. Olmsted, W. H., et al.: "Use of Synthetic Diets for Food Allergy and Typhoid," *Arch. Int. Med.,* **73:**341, 1944.
206. Rowe, P., and Sheldon, J. M.: "Synthetic Diets—Their Use as a Diagnostic Procedure in Allergic Disease," *J. Lab. & Clin. Med.,* **33:**1059, 1948.
207. Bruch, H.: "Dietary Treatment of Obesity in Childhood," *J. Am. Dietet. A.,* **20:**361, 1944.
208. Nelson, W. E.: *Textbook of Pediatrics,* 7th ed. W. B. Saunders Company, Philadelphia, 1959, p. 723.
209. Review: "Wheat Gluten and the Celiac Syndrome," *Nutrition Rev.,* **11:**199, 1953.
210. Sheldon, W., and Lawson, D.: "Management of Coeliac Disease," *Lancet,* **2:**902, 1952.
211. Anderson, C. M., et al.: "Coeliac Disease, Gastrointestinal Studies and Effect of Dietary Wheat Flour," *Lancet,* **1:**836, 1952.
212. Marble, A.: "The Future of the Child with Diabetes. Educational Value of Summer Camps," *J. Am. Dietet. A.,* **33:**569, 1957.
213. Jackson, R. L.: "Nutritional Management of Children with Diabetes Mellitus," *J.A.M.A.,* **168:**42, 1958.
214. Jacobi, H. G.: "Nutritional Studies of Juvenile Diabetics Attending Summer Camp," *J. Clin. Nutrition,* **2:**22, 1954.
215. Zellweger, H. U.: "Enzyme Deficiency Diseases. II. Phenylketonuria," *J. Am. Dietet. A.,* **34:**1045, 1958.
216. Orr, M. L., and Watt, B. K.: *Amino Acid Content of Foods.* Home Economics Research Report No. 4, U.S. Department of Agriculture, Washington, 1957.
217. Hill, L. W.: "Amino Acids as a Source of Nitrogen for Allergic Infants," *J.A.M.A.,* **116:**2133, 1941.
218. Ziegler, M. R.: "Mineral-Enriched Meats for Diets of Infants Requiring a Milk Substitute," *J. Am. Dietet. A.,* **29:**660, 1953.
219. Phelps, W. M.: "Dietary Requirements in Cerebral Palsy," *J. Am. Dietet. A.,* **27:**869, 1951.
220. Zickefoose, M.: "Feeding the Child with a Cleft Palate," *J. Am. Dietet. A.,* **36:**129, 1960.
221. Walker, G. A.: "Nutrition in Mentally Deficient Children," *J. Am. Dietet. A.,* **31:**494, 1955.
222. Adair, R.: "Home Care and Feeding of a Mentally Retarded Child," *J. Am. Dietet. A.,* **36:**133, 1960.
223. Kolmer, J. A.; Spaulding, E. H.; and Robinson, H. W.: *Approved Laboratory Technic,* 5th ed. Appleton-Century-Crofts, Inc., New York, 1951.
224. Wright, F.: "Two-Hour Renal Test—Technic and Information Obtained from the Mosenthal Modification of the Hedinger-Schlayer Test," *M. Clin. Chicago,* **2:**1029, 1917.
225. Cutler, H. H., et al.: "Concentrations of Chloride, Sodium, and Potassium in Urine and Blood; Their Diagnostic Significance in Adrenal Insufficiency," *J.A.M.A.,* **111:**117, 1938.
226. Albright, F.: *The Parathyroid Glands and Metabolic Bone Disease.* The Williams and Wilkins Company, Baltimore, 1948, p. 75.
227. Westerfeld, W. W., and Schulman, M. P.: "Metabolism and Caloric Value of Alcohol," *J.A.M.A.,* **170:**197, 1959.
228. Macy, I. G., et al.: *The Composition of Milks.* Pub. 254, Natl. Res. Council, Washington, D.C., 1953.
229. Brody, S., and Sadhu, D. P.: "The Nutritional Significance of Milk with Special Reference to Milk Sugar," *Scient. Monthly,* **64:**5, 1947.
230. *Milk Ordinance and Code,* Public Health Bulletin No. 229, U.S. Public Service, Washington, D.C., 1953.
231. Schjeide, O. A., and Urist, M. R.: "Nutritional Aspects of Egg Yolk," *Nutrition Rev.,* **17:**3, 1959.
232. Human Nutrition Research Branch: *Cooking with Dried Egg.* Home and Garden Bulletin No. 50, U.S. Department of Agriculture, Washington, D.C., 1956.

233. Behar, M., et al.: "Principles of Treatment and Prevention of Severe Protein Malnutrition in Children (Kwashiorkor)," *Ann. N.Y. Acad. Sci.,* **69:**954, 1958.
234. *Consumption of Food in the United States 1909–52,* Agriculture Handbook No. 62, and *Supplement for 1956,* U.S. Department of Agriculture, Washington, D.C.
235. Widdowson, E. M., and McCance, R. A.: "Studies on the Nutritive Value of Bread and on the Effect of Variations in the Extraction Rate of Flour on the Growth of Undernourished Children," Her Majesty's Stationary Office, Privy Council, Medical Research Council Special Report Series No. 287, London, 1954.
236. *Bread—Facts for Consumer Education,* AIB No. 142, U.S. Department of Agriculture, Washington, D.C., 1955.
237. Bradley, W. B.: "Breads for Special Dietary Purposes," Am. Institute of Baking, Chicago, 1953.
238. Vail, G. E.: "Cooking with Fats High in Polyunsaturated Fatty Acids," *J. Am. Dietet. A.,* **35:**119, 1959.
239. *Agricultural Outlook Charts 1959,* U.S. Department of Agriculture, Washington, D.C., 1958.
240. Anderson, A. W.: "Fish and the Fishing Industry," in *Food, the Yearbook of Agriculture 1959,* U.S. Department of Agriculture, 1959, p. 357.
241. Leverton, R. M., and Odell, G. V.: *The Nutritive Value of Cooked Meat.* Misc. Pub. MP-49, Oklahoma Agricultural Experiment Station, Oklahoma State University, 1958.

Additional References

One of the important objectives in any course in nutrition is to acquaint the student with authentic resource materials and to encourage the habit of reading beyond the requirements of a given course. During the introductory course in nutrition, reading assignments in addition to those of the text will be limited in number and carefully selected for their difficulty.

The references listed below vary widely in their difficulty and may be used in a wide variety of programs. Nursing students who are having clinical experience in therapeutic nutrition should be encouraged to read a number of articles pertaining to normal and therapeutic nutrition, to food habits, to methods of teaching patients, and so on. College students may use the text as a basis for course work in nutrition and supplement this material with readings in the principles of nutrition and their practical application.

GENERAL REFERENCES

Nutrition

Bogert, L. J.: *Nutrition and Physical Fitness,* 7th ed. W. B. Saunders Company, Philadelphia, 1960.

Burton, B.: *The Heinz Handbook of Nutrition.* McGraw-Hill Publishing Company, New York, 1959.

Byrd, O. E.: *Nutrition Sourcebook.* Stanford University Press, Stanford, California, 1955.

Chaney, M. S.: *Nutrition,* 6th ed. Houghton Mifflin Company, Boston, 1960.

Cooper, L. F.; Barber, E. M.; Mitchell, H. S.; and Rynbergen, H. J.: *Nutrition in Health and Disease,* 13th ed. J. B. Lippincott Company, Philadelphia, 1958.

Council on Foods and Nutrition, the American Medical Association: *Handbook of Nutrition,* 2nd ed. The Blakiston Company, Philadelphia, 1951.

Crampton, E. W., and Lloyd, L. E.: *Fundamentals of Nutrition.* W. H. Freeman and Company, San Francisco, 1959.

Davidson, S.; Meiklejohn, A. P.; and Passmore, R.: *Human Nutrition and Dietetics.* The Williams and Wilkins Company, Baltimore, 1959.

Fleck, H., and Munves, E. D.: *Everybody's Book of Modern Diet and Nutrition,** 2nd ed. Dell Publishing Company, New York, 1959.

Goodhart, R. S.: *Nutrition for You.** E. P. Dutton Company, New York, 1958.

Graubard, M.: *Man's Food: Its Rhyme or Reason.* The Macmillan Company, New York, 1943.

Hawley, E. E.; Carden, G.; and Munves, E. D.: *The Art and Science of Nutrition,* 4th ed. The C. V. Mosby Company, St. Louis, 1955.

Johnson, D.: *Modern Dietetics.* G. P. Putnam's Sons, New York, 1951.

Krause, M. V.: *Nutrition and Diet Therapy,* 2nd ed. W. B. Saunders Company, Philadelphia, 1957.

* Books marked with an asterisk are intended especially for lay readers.

Leverton, R. M.: *Food Becomes You,** 2nd ed. Iowa State University Press, Ames, 1960.

McHenry, E. W.: *Basic Nutrition.* J. B. Lippincott Company, Philadelphia, 1957.

McHenry, E. W.: *Foods without Fads.** J. B. Lippincott Company, Philadelphia, 1960.

McLester, J. S., and Darby, W. J.: *Nutrition and Diet in Health and Disease,* 6th ed. W. B. Saunders Company, Philadelphia, 1952.

Mitchell, K., and Bernard, M. C.: *Food in Health and Disease,* 6th ed. F. A. Davis Company, Philadelphia, 1958.

Mowry, L.: *Nutrition and Diet Therapy for Practical Nurses.* The C. V. Mosby Company, St. Louis, 1958.

Nasset, E. S.: *Food and You,** 2nd ed. Barnes and Noble, Inc., New York, 1958.

Peyton, A. B.: *Practical Nutrition.** J. B. Lippincott Company, Philadelphia, 1957.

Present Knowledge of Nutrition, 2nd ed. The Nutrition Foundation, New York, 1956.

Sherman, H. C.: *Chemistry of Food and Nutrition,* 8th ed. The Macmillan Company, New York, 1952.

Sherman, H. C., and Lanford, C. S.: *Essentials of Nutrition,** 4th ed. The Macmillan Company, New York, 1957.

Stefferud, A., ed.: *Food—The Yearbook of Agriculture, 1959.** U.S. Department of Agriculture, Washington, D.C., 1959.

Stevenson, G. T., and Miller, C.: *Introduction to Foods and Nutrition.* John Wiley and Sons, New York, 1960.

Taylor, C. M.; Macleod, G.; and Rose, M. S.: *Foundations of Nutrition,* 5th ed. The Macmillan Company, New York, 1956.

Wilson, E. D.; Fisher, K. H.; and Fuqua, M. E.: *Principles of Nutrition.* John Wiley and Sons, New York, 1960.

Wohl, M. G., and Goodhart, R. S.: *Modern Nutrition in Health and Disease,* 2nd ed. Lea & Febiger, Philadelphia, 1960.

Physiology

Best, C. H., and Taylor, N. B.: *The Physiological Basis of Medical Practice,* 6th ed. The Williams & Wilkins Company, Baltimore, 1955.

Greisheimer, E. M.: *Physiology and Anatomy,* 7th ed. J. B. Lippincott Company, Philadelphia, 1955.

Kimber, D. C.; Gray, C. E.; Stackpole, C. E.; and Leavell, L. C.: *Anatomy and Physiology,* 14th ed. The Macmillan Company, New York, 1961.

Ruch, T. C., and Fulton, J. F.: *Medical Physiology and Biophysics,* 18th ed. W. B. Saunders Company, Philadelphia, 1960.

Physiological chemistry

Cantarow, A., and Schepartz, B.: *Biochemistry,* 2nd ed. W. B. Saunders Company, Philadelphia, 1957.

Francis, C. A., and Morse, E. C.: *Fundamentals of Chemistry and Applications,* 4th ed. The Macmillan Company, New York, 1956.

Harper, H. A.: *Review of Physiological Chemistry,* 7th ed. Lange Medical Publications, Los Altos, California, 1959.

Peterson, W. H., and Strong, F. M.: *General Biochemistry.* Prentice-Hall, Inc., New York, 1953.

West, E. S., and Todd, W. R.: *Textbook of Biochemistry,* 3rd ed. The Macmillan Company, New York, 1961.

Journals

American Journal of Clinical Nutrition
American Journal of Digestive Diseases
American Journal of Diseases of Children
American Journal of Nursing
Annual Review of Biochemistry

Biological Abstracts—Nutrition Division
Borden's Review of Nutrition Research
Chemical Abstracts—Nutrition Division
Federation Proceedings
Food Research
Food Technology
Journal of the American Dietetic Association
Journal of the American Medical Association
Journal of Biological Chemistry
Journal of Home Economics
Journal of Nutrition
Metabolism
Nutrition Abstracts and Reviews
Nutrition Reviews
Physiological Reviews
Public Health Nursing
Public Health Reports
Science
Vitamins and Hormones
U.S. Department of Agriculture: numerous bulletins

SPECIAL REFERENCES

Chapter 1. Food and its relation to health

Brody, S.: "Facts, Fables, and Fallacies on Feeding the World Population," *Federation Proc.,* **11:**681, 1952.
Gerard, R. W.: *Food for Life.* University of Chicago Press, Chicago, 1952.
Goldsmith, G. A.: "Nutrition in Medicine," *Federation Proc.,* **17** (2):734, 1958.
Goodhart, R. S.: "Some Comments on the American Diet and Household Consumption Data," *Am. J. Clin. Nutrition,* **7:**508, 1959.
McCann, M. B., and Trulson, M. F.: "Our Changing Diet," *J. Am. Dietet. A.,* **33:**358, 1958.
Stiebeling, H. K.: "Food and Nutrient Consumption Trends and Consumer Problems," *Federation Proc.,* **17** (2):770, 1958.
Stitt, K.: "Nutritive Value of Diets Today and Fifty Years Ago," *J. Am. Dietet. A.,* **36:**433, 1960.
Todhunter, E. N.: "Role of the Home Economist and Dietitian," *Federation Proc.,* **17** (2):746, 1958.
Wells, O.V.: "Agricultural Trends and Programs," *Federation Proc.,* **17** (2):761, 1958.
See also references #1–4, page 791.

Chapter 2. History of nutrition

Arrington, L. R.: "Foods of the Bible," *J. Am. Dietet. A.,* **35:**816, 1959.
Barber, E. M.: "The Development of the American Food Pattern," *J. Am. Dietet. A.,* **24:**586, 1948.
Carpenter, T. M.: "The Historical Development of Metabolism Studies," *J. Am. Dietet. A.,* **25:**837, 1949.
Cooper, L. F.: "Florence Nightingale's Contribution to Dietetics," *J. Am. Dietet. A.,* **30:**121, 1954.
Cummings, R. O.: *The American and His Food.* University of Chicago Press, Chicago, 1941.
Jaffe, B.: *Crucibles.* Simon and Schuster, Inc., New York, 1930.
McCollum, E. V.: *A History of Nutrition.* Houghton Mifflin Company, Boston, 1957.
———: "An Adventure in Nutrition Investigation," *J. Am. Dietet. A.,* **35:**806, 1959.
Prentice, E. P.: *Hunger and History.* Harper & Brothers, New York, 1939.

Smallzreid, K. A.: *The Everlasting Pleasure.* Appleton-Century-Crofts, Inc., 1956.

Todhunter, E. N.: "Biographical Sketches," *J. Am. Dietet. A.* These excellent concise sketches appear each month.

Van Syckle, C.: "Some Pictures of Food Consumption in the United States. I. 1630–1860," *J. Am. Dietet. A.,* **21:**508, 1945; *ibid.,* "II. 1860–1941," *J. Am. Dietet. A.,* **21:** 690, 1945.

See also references #5–10, page 791.

Chapter 3. Dietary guides and their uses

Food for Fitness—A Daily Food Guide. Leaflet No. 424, Institute of Home Economics, U.S. Department of Agriculture, Washington, D.C., 1958.

Food and Nutrition Board: *Recommended Dietary Allowances—Revised 1958,* Pub. 589, National Research Council, Washington, D.C., 1958.

Heineman, H. E. O., and Bennett, E.: "The Uses of the Recommended Dietary Allowances by the Food Industry," *Am. J. Pub. Health,* **49:**1013, 1959.

Page, L., and Phipard, E. E.: *Essentials of an Adequate Diet.* Pub. ARS 62-4, U.S. Department of Agriculture, Washington, D.C., 1956.

Roberts, L. J.: "Beginnings of the Recommended Dietary Allowances," *J. Am. Dietet. A.,* **34:**903, 1958.

Shank, R. E.: "Revised Recommended Dietary Allowances—1958," *J. Am. Dietet. A.,* **34:**909, 1958.

See also references #11–15, page 791.

Tables of food composition

Bowes, A. deP., and Church, C. E.: *Food Values of Portions Commonly Used,* 8th ed. A. deP. Bowes, 7th and Delancey Sts., Philadelphia, 1956.

Goddard, V. R., and Goodall, L.: *Fatty Acids in Food Fats.* Home Economics Research Report No. 7, U.S. Department of Agriculture, Washington, D.C., 1959.

Nutritional Data, 3rd ed. H. J. Heinz Company, Pittsburgh, 1959.

Orr, M. L., and Watt, B. K.: *Amino Acid Content of Foods.* Home Economics Research Report No. 4, U.S. Department of Agriculture, Washington, D.C., 1957.

Taylor, C. M., and Macleod, G.: *Rose's Laboratory Handbook of Dietetics,* 6th ed. The Macmillan Company, New York, 1955.

Watt, B. K., and Merrill, A. L.: *Composition of Foods—Raw, Processed, Prepared.* Handbook No. 8, U.S. Department of Agriculture, Washington, D.C., 1950.

Chapter 4. Proteins and amino acids

Allison, J. B.: "Nitrogen Balance and the Nutritive Value of Proteins," *J.A.M.A.,* **164:** 283, 1957.

Autret, M., and van Veen, A. G.: "Possible Sources of Proteins for Child Feeding in Underdeveloped Countries," *Am. J. Clin. Nutrition,* **3:**234, 1955.

Block, R. J., and Weiss, K. W.: *Amino Acid Handbook.* Charles C. Thomas, Springfield, Illinois, 1956.

Flodin, N. W.: "Amino Acids and Proteins. Their Place in Human Nutrition Problems," *J. Ag. Food Chem.,* **1:**222, 1953.

Food and Nutrition Board: *Evaluation of Protein Nutrition.* Pub. 711, Nat. Acad. Sci., National Research Council, Washington, D.C., 1960.

Hartman, R. H., and Rice, E. E.: "Supplementary Relationships of Proteins," *J. Am. Dietet. A.,* **35:**34, 1958.

Hegsted, D. M.: "Theoretical Estimates of the Protein Requirements of Children," *J. Am. Dietet. A.,* **33:**225, 1957.

Howe, E. E.: "Amino Acid Supplementation," *Borden's Rev.,* **19:**19, 1958.

Jelliffe, D. B.: "Protein-Calorie Malnutrition in Tropical Pre-School Children," *J. Pediat.,* **54:**227, 1959.

Lewis, H. B.: "Fifty Years of Study of the Role of Protein in Nutrition," *J. Am. Dietet. A.,* **28:**701, 1952.

Nasset, E. S.: "Role of the Digestive Tract in the Utilization of Protein and Amino Acids," *J.A.M.A.,* **164:**172, 1957.

Olson, R. E.: "Role of Hormones in Protein Metabolism," *J.A.M.A.,* **164:**1758, 1957.

Prier, R. F., and Derse, P. H.: "Nutritive Value of a Vegetable Protein Mixture," *J. Am. Dietet. A.,* **33:**1034, 1957.

Reynolds, M. S.: "Amino Acid Requirements of Adults," *Am. J. Clin. Nutrition,* **6:**439, 1958.

Stare, F. J., Chairman: *Protein Nutrition.* A Monograph. *Ann. N. Y. Acad. Sci.,* **69:**855, 1958.

Williams, H. H.: "Amino Acid Requirements," *J. Am. Dietet. A.,* **35:**929, 1959.

See also references #16–26, page 791.

Chapter 5. Carbohydrates

Beinert, F. L.: "Growth on Cereal and Milk Diet," *J. Home Econ.,* **44:**119, 1952.

Council on Foods and Nutrition: "Some Nutritional Aspects of Sugar, Candy, and Sweetened Carbonated Beverages," *J.A.M.A.,* **120:**763, 1942.

Duncan, D. L.: "The Physiological Effect of Lactose," *Nutrition Abstracts and Rev.,* **25:**309, 1955.

Hoppert, C. A., and Clark, A. J.: "Digestibility and Effect on Laxation of Crude Fiber and Cellulose in Certain Common Foods," *J. Am. Dietet. A.,* **21:**157, 1945.

Krehl, W. A.: "The Nutritional Significance of the Carbohydrates," *Borden's Rev.,* **16:**85, 1955.

Parks, V. B., et al.: "Developing Bread of Higher Nutritive Value," *J. Am. Dietet. A.,* **30:**245, 1954.

Williams, R. R.: "Progress in Cereal Enrichment," *J. Am. Dietet. A.,* **27:**293, 1951.

See also references #27, 28, page 792.

Chapter 6. Fats and fatlike substances

Beveridge, J. M. R.: "Role of Dietary Fat in Human Nutrition. II. Role of Unsaturated Fat in Adult Nutrition," *Am. J. Pub. Health,* **47:**1370, 1957.

Bloor, W. R.: "Fat Metabolism in the Early 1900's," *Nutrition Rev.,* **10:**193, 1952.

Brewer, W. D., and Arnrich, L.: "The Role of Fat in the Diet," *J. Home Econ.,* **50:**269, 1958.

Coons, C. M.: "Fatty Acids in Foods," *J. Am. Dietet. A.,* **34:**242, 1958.

Frederickson, D. S.: "Some Biochemical Aspects of Lipid and Lipoprotein Metabolism," *J.A.M.A.,* **164:**1895, 1957.

Griffith, W. H.: "Fats in the Diet," *J.A.M.A.,* **164:**411, 1957.

Hampton, M. C., and Lee, M.: "A Study of Fat Intake and Plasma Lipids," *J. Am. Dietet. A.,* **37:**562, 1960.

Hayes, O. B., and Rose, G.: "Supplementary Food Composition Table," *J. Am. Dietet. A.,* **33:**26, 1957.

Holt, L. E.: "Dietary Fat—Its Role in Nutrition and Human Requirement," *J.A.M.A.,* **164:**1890, 1957.

Olson, R. E.: "Role of Dietary Fat in Human Nutrition," *Am. J. Pub. Health,* **47:**1537, 1957.

Review: "Cholesterol in Diet and Serum," *Nutrition Rev.,* **16:**42, 1958.

Review: "Fatty Acids and Cholesterol Metabolism," *Nutrition Rev.,* **16:**81, 1958.

Vail, G. E.: "Cooking with Fats High in Polyunsaturated Fatty Acids," *J. Am. Dietet. A.,* **35:**119, 1959.

Van Itallie, T. B.: "Role of Dietary Fat in Human Nutrition. IV. Experimental and Clinical Evidence Relating to the Effect of Dietary Fat upon Health in Man," *Am. J. Pub. Health,* **47:**1530, 1957.

Wiese, H. F., et al.: "Essential Fatty Acids in Infant Nutrition. I. Linoleic Acid Requirement in Terms of Serum Di-, Tri-, and Tetraenoic Acid Levels," *J. Nutrition,* **66:**345, 1958.

See also references #29–32 on page 792.

Stearns, G.: "Early Experiences with Vitamin D in the Nutrition of Infants and Children —A Retrospect," *Nutrition Rev.,* **12:**193, 1954.
Verner, J. V., Jr., et al.: "Vitamin D Intoxication. Report of Two Cases Treated with Cortisone," *Ann. Int. Med.,* **48:**765, 1958.

Vitamin E and vitamin K

Almquist, H. J.: "Vitamin K," *Physiol. Rev.,* **21:**194, 1941.
Mattill, H. A.: "Vitamin E—The Tocopherols," *Borden's Rev.,* **13:**109, 1952.
————: "Vitamin E," *Nutrition Rev.,* **10:**225, 1952.
Review: "Vitamin E Deficiency in Man," *Nutrition Rev.,* **15:**131, 1957.
Snell, A. M.: "Vitamin K: Its Properties, Distribution, and Clinical Importance," *J.A.M.A.,* **112:**1457, 1939.
Vietti, T. J., et al.: "Observations on the Prophylactic Use of Vitamin K in the Newborn Infant," *J. Pediat.,* **56:**343, 1960.

Ascorbic acid

Beeuwkes, A.: "The Prevalence of Scurvy among Voyageurs to America 1493–1600," *J. Am. Dietet. A.,* **24:**300, 1947.
Charles, V. R., and Van Duyne, F. O.: "Effect of Holding and Reheating on the Ascorbic Acid Content of Cooked Vegetables," *J. Home Econ.,* **50:**159, 1958.
Council on Foods and Nutrition of the American Medical Association: "Importance of Vitamin C in the Diet. Food Standards," *J.A.M.A.,* **160:**1470, 1956.
Davey, B. L., et al.: "Utilization of Ascorbic Acid in Fruits and Vegetables," *J. Am. Dietet. A.,* **32:**1064, 1069, 1956.
Ezell, B. D., and Wilcox, M. S.: "Loss of Vitamin C in Fresh Vegetables as Related to Wilting and Temperature," *J. Ag. Food Chem.,* **7:**507, 1959.
Gordon, J., and Noble, I.: "Effect of Cooking Method on Vegetables," *J. Am. Dietet. A.,* **35:**578, 1959.
King, C. G.: "Vitamin C," *J.A.M.A.,* **142:**563, 1950.
————: "Early Experiences with Ascorbic Acid—A Retrospect," *Nutrition Rev.,* **12:**1, 1954.
Lorenz, A. J.: "The Conquest of Scurvy," *J. Am. Dietet. A.,* **30:**665, 1954.
Morse, E. H., et al.: "Published vs Analyzed Values for Ascorbic Acid," *J. Am. Dietet. A.,* **34:**265, 1958.
Sabry, J. H., et al.: "Human Utilization of Dehydroascorbic Acid," *J. Nutrition,* **64:**457, 1958.
Uhl, E.: "Ascorbic Acid Requirements of Adults: 30 mg or 75 mg?" *Am. J. Clin. Nutrition,* **6:**146, 1958.
Whitacre, J., et al.: "Human Utilization of Ascorbic Acid," *J. Am. Dietet. A.,* **35:**139, 1959.
Woodruff, C.: "Infantile Scurvy," *J.A.M.A.,* **161:**448, 1956.

Thiamine

Elvehjem, C. A.: "The Vitamin B Complex," *J.A.M.A.,* **138:**960, 1948.
Griffith, R. L.: "Condition of the Heart following Beriberi and Malnutrition," *Arch. Int. Med.,* **89:**743, 1952.
Review: "The Fate of Thiamine in the Human Being," *Nutrition Rev.,* **7:**35, 1949.
Review: "Thiamine Deficiency in Infants," *Nutrition Rev.,* **16:**240, 1958.
Smith, E. B., et al.: "Planning Low-Riboflavin and Low-Thiamine Diets," *J. Am. Dietet. A.,* **34:**823, 1958.
Williams, R. R.: "Recollections of the 'Beriberi-Preventing Substance'," *Nutrition Rev.,* **11:**257, 1953.
Youmans, J. B.: "Deficiencies of the Water-Soluble Vitamins," *J.A.M.A.,* **144:**307, 1950.

Riboflavin

Bro-Rasmussen, F.: "The Riboflavin Requirements of Animals and Man and Associated Metabolic Relations," *Nutrition Abstr. & Rev.,* **28:**1, 369, 1958.

Everson, E., et al.: "Biological Availability of Certain Foods as Sources of Riboflavin," *J. Nutrition,* **46:**45, 1952.

György, P.: "Early Experiences with Riboflavin—A Retrospect," *Nutrition Rev.,* **12:**97, 1954.

Hills, O. W., et al.: "Clinical Aspects of Dietary Depletion of Riboflavin," *Arch. Int. Med.,* **87:**682, 1951.

Horwitt, M. K., et al.: "Correlation of Urinary Excretion of Riboflavin with Dietary Intake and Symptoms of Ariboflavinosis," *J. Nutrition,* **41:**247, 1950.

Morley, N. H., et al.: "Riboflavin in the Blood and Urine of Women on Controlled Diets," *J. Nutrition,* **69:**191, 1959.

Review: "Riboflavin Deficiency in Man," *Nutrition Rev.,* **8:**133, 1950.

Williams, R. R., and Cheldelin, V. H.: "Destruction of Riboflavin by Light," *Science,* **96:**22, 1942.

Niacin

Elvehjem, C. A.: "Early Experiences with Niacin—A Retrospect," *Nutrition Rev.,* **11:** 289, 1953.

Goldsmith, G. A.: "Experimental Niacin Deficiency," *J. Am. Dietet. A.,* **32:**312, 1956.

————: "Niacin-Tryptophan Relationships in Man and Niacin Requirement," *Am. J. Clin. Nutrition,* **6:**479, 1958.

Review: "Pellagra and the Cooking of Corn," *Nutrition Rev.,* **15:**53, 1957.

Sydenstricker, V. P.: "History of Pellagra, Its Recognition as a Disorder of Nutrition and Its Conquest," *Am. J. Clin. Nutrition,* **6:**409, 1958.

Youmans, J. B.: "Deficiencies of the Water-Soluble Vitamins," *J.A.M.A.,* **144:**386, 1950.

Vitamin B$_6$

György, P.: "The History of Vitamin B$_6$," *Am. J. Clin. Nutrition,* **4:**313, 1956.

Hawkins, W. W., and Barsky, J.: "An Experiment on Human Vitamin B$_6$ Deprivation," *Science,* **108:**284, 1948.

Krehl, W. A.: "Vitamin B$_6$ in Nutrition and Metabolism," *Borden's Rev.,* **18:**69, 1957.

Lepkovsky, S.: "Early Experiences with Pyridoxine—A Retrospect," *Nutrition Rev.,* **12:**257, 1954.

Review: "Role of Vitamin B$_6$ in Fat Metabolism," *Nutrition Rev.,* **10:**21, 1952.

Vilter, R. W.: "Vitamin B$_6$ in Medical Practice," *J.A.M.A.,* **159:**1210, 1955.

Wachstein, M.: "Evidence of Abnormal Vitamin B$_6$ Metabolism in Pregnancy and Various Disease States," *Am. J. Clin. Nutrition,* **4:**369, 1956.

Pantothenic acid

Hodges, R. E., et al.: "Pantothenic Acid Deficiency in Man," *J. Clin. Investigation,* **37:** 1642, 1958.

Krehl, W. A.: "Pantothenic Acid in Nutrition," *Nutrition Rev.,* **11:**225, 1953.

Review: "Pantothenic Acid Deficiency and Adrenal Insufficiency," *Nutrition Rev.,* **10:** 221, 1952.

Williams, R. J.: "Early Experiences with Pantothenic Acid—A Retrospect," *Nutrition Rev.,* **12:**65, 1954.

Biotin

Hertz, R.: "Biotin and the Avidin-Biotin Complex," *Physiol. Rev.,* **26:**479, 1946.

Lardy, H. A., and Peanasky, R.: "Metabolic Functions of Biotin," *Physiol. Rev.,* **33:**560, 1953.

Oppel, T. W.: "Studies of Biotin Metabolism in Man," *Am. J. M. Sc.,* **215:**76, 1948.

Vitamin B$_{12}$

Darby, W. J., et al.: "Vitamin B$_{12}$ Requirement of Adult Man," *Am. J. Med.,* **25:**726, 1958.

Howe, E. E.: "Effect of Vitamin B$_{12}$ on Growth-Retarded Children. A Review," *Am. J. Clin. Nutrition,* **6:**16, 1958.

Schilling, R. F.: "The Absorption and Utilization of Vitamin B₁₂," *Am. J. Clin. Nutrition,* **3:**45, 1955.

Smith, E. L.: "Vitamin B₁₂. Part I," *Nutrition Abstr. & Rev.,* **20:**795, 1951.

Ungley, C. C.: "Vitamin B₁₂. Part II. A Review of the Clinical Aspects," *Nutrition Abstr. & Rev.,* **21:**1, 1951.

Williams, J. N.: "Some Metabolic Interrelationships of Folic Acid, Vitamin B₁₂, and Ascorbic Acid," *Am. J. Clin. Nutrition,* **3:**20, 1955.

Folacin and folinic acid

Baumann, C. A.: "Citrovorum Factor. Nutrition Aspects, Associations with Leukemia and Anemia," *J. Am. Dietet. A.,* **29:**548, 1953.

Bleiler, R. E., et al.: "Metabolism of Folic Acid and Citrovorum Factor by Human Subjects," *J. Nutrition,* **56:**163, 1955.

Jukes, T. H.: "Folic Acid and Vitamin B₁₂ in the Physiology of Vertebrates," *Federation Proc.,* **12:**633, 1953.

Unglaub, W. G., and Goldsmith, G. A.: "Folic Acid and Vitamin B₁₂ in Medical Practice," *J.A.M.A.,* **161:**623, 1956.

Welch, A. D.: "Nutritional Role of Folic Acid," *Nutrition Rev.,* **15:**33, 1957.

See also references #51–65, page 792.

Chapter 14. Meal planning for the family

Hegsted, D. M.: "Establishment of Nutritional Requirements in Man," *Borden's Rev.,* **20:**13, 1959.

Institute of Home Economics, Agricultural Research Service, U.S. Department of Agriculture, Washington, D.C., bulletins as follows:
Family Fare, Home and Garden Bulletin No. 1
Food for Families with School Children, Home and Garden Bulletin No. 13
Food for the Family with Young Children, Home and Garden Bulletin No. 5

Johnston, B. J.: "The Cost of An Adequate Diet," *Am. J. Clin. Nutrition,* **5:**346, 1957.

Kinder, F.: *Meal Management.* The Macmillan Company, New York, 1956.

Monge, B., and Throssell, D.: "Good Nutrition on a Low Income," *Am. J. Nursing,* **60:**1290, 1960.

Page, L., and Phipard, E. F.: *Essentials of an Adequate Diet.* Home Economics Research Report No. 3, U.S. Department of Agriculture, Washington, D.C., 1957.

Wilmot, J. S., and Batjer, M. Q.: *Food for the Family.* J. B. Lippincott Company, Philadelphia, 1960.

See also references #66, 67, page 793.

Chapter 15. Factors influencing food habits and their modification

Babcock, C. G.: "Food and Its Emotional Significance," *J. Am. Dietet. A.,* **24:**390, 1948.

Bergevin, P.: "Telling vs Teaching—Learning by Participation," *J. Am. Dietet. A.,* **33:**781, 1957.

Eppright, E. S.: "Factors Influencing Food Acceptance," *J. Am. Dietet. A.,* **23:**579, 1947.

Fathauer, G. H.: "Food Habits—An Anthropologist's View," *J. Am. Dietet. A.,* **37:**335, 1960.

Galdston, I.: "Nutrition from the Psychiatric Viewpoint," *J. Am. Dietet. A.,* **28:**405, 1952.

Godshall, F. R.: *Nutrition in the Elementary School.* Harper & Brothers, New York, 1958.

Kreitlow, B. W.: "Teaching Adults Democratically," *J. Am. Dietet. A.,* **33:**788, 1957.

Mead, M.: "Cultural Patterning of Nutritionally Relevant Behavior," *J. Am. Dietet. A.,* **25:**677, 1949.

Norman, E. C.: "Group Discussion in Changing Food Habits," *J. Am. Dietet. A.,* **34:**1187, 1958.

Pattison, M., et al.: *Teaching Nutrition.* The Iowa State College Press, Ames, Iowa, 1957.

Pilgrim, F. J.: "The Components of Food Acceptance and Their Measurement," *Am. J. Clin. Nutrition,* **5:**171, 1957.

Pumpian-Mindlin, E.: "The Meanings of Food," *J. Am. Dietet. A.,* **30:**576, 1954.

See also references #68–70, page 793.

Chapter 16. Cultural food patterns in the United States

Adolph, W. H.: "Nutrition in the Near East," *J. Am. Dietet. A.,* **30:**753, 1954.

Bellin, M. G.: *The Jewish Cook Book.* Bloch Publishing Company, New York, 1957.

Boni, A.: *The Talisman Italian Cook Book.* (Translated by Pei, M.) Crown Publishers, New York, 1955.

Hawks, J. E.: "Preparation and Composition of Foods Served in Chinese Homes," *J. Am. Dietet. A.,* **12:**136, 1936.

Jelliffe, D. B.: "Cultural Variation and the Practical Pediatrician," *J. Pediat.,* **49:**661, 1957.

Judd, J. E.: "Century-Old Dietary Taboos in 20th Century Japan," *J. Am. Dietet. A.,* **33:**489, 1957.

Lantz, E. M., and Wood, P.: "Nutrition of New Mexican Spanish-American and 'Anglo' Adolescents. I. Food Habits and Nutrient Intakes," *J. Am. Dietet. A.,* **34:**138, 1958.

———: "———. II. Blood Findings, Height and Weight Data, and Physical Conditions," *J. Am. Dietet. A.,* **34:**145, 1958.

———: "Nutritional Condition of New Mexican Children," *J. Am. Dietet. A.,* **34:**1199, 1958.

McGuire, L. M.: *Old World Foods for New World Families.* Wayne University Press, Detroit, 1946.

Mead, M.: "Dietary Patterns and Food Habits," *J. Am. Dietet. A.,* **19:**1, 1943.

Mitchell, H. S., and Joffe, N. F.: "Food Patterns of Some European Countries: Background for Study Programs and Guidance of Relief Workers," *J. Am. Dietet. A.,* **20:**676, 1944.

Mitchell, H. S., et al.: *Selected List of References on National Food Patterns and Recipes.* The American Dietetic Association, Chicago, 1954.

Queen, G. S.: "Culture, Economics, and Food Habits," *J. Am. Dietet. A.,* **33:**1044, 1957.

Roberts, L. J.: "A Basic Food Pattern for Puerto Rico," *J. Am. Dietet. A.,* **30:**1097, 1954.

Robinson, W. D., et al.: "A Study of the Nutritional Status of a Population Group in Mexico City," *J. Am. Dietet. A.,* **20:**289, 1944.

Walker, M., et al.: "Fat, Protein, Sodium, and Calories in Diets in Hawaii," *J. Am. Dietet. A.,* **35:**122, 1959.

Wood, B. M.: *Foods of the Foreign Born in Relation to Health.* M. Barrows & Co., Inc., New York, 1929.

See also references #71–75, page 793.

Chapter 17. Nutrition during pregnancy and lactation

Bourquin, A., and Bennum, R.: "The Preconception Diet of Women Who Have Had Unsuccessful Pregnancies," *Am. J. Clin. Nutrition,* **5:**62, 1957.

Burke, B. S.: "Diet During Pregnancy," *Am. J. Clin. Nutrition,* **2:**425, 1954.

Darby, W. J., et al.: "The Vanderbilt Cooperative Study of Maternal and Infant Nutrition. I. Background. II. Methods. III. Description of the Sample and Data," *J. Nutrition,* **51:**539, 1953.

———: "The Vanderbilt Cooperative Study of Maternal and Infant Nutrition. IV. Dietary, Laboratory and Physical Findings in 2129 Delivered Pregnancies," *J. Nutrition,* **51:**565, 1953.

Ebbs, J. H., et al.: "The Influence of Prenatal Diet on the Mother and Child," *J. Nutrition,* **22:**515, 1941.

Hughes, E. C.: "Nutrition and Fetal Growth," *J. Am. Dietet. A.,* **31:**783, 1955.

Jeans, P. C., et al.: "Incidence of Prematurity in Relation to Maternal Nutrition," *J. Am. Dietet. A.,* **31:**576, 1955.

Josey, W. E.: "The Role of Nutrition in the Management of Pregnancy," *Am. J. Clinical Nutrition,* **2:**303, 1954.

Macy, I. G., et al.: "Physiological Adaptation and Nutritional Status During and After Pregnancy," *J. Nutrition,* **52** (Supplement 1): 3, 1954.

Peters, A.: *Prenatal Care.* Pub. 4, Children's Bureau, U.S. Department of Health, Education and Welfare, Washington, D.C., 1949.

Sheriff, H.: "Trends in Maternal and Child Health," *J. Am. Dietet. A.,* **34:**1304, 1958.

Toverud, K. U., et al.: *Maternal Nutrition and Child Health. An Interpretative Review.* Bull. 123, National Research Council, Washington, D.C., 1950.

Warkany, J.: "Congenital Malformations Induced by Maternal Dietary Deficiency," *Nutrition Rev.,* **13:**289, 1955.

See also references #76–82, page 793.

Chapter 18. Nutrition during infancy

Adams, S. F.: "Use of Vegetables in Infant Feeding Through the Ages," *J. Am. Dietet. A.,* **35:**692, 1959.

Barnes, G. R., Jr.: "Acceptance of Soya Food by Infants," *A.M.A. Am. J. Dis. Child.,* **98:**1, 1959.

Children's Bureau: *Infant Care,* Pub. 8, Revised. U.S. Department of Health, Education and Welfare, Washington, D.C., 1955.

György, P.: "Trends and Advances in Infant Feeding," *Nursing Outlook,* **6:**516, 1958.

Hansen, A. E.: "Essential Fatty Acids in Infant Feeding," *J. Am. Dietet. A.,* **34:**239, 1958.

Hill, L. F.: "Infant Nutrition," *Am. J. Clin. Nutrition,* **3:**75, 1955.

Holt, L. E., Jr.: "Failure to Gain Weight," *Am. J. Clin. Nutrition,* **5:**500, 1957.

Hytten, F. E.: "Is Breast Feeding Best?" *Am. J. Clin. Nutrition,* **7:**259, 1959.

Lahey, M. E.: "Iron and Copper in Infant Nutrition," *Am. J. Clin. Nutrition,* **5:**516, 1957.

Mellander, O., and Vahlquist, B.: "On the Evaluation of Artificial Feeding," *Am. J. Clin. Nutrition,* **5:**493, 1957.

Meyer, H. S.: *Infant Foods and Feeding Practice.* Charles C. Thomas, Springfield, Ill., 1960.

Nelson, W. E.: *Textbook of Pediatrics,* 7th ed. W. B. Saunders Company, Philadelphia, 1959.

Norman, F. A., and Pratt, E. L.: "Feeding of Infants and Children in Hot Weather," *J.A.M.A.,* **166:**2168, 1958.

Pratt, E. L.: "Amino Acid and Protein Requirements of Infants," *J.A.M.A.,* **164:**408, 1957.

Richmond, J. B., and Pollock, G. H.: "Psychologic Aspects of Infant Feeding," *J. Am. Dietet. A.,* **29:**656, 1953.

Salber, E. J., et al.: "Patterns of Breast Feeding. I. Factors Affecting the Frequency of Breast Feeding in the Newborn Period," *New England J. Med.,* **259:**707, 1958.

Scheinberg, I. H., ed.: *Infant Metabolism.* The Macmillan Company, New York, 1956.

Smith, C. A.: "Overuse of Milk in the Diets of Infants and Children," *J.A.M.A.,* **172:** 567, 1960.

Smith, C. S.: "Demand Feeding in the Newborn Nursery," *Nursing Outlook,* **6:**514, 1958.

Spock, B.: *Baby and Child Care.* Pocket Books, New York, 1957.

Spock, B., and Lowenberg, M. E.: *Feeding Your Baby and Child.* Pocket Books, New York, 1955.

See also references #83–88, page 794.

Chapter 19. Nutrition for children and teenagers

Beal, V. A.: "Nutritional Intake of Children. I. Calories, Carbohydrate, Fat, and Protein," *J. Nutrition,* **50:**223, 1953.

———: "———III. Thiamine, Riboflavin, and Niacin," *J. Nutrition,* **57:**183, 1955.

———: "———IV. Vitamins A and D. Ascorbic Acid." *J. Nutrition,* **60:**335, 1956.

Bowes, A. deP.: "Nutrition of Children during Their School Years," *Am. J. Clin. Nutrition,* **3:**254, 1955.

Breckenridge, M. E.: "Food Attitudes of Five-to-Twelve-Year-Old Children," *J. Am. Dietet. A.*, **35:**704, 1959.

Children's Bureau, U.S. Department of Health, Education, and Welfare, Washington, D.C., bulletins as follows:
The Adolescent in Your Family, Pub. 347, 1954.
Nutrition and Healthy Growth, Pub. 352, 1955.
Your Child from One to Six, Pub. 30, 1956.
Your Child from Six to Twelve, Pub. 324, 1949.

Everson, G. J.: "Bases for Concern about Teenagers' Diets," *J. Am. Dietet. A.*, **36:**17, 1960.

Gesell, A., et al.: *The Years from Ten to Sixteen.* Harper & Brothers, New York, 1956.

Gschneidner, M. P., and Roderuck, C. E.: "Nutriture of School Girls of Different Physiques," *J. Am. Dietet. A.*, **36:**22, 1960.

Hathaway, M.: *Heights and Weights of Children in the United States.* Home Economics Research Report No. 2, U.S. Department of Agriculture, Washington, D.C., 1958.

Ilg, F. L.: "The Child's Idea of What and How to Eat," *J. Am. Dietet. A.*, **24:**658, 1948.

Jeans, P. C.; Wright, F. H.; and Blake, F. G.: *Essentials of Pediatrics,* 6th ed. J. B. Lippincott Company, Philadelphia, 1958.

Johnston, J. A.: "Protein Requirements of Adolescents," *Ann. N. Y. Acad. Sci.*, **69:**881, 1958.

Macy, I. G., and Kelly, H. J.: *Chemical Anthropology. A New Approach to Growth in Children.* University of Chicago Press, Chicago, 1957.

Martin, E. A.: *Roberts' Nutrition Work with Children.* University of Chicago Press, Chicago, 1954.

Munro, N.: "How Do Snacks Affect Total Caloric Intake of Preschool Children?" *J. Am. Dietet. A.*, **33:**601, 1957.

The Nutritional "Ages of Man." Nutrition: Past, Present, and Future. Proc. Borden Centennial Symposium on Nutrition, The Borden Company, New York, 1958.

Roth, A.: "The Teenage Clinic," *J. Am. Dietet. A.*, **36:**27, 1960.

Stearns, G., et al.: "The Protein Requirements of Children from One to Ten Years of Age," *Ann. N. Y. Acad. Sci.*, **69:**857, 1958.

Stuart, H. C., et al.: "Protein Needs of Children. A Preliminary Report of Studies of Individual Differences," *Ann. N. Y. Acad. Sci.*, **69:**869, 1958.

Weng, L.: "Nutrition in the Pre-School Child," *Am. J. Clin. Nutrition,* **3:**150, 1955.

———: "The Child and His Food," *J. Am. Dietet. A.*, **25:**616, 1949.

See also references #89–100, page 794.

School lunch

Augustine, G., and Hunter, A.: "School Lunch Portions to Meet Children's Needs," *J. Am. Dietet. A.*, **33:**123, 1957.

Carver, A. F., and Patton, M. B.: "Plate Waste in a School Lunch. I. Overall Waste," *J. Am. Dietet. A.*, **34:**615, 1958.

Hunt, F. E., et al.: "Plate Waste in A School Lunch. III. A Vegetable Acceptance Study," *J. Am. Dietet. A.*, **34:**810, 1958.

Obert, J. C.: "The Physician's Role in the School Lunch Program," *Am. J. Clin. Nutrition,* **6:**172, 1958.

Patton, M. B., et al.: "Plate Waste in a School Lunch. II. Sources of Waste," *J. Am. Dietet. A.*, **34:**733, 1958.

School Lunch and Nutrition Education. Bull. No. 14. Office of Education, U.S. Department of Health, Education, and Welfare, Washington, D.C., 1951.

The School Lunch—Its Educational Contribution. Pamphlet No. 6. Office of Education, U.S. Department of Health, Education, and Welfare, Washington, D.C., 1954.

Scott, M. L.: *School Feeding.* FAO Nutritional Studies No. 10, Food and Agriculture Organization, Rome, Italy, 1953.

Todhunter, E. N.: "Child Feeding Problems and the School Lunch Program," *J. Am. Dietet. A.*, **24:**422, 1948.

Wells, O. V.: "Policies of National School Lunch Program," *J. Am. Dietet. A.*, **34:**805, 1958.

Chapter 20. Nutrition after fifty

Batchelder, E. L.: "Nutritional Status and Dietary Habits of Older People," *J. Am. Dietet. A.,* **33:**471, 1957.

Beeuwkes, A. M.: "Studying the Food Habits of the Elderly," *J. Am. Dietet. A.,* **37:**215, 1960.

Blumenthal, G. W.: "Emotional Aspects of Feeding the Aged," *J. Am. Dietet. A.,* **32:** 829, 1956.

Chinn, A. B.: "Some Problems of Nutrition in the Aged," *J.A.M.A.,* **162:**1511, 1956.

Daum, K., et al.: "Nitrogen Utilization in Older Men," *J. Am. Dietet. A.,* **28:**305, 1952.

Donahue, W. T.: "Psychologic Aspects of Feeding the Aged," *J. Am. Dietet. A.,* **27:**461, 1951.

Gillum, H. L., et al.: "Nutritional Status of the Aging. II. Blood Glucose Levels," *J. Nutrition,* **55:**289, 1955.

Griffith, W. H.: "Senior Citizens," *Proc. Borden Centennial Symposium on Nutrition,* The Borden Company, New York, 1958.

Heend, S.: "Serving the Aged," *J. Am. Dietet. A.,* **31:**376, 1955.

Henry, C. E.: "Feeding Elderly People in Their Homes," *J. Am. Dietet. A.,* **35:**149, 1959.

Institute of Home Economics: *Food Guide for Older Folks.* Home and Garden Bulletin No. 17, U.S. Department of Agriculture, Washington, D.C., 1959.

Kelley, L., et al.: "Food Selection and Well-Being of Aging Women," *J. Am. Dietet. A.,* **33:**466, 1957.

McCay, C. M.: "Nutritional Experiments on Longevity," *Geriatrics,* **6:**171, 1958.

Ohlson, M. A., et al.: "Utilization of an Improved Diet by Older Women," *J. Am. Dietet. A.,* **28:**1138, 1952.

Pollack, H.: "Nutritional Problems in the Aging and Aged," *J.A.M.A.,* **165:**257, 1957.

Reynolds, M. M.: "A Nutrition Program for Older People," *Geriatrics,* **14:**190, 1959.

Tucker, R. E., et al.: "Nutritive Intake of Older Institutionalized Persons," *J. Am. Dietet. A.,* **34:**819, 1958.

Waife, S. O.: "Nutritional Needs of Maturing Man," *Geriatrics,* **6:**190, 1958.

Walker, V. W., et al.: *Eating is Fun—for Older People Too.* The American Dietetic Association, Chicago, 1952.

Williams, I. F., and Smith, C. E.: "Home Delivered Meals for the Aged and Handicapped," *J. Am. Dietet. A.,* **35:**146, 1959.

See also references #101–104, page 794.

Chapter 21. Safeguarding the food supply

Anderson, O. E.: *The Health of a Nation: Harvey W. Wiley and the Fight for Pure Food.* University of Chicago Press, Chicago, 1958.

Burdon, K. L.: *Textbook of Microbiology,* 4th ed. The Macmillan Company, New York, 1958.

Coerver, R. M.: "One Man's Meat," *Am. J. Nursing,* **58:**690, 1958.

Comar, C. L.: "Radioactivity in Foods," *J.A.M.A.,* **171:**119, 1959.

Dack, G. M.: *Food Poisoning.* University of Chicago Press, Chicago, 1956.

————: "Current Status of Therapy in Microbial Food Poisoning," *J.A.M.A.,* **172:** 929, 1960.

Day, P. L.: "The Food and Drug Administration Faces New Responsibilities," *Nutrition Rev.,* **18:**1, 1960.

De Eds, F.: "Chemicals in Foods," *J. Am. Dietet. A.,* **35:**19, 1959.

Esselen, W. B.: "Food Preservation and Its Contribution to Nutrition," *Borden's Rev.,* **18:**29, 1957.

Flanagan, J. E.: "Labeling Legislation—A Summary of Recent Developments," *Am. J. Pub. Health,* **50:**637, 1960.

Food and Drug Administration: *Read the Label on Foods Drugs Devices Cosmetics.* Misc. Pub. 3, U.S. Department of Health, Education, and Welfare, Washington, D.C., 1957.

Food Protection Committee, Food and Nutrition Board: *The Safety of Artificial Sweet-*

eners for Use in Foods. Pub. 386, National Research Council, Washington, D.C., 1955.

Goresline, H. E.: "Preservation of Foods by Irradiation," *Am. J. Pub. Health,* **49:**488, 1959.

Ives, M.: "Safety Evaluation of Food Packaging Materials," *J. Am. Dietet. A.,* **33:**347, 1957.

Johnson, P. E.: "Chemicals in Foods," *J. Home Econ.,* **48:**751, 1956.

Larrick, G. P.: "The Role of the Food and Drug Administration in Nutrition," *Am. J. Clin. Nutrition,* **8:**377, 1960.

Mickelsen, O.: "Is Toxicology Enough for a Food Protection Program?" *J. Am. Dietet. A.,* **33:**341, 1957.

Nielsen, J. P.: "Effect of Processing and Handling on Foods," *J. Am. Dietet. A.,* **34:** 1313, 1958.

Pollack, H.: "Wholesomeness of Irradiated Foods," *J. Am. Dietet. A.,* **35:**235, 1959.

Tressler, D. K., and Evers, D. F.: *The Freezing Preservation of Foods.* Avi Publishing Co., Westport, 1957.

See also references #50, 105–110, page 794.

Chapter 22. Nutrition in the community

Adelson, S. L.: "Some Problems in Collecting Dietary Data from Individuals," *J. Am. Dietet. A.,* **36:**453, 1960.

Basic Course in Emergency Mass Feeding, Pocket Manual. Federal Civil Defense Administration, Washington, D.C., 1957.

Beeuwkes, A. M.: "Characteristics of the Self-Styled Scientist," *J. Am. Dietet. A.,* **32:**627, 1956.

Berry, F. B., and Schaefer, A. E.: "Program of the Interdepartmental Committee on Nutrition for National Defense," *J.A.M.A.,* **166:**775, 1958.

Bovee, D. L.: "Emergency Feeding in Disaster," *Am. J. Clin. Nutrition,* **6:**77, 1958.

Browe, J. H.: "Programs to Fit Changing Health Needs," *J. Am. Dietet. A.,* **35:**789, 1959.

Burney, L. E.: "Nutrition and Chronic Disease Control," *Nutrition Rev.,* **16:**225, 1958.

Decker, G. C.: "Insect Control vs Human Nutrition," *Nutrition Rev.,* **16:**289, 1958.

Food Facts Talk Back. The American Dietetic Association, Chicago, 1957.

Hambidge, G.: *The Story of FAO.* D. Van Nostrand Company, Inc., New York, 1955.

Hanlon, J. H.: *Principles of Public Health Administration,* 3rd ed. The C. V. Mosby Company, St. Louis, 1960.

Hawkins, M.: "The Highest Possible Level of Health," *J. Home Econ.,* **50:**416, 1958.

Heyward, E. J. R.: "Hunger is the Enemy," *J. Home Econ.,* **47:**599, 1955.

Leverton, R. M.: "Distorting Facts into Fads," *J. Am. Dietet. A.,* **33:**793, 1957.

Mustard, H. S., and Stebbins, E. L.: *An Introduction to Public Health,* 4th ed. The Macmillan Company, New York, 1959.

"Panel Discussion on Nutrition Education," *Federation Proc.,* **18** (Part II, Suppl. 3): 115, 1959.

Pate, M.: "UNICEF Goals in Maternal and Child Health," *Am. J. Pub. Health,* **50** (Suppl. June 1960):8, 1960.

Phillips, R. W.: "How Adequate is the World's Food Supply," *Scient. Monthly,* **85:**256, 1957.

The Role of Nutrition Education in Combatting Food Fads. The Nutrition Foundation, Inc., New York, 1959.

Rosenberg, R. S., "Nutritional Claims in Food Advertising," *J. Am. Dietet. A.,* **32:**631, 1956.

Thompson, W. S.: "World Population and Food Supply," *J.A.M.A.,* **172:**1647, 1960.

Trulson, M. F., and McCann, M. B.: "Comparison of Dietary Survey Methods," *J. Am. Dietet. A.,* **35:**672, 1959.

White, P. L.: "The Program of the Council on Foods and Nutrition of the American Medical Association," *Nutrition Rev.,* **16:**65, 1958.

White, P. L., and Stevenson, E. H.: "Pitfalls in the Promotion of Foods," *J. Am. Dietet. A.,* **34:**935, 1958.

Whiting, M. G., and Leverton, R. M.: "Reliability of Dietary Appraisal: Comparisons between Laboratory Analysis and Calculation from Tables of Food Values," *Am. J. Pub. Health,* **50:**815, 1960.

Wiehl, D. G., and Reed, R.: "Development of New or Improved Dietary Methods for Epidemiological Investigation," *Am. J. Pub. Health,* **50:**824, 1960.

Wilder, R. M.: "A Brief History of the Enrichment of Flour and Bread," *J.A.M.A.,* **162:** 1539, 1956.

Williams, R. R., et al.: *Cereal Enrichment in Perspective, 1958.* The Food and Nutrition Board, National Research Council, Washington, D.C., 1958.

Windemuth, A.: *The Nurse and the Outpatient Department.* The Macmillan Company, New York, 1959.

Young, C. M., and Trulson, M. F.: "Methodology for Dietary Studies in Epidemiological Surveys. II. Strengths and Weaknesses of Existing Methods," *Am. J. Pub. Health,* **50:** 803, 1960.

See also references #111–115, page 794.

Therapeutic nutrition. Books

Duncan, G. G.: *Diseases of Metabolism,* 4th ed. W. B. Saunders Company, Philadelphia, 1959.

Jolliffe, N., et al.: *Clinical Nutrition.* Paul B. Hoeber, Inc., New York, 1950.

National League for Nursing: *Bibliographies on Nursing. II. Nutrition and Diet; Pharmacology.* National League for Nursing, New York, 1957.

Pollack, H., and Halpern, S. L.: *Therapeutic Nutrition.* Pub. 234, Food and Nutrition Board, National Research Council, Washington, D.C., 1952.

Practical Diet Therapy. Reprints of papers in diet therapy. The American Journal of Clinical Nutrition, New York, 1956.

Stern, F.: *Applied Dietetics,* 3rd ed., edited by H. Rosenthal, et al. The Williams & Wilkins Company, Baltimore, 1949.

Turner, D. F.: *Handbook of Diet Therapy,* 3rd ed. University of Chicago Press, Chicago, 1959.

See also General References: Nutrition, page 800.

Chapter 23. Therapeutic nutrition: factors in patient care

Aldrich, C. K.: "Prescribing a Diet Is Not Enough," *J. Am. Dietet. A.,* **33:**785, 1957.

Babcock, C. G.: "Comments on Human Interrelations," *J. Am. Dietet. A.,* **33:**871, 1957.

English, O. S.: "Psychosomatic Medicine and Dietetics," *J. Am. Dietet. A.,* **27:**721, 1951.

Fogelman, M. J., and Crasilneck, H. B.: "Food Intake and Hypnosis," *J. Am. Dietet. A.,* **32:**519, 1956.

Kaufman, M., and Bryan, M. S.: "The Nutritionist in Organized Home Care," *Pub. Health Rep.,* **74:**923, 1959.

Legant, J., and Baiano, M. J.: "The Dietitian and Nutritionist as Members of a Home Care Rehabilitation Team," *J. Home Econ.,* **51:**209, 1959.

Morris, E.: "How Does a Nurse Teach Nutrition to Patients?" *Am. J. Nursing,* **60:**67, 1960.

Pennell, M. Y., and Smith, L. M.: "Characteristics of Families Served by Homemakers," *Am. J. Pub. Health,* **49:**1467, 1959.

Reams, A.: "Education of the Patient," *J. Home Econ.,* **51:**207, 1959.

Robinson, C.: "Dietary Nomenclature," *J. Am. Dietet. A.,* **28:**640, 1952.

———: "Food Therapy Begins with the Normal Diet," *J. Clin. Nutrition,* **1:**150, 1953.

Robinson, C. H., and Proudfit, F. T.: "Development of Positive Food Therapy. Changing Concepts Lead to Better Health," *J. Am. Dietet. A.,* **25:**497, 1949.

Sailor, N. M.: "Nutrition in Rehabilitation of the Handicapped," *J. Home Econ.,* **51:**208, 1959.

Seifrit, E.: "Bookshelf on Nutrition and Diet Therapy," *Am. J. Clin. Nutrition,* **7:**98, 1959.

White, G.: "The Patient as the Focus of Attention," *J. Am. Dietet. A.,* **30:**25, 1954.

Wood, C. L.: "How the Chaplain and the Dietitian Can Cooperate," *J. Am. Dietet. A.,* **35:**821, 1959.

Wright, E. G., et al.: "Do Spices Increase the Acceptability of Therapeutic Diets?" *J. Am. Dietet. A.,* **33:**895, 1957.

See also references #116–120, page 795; and on Food Habits, page 809.

Chapter 26. Nutritional deficiencies

Brock, J. F., and Autret, M.: *Kwashiorkor in Africa.* FAO Nutrition Studies No. 8, Rome, Italy, 1952.

Brozek, J.: "Starvation and Nutritional Rehabilitation. A Quantitative Case Study," *J. Am. Dietet. A.,* **28:**917, 1952.

Kinney, T. D., and Follis, R. H., Jr., ed.: *Nutritional Disease.* Proc. of Conference on Beriberi, Endemic Goiter, Hypovitaminosis A., *Federation Proc.,* **17:**1–162, 1958.

Spies, T. D.: "Some Recent Advances in Nutrition," *J.A.M.A.,* **167:**675, 1958.

Stare, F. J., and Thorn, G. W.: "Protein Nutrition in Problems of Medical Interest," *J.A.M.A.,* **127:**1120, 1945.

See also references for the various nutrients, Chaps. 4–11, pages 803–9.

Chapter 27. Overweight and underweight

Ayers, W. M.: "Changing Attitudes toward Overweight and Reducing," *J. Am. Dietet. A.,* **34:**23, 1958.

Barnes, R. H.: "Weight Control—A Practical Office Approach," *J.A.M.A.,* **166:**898, 1958.

Berryman, G. H.: " 'Simple' Obesity. A Current Review," *J. Am. Dietet. A.,* **31:**347, 1955.

Bruch, H.: "The Emotional Significance of the Preferred Weight," *Am. J. Clin. Nutrition,* **5:**192, 1957.

Conrad, S. W.: "Resistance of the Obese to Reducing," *J. Am. Dietet. A.,* **30:**581, 1954.

Fryer, J. H.: "The Effects of a Late-night Caloric Supplement upon Body Weight and Food Intake in Man," *Am. J. Clin. Nutrition,* **6:**354, 1958.

Fryer, J. H., et al.: "Satiety Values of Isocaloric Diets for Reducing," *J. Am. Dietet. A.,* **31:**868, 1955.

Goldsmith, G. A.: "Nutritional Pitfalls of Prosperity," in *Proceedings of the Borden Centennial Symposium on Nutrition,* The Borden Company Foundation, New York, 1958, p. 71.

Hamburger, W. W.: "The Psychology of Weight Reduction," *J. Am. Dietet. A.,* **34:**17, 1958.

Mayer J.: "Obesity: Causes and Treatment," *Am. J. Nursing,* **59:**1732, 1959.

Page, L., and Fincher, L. J.: *Food and Your Weight.* Home and Garden Bulletin No. 74, U.S. Department of Agriculture, Washington, D.C., 1960.

Pangborn, R. M., and Simone, M.: "Body Size and Sweetness Preference," *J. Am. Dietet. A.,* **34:**924, 1958.

Passmore, R., et al.: "The Chemical Composition of the Tissue Lost by Obese Patients on a Reducing Regimen," *Brit. J. Nutrition,* **12:**113, 1958.

————: "Water and Electrolyte Exchanges of Obese Patients on a Reducing Regimen," *Brit. J. Nutrition,* **13:**17, 1959.

Pollack, H., et al.: "Metabolic Demands as a Factor in Weight Control," *J.A.M.A.,* **167:**216, 1958.

Salzano, J., et al.: "Effect of Weight Loss on Respiratory Functions," *J. Am. Dietet. A.,* **34:**258, 1958.

————: "Effect of Weight Loss on Blood Pressure," *J. Am. Dietet. A.,* **34:**1309, 1958.

Sebrell, W. H., Jr.: "Weight Control through Prevention of Obesity," *J. Am. Dietet. A.,* **34:**920, 1958.

Strong, J. A., et al.: "Clinical Observations on Obese Patients during a Strict Reducing Regimen," *Brit. J. Nutrition,* **12:**105, 1958.

Stunkard, A. J., et al.: "The Night-eating Syndrome," *Am. J. Med.,* **19:**78, 1955.

Stunkard, A. J.: "The 'Dieting Depression.' Incidence and Clinical Characteristics of Untoward Responses to Weight Reduction Regimens," *Am. J. Med.*, **23:**77, 1957.

Sussman, M. B.: "Psychosocial Correlates of Obesity," *J. Am. Dietet. A.*, **32:**423, 1956.

Weight Control, a collection of papers presented at the *Weight Control Colloquium*, Iowa State College Press, Ames, Iowa, 1955.

Wolf, J. L.: "On-the-job Weight Watching," *Nursing Outlook*, **5:**406, 1957.

Young, C. M., et al.: "Psychologic Factors in Weight Control," *Am. J. Clin. Nutrition*, **5:**186, 1957.

————: "Stepwise Weight Reduction in Obese Young Men. Nitrogen, Calcium, and Phosphorus Balances," *J. Nutrition*, **64:**203, 1958.

Yule, J. B., et al.: "Weight Control. A Community Program," *J. Am. Dietet. A.*, **33:**47, 1957.

See also references #125–134, page 795.

Chapter 28. Fevers and infections

Brewer, W. D., et al.: "Studies of Food Intake and Requirements of Women with Active and Arrested Tuberculosis," *Am. Rev. Tuberc.*, **60:**455, 1949.

Coburn, A. F., and Moore, L. V.: "Nutrition as a Conditioning Factor in the Rheumatic State," *Am. J. Dis. Child*, **65:**744, 1943.

Dingledine, M. J., et al.: "High Protein Diets in Therapy of Rocky Mountain Spotted Fever," *J. Am. Dietet. A.*, **22:**389, 1946.

Edwards, H. R., and Turner, J.: "Diet Suggestions for the Tuberculous on Low Income," *Pub. Health Nursing*, **43:**681, 1951.

Goodman, J. I., and Garvin, R. O.: "Results of High Caloric Feeding," *Gastroenterology*, **6:**537, 1946.

Jackson, R. L., and Kelly, H. G.: "Nutrition in Rheumatic Fever," *J. Am. Dietet. A.*, **25:**392, 1949.

Jacobs, A. L., et al.: "Vitamin A in Rheumatic Fever," *J. Clin. Nutrition*, **2:**155, 1954.

Pottenger, F. M., and Pottenger, F. M., Jr.: "Adequate Diet in Tuberculosis," *Am. Rev. Tuberc.*, **54:**213, 1946.

Review: "Nutrition and Susceptibility to Tuberculosis," *Nutrition Rev.*, **10:**141, 1952.

See also references #135–138, page 795.

Chapter 29. Nutrition in surgical conditions

Artz, C. P., et al.: "Some Recent Developments in Oral Feedings for Optimal Nutrition in Burns," *Am. J. Clin. Nutrition*, **4:**642, 1956.

Barker, H. G.: "Supplementation of Protein and Caloric Needs in the Surgical Patient," *Am. J. Clin. Nutrition*, **3:**466, 1955.

Biggar, B. L., et al.: "Nutrition Following Gastric Resection," *J. Am. Dietet. A.*, **37:**344, 1960.

Elman, R.: "Protein Needs in Surgical Patients," *J. Am. Dietet. A.*, **32:**524, 1956.

Esson, M. H.: "Standard Formula for Tube Feedings Saves Time and Labor," *Hospitals*, **33:**71 (Feb.) 1959.

Fisher, J. A.: "The Dumping Syndrome," *Am. J. Nursing*, **58:**1126, 1958.

Hayes, M. A.: "Dietary Control of the Post-Gastrectomy 'Dumping Syndrome,'" *J. Am. Dietet. A.*, **31:**133, 1955.

Jordan, G. L., Jr.: "Treatment of the Dumping Syndrome," *J.A.M.A.*, **167:**1062, 1958.

Mccray, P., Jr.: "Nutrition and Wound Healing," *Am. J. Clin. Nutrition*, **3:**461, 1955.

Pareira, M. D., et al.: "Therapeutic Nutrition with Tube Feeding," *J.A.M.A.*, **156:**810, 1954.

Pearson, E., et al.: "Metabolic Derangements in Burns," *J. Am. Dietet. A.*, **32:**223, 1956.

Pittman, A. C., and Robinson, F. W.: "Dumping Syndrome—Control by Diet," *J. Am. Dietet. A.*, **34:**596, 1958.

Review: "Nutritional State Following Surgery," *Nutrition Rev.*, **15:**102, 1957.

Rhoads, J. E.: "Supranormal Dietary Requirements of Acutely Ill Patients," *J. Am. Dietet. A.*, **29:**897, 1953.

Zollinger, R. M., and Stewart, W. R. C.: "Surgical Management of Gastric Ulcer," *J.A.M.A.,* **171:**2056, 1959.
See also references #139–146, page 795.

Chapter 30. Diseases of the stomach and duodenum

Barborka, C. J., and Texter, E. C., Jr.: *Peptic Ulcer: Diagnosis and Treatment.* Little Brown, Boston, 1955.
Caravati, C.: "Management of Peptic Ulcer. Clinical Appraisal of Therapeutic Measures," *Am. J. Digest. Dis.,* **4:**959, 1959.
Doll, R., et al.: "Dietetic Treatment of Peptic Ulcer," *Lancet,* **1:**5, 1956.
Editorial: "Value of Diet in Treatment of Peptic Ulcer," *Am. J. Digest. Dis.,* **2** (N.S.): 130, 1957.
———: "Is There a Rationale for the Bland Diet," *J. Am. Dietet. A.,* **33:**608, 1957.
Johnson, D.: "The Bland Diet in Ulcer Therapy," *J. Am. Dietet. A.,* **23:**686, 1947.
Jordan, S. M., and Hibben, S.: *Good Food for Bad Stomachs.* Doubleday & Co., Inc., Garden City, New York, 1951.
Marshall, E. A., and Sass, M.: "Treatment of Peptic Ulcer in the Aged with Unrestricted Diet," *Geriatrics,* **4:**498, 1956.
Miller, T. G., and Berkowitz, D.: "Analysis of Results of Conservative Peptic Ulcer Therapy," *Gastroenterology,* **20:**353, 1955.
Miller, T., and Cantwell, A. E.: "Gastric Cancer," *Am. J. Nursing,* **56:**1420, 1956.
Palmer, E. D.: *Clinical Gastroenterology.* Paul H. Hoeber, Inc., New York, 1957.
Robinson, C. H.: "The Bland Diet," *J. Clin. Nutrition,* **2:**206, 1954.
Seymour, C. T., and Weinberg, J. A.: "Emotion and Gastric Activity," *J.A.M.A.,* **171:** 1193, 1959.
For additional references, see #147–156, page 796.

Chapter 31. Diet in disturbances of the small intestine and colon

Adlersberg, D.: "Problems of Management of Idiopathic Sprue," *New York J. Med.,* **55:**3575, 1955.
Adlersberg, D., and Rabinowitz, D.: "The Sprue Syndrome—Improved Dietary Management," *J. Am. Dietet. A.,* **26:**879, 1950.
Bercowitz, Z. T.: "A Long-Range Evaluation of Modern Methods in the Treatment of Chronic Ulcerative Colitis," *New York J. Med.,* **53:**2200, 1953.
Comfort, M. W., and Wollaeger, E. E.: "Nontropical Sprue. Pathologic Physiology, Diagnosis, and Therapy," *Arch. Int. Med.,* **98:**807, 1956.
Crohn, B. B.: "Current Status of Therapy in Regional Ileitis," *J.A.M.A.,* **166:**1479, 1958.
Flood, C. A., and Lepore, M. J.: "Medical Management of Chronic Ulcerative Colitis," *New York J. Med.,* **52:**2265, 1952.
Friedlander, P. H.: "Food and Indigestion. An Investigation of Possible Relationships," *Brit. M. J.,* **5164:**1454, 1959.
Frohman, I. P.: "Constipation," *Am. J. Nursing,* **55:**65, 1955.
Green, P. A., et al.: "Nontropical Sprue," *J.A.M.A.,* **171:**2157, 1959.
Jay, A. N.: "Colitis," *Am J. Nursing,* **59:**1133, 1959.
Kiefer, E. D.: "The Management of Chronic Ulcerative Colitis," *S. Clin. North America,* **35:**809, 1955.
Review: "Absorption and Metabolism in Nontropical Sprue," *Nutrition Rev.,* **11:**261, 1953.
Robinson, C. H.: "Fiber in the Diet," *Am. J. Clin. Nutrition,* **4:**288, 1956.
Ruffin, J. M., et al.: " 'Wheat-free' Diet in the Treatment of Sprue," *New England J. Med.,* **250:**281, 1954.
Sleisenger, M. H., et al.: "A Wheat-, Rye-, and Oat-Free Diet," *J. Am. Dietet. A.,* **33:** 1137, 1957.
See also references #157–161, page 796.

Chapter 32. Diseases of the liver and gallbladder

Chambers, T. C., et al.: "Treatment of Acute Infectious Hepatitis," *J. Clin. Investigation,* **34:**1163, 1955.
Davidson, C. S.: "Cirrhosis in Alcoholics. Protein Nutrition and Hepatic Coma," *J.A.M.A.,* **160:**390, 1956.
————: "Diet in the Treatment of Liver Disease," *Am. J. Med.,* **25:**690, 1958.
Gabuzda, G. J.: "Clinical and Nutritional Aspects of Lipotropic Agents," *J.A.M.A.,* **160:**969, 1956.
Klatskin, G.: "Effect of Alcohol on the Liver," *J.A.M.A.,* **170:**1671, 1959.
Lambert, M.: "Fundamental Concepts of Liver Disease," *J. Am. Dietet. A.,* **33:**1005, 1957.
Leevy, C. M.: "Nutritional Factors in Liver Disease in Man," *Am. J. Clin. Nutrition,* **7:**146, 1959.
Patek, A. J.: "Relation of Nutrition to Etiology and Treatment of Laennec's Cirrhosis," *J. Chron. Dis.,* **3:**560, 1956.
Review: "Dietary Protein and Hepatic Coma," *Nutrition Rev.,* **14:**74, 1956.
Robinson, C.: "Diets Restricted in Fat," *Am. J. Clin. Nutrition,* **2:**47, 1954.
————: "The Low Cholesterol, Low Fat Diet," *Am. J. Clin. Nutrition,* **2:**353, 1954.
Snell, A. M., et al.: "Panel on Liver Disease," *J.A.M.A.,* **158:**116, 1955.
Watson, C.: "Current Status of Treatment of Cirrhosis of the Liver," *J.A.M.A.,* **166:**764, 1958.
See also references #163–165, page 796.

Chapter 33. Diabetes mellitus

Books and manuals for the patient

American Dietetic Association: *ADA Meal Plans No. 1 through 9.* The American Dietetic Association, Chicago, 1956.
Beardwood, J. T., Jr., and Kelly, H. T.: *Simplified Diabetic Management,* 6th ed. J. B. Lippincott Company, Philadelphia, 1954.
Behrman, Deaconess M.: *A Cookbook for Diabetics.* The American Diabetes Association, New York, 1959.
Duncan, G.: *A Modern Pilgrim's Progress for Diabetics.* W. B. Saunders Company, Philadelphia, 1956.
Joslin, E. P.: *A Diabetic Manual.* 10th ed. Lea & Febiger, Philadelphia, 1959.
Pollack, H., and Krause, M. V.: *Your Diabetes—A Manual for the Patient,* rev. ed. Harper & Brothers, New York, 1951.
Rosenthal, H., et al.: *Diabetic Care in Pictures.* 2nd ed. J. B. Lippincott Company, Philadelphia, 1953.
Strachan, C. B.: *The Diabetic's Cookbook.* The Medical Arts Publishing Foundation, Houston, Texas, 1955.

References

Adlersberg, D.: "Obesity, Fat Metabolism and Diabetes," *Diabetes,* **7:**236, 1958.
Beaser, S. B.: "Diabetes Mellitus," *New England J. Med.,* **259:**525, 573, 1958.
Breneman, J. C.: "Clinical Use of Tolbutamide (Orinase) in Office and Home Care of Diabetics," *J.A.M.A.,* **164:**627, 1957.
Caso, E. K.: "Calculation of Diabetic Diets," *J. Am. Dietet. A.,* **26:**575, 1950.
————: "Supplements to Diabetic Diet Material," *J. Am. Dietet. A.,* **32:**929, 1956.
Caso, E. K., and Youland, D. M.: "An Apple for an Orange," *Am. J. Nursing,* **55:**942, 1955.
"Current Concepts in Therapy. Hypoglycemic Agents for Oral Administration," *New England J. Med.,* **262:**297, 1960.
DeLawter, D. E., and Moss, J. M.: "Tolbutamide—Orally Effective Drug for Diabetes Mellitus," *Am. J. Nursing,* **58:**1106, 1958.

Diabetes Guide Book for the Physician, 2nd ed. American Diabetes Association, New York, 1956.

Elrick, H., et al.: "Glucagon Treatment of Insulin Reactions," *New England J. Med.,* **258:**476, 1958.

Jenne, F. H.: "Working Together to Meet the Needs of Diabetes Patients," *Pub. Health Nursing,* **44:**451, 1952.

Johnson, D.: "Planning the Modern Diabetic Diet," *J. Clin. Nutrition,* **1:**309, 1953.

Joslin, E. P.: "Development of the Present Treatment of Diabetes," *J. Am. Dietet. A.,* **25:**213, 1949.

Marble, A., et al.: "Unstable Diabetes," *Diabetes,* **5:**475, 1956.

Pollack, H.: "Dietary Management of Diabetes Mellitus," *Am. J. Med.,* **25:**708, 1958.

Ricketts, H. T.: *Diabetes Mellitus.* Charles C. Thomas, Springfield, Ill., 1955.

Wagner, D. H.: "The Preparation and Care of Diabetic Patients Requiring Surgery," *Surg. Clin. N.A.,* **39:**161, 1959.

Wilder, R. M.: "Adventures among the Islands of Langerhans," *J. Am. Dietet. A.,* **36:** 309, 1960.

Wilson, J. L., et al.: "Controlled versus Free Diet Management of Diabetes," *J.A.M.A.,* **147:**1526, 1951.

See also references #166–170, page 796.

Chapter 34. Various metabolic disturbances

Cochrane, W. A., et al.: "Familial Hypoglycemia Precipitated by Amino Acids," *J. Clin. Investigation,* **35:**411, 1956.

Conn, J. W., and Seltzer, H.: "Spontaneous Hypoglycemia," *Am. J. Med.,* **19:**460, 1955.

Eisenstein, A. B.: "Effects of Dietary Factors on Production of Adrenal Steroid Hormones," *Am. J. Clin. Nutrition,* **5:**369, 1957.

Hart, F. D.: "Treatment of Adrenocortical Deficiency States," *Brit. M. J.,* **5016:**417, 1957.

Hoffman, W. S.: "Metabolism of Uric Acid and Its Relation to Gout," *J.A.M.A.,* **154:** 213, 1954.

Lockie, L. M.: "Steroid Therapy in Rheumatoid Diseases," *J.A.M.A.,* **170:**1063, 1959.

Reich, B. H., and Ault, L. P.: "Nursing Care of the Patient with Addison's Disease," *Am. J. Nursing,* **60:**1252, 1960.

Review: "Calcium Metabolism and Hyperthyroidism," *Nutrition Rev.,* **16:**269, 1958.

Robinson, C. H.: "The Low Purine Diet," *Am. J. Clin. Nutrition,* **2:**276, 1954.

Robinson, W. D.: "Current Status of the Treatment of Gout," *J.A.M.A.,* **164:**1670, 1957.

Talbott, J. H., and Ricketts, A.: "Gout and Gouty Arthritis," *Am. J. Nursing,* **59:**1405, 1959.

See also references #171–177, page 796.

Chapter 35. Diet in nervous disturbances

Brozek, J.: "Experimental Studies on the Impact of Deficient Diet on Behavior," *Borden's Rev.,* **20:**75, 1959.

Cherescavich, G., and Tieger, M. E.: "Coffee Break Therapy," *Nursing Outlook,* **5:**227, 1957.

Crawfis, E. H.: "The Dietitian in the Mental Hospital," *J. Am. Dietet. A.,* **30:**464, 1954.

Donahue, H. H., and Fowler, P. A.: "Some Problems of Feeding Mental Patients," *Am. J. Clin. Nutrition,* **5:**180, 1957.

Miller, V.: "Role of the Dietetic Service in a Neuropsychiatric Hospital," *J. Am. Dietet. A.,* **30:**465, 1954.

O'Brien, F. M.: "The Dietitian on the Mental Health Team," *J. Am. Dietet. A.,* **32:**450, 1956.

Owens, L., and White, G. S.: "Observations on Food Acceptance during Mental Illness," *J. Am. Dietet. A.,* **30:**1110, 1954.

Ralli, F. M.: "Selective Menus in a Psychiatric Hospital," *J. Am. Dietet. A.,* **33:**1172, 1957.

Waide, S. E., and Hastings, D. W.: "Diet in Insulin Shock Therapy," *J. Am. Dietet. A.,* **14**:261, 1938.

See also references #178–184, page 797.

Chapter 36. Diet in diseases of the cardiovascular system

Atherosclerosis. Modified-fat diets

Ahrens, E. H., et al.: "Dietary Control of Serum Lipids in Relation to Atherosclerosis," *J.A.M.A.,* **164**:1905, 1957.

Brandt, M. B.: "Palatable Ways to Combine Oil with Egg-Milk Mixtures," *J. Am. Dietet. A.,* **35**:121, 1959.

Brown, H. B., and Page, I. H.: "Lowering Blood Lipid Levels by Changing Food Patterns," *J.A.M.A.,* **168**:1989, 1958.

Council on Foods and Nutrition: "Symposium on Significance of Lowered Cholesterol Levels," *J.A.M.A.,* **170**:2198, 1958.

Gofman, J. W.; Nichols, A. V.; and Dobbin, E. V.: *Dietary Prevention and Treatment of Heart Disease.* G. P. Putnam's Sons, New York, 1958.

Hartroft, W. S., and Thomas, W. A.: "Pathological Lesions Related to Disturbances of Fat and Cholesterol Metabolism in Man," *J.A.M.A.,* **164**:1899, 1957.

Hashim, S. A., and Clancy, R. E.: "Dietary Fats and Blood Coagulation," *New England J. Med.,* **259**:1115, 1958.

Hayes, O. B., and Rose, G.: "Supplementary Food Composition Table," *J. Am. Dietet. A.,* **33**:26, 1957.

Houk, T. W.: "Palatable Vegetable-Oil Milk," *J.A.M.A.,* **172**:1387, 1960.

Jolliffe, N., et al.: "The Anti-Coronary Club; Including a Discussion of the Effects of a Prudent Diet on the Serum Cholesterol Level of Middle-Aged Men," *Am. J. Clin. Nutrition,* **7**:451, 1959.

Kuo, P. T.: "Lipemia in Patients with Coronary Heart Disease," *J. Am. Dietet. A.,* **33**:22, 1957.

Mayer, J.: "Nutrition and Heart Disease," *Am. J. Pub. Health,* **50** (Part II, No. 3):5, 1960.

Okey, R., et al.: "Dietary Fat and Cholesterol Metabolism. Effects of Unsaturation of Dietary Fats on Liver and Serum Lipids," *Metabolism,* **8**:241, 1959.

Portman, O. W., et al.: "Dietary Regulation of Serum Cholesterol Levels," *Physiol. Rev.,* **39**:407, 1959.

Stamler, J.: "The Problem of Elevated Blood Cholesterol," *Am. J. Pub. Health,* **50** (Pt. II, No. 3): 14, 1960.

Stare, F. J., et al.: "Nutritional Studies Relating to Serum Lipids and Atherosclerosis, Therapeutic Implications," *J.A.M.A.,* **164**:1920, 1957.

Stefanik, P. A., and Trulson, M. F.: "Modifying the Fatty Acid Content of the Diet," *J. Am. Dietet. A.,* **34**:591, 1958.

Vail, G. E.: "Cooking with Fats High in Polyunsaturated Fatty Acids," *J. Am. Dietet. A.,* **35**:119, 1959.

See also references #185, 186, page 797, and on Fats, page 804.

Sodium-restricted diets

Beychok, S., et al.: "Practical Methods for Preparing Diets Low in Sodium and High in Protein," *Am. J. Clin. Nutrition,* **4**:254, 1956.

Black, D. A. K.: *Sodium Metabolism in Health and Disease.* Charles C. Thomas, Springfield, Ill., 1952.

Dahl, L. K.: "Role of Dietary Sodium in Essential Hypertension," *J. Am. Dietet. A.,* **34**:585, 1958.

————: "Sodium in Foods for a 100-mg Sodium Diet," *J. Am. Dietet. A.,* **34**:717, 1958.

Danowski, T. S.: "Low-Sodium Diets—Physiological Adaptation and Clinical Usefulness," *J.A.M.A.,* **168**:1886, 1958.

Davidson, C. S., et al.: *Sodium Restricted Diets. The Rationale, Complications, and Practical Aspects of Their Use.* Pub. 325, Food and Nutrition Board, National Research Council, Washington, D.C., 1954.

Franz, M., et al.: "Composition of 95 Foods. Calcium, Phosphorus, Magnesium, Sodium, and Potassium," *J. Am. Dietet. A.,* **35:**1170, 1959.

Heap, B., and Robinson, C.: "New Booklets for Patients on Sodium Restriction," *J. Am. Dietet. A.,* **34:**277, 1958.

Johnson, D.: "Planning a Restricted Sodium Diet and Bland, Low-Fiber Diet for the Diabetic Patient," *Am. J. Clin. Nutrition,* **5:**569, 1957.

Reimer, A., et al.: "Sodium-Restricted Diets. A Bookshelf," *J. Am. Dietet. A.,* **33:**104, 1957.

Robinson, C. H.: "Planning the Sodium-Restricted Diet," *J. Am. Dietet. A.,* **31:**28, 1955.

Seifrit, E.: "Low-Sodium Milk. Growth and Consumption Studies with Rats," *J. Am. Dietet. A.,* **32:**1167, 1956.

Wacker, W. E. C., et al.: "Bananas as a Low Sodium Dietary Staple," *New England J. Med.,* **259:**901, 1958.

Weller, J. M., and Hoobler, S. W.: "Salt Metabolism in Hypertension," *Ann. Int. Med.,* **50:**106, 1958.

Your Sodium-Restricted Diet: 500 mg, 1000 mg, Mild Restriction. American Heart Association, New York, 1958.

See also references #187–190, page 797.

Chapter 37. Diseases of the kidney

Boyce, W. H., et al.: "Abnormalities of Calcium Metabolism in Patients with 'Idiopathic' Urinary Calculi. Effect of Oral Administration of Sodium Phytate," *J.A.M.A.,* **166:** 1577, 1958.

Boyce, W. H.: "Nutrition and the Formation of Urinary Calculi," *Borden's Rev. Nutrition Research,* **21:**27, 1960.

Hughes, J., et al.: "Oxalate Urinary Tract Stones," *J.A.M.A.,* **172:**774, 1960.

Kark, R. M., et al.: "Nephrotic Syndrome in Adults. Common Disorder with Many Causes," *Ann. Int. Med.,* **49:**751, 1958.

Kolff, W. J.: "Treatment of Uremia with Forced High Calorie-Low Protein Diet," *Nutrition Rev.,* **11:**193, 1953.

Lowe, K. G., and Valtin, H.: "Dietary Treatment in Acute Anuria," *Am. J. Clin. Nutrition,* **4:**486, 1956.

Merrill, A. J.: "Nutrition in Chronic Renal Failure," *J.A.M.A.,* **173:**905, 1960.

Palmer, R. A.: "The Management of Acute Renal Failure," *Canad. M.A.J.,* **77:**11, 1957.

Rantz, L. A.: "Current Status of Therapy in Glomerulonephritis," *J.A.M.A.,* **170:**948, 1959.

Squire, J. R.: "Nutrition and the Nephrotic Syndrome in Adults," *Am. J. Clin. Nutrition,* **4:**509, 1956.

Winer, J. H.: "Practical Value of Analysis of Urinary Calculi," *J.A.M.A.,* **169:**1715, 1959.

Winters, R. W.: "Nutrition and Renal Disease," *Borden's Rev. Nutrition Research,* **19:** 75, 91, 1958.

See also references #191–196, page 797.

Chapter 38. Anemia

Crafts, R. C.: "Relationships of Hormones to the Utilization of Essential Nutrients in Erythropoiesis," *Am. J. Clin. Nutrition,* **3:**52, 1955.

Goldsmith, G. A.: "Nutritional Anemias with Especial Reference to Vitamin B_{12}," *Am. J. Med.,* **25:**680, 1958.

Heathcote, J. G., and Mooney, F. S.: "The Oral Treatment of Pernicious Anemia. A New Approach," *Lancet,* No. **7028:**982, 1958.

Jacobs, A.: "Pernicious Anemia—1822–1929," *Arch. Int. Med.,* **103:**329, 1959.

Johnson, A. C.: "Iron Equilibrium. Clinical Observations in Nutritional Anemia," *Am. J. Digest. Dis.,* **20:**179, 1953.

Mueller, J. F., and Will, J. J.: "Interrelationship of Folic Acid, Vitamin B_{12} and Ascorbic Acid in Patients with Megaloblastic Anemia," *Am. J. Clin. Nutrition,* **3:**30, 1955.

Murphy, W. P.: "Twenty-five Years Experience in Treatment and Management of Pernicious Anemia," *J.A.M.A.*, **149**:907, 1952.
Rundles, R. W.: "Hematopoietic Effects of Folic Acid Metabolites in the Megaloblastic Anemias," *Am. J. Clin. Nutrition*, **7**:385, 1959.
Vilter, R. W.: "Essential Nutrients in the Management of Hematopoietic Disorders of Human Beings. A Resumé," *Am. J. Clin. Nutrition*, **3**:72, 1955.
Wiener, J. S., and Hope, J. M.: "Cerebral Manifestations of Vitamin B₁₂ Deficiency," *J.A.M.A.*, **170**:1038, 1959.
Wintrobe, M. M.: *Clinical Hematology*, 4th ed. Lea & Febiger, Philadelphia, 1956.
See also references #197–201, page 797.

Chapter 39. Diet in allergic and skin disturbances

Allergy Recipes. The American Dietetic Association, Chicago, 1957.
Alvarez, W. C.: "The Production of Food Allergy," *Gastroenterology*, **30**:325, 1956.
Bereston, E. S.: "Vitamins in Dermatology," *J. Clin. Nutrition*, **2**:133, 1954.
Derlacki, E.: "Food Sensitization as a Cause of Perennial Nasal Allergy," *Ann. Allergy*, **13**:82, 1956.
Krehl, W. A.: "Nutrition and Skin Disease," *Borden's Rev. Nutrition Research*, **18**:1, 1957.
Lorincz, A. L.: "Nutrition in Relation to Dermatology," *J.A.M.A.*, **166**:1862, 1958.
Markow, H.: "Food Allergy," *New York J. Med.*, **56**:3735, 1956.
Randolph, T. G.: "Concepts of Food Allergy Important in Specific Diagnosis," *J. Allergy*, **21**:471, 1950.
Rinkel, R., and Zeller, M.: *Food Allergy*. Charles C. Thomas, Springfield, Ill., 1950.
Robert, J. H.: "Gastrointestinal Wheat Allergy," *J. Allergy*, **27**:523, 1956.
Rowe, A. H.: *Elimination Diets and the Patient's Allergies*, 2nd ed. Lea & Febiger, Philadelphia, 1944.
Rowe, A. H., et al.: "Diarrhea Caused by Food Allergy," *J. Allergy*, **27**:424, 1956.
Sammis, F. E.: *The Allergic Patient and His World*. Charles C. Thomas, Springfield, Ill., 1953.
Vaughan, W. T., and Black, J. H.: *Primer of Allergy*, 4th ed. The C. V. Mosby Company, St. Louis, 1954.
Wilkinson, D. S.: *The Nursing and Management of Skin Diseases*. The Macmillan Company, New York, 1958.
See references #202–206, page 797.

Chapter 40. Nutrition in children's diseases

General references

Jordan, I. M.: "The Nurse's Approach to the Feeding of Children," *J. Am. Dietet. A.*, **25**:626, 1949.
Nelson, W. E.: *Textbook of Pediatrics*, 7th ed. W. B. Saunders Company, Philadelphia, 1959.
Southmayd, E. B., and Marioka, M.: "Vegetables in the Child's Menu at the Hospital," *J. Am. Dietet. A.*, **30**:450, 1954.
Stitt, P. G.: "The Family Approach to Feeding Chronically Ill Children," *Children*, **5**:213, 1958.
Wallace, M. V.: "Feeding the Hospitalized Child. A Developmental Approach," *J. Am. Dietet. A.*, **29**:449, 1953.
Weng, L.: "Group Feeding for Hospitalized Children," *J. Am. Dietet. A.*, **25**:620, 1949.
Ylvisaker, E. N.: "Feeding Practices for Children in Ohio Hospitals," *J. Am. Dietet. A.*, **29**:454, 1953.
See references #207–222, page 798.
See also references on Infant and Child Feeding, pages 811–12.

Obesity

Bruch, H.: "Psychological Aspects of Obesity in Adolescence," *Am. J. Pub. Health*, **48**:1349, 1958.

Flack, H.: "Britain's New School Health Problem—The Fat Child," *Am. J. Pub. Health,* **50** (Suppl. to June 1960): 79, 1960.
Forbes, G. B.: "Overnutrition for the Child—Blessing or Curse?" *Nutrition Rev.,* **15:** 193, 1957.
Hoffman, R. H.: "Obesity in Childhood and Adolescence," *Am. J. Clin. Nutrition,* **5:**1, 1957.
Johnson, M. L., et al.: "Relative Importance of Inactivity and Overeating in the Energy Balance of Obese High School Girls," *Am. J. Clin. Nutrition,* **4:**37, 1956.
————: "The Prevalence and Incidence of Obesity in a Cross-section of Elementary and Secondary School Children," *Am. J. Clin. Nutrition,* **4:**231, 1956.
Lowry, G. H.: "Obesity in the Adolescent," *Am. J. Pub. Health,* **48:**1354, 1958.
Norman, J. M.: "Treating Obesity in Children," *J. Am. Dietet. A.,* **30:**695, 1954.
Stefanik, P. A., et al.: "Caloric Intake in Relation to Energy Output of Obese and Non-Obese Adolescent Boys," *Am. J. Clin. Nutrition,* **7:**55, 1959.
See also references on Overweight and Underweight, page 816.

Celiac syndrome

Andersen, D. H.: "Cystic Fibrosis of the Pancreas and Its Relation to Celiac Disease," *Am. J. Dis. Child.,* **56:**344, 1938.
————: "Cystic Fibrosis and Family Stress," *Children,* **7** (No. 1):9, 1960.
Andersen, D. H., and Mike, E. M.: "Diet Therapy in the Celiac Syndrome," *J. Am. Dietet. A.,* **31:**340, 1955.
Anderson, D. M.: "History of Celiac Disease," *J. Am. Dietet. A.,* **35:**1158, 1959.
Barnes, R. H.: "The Wheat Protein Effect in Celiac Disease," *New York J. Med.,* **58:** 1926, 1958.
Brown, A.: "Effect of a Gluten-Free Diet in Idiopathic Steatorrhea," *Brit. M.J.,* **2:**237, 1957.
di Sant' Agnese, P. A.: "Fibrocystic Disease of the Pancreas with Normal or Partial Pancreatic Function. Current Views on Pathogenesis and Diagnosis," *Pediatrics,* **15:** 683, 1955.
Holt, L. E., Jr.: "Celiac Disease—What Is It?" *J. Pediat.,* **46:**369, 1955.
Mike, E. M.: "Practical Dietary Management of Patients with the Celiac Syndrome," *Am. J. Clin. Nutrition,* **7:**463, 1959.
Mudge, G. H., ed.: "Combined Staff Clinic. Malabsorption Syndrome," *Am. J. Med.,* **15:**790, 1953.
Ross, C. A., et al.: "Coeliac Disease, the Relative Importance of Wheat Gluten," *Lancet,* **28:**1087, 1955.
Weijers, H. A., and van de Kamer, J. H.: "Some Biochemical Investigations into the Cause of Wheat Sensitivity in Celiac Disease," *Gastroenterology,* **38:**587, 1960.

Diabetes

Chute, A. L.: "Survey of Patients with Juvenile Diabetes Mellitus," *Am. J. Dis. Child.,* **75:**1, 1948.
Fajans, S. S., and Conn, J. W.: "Tolbutamide-Induced Improvement in Carbohydrate Tolerance of Young People with Mild Diabetes Mellitus," *Diabetes,* **9:**83, 1960.
Hooker, A. D.: "Camping and the Diabetic Child," *J. Am. Dietet. A.,* **37:**143, 1960.
Jackson, R. L., and Beckett, S. W.: "Dietary Management of Children with Diabetes," *J. Am. Dietet. A.,* **32:**528, 1956.
Payne, W. W.: "A Study of the Late Complications of Juvenile Diabetes in Approximately One Hundred Cases Using a "Free" Diet," *A.M.A. Am. J. Dis. Child.,* **90:**550, 1955.
White, P.: "Natural Course and Prognosis of Juvenile Diabetes," *Diabetes,* **5:**445, 1956.
See also references for Diabetes Mellitus, page 819.

Errors of metabolism

Acosta, P. B., and Centerwall, W. R.: "Phenylketonuria-Dietary Management. Special Low-Phenylalanine Recipes," *J. Am. Dietet. A.,* **36:**206, 1960.

Armstrong, M. D., et al.: "Studies on Phenylketonuria. IX. Further Observations on the Effect of Phenylalanine-Restricted Diet on Patients with Phenylketonuria," *Am. J. Clin. Nutrition,* **5:**543, 1957.

Centerwall, W. R.: "Phenylketonuria and Special Diet," *J.A.M.A.,* **166:**1507, 1958.

————: "Phenylketonuria. A General Review," *J. Am. Dietet. A.,* **36:**201, 1960.

"Galactosemia: Clinical Staff Conference at National Institutes of Health," *Ann. Int. Med.,* **46:**773, 1957.

Guest, G. M.: "Hereditary Galactose Disease," *J.A.M.A.,* **168:**2015, 1958.

Hsia, D. Y. Y., et al.: "A One-Year Controlled Study of the Effect of Low-Phenylalanine Diet on Phenylketonuria," *Pediatrics,* **21:**178, 1958.

Isselbacher, K. J.: "Clinical and Biochemical Observations in Galactosemia," *Am. J. Clin. Nutrition,* **5:**527, 1957.

Karle, I. P., et al.: "Enzyme Deficiency Diseases. II. Phenylketonuria," *J. Am. Dietet. A.,* **34:**1051, 1958.

Kretchmer, N., and Etzwiler, D. D.: "Disorders Associated with the Metabolism of Phenylalanine and Tyrosine," *Pediatrics,* **21:**445, 1958.

Review: "Genetic Aspects of Metabolic Disease in Childhood," *Nutrition Rev.,* **16:**323, 1958; **17:**3, 1959.

Review: "Maple Syrup Urine Disease," *Nutrition Rev.,* **17:**165, 1959.

Review: "Urinary Amino Acid Excretion in Disease," *Nutrition Rev.,* **16:**39, 1958.

Wright, S. W.: "Phenylketonuria," *J.A.M.A.,* **165:**2079, 1957.

Feeding the handicapped

Dittman, L. L.: *The Mentally Retarded Child at Home.* Children's Bureau, U.S. Department of Health, Education, and Welfare, Washington, D.C., 1959.

Flory, M. C.: "Training the Mentally Retarded Child," *Nursing Outlook,* **5:**344, 1957.

Leamy, C. M.: "A Study of the Food Intake of a Group of Children with Cerebral Palsy in the Lakeville Sanatorium," *Am. J. Pub. Health,* **43:**1310, 1953.

Martin, E. A.: "Planning Good Eating for the Handicapped Child," *The Crippled Child,* **34,** 6, 1956 (December).

Wright, S. W., et al.: "Etiologic Factors in Mental Deficiency; Errors of Metabolism That May Lead to Mental Deficiency," *A.M.A. Am. J. Dis. Child.,* **95:**541, 1958.

Chapters 41–54. Foods and food preparation

Better Homes and Gardens New Cookbook. Meredith Publishing Co., Des Moines, 1953.

General Foods Kitchens Cookbook. Random House, Inc., New York, 1959.

Halliday, E. G., and Noble, I. T.: *Hows and Whys of Cooking,* 3rd ed. University of Chicago Press, Chicago, 1946.

Handbook of Food Preparation. American Home Economics Association, Washington, D.C., 1959.

Harris, R. S., and Loesecke, H.: *Nutritional Evaluation of Food Processing.* John Wiley & Sons, Inc., New York, 1960.

Heseltine, M., and Dow, U. M.: *The New Basic Cook Book.* Houghton Mifflin Company, Boston, 1957.

Hughes, O.: *Introductory Foods,* 3rd ed. The Macmillan Company, New York, 1955.

Johnson, D.: *A Laboratory Manual in Cooking.* 2nd ed. G. P. Putnam's Sons, New York, 1950.

Justin, M. M.; Rust, L. O.; and Vail, G.: *Foods,* 4th ed. Houghton Mifflin Company, Boston, 1956.

Lowe, B.: *Experimental Cookery from the Chemical and Physical Standpoint,* 4th ed., John Wiley & Sons, New York, 1955.

Nichols, N. B.: *Farm Journal's Country Cookbook.* Doubleday & Company, Garden City, 1959.

Rombauer, I. S., and Becker, M. R.: *The Joy of Cooking.* Bobbs Merrill Company, New York, 1951.

Shackelton, A. D.: *Nutrition Manual for Nurses.* The Author, 914 E. State St., Ithaca, New York, 1957.

Sherman, H. C.: *Foods: Their Values and Management*. Columbia University Press, New York, 1947.

————: *Food Products*. The Macmillan Company, New York, 1948.

Stanley, L., and Cline, J. A.: *Foods: Their Selection and Preparation*. Ginn and Company, Boston, 1950.

Stefferud, A., ed.: *Food, the Yearbook of Agriculture 1959*. U.S. Department of Agriculture, Washington, D.C., 1959.

Sweetman, M. D., and MacKellar, I.: *Food Selection and Preparation,* 4th ed. John Wiley & Sons, Inc., New York, 1954.

Truax, C. (ed.): *Ladies' Home Journal Cookbook*. Doubleday & Company, Inc., New York, 1960.

Wilmot, J. S., and Batjer, M. Q.: *Food for the Family,* 5th ed. J. B. Lippincott Company, Philadelphia, 1960.

Pamphlets pertaining to menu planning and food preparation are available from:
Institute of Home Economics, U.S. Department of Agriculture
Extension services of state departments of agriculture

INDEX

Illustrations are indicated by numbers which appear in bold face type.

827

Carbohydrate — 1 gm. yields 4 calories.
Protein — 1 " " 4 calories.
Fat — 1 " " 9 "

B.M.R — 1 L. O₂ will generate 4.825 Calories heat

16 pp per day — 80 per wk

	AGE Years	WEIGHT kg (lb.)	HEIGHT cm (in.)	CALORIES	PROTEIN gm
Men	25	70 (154)	175 (69)	3200 [3]	70
	45	70 (154)	175 (69)	3000	70
	65	70 (154)	175 (69)	2550	70
Women	25	58 (128)	163 (64)	2300	58
	45	58 (128)	163 (64)	2200	58
	65	58 (128)	163 (64)	1800	58
	Pregnant (second half)			+300	+20
	Lactating (850 ml daily)			+1000	+40
Infants [4]	0–1/12 [4]				See
	2/12–6/12	6 (13)	60 (24)	kg × 120	Footnote
	7/12–12/12	9 (20)	70 (28)	kg × 100	4
Children	1 – 3	12 (27)	87 (34)	1300	40
	4 – 6	18 (40)	109 (43)	1700	50
	7 – 9	27 (60)	129 (51)	2100	60
	10–12	36 (79)	144 (57)	2500	70
Boys	13–15	49 (108)	163 (64)	3100	85
	16–19	63 (139)	175 (69)	3600	100
Girls	13–15	49 (108)	160 (63)	2600	80
	16–19	54 (120)	162 (64)	2400	75

[1] The allowance levels are intended to cover individual variations among most normal persons as they live in the United States under usual environmental stresses. The recommended allowances can be attained with a variety of common foods, providing other nutrients for which human requirements have been less well defined. See text for more detailed discussion of allowances and of nutrients not tabulated.

[2] Niacin equivalents include dietary sources of the preformed vitamin and the precursor, tryptophan. 60 milligrams tryptophan equals 1 milligram niacin.

[3] Calorie allowances apply to individuals usually engaged in moderate physical activity. For office workers or others in sedentary occupations they are excessive. Adjustments must be made for variations in body size, age, physical activity, and environmental temperature.